Other Best-selling Books

CASE STUDIES IN UNCOMMON HEADACHE DISORDERS

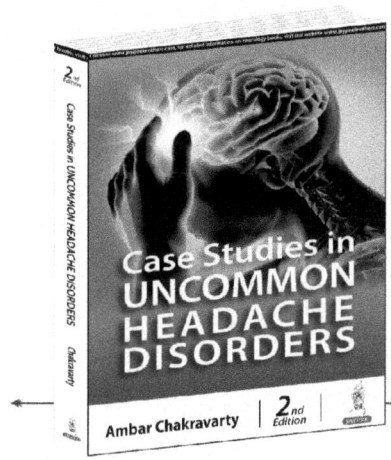

Ambar Chakravarty
Single Color | Hard Cover | 2/e, 2024
6.25" x 9.5" | 444 Pages | 9789356963160

VERTIGO AND DIZZINESS: A CASE-BASED STUDY

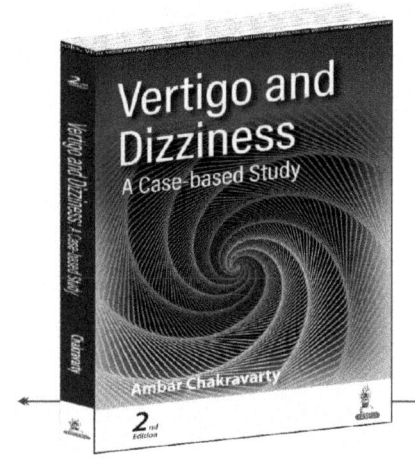

Ambar Chakravarty
Single Color | Hard Cover | 2/e, 2023
6.25" x 9.5" | 342 Pages | 9789356962064

PITFALLS IN THE DIAGNOSIS OF NEUROLOGICAL DISORDERS

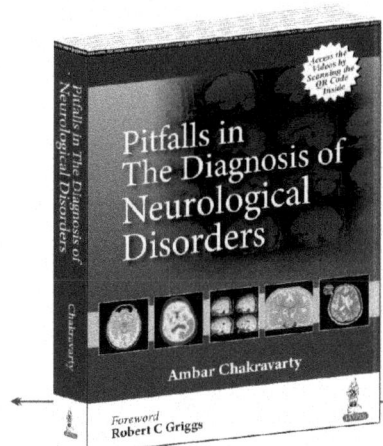

Ambar Chakravarty
Two Color | Soft Cover | 1/e, 2022
8.5" x 11" | 716 Pages | 9789354656668

JAYPEE
The Health Sciences Publisher

Please visit our website
www.jaypeebrothers.com or Scan the QR Code

Essentials of
CLINICAL NEUROLOGY
for The Psychiatrist

Essentials of
CLINICAL NEUROLOGY
for The Psychiatrist

Editor

Ambar Chakravarty
MD FRCPC FRCP FRCPE FICP FIAN
Honorary Professor and Emeritus Consultant
Department of Neurology
Vivekananda Institute of Medical Science
Kolkata, West Bengal, India
Past President, Indian Academy of Neurology (2005–2006)

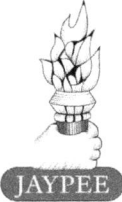

JAYPEE BROTHERS MEDICAL PUBLISHERS
The Health Sciences Publisher
New Delhi | London

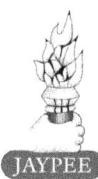 **Jaypee Brothers Medical Publishers (P) Ltd**

Headquarters
EMCA House
23/23-B, Ansari Road, Daryaganj
New Delhi 110 002, India
Landline: +91-11-23272143, +91-11-23272703
+91-11-23282021, +91-11-23245672
E-mail: jaypee@jaypeebrothers.com

Corporate Office
Jaypee Brothers Medical Publishers (P) Ltd.
4838/24, Ansari Road, Daryaganj
New Delhi 110 002, India
Phone: +91-11-43574357
Fax: +91-11-43574314
E-mail: jaypee@jaypeebrothers.com

Overseas Office
JP Medical Ltd.
83, Victoria Street, London
SW1H 0HW (UK)
Phone: +44-20 3170 8910
Fax: +44(0)20 3008 6180
E-mail: info@jpmedpub.com

Website: www.jaypeebrothers.com
Website: www.jaypeedigital.com

© 2025, Jaypee Brothers Medical Publishers

The views and opinions expressed in this book are solely those of the original contributor(s)/author(s) and do not necessarily represent those of editor(s) or publisher of the book.

All rights reserved. No part of this publication may be reproduced, stored or transmitted in any form or by any means, electronic, mechanical, photocopying, recording or otherwise, without the prior permission in writing of the publishers.

All brand names and product names used in this book are trade names, service marks, trademarks or registered trademarks of their respective owners. The publisher is not associated with any product or vendor mentioned in this book.

Medical knowledge and practice change constantly. This book is designed to provide accurate, authoritative information about the subject matter in question. However, readers are advised to check the most current information available on procedures included and check information from the manufacturer of each product to be administered, to verify the recommended dose, formula, method and duration of administration, adverse effects and contraindications. It is the responsibility of the practitioner to take all appropriate safety precautions. Neither the publisher nor the author(s)/editor(s) assume any liability for any injury and/or damage to persons or property arising from or related to use of material in this book.

This book is sold on the understanding that the publisher is not engaged in providing professional medical services. If such advice or services are required, the services of a competent medical professional should be sought.

Every effort has been made where necessary to contact holders of copyright to obtain permission to reproduce copyright material. If any have been inadvertently overlooked, the publisher will be pleased to make the necessary arrangements at the first opportunity.

Inquiries for bulk sales may be solicited at: jaypee@jaypeebrothers.com

Essentials of Clinical Neurology for The Psychiatrist / Ambar Chakravarty

First Edition: **2025**

ISBN: 978-93-5696-550-8

In Memorium

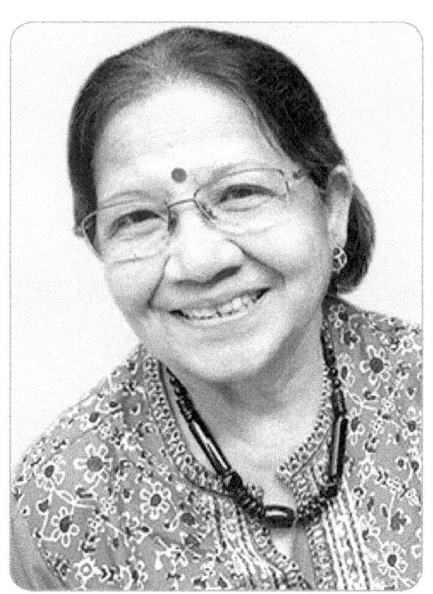

Dr (Mrs) Srilekha Chakravarty
(27 December 1948 – 7 January 2024)

*A life full of sacrifices made towards whatever I could achieve
in my academic and professional life.*

Dedication

Professor Jose Biller

For his continued guidance and mentoring

Contributors

Venkatesh Aiyagari DM FAHA
Professor
Division Chief, Neurocritical Care
Departments of Neurological Surgery
and Neurology
University of Texas Southwestern
Medical Center
Dallas, Texas, USA

Santosh Sriram Andugulapati
MD DM
Senior Resident
Department of Neurology
Seth GS Medical College and
KEM Hospital
Mumbai, Maharashtra, India

Neenu Alexander MD DM
Consultant Neurologist
Zydus Hospital
Vadodara, Gujarat, India

Joshua Battley MD
Assistant Professor
Division of Neurocritical Care
Departments of Neurology and
Neurological Surgery
University of Texas Southwestern
Medical Center
Dallas, Texas, USA

Atanu Biswas MD DM
Professor
Department of Neurology
Institute of Post Graduate Medical
Education and Research (IPGME&R)
Bangur Institute of Neurosciences
Kolkata, West Bengal, India

Niloy Biswas MS MCh
Consultant Neurosurgeon
Park Neurosciences Centre
Kolkata, West Bengal, India

Ambar Chakravarty MD FRCPC FRCP
FRCPE FICP FIAN
Honorary Professor and Emeritus
Consultant
Department of Neurology
Vivekananda Institute of Medical
Science
Kolkata, West Bengal, India
Past President, Indian Academy of
Neurology (2005–2006)

Sandip Chatterjee DNB FRCS
DNB(Neurosurg) FRCS(SN)
Professor of Neurosurgery
Vivekananda Institute of Medical
Sciences
Senior Consultant Neurosurgeon
Park Neuroscience Centre
Kolkata, West Bengal, India

Gautam Das MD DM
Consultant Neurologist
Department of Neurology
Ramrik Das Harlalka Hospital, Bangur
Institute of Neurosciences
Kolkata, West Bengal, India

Soumik Das MD DM
Assistant Professor
Department of Radiodiagnosis
Raiganj Government Medical College
and Hospital
Kolkata, West Bengal, India

Joy D Desai MD DNB
Director of Neurology
Jaslok Hospital and Research Center
Mumbai, Maharashtra, India

Rishikesh Deshpande MD DM
Consultant Neurologist
Deenanath Mangeshkar Hospital and
Research Center
Pune, Maharashtra, India

Omkar P Hajirnis DNB MRCPCH(UK)
Fellowship in Pediatrics Neurology
Consultant
Department of Paediatric Neurology
Fortis Mulund
Mumbai, Maharashtra, India

Hiral Halani MD DM DrNB
Associate Consultant in Neurology
Bombay Hospital Institute of
Medical Sciences
Mumbai, Maharashtra, India

Amit Halder MD DM
Associate Professor
Department of Neurology
Vivekananda Institute of Medical
Science
Consultant Neurologist
Fortis Hospital
Kolkata, West Bengal, India

Anaita Udwadia Hegde DCH
MD(Pediatrics) MRCPCH(London) Fellowship in
Pediatric Neurosciences
Consultant Pediatric Neurologist
SRCC Narayana Health Children's
Hospital
Jaslok Hospital and Research Center
Wadia Childrens Hospital
Mumbai, Maharashtra, India

Shashank Jaiswal MD DM
Consultant
CARE Hospitals
Banjara Hills, Hyderabad, India

Sarosh M Katrak MD DM FRCP FIAN
Emeritus Professor
Department of Neurology
Grant Medical College
Mumbai, Maharashtra, India

Contributors

Subhash Kaul MD DM FIAN
Senior Neurologist
Krishna Institute of Medical Sciences
Hyderabad, Telangana, India

Satish V Khadilkar MD DM DNBE FIAN FICP FAMS FRCP
Dean, Professor and Head
Department of Neurology
Bombay Hospital Institute of Medical Sciences
Mumbai, Maharashtra, India

Rahul Kulkarni MD DM DNB FAAN
Consultant Neurologist
Deenanath Mangeshkar Hospital and Research Center
Pune, Maharashtra, India

Sayan Malakar MD
Senior Resident
Department of Medicine
Vivekananda Institute of Medical Sciences
Kolkata, West Bengal, India

Adreesh Mukherjee MD DM
Assistant Professor
Department of Neurology
Bangur Institute of Neurosciences
Kolkata, West Bengal, India

Madhu Nagappa MD DM
Centre Co-Investigator and ICGNMD Faculty PI Fellow
National Institute of Mental Health and Neurosciences (NIMHANS)
Bengaluru, Karnataka, India

Amitkumar V Pande MD DM
Consultant Neurologist
Dr Pande's Neuro and Physio Clinic
Pune, Maharashtra, India

Varsha A Patil MD DM
Assistant Professor
Department of Neurology
Bombay Hospital and Medical Research Centre
Mumbai, Maharashtra, India

Sanjay Prakash MD DM
Professor and Head
Department of Neurology
Smt BK Shah Medical Institute and Research Centre
Vadodara, Gujarat, India

Shripad Pujari MD DM DNB FRCP
Consultant Neurologist
Deenanath Mangeshkar Hospital and Research Center
Noble Hospital
Pune, Maharashtra, India

Sukalyan Purakayastha MD DM
Head
Department of Neurointervention and Endovascular Surgery
Consultant Neuroradiologist
Institute of Neurosciences Kolkata
Kolkata, West Bengal, India

Neetu Ramrakhiani MD DM
Consultant Neurologist
Fortis Escorts Hospital
Jaipur, Rajasthan, India

Chaturbhuj Rathore MD DM
Professor, Department of Neurology
Smt BK Shah Medical Institute and Research Centre
Vadodara, Gujarat, India

Parthvi Ravat MD(Medicine) DNB(Neurology)
Senior Clinical Associate
PD Hinduja Hospital
Mumbai, Maharashtra, India

Sangeeta Ravat MD DM FIAN
Dean and Professor of Neurology
Seth GS Medical College and KEM Hospital
Mumbai, Maharashtra, India

Bappaditya Ray MD
Associate Professor
Division of Neurocritical Care
Departments of Neurology and Neurological Surgery
University of Texas Southwestern Medical Center Dallas, Texas, USA

Debasish Roy MD DNB DM
Professor
Department of Neurology
Vivekananda Institute of Medical Science
Kolkata, West Bengal, India

Sanjib Sinha MD DM
Professor and Head
Department of Neurology
National Institute of Mental Health and Neurosciences
Bengaluru, Karnataka, India

Mayur Thakkar MD DM
Assistant Professor
Department of Neurology
Seth GS Medical College and KEM Hospital
Mumbai, Maharashtra, India

Sweety Tribedi MD DM
Post-doctoral Fellow
Department of Neurology
Sanjay Gandhi Postgraduate Medical Institute of Medical Sciences
Lucknow, Uttar Pradesh, India

Varoon Vadodaria DNB(Neurology)
Assistant Professor
Department of Neurology
Smt BK Shah Medical Institute and Research Centre
Vadodara Gujarat, India

LG Viswanathan DM
Assistant Professor
Department of Neurology
National Institute of Mental Health and Neurosciences
Bengaluru, Karnataka, India

Preface

Neurology and psychiatry are indeed allied disciplines, but the gap between the two seems wide, especially among the specialists but not perhaps amongst the lay public. While neurologists try to explain a patient's symptoms on the basis of structural changes in the central or peripheral nervous system which can be detected in life through imaging, biopsy, and microscopy or after death through postmortem studies and subsequently through histopathological means, psychiatrists deal with an abstract concept, namely disorders of the mind. Lishman wrote in the Preface to the first edition of his book Organic Psychiatry—"*Neurology deals directly with the apparatus of mind by investigating malfunction of the brain. Yet paradoxically it has often paid scant attention to mental disorder itself. Psychiatry on its part deals essentially with mental disorder, yet has had little in relative terms to do with the hardware upon which mind depends. The rich complexity of human behavior and the multitude of factors which can shape and distort it have clearly demanded a multifaceted growth of clinical psychiatry; the subject had profited from psychodynamic, psychosocial and pharmacological approaches to mental disorder, but with the expert neurologist waiting in the wings the factor of brain malfunction has sometimes tended to be eclipsed………"*

With advancement in neurosciences and molecular sciences, this gap between the two disciplines is seemingly becoming narrower and narrower. Structural neurological disorders result from dysfunctioning at the cellular level at the diseased site, which in its turn produces clinically recognizable abnormalities through excessive or decreased release of chemicals called neurotransmitters, which generally act at the synaptic sites in the neural network that controls the appropriate function of the diseased brain part. This basic mechanism is also applicable in relation to the disorders of the peripheral nervous system as well. Mind, on the other hand, can be viewed as an abstract function of the brain, which is totally dependent on the neural networking in the brain made up of axons and dendrites of the brain cells (hence structural elements), and the activities of the various neurotransmitters released by the brain cells (again structural elements). Modern-day technologies have made it possible to visualize these changes histopathologically as well as in life through functional and molecular neuroimaging. The gap, thus, between neurology and psychiatry can be bridged. The result had been greater understanding of the psychiatric manifestations of essentially structural neurological disorders and for the psychiatrists to look for stigmata of underlying structural brain disorders in patients presenting with apparently disorders of mind like emotional and behavioral alterations and also to identify neurological phenomena developing as a result of treatment with various drugs commonly used by them to treat such aberrations of mental functions. The bottom line is that neurologists must have some basic knowledge of psychiatric illnesses and the vice versa. In an ideal situation, basics of both the subjects need to be incorporated in the curriculum of either through practical clinical training. And this is indeed practiced in a handful of premier institutions of the country.

My interest in neuropsychiatry was lit after listening to some lectures of Professor Alwyn Lishman during my training days in neurology in the North of England, and I did purchase a copy of the first edition of his book "*Organic Psychiatry*", which helped me immensely to learn the higher cortical functions of the brain. Later reading Howard Kishner's Behavioral Neurology and Kaufman's voluminous text, my knowledge was much enriched. As I was, at some stage of my clinical career in this country, involved in conducting teaching sessions organized by the Psychiatric Societies, I felt the need of enriching the knowledge of specialist psychiatrics about the fundamental principles of clinical neurology, which I feel an absolutely necessity for a comprehensive evaluation of a patient with a mental illness. There indeed are a host of systemic and neurological conditions, which manifest psychiatric symptoms, at times as the first presenting symptom. Early identification of these is essential for appropriate treatment. Furthermore, such neurological conditions need not always be of central nervous system in origin. Peripheral neuromuscular disorders, though only rarely may manifest behavioral disorders, may concurrently occur along with a primarily psychiatric disorder like depression, which may be of reactive type, but not necessarily.

Long back I felt the need of a comprehensive text on the subject of Clinical Neurology meant for Psychiatrists. Kaufman's book, though an ideal for this, is too vast to be attractive to busy practicing psychiatrists and especially trainees in Psychiatry. I could find none easily available in this country nor in the international market.

The present volume would hopefully be able to meet the needs of both trained and trainee psychiatrists in enriching their knowledge about the various clinical neurological conditions, which they would be encountering in their daily clinical practice. Indeed the neuropsychiatric aspects of these neurological disorders and some systemic illnesses as have been highlighted in this book, enough informations have been provided for their recognitions and at times management. Borderland conditions like dementias have also been discussed in as practice-oriented way as possible.

Apart from myself, many leading neurologists of the country have contributed to this book making it as comprehensive as possible. Additionally, many chapters have been followed by Editorial Commentaries wherein I have tried to highlight on finer clinical and pathological issues related to the subject discussed in the chapter. Many chapters and commentaries are supplemented with Case Vignettes, which would make reading more interesting. The first two chapters would be of much interest to those who are interested in the historical aspects of the two sister disciplines of Neurology and Psychiatry. I sincerely hope that the book would be much appreciated by the Psychiatric community of this country and abroad.

I would like to thank profusely the contributing authors, some of whom are world renowned authorities, for kindly writing for this book in the midst of their numerous commitments. Special mention needs to be made of Drs Sarosh M Katrak, Satish V Khadilkar, Sanjib Sinha, Subhash Kaul, Sangeeta Ravat, Joy D Desai, Sulalyan Purkayastha, and Sandip Chatterjee for their contributions. Special thanks would go to Dr Sayan Malakar, Senior Resident at VIMS for helping me to write the opening Chapter and to edit a few more ones.

My sincerest thanks go to my long time patient and family friend Anuradha for inspiring me to put back the wheels on the track during the period of a devastating family medical crisis. This book would not have seen the light of the day without her help.

I am indebted to the publishers for their co-operation to bring out the book in time even in the midst of the post pandemic hard days. Thank you to the team of M/s Jaypee Brothers Medical Publishers (P) Ltd, New Delhi, India and especially to Sabyasachi Hazra [Associate Director (Publishing) and Team lead—East (Diginerve)] for standing with my vision of this book and taking the initial lead and Priyansh Saxena (Development Editor) for very prompt in text work and all the collaborations.

Lastly, I wish and pray that the book becomes really useful to all those for whom it had been written.

Ambar Chakravarty

Contents

CHAPTER 1: **The Evolution of Neuropsychiatry: From Antiquity to Current Time**   1
Sayan Malakar, Ambar Chakravarty

CHAPTER 2: **Hysteria: Through the Ages**   9
Ambar Chakravarty

    Commentary 1: Somatic Symptom Disorder: A Brief Note   *17*
    Ambar Chakravarty

CHAPTER 3: **Functional Neurological Disorders: An Overview—Pathophysiology, Clinical Recognition, and Outlines of Management**   19
Amit Halder, Ambar Chakravarty

CHAPTER 4: **Systemic and Neurological Red Flags in the Diagnosis of Psychiatric Diseases**   26
Sarosh M Katrak

    Commentary 2: A Truly Neuropsychiatric Problem!   *38*
    Ambar Chakravarty

CHAPTER 5: **Cognition Testing at the Bedside**   42
Amit Halder, Ambar Chakravarty

    Commentary 3: A Relook at Acute Onset Amnesia Syndromes   *58*
    Ambar Chakravarty

CHAPTER 6: **Pitfalls in Neuropsychological Testing in Adults with Suspected Dementias**   64
Atanu Biswas

CHAPTER 7: **Cornerstones in the Diagnosis of Epileptic Seizures in Children and Adolescents: Their Pitfalls and Mimics**   70
Ambar Chakravarty

    Appendix 1: Epilepsy Imitators   *79*

    Commentary 4: Utility of Sleep in Seizure Diagnosis   *80*
    Ambar Chakravarty

    Commentary 5: Geriatric Seizure Mimics: A Problem Oriented Approach   *84*
    Ambar Chakravarty

CHAPTER 8: **Seizures and Epilepsy Syndromes: What a Psychiatrist should Know?**   87
Neenu Alexander, Chaturbhuj Rathore

CHAPTER 9: **Neuropsychiatric Aspects of Epilepsy**   109
Ambar Chakravarty

| CHAPTER 10: | **Psychogenic Nonepileptic Seizures: Psychobiology, Clinical Aspects, and Management** | **116** |

LG Viswanathan, Sanjib Sinha

Commentary 6: Psychogenic Nonepileptic Seizure and Psychogenic Movement Disorder: Are they Really Different? *123*
Ambar Chakravarty

Commentary 7: Psychogenic Nonepileptic Seizures: Is it All in the Mind? *125*
Ambar Chakravarty

| CHAPTER 11: | **Psychiatric Mimics of Epileptic Seizures: Part 1—Episodic Dyscontrol Syndrome: The Concept** | **127** |

Ambar Chakravarty

| CHAPTER 12: | **Psychiatric Mimics of Epileptic Seizures: Part 2—Epilepsy, Rage, Tantrums, and Violence** | **131** |

Ambar Chakravarty

| CHAPTER 13: | **An Overview of Stroke Medicine for the Psychiatrist** | **135** |

Neetu Ramrakhiani

Commentary 8: Stroke Mimics and Chameleons *143*
Ambar Chakravarty

| CHAPTER 14: | **Neuropsychiatric Aspects of Cerebrovascular Disorders** | **147** |

Shashank Jaiswal, Subhash Kaul

| CHAPTER 15: | **An Overview of Movement Disorders for the Psychiatrist** | **156** |

Adreesh Mukherjee

Commentary 9: Psychogenic Gait Disorders *167*
Ambar Chakravarty

Commentary 10: Astasia–Abasia: Neurologic or Functional? *170*
Ambar Chakravarty

Commentary 11: Diagnosis of Vascular Parkinsonism *172*
Ambar Chakravarty

Commentary 12: Alcohol and Movement Disorders *176*
Ambar Chakravarty

| CHAPTER 16: | **Neuropsychiatric Manifestations of Parkinson's Disease** | **178** |

Ambar Chakravarty

Commentary 13: Neural Basis of Impulsive Control Disorders *188*
Ambar Chakravarty

Commentary 14: A Note on Wilson's Disease and its Psychiatric Aspects *192*
Ambar Chakravarty

| CHAPTER 17: | **An Overview of Headache Disorders and their Neuropsychiatric Aspects** | **195** |

Sanjay Prakash, Varoon Vadodaria

Commentary 15: A Note on Medication Overuse Headache *206*
Ambar Chakravarty

CHAPTER 18:	**An Overview of Neuromuscular Diseases for the Psychiatrists**	**210**
	Satish V Khadilkar, Varsha A Patil	
CHAPTER 19:	**Chronic Pain and Chronic Fatigue: A Diagnostic and Therapeutic Challenge**	**222**
	Satish V Khadilkar, Hiral Halani	
CHAPTER 20:	**Neuropsychiatric Manifestations of Demyelinating Disorders**	**234**
	Parthvi Ravat, Santosh Sriram Andugulapati, Sangeeta Ravat, Mayur Thakkar	
CHAPTER 21:	**Neuropsychiatric Aspects of Autoimmune Encephalitis**	**243**
	Rahul Kulkarni, Rishikesh Deshpande, Shripad Pujari	
	Commentary 16: Autoimmune Encephalitis: Some Current Thoughts *253*	
	Ambar Chakravarty	
CHAPTER 22:	**Neuropsychiatric Aspects of Central Nervous System Infections**	**255**
	Madhu Nagappa, Sanjib Sinha	
CHAPTER 23:	**Essentials of Sleep Medicine for the Psychiatrist**	**267**
	Joy D Desai	
CHAPTER 24:	**Clinical and Radiological Pitfalls in the Diagnosis of Dementias**	**275**
	Gautam Das, Atanu Biswas	
	Commentary 17: Pseudodementia and Pseudodepression: Two Sides of the Coin *283*	
	Ambar Chakravarty	
CHAPTER 25:	**Young-onset Rapidly Progressive Dementias: Recognition and Red Flags**	**287**
	Ambar Chakravarty	
CHAPTER 26:	**Neuroimaging in the Diagnosis of Dementias**	**297**
	Sukalyan Purakayastha, Soumik Das	
	Commentary 18: Utility and Limitations of Neuroimaging and Cerebrospinal Fluid Biomarkers in Diagnosis of Dementia Subtypes *312*	
	Ambar Chakravarty	
CHAPTER 27:	**Neurological Aspects of Autism Spectrum Disorder**	**314**
	Anaita Udwadia Hegde, Omkar P Hajirnis	
CHAPTER 28:	**Hyperventilation Syndrome, Panic Disorders, and Related Conditions**	**323**
	Debasish Roy, Ambar Chakravarty	
CHAPTER 29:	**Psychiatric Emergencies in Critical Care Units: Recognition and Management**	**336**
	Joshua Battley, Bappaditya Ray, Venkatesh Aiyagari	
CHAPTER 30:	**Exploring the Neurobiology of Human Sexuality**	**348**
	Joy D Desai	
CHAPTER 31:	**Neuropsychological Aspects of Traumatic Brain Injury**	**355**
	Sandip Chatterjee, Niloy Biswas	
	Commentary 19: Chronic Traumatic Encephalopathy *359*	
	Ambar Chakravarty	

CHAPTER 32:	**Neurological Side Effects of Psychiatric Medications** *Shripad Pujari, Amitkumar V Pande, Rahul Kulkarni*	**362**
CHAPTER 33:	**Central Neurological Manifestations of Alcoholism and Substance Abuse** *Sweety Tribedi, Ambar Chakravarty*	**371**
CHAPTER 34:	**Visual Illusions and Hallucinations of Central Origin and their Differentials** *Ambar Chakravarty*	**386**
	Commentary 20: A Note on Auditory Hallucinations *395* *Ambar Chakravarty*	

Index   **399**

CHAPTER 1

The Evolution of Neuropsychiatry: From Antiquity to Current Time

Sayan Malakar, Ambar Chakravarty

INTRODUCTION

Neuropsychiatry, also known as organic psychiatry, is a specialized branch of medicine that explores the intersection between psychiatry and neurology. Its primary goal is to comprehend and attribute human behavior to the complex interplay of neurobiology and social psychology factors. Unlike other fields within behavioral and neurological specialties, which often treat the mind and brain as separate entities, neuropsychiatry views the mind as an emergent property of the brain. It is important to note that neuropsychiatry predates the current disciplines of psychiatry and neurology, which were previously integrated in terms of training. However, these disciplines have since diverged and are typically practiced independently.

In recent years, neuropsychiatry has emerged as a growing subspecialty within psychiatry due to its close association with neuropsychology and behavioral neurology. Its aim is to apply this interdisciplinary knowledge to improve the treatment of disorders that encompass both neurological and mental health classifications.

HISTORICAL ASPECTS

To trace the origins of neuropsychiatry, one must turn to ancient Greece and the influential works of Hippocrates. He boldly challenged the prevailing belief that epilepsy was caused by the gods, asserting instead that it originated from the brain. Hippocrates recognized the profound influence of the brain, stating, "...men ought to know that from nothing else but thence (from the brain) comes joys, delights, laughter and sports and sorrows, griefs, despondency, and lamentations... And by the same organ, we become mad and delirious, and fears and terrors assail us...".[1]

The brain itself did not garner significant scientific interest until the Renaissance and the early Enlightenment period.[2] A major breakthrough occurred in 1543 when Andreas Vesalius published his work, De Humani Corporis Fabrica, coinciding with Copernicus' publication of De revolutionibus orbium coelestium (**Fig. 1**). Thomas Willis, a prominent figure in this field (1621-1675), made significant contributions by rectifying anatomical inaccuracies related to the brain's structure that had persisted since Galen's time (**Fig. 2**). Willis focused extensively on the basal ganglia and cerebral circulation but curiously overlooked the cerebral cortex. Much like Hippocrates, Willis was preoccupied with distinguishing epilepsy from certain seizure variants, now known as psychogenic nonepileptic seizures (PNES). However, a recurring challenge throughout the literature on brain function has been the intricate relationship between the mind and the brain, as well as the enigmatic nature of the soul and its functions. The ancient Greeks did not offer any definitive solutions, and Willis, despite his religious beliefs, also lacked answers. It was philosopher-scientist René Descartes (1596-1650) who profoundly influenced our perspectives on this matter. Descartes

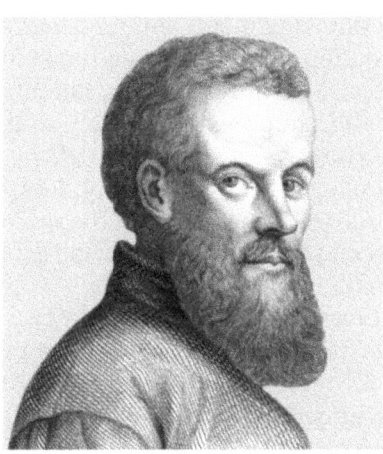

FIG. 1: Andreas Vesalius (1514–1564) was a 16th century anatomist, physician, and author of one of the most influential books on human anatomy.

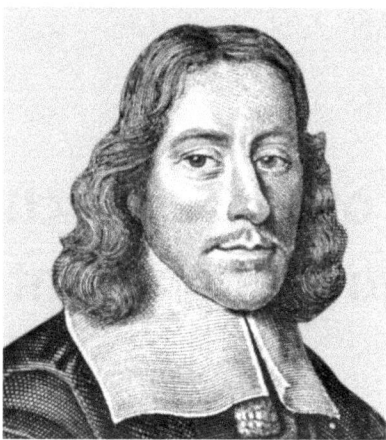

FIG. 2: Thomas Willis (1621–1625) was a pioneer in research into the anatomy of the brain, nervous system, and muscles. His most notable discovery was the "Circle of Willis".

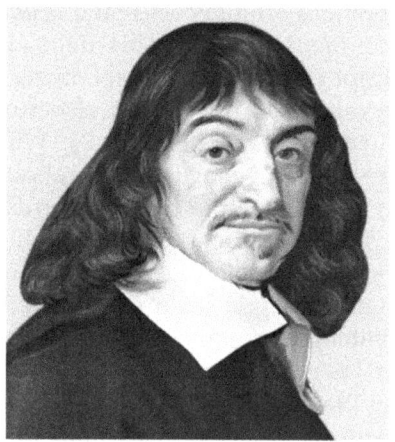

FIG. 3: René Descartes (1596–1650) was a French philosopher, scientist, and mathematician, widely considered a seminal figure in the emergence of modern philosophy and science.

sought a new approach to explore the nature of the mind, considering humans as composed of two substances: Res cogitans (thinking mind) and res extensa (the body) **(Fig. 3)**. According to Descartes, our humanity could not be solely derived from the body or, notably, the brain. However, he did not provide a solution to the enduring conundrum known as Cartesian dualism, which has plagued neurology, psychiatry, and philosophy. Despite Descartes' brilliance, his views on the mind and reflex theory further emphasized by Willis came to be referred to as neurologie.[2,3]

Samuel Taylor Coleridge (1772–1834), a prominent figure of his time, had a revolutionary mindset that aligned with the revolutionary era he lived in. Coping with neuralgia, he turned to opium and found inspiration in a mythical place called Kubla Khan, a realm of abundance **(Fig. 4)**. Coleridge recognized that the materialistic and empirical philosophies of the Enlightenment could not adequately explain the works of literary giants like Milton, Shakespeare, or Wordsworth. He rejected John Locke's notion of the mind as a blank slate (tabula rasa) and instead embraced the concept of a creative mind with active powers that shape individual experiences. These ideas that sparked the imagination of poets also resonated with certain neuroscientists of the time.[3]

Alan Richardson explored the origins of what he termed "neural Romanticism," attributing it to influential scientists such as Erasmus Darwin (1731–1802), Franz Gall (1758–1828), Pierre Cabanis (1757–1808), and Charles Bell (1774–1842) **(Figs. 5 to 7)**.[2] Erasmus Darwin's comprehensive book, Zoonomia, covered a wide range of medical knowledge at the time, including anatomy, physiology, natural science, and connections to contemporary philosophies. Bell, in his work titled Idea of a New Anatomy of the Brain (1811), presented an early summary of his ideas on brain and spinal cord functions

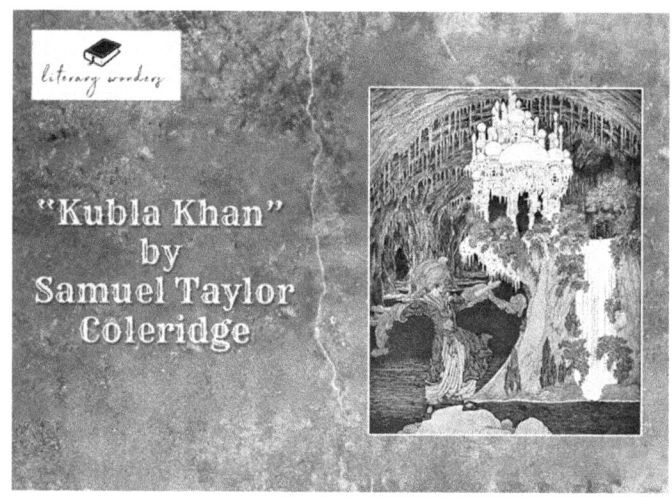

FIG. 4: Kubla Khan, a realm of abundance.

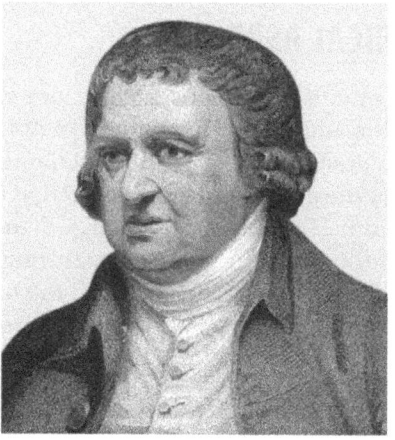

FIG. 5: Erasmus Darwin (1731–1802).

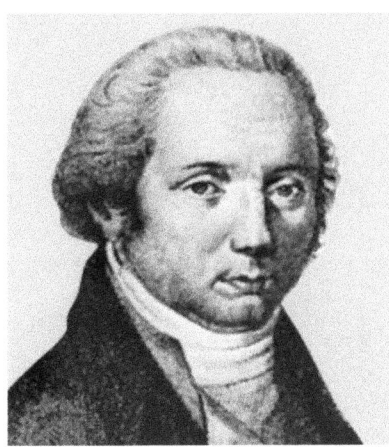

FIG. 6: Franz Gall (1758–1828).

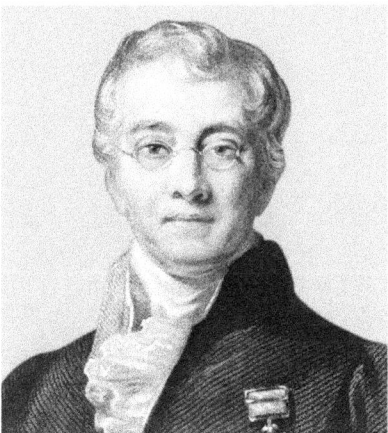

FIG. 7: Charles Bell (1774–1842).

based on meticulous dissections. He posited that the cerebrum and cerebellum had distinct functions, with the former being the seat of intellectual faculties and the mind.[2,3]

Gall, along with his pupil and collaborator Johann Spurzheim (1776-1832), is best known for developing phrenology, which, despite being trivialized and misused in the public eye, made significant contributions to neuroscience. Gall examined animal brains, studying the evolutionary development of brain shapes and sizes in relation to different natural skills. He was fascinated by the increasing complexity of cerebral convolutions in correlation with phylogeny. Rather than using horizontal and vertical brain slices, Gall dissected along the white matter, revealing its connection to the gray matter. He proposed that the brain is the organ of the mind and can be analyzed into distinct faculties, which are innate and reside in the cortex. However, his downfall was his suggestion of a correlation between the shape of the skull and the cortex of the brain, leading to the idea that the size of specific brain organs and their potential role in psychological makeup could be determined by cranial inspection. Gall's approach displayed a Romantic inclination, seeking to understand unity within diversity, not only from an evolutionary standpoint but also within an individual's brain.[4]

The study of dreams, drugs, and mental disorders prompted scientists like Erasmus Darwin and Gall to present a new perspective on the mind, with a focus on emotions and feelings rather than reason. For John Hughlings Jackson, the brain evolved from an undifferentiated, simple, and homogeneous state to a differentiated, complex, and heterogeneous structure with integrated specialized parts **(Fig. 8)**. He conceptualized the brain's structure and function hierarchically, with interactions between different levels, placing the prefrontal cortex at the highest level. This principle, based on the concepts of inhibition and release, emphasized that clinical signs involve both processes simultaneously. Jackson introduced the notions of negative and positive symptoms, suggesting their presence in every neuropsychiatric case. He argued that lesions could not precisely localize a function but rather impair a system, and the effects reflected the ongoing activity of the brain parts unaffected by the lesion. His studies on aphasia led him to challenge the growing idea of strict localization of function. While acknowledging the left hemisphere's prominence in language production and conscious acts, he also emphasized the significant role of the right hemisphere, particularly in language production and emotional aspects.

Sigmund Freud was greatly influenced by John Hughlings Jackson, as evident in his work "On Aphasia" (1891), which he wrote before his psychoanalytic period and is now often overlooked **(Fig. 9)**. Both Jackson and

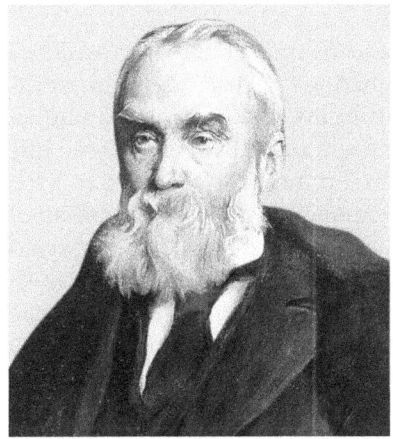

FIG. 8: John Hughlings Jackson (1835–1911).

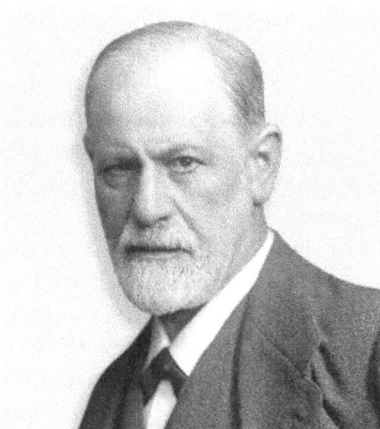

FIG. 9: Sigmund Freud (1856–1939).

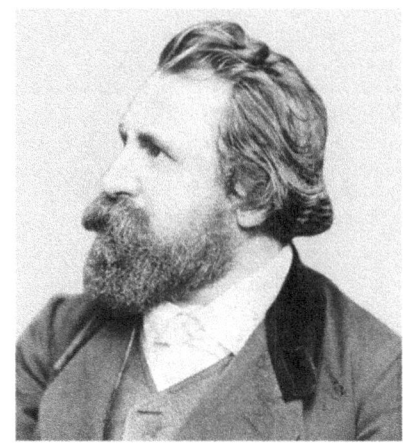

FIG. 10: Theodor Meynert (1833–1892).

Freud rejected the idea of a distinct "faculty" of language and instead incorporated concepts of "dissolution" (the opposite of evolution) and hierarchical neurological and psychological processes into their theories.[5]

Meanwhile, Theodor Meynert (1833–1892) and his student Carl Wernicke (1848–1905) were taking the understanding of the relationship between mental disorders and brain pathology in a different direction **(Figs. 10 and 11)**. Wernicke observed that not all cases of aphasia had lesions in the areas identified by Paul Broca (1824–1880). He described a different form of aphasia associated with lesions in the left superior temporal areas, which is now known as Wernicke's aphasia. Wernicke also described cases of alexia and agraphia. His classification of aphasic disorders gained wide acceptance, and other cortical syndromes, such as alexia without agraphia (Joseph Jules Dejerine, 1849–1917), ideomotor and other forms of apraxia (Hugo Liepmann, 1863–1925), and visual agnosia (Heinrich Lissauer, 1861–1891), were subsequently described. These disorders were rediscovered in the 20th century and formed the foundation of behavioral neurology.[6,7]

Freud was not impressed by Wernicke's reduction of cortical functions to discrete brain areas depicted in diagrams. During his education, Freud studied philosophy under Franz Brentano (1838–1917), who introduced the concept of intentionality. According to Brentano, every mental phenomenon is directed toward an object, which laid the groundwork for Freud's object relations theory. Freud's ideas of cathexis and libidinal investment also stemmed from this concept. These ideas had significant implications for the development of 20th-century neuropsychiatry.[7]

In the first half of the 20th century, several neuropsychiatrists sought to bridge the gap between brain-based neurology and Freudian psychology. Notable figures

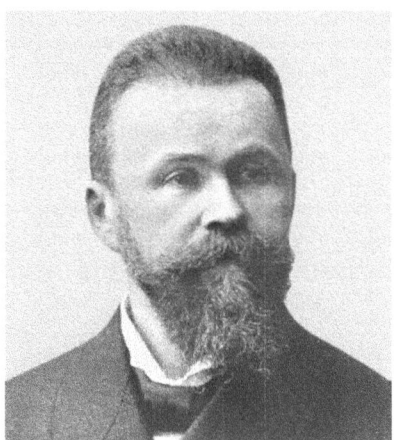

FIG. 11: Carl Wernicke (1848–1905).

included Smith Ely Jelliffe (1866–1945) and William White (1870–1937), whose book "Diseases of the Nervous System: A Text-book of Neurology and Psychiatry" (1915) provided comprehensive information on neuropsychiatry.[7]

Adolf Meyer (1866–1950) approached psychiatry through the autopsy room and had extensive knowledge of European ideas in neurology and psychiatry **(Fig. 12)**. His interest in patients' social environments and personalities led him to develop a "psychobiological" approach to mental illness. Meyer emphasized the need for an understanding of both the structure and function of the central nervous system, referring to conscious activity and bringing a "psychobiological" organization to the integrated functioning of the brain and the organism as a whole.[5]

In Meyer's words: "We want neuropsychiatrists—not just neurologists or psychologists, but primarily physicians capable of studying the entire organism, its functions, behaviors, and particularly the involvement of the nervous system and the challenges of adaptation."[5]

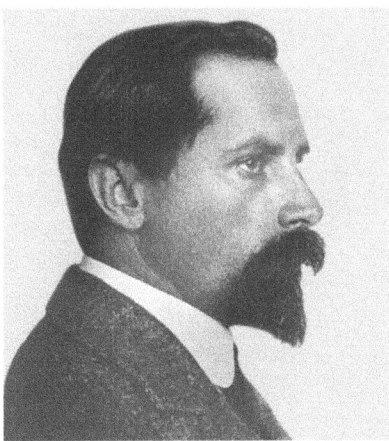

FIG. 12: Adolf Meyer (1866–1950).

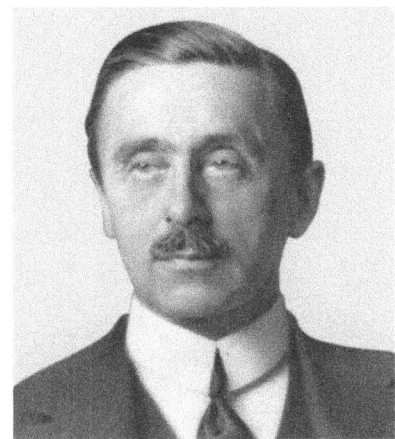

FIG. 14: Constantin von Economo (1876–1931).

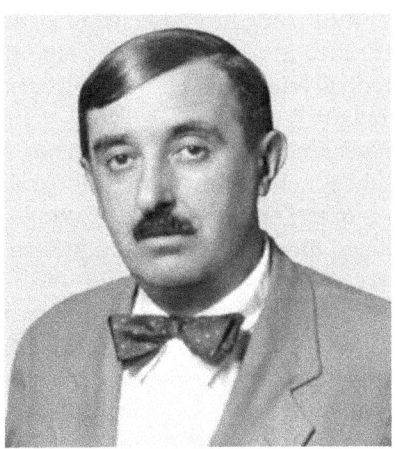

FIG. 13: Paul Schilder (1886–1940).

Paul Schilder (1886–1940), a follower of Wagner-Jauregg and a proponent of psychoanalytic ideas, developed a philosophical and psychological framework based on phenomenology **(Fig. 13)**. He aimed to establish a methodological foundation that encompassed all realms of experience and being, integrating it within a scientific and biological framework.

In 1916, Constantin von Economo (1876–1931) reported on a group of patients who exhibited a distinctive range of symptoms following an influenza-like prodrome **(Fig. 14)**. Some experienced severe lethargy and eye movement disturbances, and postmortem examinations revealed inflammatory changes primarily localized in the gray matter of the midbrain. Von Economo termed this condition "encephalitis lethargica" (commonly known as von Economo's disease), and it soon became recognized as an encephalitis linked to the influenza pandemics that occurred in Europe during the early 20th century. Survivors presented with various clinical manifestations, including motor disorders such as dystonias and Parkinsonism, as well as anxiety, obsessive-compulsive disorders, and psychoses.[6]

Von Economo emphasized the significance of these findings, stating: "The dialectic combinations and psychological constructions of many ideologists will collapse like a pack of cards if they do not consider these new fundamental facts in the future. Any psychiatrist seeking to understand disturbed motility, changes in character, psychological mechanisms of mental inaccessibility, neuroses, and more, must have a thorough understanding of the experiences gained from encephalitis lethargica... Those who do not familiarize themselves with the appropriate observations on encephalitic patients, the descriptions of severe mental symptoms in the original papers, will be building their understanding on shaky ground."

These developments in the understanding of encephalitis lethargica led to the revelation of an underlying neuroanatomy associated with neuropsychiatric disorders. It also facilitated the exploration of a unified understanding of movement and emotional disorders.[6]

The concept of the "integrated action" of the human organism, brain, and mind was central to the work of Charles Sherrington (1857–1952), a prominent neuroscientist **(Fig. 15)**. Sherrington emphasized the significance of the instinctive drive to live and reproduce, which he referred to as "zest," as the foundation of the mind. He disagreed with Descartes' view of humans as mere automatons, operating solely on stimulus-response mechanisms and disconnected from the mind and soul.[7]

In the field of neuroscience, Hans Berger (1873–1941) made a groundbreaking discovery **(Fig. 16)**. He demonstrated the possibility of recording electrical brain potentials from the surface of the skull, which he termed the electroencephalogram (EEG). Advancements in technology enabled more sophisticated EEG recordings,

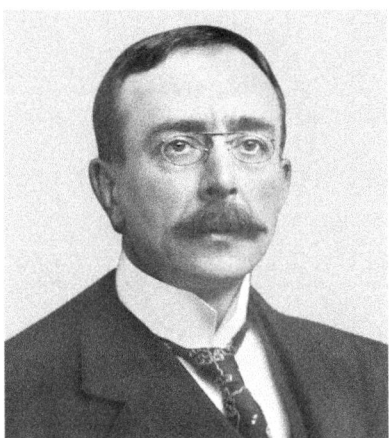

FIG. 15: Charles Sherrington (1857–1952).

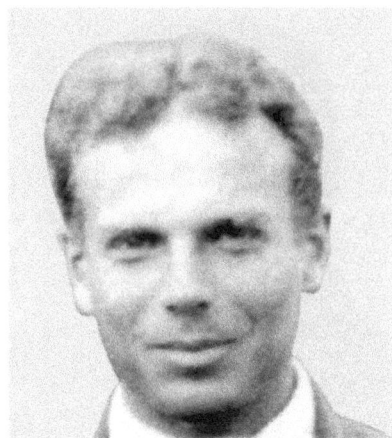

FIG. 17: Stanley Cobb (1887–1968).

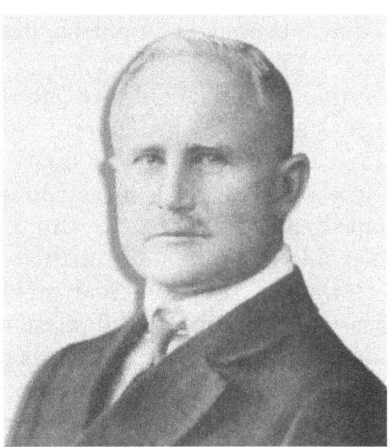

FIG. 16: Hans Berger (1873–1941).

and the contributions of pioneers such as Stanley Cobb (1887-1968), George Engel (1913-1999), Fred (1903-1992) and Erna (1904-1987) Gibbs, and John Romano (1908-1994) played a crucial role in the development of modern neuropsychiatry.[7-9]

Cobb made significant contributions to the field of neuropsychiatry with his book "Foundations of Neuropsychiatry" (1936) **(Fig. 17)**. The book underwent four editions, with each edition incorporating new insights into anatomy and physiology. Cobb consistently stressed the importance of maintaining integration between neurology and psychiatry. He rejected the dichotomy between "functional" and "organic" disorders, considering it misleading, as he believed that the division between the "physical" and the "mental" realms was arbitrary.[7]

Fred and Erna Gibbs conducted research on epilepsy and found that anterior temporal lobe foci were associated with a higher frequency of psychiatric disorders, particularly severe personality disorders and psychoses. Their emphasis on neuroanatomy and the underlying brain structures influenced the field. Similarly, George Engel and John Romano utilized EEG to study organic brain syndromes and played a significant role in advancing medical education with a comprehensive focus on neuropsychiatry.[8]

A groundbreaking development in neurology was the recognition that specific brain structures could constitute the foundation of an "emotional brain". Pioneers like Paul MacLean utilized new staining techniques to explore the neuroanatomy of the basal forebrain and revealed the extensive connectivity between limbic structures, the basal ganglia, and the neocortex. MacLean challenged the prevailing notion of a strict separation between cortical and subcortical systems and highlighted the integration of limbic and neocortical activity in shaping the sense of self. He also discussed how the limbic cortex generates free-floating affective feelings, which provide a subjective sense of reality and truth for individuals but cannot be expressed verbally. MacLean initially referred to these feelings as "visceral".[7,9]

In the 21st century, the field of neuropsychiatry has witnessed the convergence of ideas and investigations that are crucial to its modern understanding. Departing from Cartesian principles, post-Kantian concepts like intentionality challenged the objective necessity of empirical philosophy and instead sought to comprehend the relationship between our inner world and the external world. This shift did not advocate for introspection but aimed to understand the connection between subject and object. Inner perception, characterized by immediacy, ineffability, and self-evidence, constitutes our constant consciousness of something.[10]

Karl Jaspers, renowned for his work Allgemeine Psychopathologie (General Psychopathology), published in 1913, is closely associated with phenomenology—a term often misused by psychiatrists. Jaspers sought to explore the interconnectedness of reality as experienced in the mind and revealed through mental associations.

He distinguished between explaining nature and understanding mental life, emphasizing the quest to capture the essences of mental states through an "objective" descriptive psychology that transcended outdated psychological constructs and biases, including Freudian theories. Jaspers' descriptions of variously classified mental phenomena still underpin many contemporary psychopathological terms and inform diagnostic manuals such as later editions of the ICD and DSM. Regrettably, the concept of phenomenology and Jaspers' insightful constructs, which hold relevance for neuropsychiatry, have been reduced to mere descriptions of signs and symptoms assigned to often unvalidated rating scales of psychopathology, further diluted by computer-generated patient diagnoses. This approach does not align with the essence of neuropsychiatry.[10-14]

The term "neurophenomenology" reflects attempts to understand the intricate connections, contradictions, and puzzles pertaining to the relationship between neurobiological findings and mental states, going beyond the empirical limitations of diagnostic classifications determined by committees. As previously mentioned, modern neuropsychiatry is a distinct discipline within the clinical neurosciences that necessitates specialized expertise encompassing fundamental knowledge of the brain, its structure, and functions, as well as the consequences of their alterations in health and disease. It also requires a philosophy firmly rooted in phenomenology, embodiment, and empathy. Above all, the emergence of neuropsychiatry within the clinical neurosciences stems from the clinical need that arose due to the historical division between neurology and psychiatry, leaving many patients without effective understanding and management.[14]

In the field of neuropsychiatry, practitioners aim to effectively address psychiatric and neurological symptoms by integrating research from various disciplines, including neuropsychopharmacology, electroencephalography (EEG), clinical neurogenetics, neural network theory, medical informatics, and neuroimaging. Neuroimaging techniques, such as single-photon emission computed tomography (SPECT), functional magnetic resonance imaging (fMRI), magnetic resonance angiography, diffusion tensor imaging, and positron emission tomography (PET), play a significant role in the advancement of diagnostic and treatment approaches.

To utilize these tools in a clinical setting, neuropsychiatrists often collaborate with established professionals such as neuroradiologists and electrophysiologists. However, due to their comprehensive understanding of the patient's medical history, psychosocial context, and more extensive interaction with the patient during clinical sessions, it becomes the responsibility of the neuropsychiatrist to make optimal use of this information in guiding the overall treatment plan. This holistic approach allows them to consider both the biological and psychosocial factors influencing the patient's condition.

CLINICAL CONDITIONS ADDRESSED IN NEUROPSYCHIATRY

Here are examples of clinical problems that may be addressed by a neuropsychiatrist:
- A patient with Parkinson's disease who develops delusions and hallucinations as a side effect of dopamine-enhancing medications
- A patient with Huntington's disease exhibiting personality changes and violent behavior
- A developmentally disabled patient displaying self-injurious behavior
- A dementia patient causing behavioral disturbances and social disruptions
- A postoperative neurosurgical patient experiencing delirium and speech impairment
- A seizure patient presenting with psychosis or depression
- A patient with recurrent seizures requiring management
- A patient with chronic fatigue syndrome and cognitive decline
- A patient with a traumatic brain injury, unstable mood, and cognitive impairments
- A poststroke patient demonstrating apathy
- A patient with both schizophrenia and dementia
- A patient with Tourette syndrome and severe obsessive-compulsive disorder

Neuropsychiatry has played a crucial role in managing violent behavior in patients with known brain diseases. Neuropsychiatrists have been involved in treating individuals who exhibit violence patterns associated with various brain lesions. These include violence stemming from manic behavior after right parietal stroke, impulsive aggression in cases of congenital brain abnormalities or diencephalic injury, reflexive aggression triggered by transient environmental stimuli in dementia patients, violence resulting from a dysexecutive syndrome due to prefrontal cortical disease, and violence in individuals who experienced traumatic brain injury as victims of childhood abuse. The use of carefully selected combinations of medications such as beta-blockers, anticonvulsants, antipsychotics, antidepressants, and psychostimulants has been employed to improve brain function and reduce the frequency and intensity of violent behavior. This is crucial for effective nursing care, rehabilitation, and outpatient management.

FUTURE THOUGHTS: BRIDGING THE GREAT DIVIDE

In recent years, there has been renewed interest and debate surrounding neuropsychiatry in academic circles.[15,16] This resurgence has led to arguments for the integration of neurology and psychiatry as a unified specialty, transcending their previous status as separate subspecialties within psychiatry. Proponents of this viewpoint argue that the division between brain and mind, which has long characterized the differences between the two fields, is arbitrary and unsupported by scientific evidence. Research conducted over the past century has demonstrated that our mental experiences are rooted in the brain, challenging the notion of a distinct separation between brain and mind.[4]

Embracing the concept of mind/brain monism, or the idea that mind and brain are different perspectives of the same system, is seen as advantageous for several reasons. Firstly, it promotes the understanding that all mental processes have a biological basis, providing a common research framework for advancing our knowledge and treatment of mental disorders. Secondly, it helps alleviate confusion regarding the legitimacy of mental illnesses by suggesting that all disorders should manifest in the brain.

The traditional division between neurology and psychiatry has been attributed to their differing approaches to understanding the causes of disorders. Neurology has historically focused on internal factors such as neuropathology and genetics, while psychiatry has examined external factors such as personal, interpersonal, and cultural influences. However, it is debated that this dichotomy is not instructive and can be better understood as two ends of a spectrum. This expanded perspective on etiology allows for a more comprehensive understanding of the complex interactions between the brain and the environment.

This enhanced understanding of etiology can also lead to more effective remediation and rehabilitation strategies by identifying different points of intervention in the causal process. Nonorganic interventions such as cognitive-behavioral therapy (CBT) may be particularly effective in attenuating disorders either alone or in combination with pharmacotherapy. Studies have demonstrated neurobiological commonalities between psychotherapy and pharmacotherapy, highlighting the potential benefits of incorporating both approaches to improve patient outcomes and reduce side effects while increasing self-efficacy.

Furthermore, merging neurology and psychiatry is expected to facilitate the development of a more precise classification of mental illnesses, which in turn can enhance remediation and rehabilitation strategies. The current approach often groups together various symptoms, while a refined taxonomy would allow for more tailored interventions. Conversely, traditionally neurological disorders such as Parkinson's disease are increasingly recognized for their high incidence of psychiatric symptoms such as psychosis and depression, which are often overlooked in neurology. Neuropsychiatry can address these symptoms and contribute to improved patient care.

CONCLUDING REMARKS

The argument asserts that a comprehensive understanding of mental disorders requires knowledge not only of brain constituents and genetics but also of the contextual factors in which these components operate. By integrating neurology and psychiatry, this interconnectedness can be utilized to alleviate human suffering.

REFERENCES

1. Adams F. The Genuine Works of Hippocrates. Baltimore, MD: Williams and Wilkins; 1939.
2. Richardson A. British Romanticism and the Science of the Mind. Cambridge, UK: Cambridge University Press; 2001.
3. Massey I. Review. British Romanticism and the Science of the Mind.Criticism. 2002;44(1):78, 227.
4. Harrington A. Medicine, Mind, and the Double Brain. Princeton, NJ: Princeton University Press; 1989.
5. Lief A. The Commonsense Psychiatry of Dr Adolf Meyer. New York: McGraw Hill; 1948: 574.
6. Von Economo C. Encephalitis Lethargica [Trans. Newman KO]. Oxford, UK: Oxford University Press; 1931: p. 167.
7. Cobb S. Foundations of Neuropsychiatry, 3rd ed. Baltimore, MD: Williams and Wilkins; 1944: pp. 1-4.
8. Gibbs FA, Stamps FW. Epilepsy Handbook. Thomas Springfield; 1953.
9. Bergson H. Creative Evolution. New York: Henry Holt & Co.; 1911.
10. Merleau-Ponty M. The Phenomenology of Perception [Trans Smith C]. London: Routledge; 2002.
11. Jeannerod M. Motor Cognition: What Actions Tell the Self. Oxford, UK: Oxford University Press; 2006: vi.
12. Damasio A. The Feeling of What Happens. London: Heinemann; 2003:128.
13. Dilthey W. Ideas about a descriptive and analytical psychology. In: Dilthey W (Ed). Selected Writings [Trans. Ed Rickman HP]. Cambridge: Cambridge University Press;1894/1976. pp. 88-97.
14. Varela FJ. Neurophenomenology: A Methodological Remedy for the Hard Problem. J Consciousness Studies. 1996;3(4):330-50.
15. Saschev P. Whither Neuropsychiatry? J Neuropsychiatry Clin Neurosci. 2005;17:2.
16. Saschev P, Mohan A. Neuropsychiatry: Where Are We And Where Do We Go From Here? Mens Sana Monogr. 2013;11:4-15.

CHAPTER 2

Hysteria: Through the Ages

Ambar Chakravarty

INTRODUCTION

The term hysteria has been in use for long to denote a psychological disorder characterized by conversion of psychological stress into physical symptoms (somatization) or a change in self-awareness (such as a fugue state or selective amnesia).

Hysteria has historically been confusing to physicians because of its lack of easily measurable signs and symptoms. There is no standard presentation for this disease. Many centuries of neurologic and psychiatric observations have resulted in the incorporation of tests for hysteria into the bedside examination. This term had been omitted from the Mental Disorders Diagnostic Manual of the American Psychiatric Association in 1952[1] and replaced by Conversion Disorder which was described back in 1920 by Poul Bjerre as an unconscious emotional tension that arose from an unconscious source which may be converted into a physical ailment.[2] The present author feels that somatization, factitious disorder, malingering, conversion disorder, pseudoseizure, pseudomovement disorder, and functional illness to all have potential hysterical manifestations in the neurological examination. Pierre Janet poignantly commented, *"the word hysteria should be preserved although its primitive meaning has much changed. It would be very difficult to modify it nowadays, and truly it has so great and beautiful a history that it would be painful to give it up."*[3]

The word "Hysteria" is derived from the Greek word "hysteros" meaning uterus. Hysteria was originally recognized to occur exclusively in women and it was therefore thought that the illness was related to the womb. Katz wrote: *"When not satisfied with the body's desire to have children the womb wandered through it like a restless animal"* It would make sense that one of the first treatment was pregnancy.[4] From 1900 BC to AD 1600, the explanation of hysteria remained the wandering womb. In 1900 BC the Kahun papyrus explained the hysteria as a result of displacement of the uterus. The fragment of the papyrus that survived, described a series of morbid states that included hysteria and its early treatment with aromatic substances.[5] About 300 years ago, a German Egyptologist, Ebers, discovered a completely preserved document which contained a chapter on diseases of women. We learned from the Ebers Papyrus that there were several treatments to enable the uterus to descend. These included ingesting tar from the wood of a ship as well as imbibing from dregs of beer, or eating dry excrement moistened with beer. Popular treatments also included fragrances and aromatics.[6] Hippocrates, who was born in 460 BC, wrote about the displaced uterus in *"On the Nature of Women"*.[7] He expanded on this concept by stating in his 35th aphorism that those suffering from hysteria, but not those afflicted with epilepsy, felt digital pressure on the uterus. The theory was not challenged until Galen, born in AD 129, modified the understanding of hysteria by teaching that it was not a result of failure of the uterus to descend but rather it was due to a lack of sexual activity. Galen's treatment was marriage.[8] The philosophy of the Greeks also included looking to Gods such as Aesculapius, the God of healing. There were over 300 Aesculapian temples in existence during the reign of Alexander the Great (336-323 BC).[1] The great Roman encyclopedian Celsus was among the first to recommend bloodletting for the hysterical affliction.[1]

Galen's teachings on hysteria were the preferred view until the Middle Ages (AD 500-1500) when the church offered an alternative explanation for the sickness. It taught that the abnormal behavior was due to a lapse in faith. The era was filled with religious fervor and consequently drove a worldwide epidemic of the dancing mania.[9] New explanations of hysteria in this time period expanded to include demonic possession. This premise of hysteria inspired by demons was outlined by St Augustine (AD 354–430), whose ideas spurred a powerful movement that resulted in the persecution of many innocent victims.[10] The organized persecution for hysteria actually began earlier in the 9th century when Charlemagne banished citizens suspected of witchcraft.[1] This excessively violent attitude toward hysterical women culminated when Pope Innocent VIII commissioned Heinrich Kramer and James Sprenger to travel through Germany and enforce the views of their new book entitled Malleus Maleficarum (The Witches Hammer).[11] As a result, in late 15th century in Germany, approximately 600 persons a year suffering from the symptoms of hysteria were executed.[11] A new profession evolved in this era. Professional "prickers," screened the population testing for anesthetic spots as stigmata of the devil.[12] In England witchcraft became a statutory crime in 1541, although John Webster and others lobbied that witchcraft was really hysteria with melancholic dreams and hysterical imaginings.[1] Hutchinson, in a historic essay concerning witchcraft dispelled previous ridiculous notions and coined the term "vapors" to describe hysteria.[1] While Europe and the new colonies aggressively persecuted hysterics, the people of the Far East took a much more civilized position believing hysteria to be due to the protean powers of the fox, which was the messenger of the rice goddess and they did not persecute hysterics.[13]

Even the great Paracelsus felt that nature was the origin of all diseases and not Gods or ghosts.[14] Later Francois Rabelais (French novelist and physician) would observe that hysteria was susceptible to voluntary motor control[15] and his contemporary Johann Weyer, the father of modern psychiatry, declared of hysterics, *"if they do seem to merit punishment, illness alone is enough"*.[16] The 16th century also brought invention to the field of hysteria. The French surgeon Parey designed a pessaire of gold or silver to get fumes into the vagina. He also sent virgins into the woods on horseback as a modern treatment.[17]

The 1700's were marked by the birth of Mesmerism. Anton Mesmer (1734-1815) felt that all humans possessed an animal magnetism. He expressed the view that man was bipolar like a magnet. Mesmer explained that a person's magnetism could be manipulated and therefore he reasoned that hysteria was suggestible. In addition, Mesmer employed hypnotism and introduced group therapy. Mesmer would wear a robe and carry a magnetic wand in traditional ceremonies that included a tub of iron filings. His teachings led to mass hysteria and exorcisms and were condemned by a French commission appointed by Louis XVI of whom Benjamin Franklin, the chemist Lavoisier, and the astronomer Baillie were members.[18] The 1700's also brought important new acceptance to the understanding of hysteria. The American, Benjamin Rush, influenced by the Revolutionary War advocated a change of environment for hysterics. He also wrote of hysteria being a token of social distinction rarely occurring in servants and laborers.[19] The Frenchman, Pinel, influenced by his close friend who had gone insane, lobbied for the humane treatment of the hysterics in Salpetriere in Paris. He often used to see chronic patients free, and advocated putting patients back to useful labor.[20]

Earlier in 1681, Thomas Sydenham proposed that hysteria was due to psychological and emotional causes. He wrote in his Epistolary Dissertation that *"the frequency of hysteria is no less remarkable than the multiformity of the shapes which it puts on".*[21] Sydenham recognized the protean nature of the malady. He described hysteria to be polysymptomatic. Since Sydenham discovered this disorder in men, where, by definition it could not be found (*historically it should be a disorder only to be found in women, as the term was linked to "hysteros" meaning uterus*), a separate diagnostic term was required. He used the word "hypochondriasis", linking somatic disturbance with a disorder of emotional life, since the hypochondrium was supposed by the ancients to be the seat of melancholy In the late 18th century William Cullen classified hysteria as neurosis. It was a disorder of the nervous system that lacked an anatomical site or lesion.[22] Cullen is generally credited for introducing hysteria as a neurosis.

Two conflicting views of mental illness emerged in the 19th century. Moral theorists led by Philippe Pinel, felt that there was a defect in spirituality and that patients could be treated by kindness and appeal to the intellect. The physicalists disagreed with the moralists, arguing that mental illness was due to a defective brain, and therefore proposed somatic treatments.[23] One of the treatments was championed by Victor Burq. Burquism was the application of metals internally and to the body surface.[24]

By the mid-19th century, hysteria remained a marginal and somewhat awkward category of illness for both patients and physicians. Later in the 19th century RB Carter, in his book *"On the Pathology and Treatment of Hysteria"*, introduced a new understanding of hysteria. He recognized that there was a psychological basis for symptomatology and also was one of the first persons to point out that hysteria could affect men.[25] Carter was the first to choose different forms of psychotherapy for different kinds of hysteria. Briquet, a student of Charcot, published epidemiological and clinical data on 430 patients including seven mens. There were many symptoms which included many pains and also those symptoms of loss of neurological function classically associated with hysteria. Regarding etiology, he found no evidence in favor of sexual causes. Briquet outlined the factors predisposing to hysteria. Among them, were—youth, female gender, affective temperament, family history, low socioeconomic class, migration, sexual licentiousness, situational factors, and poor overall health. He believed that there was an affective part of the brain, which mediated all of the causative agents.[26] The term Briquet's syndrome was

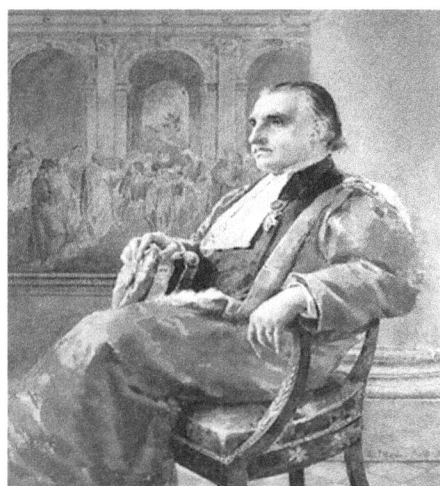

FIG. 1: Jean–Martin Charcot (1825–1893).

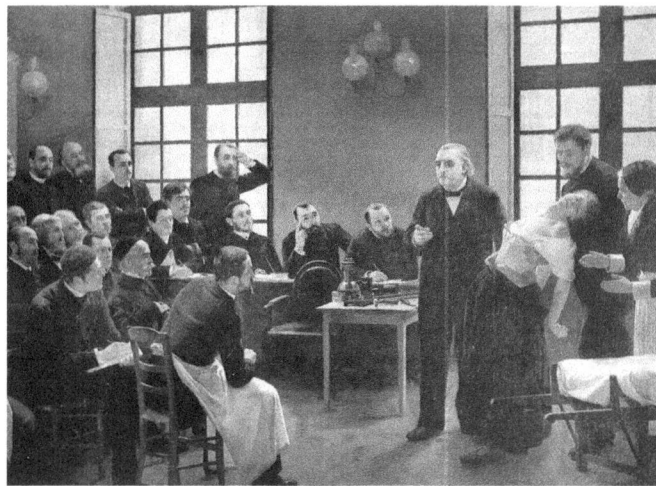

FIG. 2: Charcot's Tuesday Lesson at the Salpetriere, Paris: Demonstrating a lady with hysteria; the gentleman holding the lady is Josef Babinski.

subsequently used to denote somatic symptoms arising out of an underlying psychological cause.

A large part of our understanding of both neurology and psychiatry came from 19th century teachings of Jean-Martin Charcot (1825–1893) **(Fig. 1)**. He drew much of his knowledge from the British literature including the 1837 lessons on local hysteria and paralysis by the surgeon Benjamin Brodie. He also drew on other English works including Laycock (1840), Skey (1867), Todd (1867), and Reynolds (1869). Charcot took care of and became extremely interested in patients exhibiting hysteria. He is most famous for his teachings on the subject and often used hypnosis and suggestibility as part of his bedside examination and the "Tuesday lessons".[27,28] He derived much of his knowledge of hypnotism from the teachings of James Braid who invented neurohypnology. Braid was a surgeon who used the technique to eliminate pain.[29] Charcot used hypnosis in diagnosis of hysterics while his Nancy School rivals Bernheim and Liebault advocated its use as a therapeutic tool **(Fig. 2)**.[1] He added many facts to the modern neurological examination for hysteria, and it was in his era that the neurological examination began to expand to include tests for hysteria. Unfortunately at this time, two German physicians began to perform surgical procedures for the treatment of hysteria. Alfred Hegart pioneered ovariectomy, and Nikolaus Friedrick began cauterizing the clitoris.[1]

Charcot's famous patient Justine Etcheverry (depicted in Iconographie Photographique de la Salpetriere—edited by Bourneville) served as a kind of lexicon to many of Charcot's early views on the ingrained yet paradoxically evanescent clinical signs of "local" hysteria that persisted as stigmata between her convulsive attacks (hysteron-epilepsy). The classic ovarian sign, presence of an area of hypersensitivity over the region of the ovary, could be elicited in her. Charcot insisted on the diagnostic importance of the ovarian sign and the reference to that organ itself. He noted that the hysteron-epileptic attack could sometimes be terminated (as well as provoked) by exerting pressure on the ovarian region, a distinguishing feature from true epilepsy. Etcheverry also displayed a pattern of paralyses, contractures, and anesthesias distinct from those associated with organic disease of the brain; her contractures and other symptoms persisted while asleep, resisting even chloroform induced sleep except when taken to the last limits.[28]

Charcot reviewed a number of criteria by which true epileptic seizures could be distinguished from hystero-epileptic attacks. He gave maximum importance to clinical thermometry where he claimed to be the first to observe characteristic difference between epilepsy and hysteria. Dangerous temperature elevations were noted in true epileptic attacks but not in hysteria.[28]

Charcot illustrated convulsive hysteria with the case of Rosalie Leroux, a patient who had been a subject of for nearly 40 years to the most violent form of "epileptiform hysteria" (later called by him la grande hysteria—hysteria major). This lady had been suffering from violent convulsions, but she had no mental impairment. This was thought to be an important distinguishing feature from epilepsy proper. She also developed a right-sided "hemiplegia" from which she recovered "fully" **(Figs. 3A to E)**.[28]

There was no dearth of criticism of Charcot's views on ovarian hysteria. At a Cambridge meeting, Mathews Duncan (1826–1890) a leading London obstetrician, questioned Charcot's views on ovarian hysteria and trigger zone *"with expressions by word and gesture of lively*

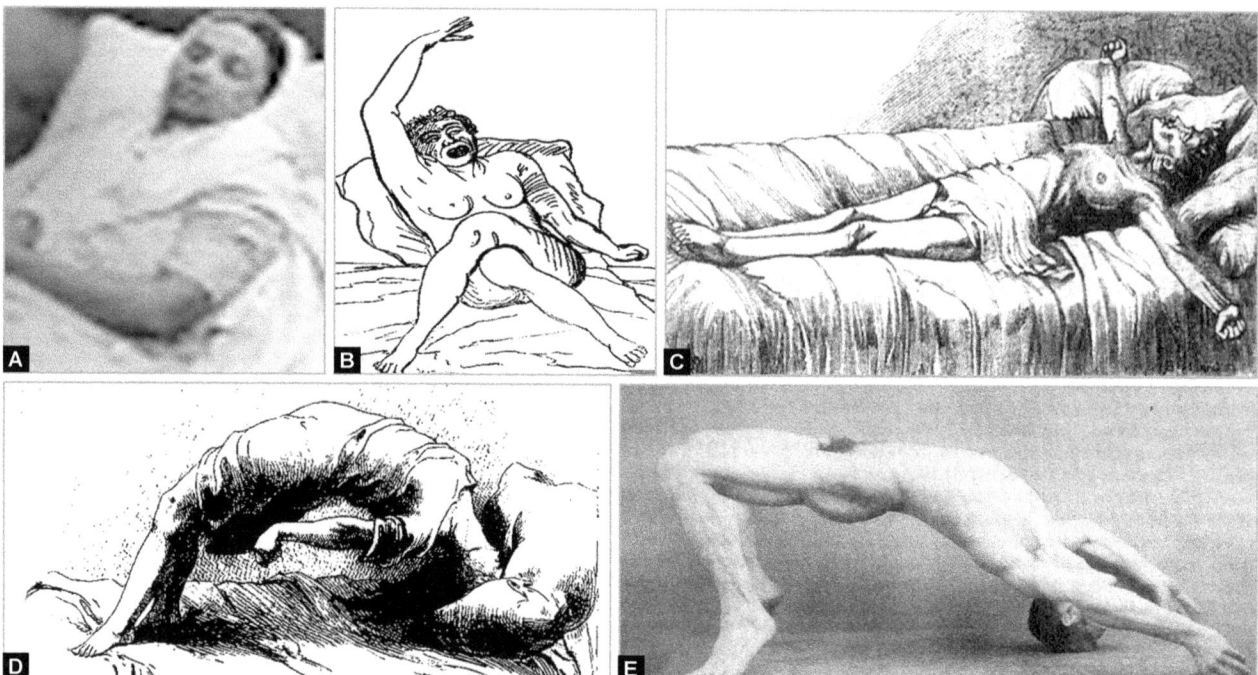

FIGS. 3A TO E: Charcot's famous patients: (A) Justine Etcheverry—note fixed dystonia in her left hand; (B and C) Rosalie Leroux—note great hysterical forms; (B) period of contortions; (C) attack of crucification in form of crucification; (D) La grande courbure—acute opisthotonus of body: (E) Traumatic male hysteria with arc-en-circle posturing.

contempt" (The Lancet 1880, Aug 14). Charcot, of course, denounced his *"adversary"* as *"a madman and a maniac"* and other critics as *"working to devalue me at every chance they get"*.[28]

Two of Charcot's pupils, both hailing from Vienna, Austria, Pierre Janet, and Sigmund Freud made very significant contributions to our understanding of hysteria—views that were significantly different from those of Charcot himself **(Fig. 4)**.

Janet[29,30] proposed a certain limited number of symptoms, by which hysteria must be identified and these he called the *"stigmata"*. These included typical symptoms of altered neurological function, namely paralysis, anesthesia, memory loss, unconsciousness, and loss of special senses functions. Janet excluded symptoms such as pain, tremor, dystonia, and ataxia. In addition Janet mentioned a group of symptoms which he labeled as *"accidents"* since they were not essential to the diagnosis and often were indicative of the psychic trauma.

This had been an important concept which influenced early psychoanalytic thinking. Janet's observations led him to conclude that the *"stigmata"* or *"accidents"* (basically conversion reactions) do not represent psychic trauma. They are *"precipitated"*, as he wrote, by many provocative agents such as *"physical and moral shocks"* and were increased by stress. Conversion reactions according to Janet's view were not directly or indirectly

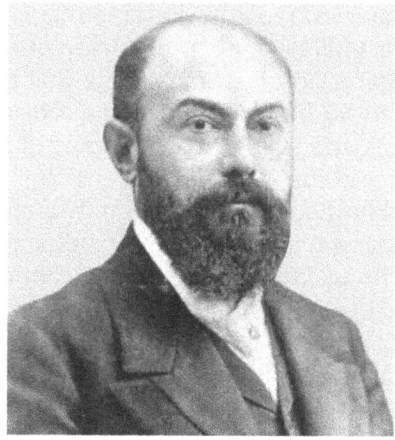

FIG. 4: Pierre Marie Félix Janet (1859–1947).

symbolic of psychic trauma. Janet also felt that the psychic trauma underlying the "accident", was *"repressed below the horizon of consciousness"*.

He postulated that certain individuals are constitutionally predisposed to hysterical symptoms; and he rejected the theory of a sexual cause. Janet elaborated on the type of personality which predisposes to the development of conversion and dissociative phenomena. The predisposed person was generally supposed to be coquettish and vain, quite akin to the hysterical personality disorder of modern times. More specifically, it resembles

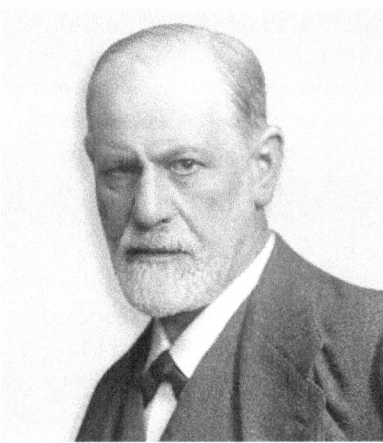

FIG. 5: Sigmund Freud (1856–1939).

the modern concept of the borderline personality. In many ways, Janet's work was revolutionary and very different from the then commonly held notions about hysteria. Not only did he reject the sexual theory outrightedly, but he also contradicted the prevailing view that hysteria was a most variable and protean malady.

The most influential of those rejecting Janet's ideas was Sigmund Freud, another of Charcot's pupils. *Studies in hysteria*,[30,31] published with Breuer in 1895, include four of Freud's cases **(Fig. 5)**. In this book, Janet's diagnostic recommendations are implicitly rejected and his theory of constitutional predisposition explicitly contradicted. The theory of sexual etiology was revived, but in an altered form. Freud opined that *"sexuality plays the principal role in the pathogenesis of hysteria as a source of psychic traumas"*.

The symptom complex of hysteria, was thought to symbolize the *"unconscious conflict surrounding unconscious, unacceptable, and sexual drives"*. Why did Freud's views were more acceptable than those of Janet's? Perhaps the long prevailing view that hysteria had a sexual basis, might have influenced the choice. Also, the suggestion that repression of sex-centered ideas might have an enormous malign consequence on mental health seemed peculiarly attractive to common people.

20TH CENTURY

In the English-speaking world, many disorders of unknown, but presumably psychological origin were viewed as if they were hysteria, and as if the symptoms symbolized unconscious conflict, usually of an Oedipal kind. Spasmodic torticollis, now considered a form of cervical dystonia, had been a classic example. It was felt in earlier times, that the head and neck "symbolized" an erect penis, and that the distressing intermittent twisting movements reflected castration anxiety.

The result of this conceptual and diagnostic confusion came with Slater's publication in 1965[32] of a follow-up of patients given the diagnosis of hysteria at Queen Square, London. He noted that after 10 years, a third of these patients had an organic diagnosis such as multiple (then called "disseminated") sclerosis; one-third already had such a diagnosis and hence the additional diagnosis of hysteria seemed superfluous; the remainder had a variety of psychiatric illnesses. Since the diagnosis changed over time, Slater postulated hysteria not only a "delusion but also a snare". His view that hysteria did not exist was supported by some contemporary psychiatrists as well.

Serious opposition to Charcot's views was expressed from both Germany and England. From Germany,[30] Oppenheim, based on his observations on cases diagnosed as hysteria, at Charité Hospital in Berlin, postulated that hysteria results from a psychic trauma to some undetectable brain structures which could explain the various somatic symptoms coupled with psychic symptoms in subjects with hysteria. He suggested a clear distinction between traumatic neurosis (resulting from physical trauma) and hysterical symptoms resulting from psychic trauma. Two great British neurologists, Hughlings Jackson and Gordon Holmes, from National Hospital, Queen Square, ascribed hysteria resulting as a consequence of *"dissolution of the highest level of function of the brain"*. William Gowers noted that the standard French practice of ovarian compression (introduced by Charcot) did not help British women with hysteria.[33] However, still several British physicians could not get over the feminine connection to hysteria and were still inclined to consider hysteria as a form of sexual dysfunction. A typical treatment, particularly, for high social class English women was the massage of the patient's genitalia by the physician and, later, by vibrators to cause orgasms (defined at that time "hysterical paroxysms").

It would be interesting at this stage to briefly discuss Charcot's most favorite pupil Josef Babinski's concept of hysteria and how it deviated from that of his Master.[34] Joseph Jules François Félix Babinski (1857–1932) had at the beginning of his career, was influenced by the concept of hysteria proposed by his Master Jean–Martin Charcot **(Fig. 6)**. However, from 1901 on, he presented his own theory about the malady, as well as several approaches to differentiate organic from hysterical symptomatology expressing the same in a number of publications (1893–1917/8). including his last book *Reponse à Radovici. Sur l'Hystérie* (1930). From the 1920s on, there arose not only a growing criticism of the theories of Charcot, but also a change in the conceptualization of hysteria, by neurologists mostly based on theories proposed by Babinski. He was a great semiologist; his greatest contribution in neurosemiology, was perhaps description

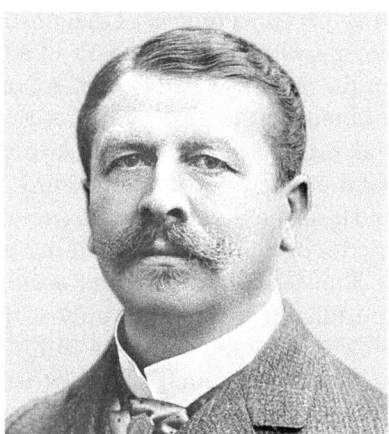

FIG. 6: Joseph Babinski (1857–1932).

of the Toe Phenomenon, written in only 28 lines, to explain its great importance in bedside clinical neurology.

In 1901, he launched his *Définition de' hystérie*, in which he spelt out his concepts on hysteria. Babinski proposed that hysteria was a psychical state in which the patient had a predisposition to self-suggestion, and hence he suggested the term *"pithiatism"* (from the Greek: Meaning created by suggestion and curable by persuasion) Babinski's concept of importance of suggestion was subsequently rejected by neurologists like Dejerine and Raymond, but was widely accepted in different parts of the world.

World War I, brought in to focus the syndrome of "traumatic hysteria", which was first proposed by Charcot himself. Several of Charcot's students were involved in medical military care, Babinski himself was involved and working with Jules Froment (1878–1946) of Lyon, was engaged in distinguishing patients with nervous organic diseases from those with "pithiatism" and malingering.

Clovis Vincent, a neurosurgeon of the time and close to Babinski, developed a treatment called torpillage (torpedoing) for war hysteria: Painful galvanic current discharges with "persuasion".

Major contribution in conceptualizing hysteria came from Brazil by Antônio Austregesilo.[35] He viewed hysteria as a *"diagnosis of the facility, above all when dealing with females"*. He defended a division of true hysteria (hysterical syndrome or pithiatism) and a pseudohysteria (hysteroid syndrome or false hysteria due to other physical or mental disorders).[34] In his *"New concepts on hysteria"*, his first work on the subject (1908), he stated, in line with Babinski's concept, that the phenomenon was produced by suggestion. Austregesilo argued that hysteria, be placed, in the field of Psychiatry. He admitted that hysteria was a psychoneurosis that developed from a preexisting diathesis: "nervousness". This was somewhat akin to the modern day concept of the term *Hysterical personality*.

Charcot probably changed his views about ovarian hysteria toward the fag end of his life. The last number of the Archives de Neurologie (July 1893) to appear before Charcot's death, contained innovative pragmatic essays on the psychological aspects of hysteria by Janet and Sigmund Freud; and private correspondences with his enthusiastic Viennese disciple (Pierre Janet) indicate that Charcot was receptive to Freud's earliest formulation of a psychogenic mechanism for the hysterical attack.[28]

Silas Weir Mitchell, during the American Civil War, had the unique opportunity at Turner's Lane to observe soldiers with exclusively neurologic and psychiatric disease. It was from this experience that Mitchell began to advocate noninstitutionalized care for hysterics. He opposed psychoanalysis, and based on his observations of nostalgia in soldiers, he advocated a rest cure.[36,37]

19TH AND 20TH CENTURY ADDITIONS TO THE NEUROLOGICAL EXAMINATION

It has been in the last 200 years that the traditional modern neurological examination has taken shape. From Charcot and the French school of neurological teachings much of the specialty of modern neurology has evolved. Many important observations were made in the 19th and 20th centuries that led to an understanding of how to separate organic from hysterical illness. Clinicians not only in France, but also in Germany, Great Britain, The Netherlands, Vienna, America, and from throughout the world added important signs to neurological examination to distinguish hysterical illness. Among the most important additions were tests for hysterical hemianesthesia, hemisensory loss, hemiplegia, astasia abasia and visual loss. Significant contribution to the history of hysterical signs in neurology is the observation by Buzzard that *"the figure of hysteria shrinks in proportion as the various forms of organic disease acquire greater solidity and sharper definition"*.[38] Detailing of bedside neurological examination techniques to differentiate between organic and hysterical or functional somatic complaints of patients would be beyond the scope of this commentary. Descriptions of such tests carry tremendous historical value and are fascinating to read and practice at the bedside.

PRESENT DAY CONCEPT OF HYSTERIA, DISSOCIATIVE DISORDERS AND CONVERSION DISORDERS: ARE THEY ALL SYNONYMOUS ?

The term, hysteria, with its multitude of symptom complex, was no longer included in the DSM-III (1980) and following editions. Newer terms such as "Somatoform Disorders" and "Dissociative Disorders", have come into use. Terms such as "somatization disorder" and Briquet's syndrome, have fallen into disrepute. In short, the old Freudian concept of conversion neurosis (unconscious conflicts become converted to bodily manifestations) is called now somatoform (such as conversion and somatization). This somatization concept became characterized by a multitude of somatic symptoms affecting different organ systems. Five symptom complexes constituting the somatization concept include—(1) somatoform disorders, (2) conversion, (3) pain, (4) hypochondria, and (5) dysmorphophobic disorders. Conversion disorder (DSM-IV) involves "one or more symptoms affecting voluntary motor or sensory function related to psychological factors, unintentional and unfeigned, and resembling neurological or medical ailments". However, its nomenclature suffered changes over the time—in 1952 (DSM-I), the used term was conversion reaction; in 1968 (DSM-II), hysterical neurosis (conversion type); and in 1980 (DSM-III), conversion disorder.

Henceforth, the label "dissociation" and "conversion" disorders began to be used. In ICD-10 (1992), conversion disorder is discussed under the category of dissociative (conversion) disorders, together with dissociative amnesia and fugue states. Confusion continues to linger on. The currently in vogue DSM V (2013)[39] includes the following to cover the entire spectrum of disorders which were included under the broad concept of hysterical disorders prior to 1980:
- Trauma- and stressor-related disorders
- Dissociative disorders
- Somatic symptom disorder (SSD) and other related disorders (including conversion disorder)
- Psychological factors affecting other medical conditions

THE WAY FORWARD—ONTO 21ST CENTURY

"Hysteria" has transformed in name, but not in nature. What was deemed to be dysfunction of the uterus is now deemed as neurological manifestations of underlying psychological conflicts or stressors. Somatoform and conversion disorders are just as prevalent today in developed and developing countries as it was centuries ago. Increased attention and awareness toward somatoform disorders include both improvements in diagnosis and improvements in treatments. Insight advances in functional neuroimaging and neurophysiology would help progress in our understanding of the pathophysiology of conversion disorders.[40]

To explore neurophysiology from a functional neuroanatomic perspective, recent studies are more directed toward functional neuroimaging than structural imaging. Much has been done in functional neuroimaging in psychogenic movement disorders and psychogenic nonepileptic seizure (PNES). Conversion disorder subjects with positive motor symptoms show greater amygdala activity to arousing facial stimuli compared to healthy volunteers. Arousing stimuli were also associated with enhanced functional connectivity between the amygdala and supplementary motor area in conversion disorder subjects. Abnormalities in connectivity and neural networks in PNES have been investigated using electroencephalogram (EEG) and resting state functional magnetic resonance imaging (MRI). Scientists have found decreased prefrontal and parietal synchronization with a greater number of PNES events. Using resting state functional MRI, it had been noted that PNES subjects had greater functional correlation between regions implicated in emotion and self-perception (insula) and motor preparation (precentral and central sulcus), and that dissociation scores were positively correlated with this connectivity. Structural neuroimaging (morphometric MRI) in small subset of patients with conversion disorder compared to healthy controls, revealed smaller mean volumes of the left and right basal ganglia and a smaller right thalamus in the conversion patients. How relevant or helpful these studies would be in clarifying diagnosis of somatoform disorders and conversion disorders (in particular in PNES), can only be known once such studies are extended to larger number of subjects and research moves from the bench to the bedside.

Treatment modalities are undergoing sea change. Prior "treatments" for hysteria documented in the medical literature included hydrotherapy (a jugful of water to an open mouth), faradization (electric current applied to the skin), and a vigorous tug at the pubic hair, used in England, or the ovarian compression belt, used in France. Hypnosis and psychoanalysis were commonly used in the early and mid-20th century for conversion treatment. Over the past 10 years, however, rigorous trials comparing pharmacotherapies and psychotherapies (psychotropic medicines , cognitive behavioral therapy) have been conducted providing an evidence-based medicine approach to somatoform disorders.

In a 2000 report in Lancet, Halligan et al.[41] cited one patient with hypnotic paralysis who underwent a PET study. Results revealed that similar brain regions as in conversion disorder were activated suggesting that hypnosis and hysteria may share common neurophysiological mechanism. Could hysteria then be a form of self-hypnotism? One wonders!

REFERENCES

1. Veith I. Hysteria: The History of a Disease. Chicago: University of Chicago Press; 1965; pp. 1–58.
2. Bjerre P. The History and practice of psychoanalysis. Boston : Richard G Badger 1920:95-96
3. Janet P. The Mental state of hystericals: A Study of Mental Stigmata and Mental Accidents (Trans. CR Carson). New York: Putnam and Sons; 1901. p. 527.
4. Pryse-Phillips W. Companion to Clinical Neurology. Philadelphia: Lippincott Williams and Wilkins; 1995. p. 437.
5. Griffith F. The Petri Papyri, Hieratic Papyri from Kahum and Gurob. London: Bernard Quaritch; 1897. pp. 5-11.
6. Sigerist E. A History of medicine Volume I of Primitive and Archaic Medicine. New York: Oxford University Press: 1951. p. 102
7. Hippocrates. On the Diseases of Women [Trans. Littre E]. Paris: Bailliere; 1851.
8. Galen. De Locis affectis, Lib. VI. In : Histoir critique de l'hysterie, Paris : Asselin et Houzean 1909.
9. Sigerst HE. Four Treatise of Theophrastus Von Hohenheim called Paracelsus. Baltimore : The Johns Hopkins Press; 1941. pp. 127-212.
10. Brown P. Augustine of Hippo. London and Berkeley: Faber and Faber; 1967.
11. Institoris H. Malleus Maleficarum [translated with an introduction, bibliography and notes by the Rev. Montague Summers]. London: Pushkin Press; 1951.
12. Pusey EB. The Confessions of St. Augustine. Oxford: John Henry Parker; 1853.
13. Veith I. Psychiatric thought in Chinese Medicine. J History Med Allied Sci.1955;3:262-3.
14. Goodrick-Clark N. Paracelsus. Wellingborough: Aquarian Press; 1990.
15. Rabelais F. Pantagruel in the Portable Rabelais [Trans. Samuel Putnam]. New York: The Viking Press; 1946. p. 477-8.
16. Zillboorg G. The Medical Man and the Witch during the Renaissance. Baltimore: Johns Hopkins Press; 1935. p. 109.
17. Johnson T. The Works of the famous Ambrose Parey. London: R Cotes and W. Du-Gard: 1649.
18. Spanos NP, Gottlieb J. Demonic possession, mesmerism, and hysteria—a social psychological perspective on their historical interrelations. J Abnormal Psychol. 1979;88:527-46.
19. Rush B. Medical Enquiries and Observations Upon the Diseases of Mind. Philadelphia: Kimber and Richardson; 1812.
20. Pinel P. Tratte medico-philosophique sur l'alienation mentale ou la manie. Paris. Richard, Caille and Ravier; 1801.
21. Sydenham T. The Works of Thomas Sydenham, M.D [Translated by R.G. Latham]. London. Birmingham: The Classics of Medicine Library; 1979.
22. Cullen W. Of the Hysteria or the hysteric disease. Edinburgh: Bell, Brafute; 1796.
23. Finger S. Origins of Neuroscience. New York: Oxford University Press; 1994. p. 389.
24. Burq V. Metallotherapie. Paris: Balliere; 1853.
25. Carter RB. On the Pathology and Treatment of Hysteria. London; Churchill; 1853.
26. Briquet P. Traite Clinique et therapeutique de l'hysterie. Paris: JB Baillerie; 1859:200-304.
27. Charcot JM. Lectures on the diseases of the nervous system, delivered at the Saltpetrierre [translated by George Sigerson]. Philadelphia: Henry C. Lea; 1879.
28. Goetz CG, Bonduelle M, Gelfond T. Charcot Constructing Neurology. New York: Oxford University Press; 1995. pp. 172-216.
29. Janet P. Major symptoms of hysteria, fifteen lectures given in the medical school of Harvard University. New York: MacMillan; 1920.
30. Carota A, Calabrese P. Hysteria around the World. In: Bogousslavsky J (ed). Hysteria: The Rise of an Enigma. Basel: Karger; 2014. pp. 169-80.
31. Freud S, Breuer J, Luckhurst N, Bowlby R. Studies in Hysteria. London: Penguin Classics; 2004.
32. Slater ET, Glithero E. A follow-up of patients diagnosed as suffering from "hysteria". J Psychosom Res. 1965;9(1):9-13.
33. Gowers WR. Epilepsy and Other Chronic Convulsive Diseases, 2nd edition. London: Churchill; 1901.
34. Gomes MM, Engelhardt E. Hysteria to conversion disorders: Babinski's Contributions. Arq Neuropsiquiatr. 2014;72(4): 318-21.
35. Gomes Mda M, Cavalcanti JL. The Brazilian Neurology centenary (1912-2012) and the common origin of the fields of Neurology and Psychiatry. Arq Neuropsiquiatr. 2013;71(1):63-5.
36. Pearce JM. Silas Weir Mitchell and the "rest cure". J Neurol Neurosurg Psychiatry. 2004;75(3):381.
37. Mitchell SW. Fat and Blood: And how to make them. Philadelphia: JB Lippincott; 1877.
38. Buzzard T. Remarks on the Differential Diagnosis of Insular Sclerosis from Hysteria. Br Med J. 1899;1(2001):1077-9.
39. American Psychiatric Association. Diagnostic and Statistical Manual of Mental Health (DSM5). Washington DC: American Psychiatric Association; 2013.
40. LaFrance Jr WC. 'Hysteria' Today and Tomorrow. Bogousslavsky J (ed): Hysteria: The Rise of an Enigma. Basel: Karger; 2014. pp. 198-204.
41. Halligan PW, Athwal BS, Oakley DA, Frachowiak RS. Imaging hypnotic paralysis: implications for conversion hysteria. Lancet. 2000;355:986-7.

Somatic Symptom Disorder: A Brief Note

Ambar Chakravarty

INTRODUCTION

Somatization may be defined as a constellation of bodily symptoms recurring or persisting for >6 months affecting well-being and activities of daily living. In the Diagnostic and Statistical Manual of Mental Disorders, Fifth Edition (DSM-5), the term "Somatic Symptom Disorder" is preferred and the concept has been changed from one which had been a negative one[1] (absence of physical signs or medically detectable cause) to one which is more positive with some detailing of specific symptoms which patients perceive. The current diagnostic criteria include:

"A. One or more somatic symptoms that are distressing or result in significant disruption of daily life.
B. Excessive thoughts, feelings, or behaviors related to the somatic symptoms or associated health concerns as manifested by at least one of the following:
- Disproportionate and persistent thoughts about the seriousness of one's symptoms.
- Persistently, high level of anxiety about health or symptoms.
- Excessive time and energy devoted to these symptoms or health concerns.
C. Although any one somatic symptom may not be continuously present, the state of being symptomatic is persistent (typically >6 months)".

In the DSM-5, two other conditions are included within the rubric of "somatic symptom disorder" and these include "illness anxiety disorder" and "factitious disorder".[1] The illness anxiety disorder is characterized by:

"A. Preoccupation with having or acquiring a serious illness.
B. Somatic symptoms are not present or if present, are only mild in intensity. If another medical condition is present or there is a high risk for developing a medical condition (e.g., strong family history is present), the preoccupation is clearly excessive or disproportionate.
C. There is a high level of anxiety about health, and the individual is easily alarmed about personal health status.
D. The individual performs excessive health-related behaviors (e.g., repeatedly checks his or her body for signs of illness) or exhibits maladaptive avoidance (e.g., avoids doctor appointments and hospitals).
E. Illness preoccupation has been present for at least 6 months, but the specific illness that is feared may change over that period of time.
F. The illness-related preoccupation is not better explained by another mental disorder, such as *somatic symptom disorder, panic disorder, generalized anxiety disorder, body dysmorphic disorder, obsessive-compulsive disorder,* or *delusional disorder, somatic type.*"

Patients with factitious (Latin for *artificial*), disorder present with multitude symptoms of mimicking those several disease processes, that are essentially intentionally produced to assume the role of a sick person. Such symptoms and features are produced voluntarily and with full awareness but with no intention of secondary gain. These people assume the role of a sick person to receive appropriate care and attention from friends and relatives to cope with their emotional or psychological distress. Factitious disorder is more prevalent in females, especially those having some experience in health care practices, with age at onset around mid-20s for both sexes. Symptoms may develop in childhood as means to receive care, attention, and protection from medical personnel to compensate for an unhealthy home environment. Warning signs for early recognition of factitious disorders include patients seeking treatment and testing at multiple sites, inconsistent histories, and discrepancies between patient behavior, symptoms, and history.

In clinical practice, clear differentiation between somatic symptom disorders, malingering, conversion disorder, illness anxiety disorder, generalized anxiety disorders, and factitious disorders are often difficult unless an obvious secondary gain can be identified or features like obsessive compulsive nature or delusional thought processes can be identified. For a neurologist, exclusion of an organic disorder is of utmost importance, and it would be safer to designate nearly all nonorganic psychogenic disorders as "functional disorders".

There are two important facets to the diagnosis of functional neurological disorders. The first is elicitation of a detailed history about the subject's problems. However, convinced a doctor is about the patients' symptoms being nonorganic in origin in the first few minutes of interview, he should continue interviewing the patient for an adequate time. This, on one hand, would lessen the chance of missing any organic pathology which may present initially with a multitude of and apparently unrelated symptoms, and on the other would help to convince the patient that the doctor is taking his/her problems seriously and genuinely taxing his brain to find the root cause of the problems and is sympathetic to his/her symptoms and trying hard to relieve them. Secondly, these patients must be examined very thoroughly to be absolutely sure that nothing organic is being missed and this would help in boosting the patients' confidence in the doctor. Patients with multitude of symptoms very often visit multitude of doctors, which only make themselves more and more anxious about their physical condition. The principal reason for this practice is failure to acquire adequate confidence on one individual doctor that he would be able to lessen or cure his/her problems.

Having being confident himself that nothing organic is at miss, the doctor should proceed to explain to the patient in simple terms the nature of his/her problem and assure the patient that there is nothing very seriously wrong which cannot be cured. It is extremely unwise to mention to the patient that his/her symptoms are all in the mind. Diagnostic tests should be kept at the minimum essentials which are absolutely needed to exclude an organic pathology because more the patient undergoes through more tests, he/she gets more convinced that he/she is harboring a serious illness which the doctor is unable to pinpoint.

Apart from excluding any organic pathology, through a detailed history, the doctor should try hard to assess the underlying psychiatric condition of the patient.[2-5] As mentioned earlier, these generally include anxiety disorders and depression, at times mixed with personality disorders. Body dysmorphic disorders are often present. Factitious disorders and malingering are on the whole, uncommon, and these should not be mentioned directly to the patients. Psychiatric help may at times be needed but should only be reserved for a very limited number of patients, as such referrals often have a negative impact on their minds (especially Indian subjects) and often results in a change of the primary treating physician. It is often more helpful to refer patients to support groups or mental health providers like counselors. Physicians themselves may try their patients on a small dose of a selective serotonin reuptake inhibitor (SSRI) like sertraline or fluoxetine. But, the most essential part of treatment is to alter the psyche of the patient so that they can:

- Avoid disproportionate and persistent thoughts about the seriousness of the symptoms.
- Avoid persistent high level of anxiety about health or symptoms.
- Avoid excessive time or energy devoted to symptoms or health concerns.

Perhaps the best ways to achieve the above include:
- Regular supervised physical training
- Swimming sessions
- Traveling
- Spending time in any activity that the patient enjoys.

Patients need to be informed that theirs is not an uncommon rare disease; hundreds and hundreds of people around the world suffer from similar conditions and that most of them improve or get cured following some simple forms of therapy but at times these may take time to work.

REFERENCES

1. American Psychiatric Association, DSM-5 Task Force. Diagnostic and statistical manual of mental disorders: DSM-5™ (5th edition). United States: American Psychiatric Publishing, Inc.; 2013.
2. Sharma MP, Manjula M. Behavioural and psychological management of somatic symptom disorders: an overview. Int Rev Psychiatry. 2013;25(1):116-24.
3. Heijmans M, Olde Hartman TC, van Weel-Baumgarten E, Dowrick C, Lucassen PL, van Weel C. Experts' opinions on the management of medically unexplained symptoms in primary care. A qualitative analysis of narrative reviews and scientific editorials. Fam Pract. 2011;28(4):444-55.
4. Fallon BA, Ahern DK, Pavlicova M, Slavov I, Skritskya N, Barsky AJ. A randomized controlled trial of medication and cognitive-behavioral therapy for hypochondriasis. Am J Psychiatry. 2017;174(8):756-64.
5. Somashekar B, Jainer A, Wuntakal B. Psychopharmacotherapy of somatic symptoms disorders. Int Rev Psychiatry. 2013;25(1):107-15.

CHAPTER 3

Functional Neurological Disorders: An Overview—Pathophysiology, Clinical Recognition, and Outlines of Management

Amit Halder, Ambar Chakravarty

INTRODUCTION

Functional neurological disorders (FNDs) have remained an enigma through the ages. A variety of terms such as hysteria, nervous system disorder, conversion disorder, and psychogenic or nonorganic illness have been used in various contexts to essentially mean the same condition. The plethora of terms used to mean the same phenomenon highlights the difficulty in explaining the condition.

The disorder is more common in females in general. However, some peculiar types of FNDs such as myoclonus and parkinsonism may be more common in males.

The last couple of decades have seen a substantial increase in research interest across many areas of FNDs. Newer insights into the underlying mechanisms of FNDs have been gained. Several well-conducted randomized controlled trials (RCTs) added much needed evidence base to treatment approaches.

NOSOLOGY

There have been substantial changes in the classification and nosology of the FNDs. The fundamental change in approach has been the emphasis on demonstration of "typical positive signs" for diagnosis (e.g., Hoover's sign). FNDs are thus not a diagnosis of exclusion; nor can they be diagnosed on the basis of associated psychosocial factors.

The Diagnostic and Statistical Manual of Mental Disorders, fifth edition (DSM-5) criteria published in 2013 thus removed both the requirement for a "recent psychological stressor" as well as the need to exclude feigning (which is not possible in practice). The criteria include:
- One or more symptoms of altered voluntary motor or sensory function
- Clinical findings provide evidence of incompatibility between the symptom and recognized neurological or medical conditions
- The symptom or deficit is not better explained by another medical or mental disorder
- The symptom or deficit causes clinically significant distress or impairment in social, occupational, or other important areas of functioning or warrants medical evaluation.

The term "functional neurological symptom disorder" has been added to the previous term "conversion disorder".

FUNCTIONAL NEUROLOGICAL DISORDERS: EVOLUTION OF THE CONCEPTS

Role of Supernatural Forces

In ancient times, whatever that could not be explained rationally was ascribed to the supernatural forces. FND was no exception to this rule. Epizelus, an Athenian soldier who fought the Battle of Marathon at 490 BCE was said to have lost both his vision after witnessing the death of a fellow soldier. This eyesight loss was believed to be caused by "divine intervention". Citizens sought treatment for such FNDs at the "Temple of Aesculapius".[1]

This practice continued through the middle ages. Sickness was ascribed to the devil's influence or as punishment for some past actions. Some of them were tortured and even executed after being accused of witchcraft. On the other end of the spectrum were some who got worshipped as saints due to their distortions in perception and sense.

Role of Reproductive Organs

Texts as old as the 1900 BC Egyptian Kahun Medical Papyrus referred to a collection of otherwise unexplained symptoms attributed to uterine dysfunction. The term "hysteria" owed its origin to ancient Greek philosophers and physicians, with its root meaning associated with the womb or uterus.[2] It was hypothesized that the displaced uterus (or testes) interfered with the function of the other organs. Both Hippocrates and Galen tried to explain the functional symptoms of other organs with this reproductive organ hypothesis. The subsequent changing concepts in the genesis of FNDs, the so called hysteria,[3,4] have been discussed in detail elsewhere in this volume.

NEUROBIOLOGICAL BASIS

The traditional model of psychological distress being converted into physical symptoms has also existed for centuries. They however could not account for the long latency between the experience and the onset of FNDs. They also could not explain why similar experience created different symptoms in different individuals.[5]

Edwards et al. suggested a "Bayesian model" to account for the symptoms. They suggest the common abnormality that produces functional motor and sensory symptoms is the emergence of *abnormal prior beliefs* that are afforded *excessive precision by attention*. They do not distinguish between a primary pathology in neuronal populations encoding prior beliefs that could misappropriate attention or a primary pathology of attention that produces prior beliefs held with undue conviction (precision).

The consequences of endowing beliefs about sensations or movements with undue precision (certainty) are two-fold. First, there will be false perceptual inference as top-down prior beliefs overwhelm bottom-up sensory evidence from lower levels. Second, higher levels now have to explain the emergence of the belief, leading to a misattribution of agency in the sense that top-down attentional processes induced the belief but did not predict its content.

The role of attention is emphasized by the role of suppression of symptoms of FNDs on distraction. This can also be used in therapy of such patients.

Regardless of the triggering mechanism, once the symptoms start it is propagated by a variety of factors. Phobic avoidance, affective disorders, and ultimately brain plasticity may all be involved.

NEUROIMAGING PERSPECTIVES

Functional neuroimaging has shown changes in brain metabolism in specific anatomical areas. Altered activity and connectivity of brain networks can differentiate between feigned and functional weakness. In patients with functional tremors, dystonia, or gait disorders there is hypoactivation of the supplementary motor area, a key structure involved in action selection and movement preparation. There is also abnormal connectivity between the supplementary motor area and limbic areas. They may be associated with abnormally increased activation in areas involved in emotion recognition and self-awareness (primarily the amygdalae and cingulate gyrus). In psychogenic nonepileptic seizure (PNES), resting functional MRI shows areas involved in emotion (insula), executive control (inferior frontal gyrus and parietal cortex), and movements (precentral sulcus) having strong functional connectivity.

CLINICAL SIGNS

Joseph Babinski, the famous French neurologist, devised many signs to distinguish between these two groups of disorders. His most famous sign being the "le phenoméne des orteil" ("the phenomenon of the toes"). It must be remembered that absence of positive signs does not exclude organic disease. On the other hand, presence of certain "positive signs" can add to the value of the diagnosis of FNDs.[6]

POSITIVE SIGNS OF LOWER LIMB FUNCTIONAL WEAKNESS

Hoover's Sign

Charles Franklin Hoover in 1908 described a sign that utilizes the principal of contralateral synergistic movement resembling the earlier "Ersatzbewegungen" ("substitution movements") formulated by Babinski who described the trunk–thigh test, also known as "the rising sign". The key concept enabling Hoover to come up with his sign was probably the "Ersatzphenomän", or "substitution phenomenon" of Bychowski. These concepts are related to the clinical observation of synkinetic oppositional movements during the execution of specific maneuvers in hemiplegic patients.

Hoover's sign is characterized by an involuntary extension of the weak leg when the contralateral limb is forced to flex against resistance and it is perceived by the examiner's hand placed under the heel. There's a complementary way of eliciting the Hoover's sign. The examiner asks the subject to lift the "weak leg". If the examiner does not perceive pressure from the heel on the good side, while trying to lift the weak leg, the sign is demonstrated. Hoover himself reported the possibility of inverting the procedure in order to obtain similar information by asking the patient to press his/her leg against the couch instead of lifting it.

A UK-based study on hemiplegic patients found that Hoover's sign displayed moderate sensitivity (63%) and high specificity (100%).[7]

Hoover's sign does have some limitations. This is regarding the correct interpretation of mildly positive signs, especially in the setting of marked spasticity, pain, cortical neglect, or even in a normal individual.

Abductor Sign

This is elicited when both legs are initially abducted against resistance, and regardless of the cause of weakness the weak leg will be always adducted by the force imposed by the examiner. This relies on contralateral synergistic movement.

Next, the patient is asked again to abduct against resistance. This time the patient concentrates on each leg separately, keeping the other leg in an adducted position along the midline. Weakness of abduction in the affected leg returns to normal during contralateral abduction against resistance in functional cases.

A comparison of the two signs in an unblinded trial of organic and functional patients clearly demonstrated the superiority of "abductor sign".

Other Leg Signs

Raimiste's Leg sign and its modified version resemble the abductor sign in testing for leg movements. However, the main difference with the abductor sign was the fact that in the modified test the examiner does not ask the patient to adduct–abduct each leg separately.

The Spinal Injuries Centre (SIC, Izuka, Japan) devised a SIC test for lower limb functional weakness. The patient is tested in supine position and the examiner lifts up the patient's knees, and then gently releases them. If the lifted position is maintained, the SIC test is positive. In cases of severe organic paralysis, the test is negative. On the other hand, the test is positive in cases of "functional paralysis".

The *dragging monoplegic gait* is observed by spontaneous leg dragging at the hip behind the body instead of performing a circumduction seen in organic cases.

Waddell Signs

Professor Gordon Waddell was an orthopedic surgeon who worked principally in Scotland and Wales. He was running a clinic in Western Infirmary, Glasgow and wondered why some patients were far more disabled by back pain than others. In what was a highly unusual move at the time (1970s), he formed a partnership with a young clinical psychology researcher, Chris Main, and together they investigated why some patients could hardly walk while others were walking reasonably well, despite looking the same on physical examination. Waddell asked three doctors to examine the same patient and found that they came up with differing degrees of disability. Based on his observations on 350 patients with low back pain, Waddell and his colleagues described the physical signs associated with nonorganic low back pain. He found nonorganic signs of low back pain that were clearly distinguishable from the standard clinical signs of organic disorders causing back pain.

Waddell's signs consist of eight clinical signs that are divided into five broad categories that include:
1. Superficial and nonanatomic tenderness
2. Axial loading and acetabular rotation simulation
3. Distraction
4. Regional sensory disturbance and weakness
5. Overreaction

Waddell signs include:
- *Superficial tenderness*: Tenderness over a wide area of lumbar skin to light touch or pinch.
- *Nonanatomic tenderness*: Deep tenderness over a wide area that crosses over nonanatomic boundaries.
- *Axial loading*: In axial loading patient stands and the examiner presses downward vertically on the patient's head, eliciting lumbar pain.
- *Acetabular rotation*: The examiner rotates the shoulder and the pelvis passively in the same plane while the patient is standing. It is a positive sign if pain is elicited in the first 30° of rotation.
- *Distracted straight leg raise (SLR) discrepancy*: Straight leg raising test can be used as a distraction test by using its variations. The test is positive when the patient reports pain on formal SLR examination such as on supine and the pain markedly decrease on performing the distracted SLR when the examiner extends the knee with the patient sitting.
- *Regional sensory disturbance*: The patient's reports pain that follows a stocking-like disturbance and does not follow a dermatomal pattern.
- *Regional weakness*: Weakness or cogwheel "giving away" that cannot be explained on neuroanatomical basis.
- *Overreaction*: Which is exaggerated painful response to a stimulus that is not reproduced when the same stimulus is given later.

A score of 3 or more out of the five categories is considered significant and the test is positive.[8]

POSITIVE SIGNS OF UPPER LIMB FUNCTIONAL WEAKNESS

Signs of functional upper limb weakness have been neglected for long. Lombardi and colleagues utilized the same principle of synergistic oppositional movements to develop the "elbow flex-ex" sign. This is performed by testing contralateral elbow extension strength while opposing resistance to elbow flexion of the arm, on both the nonaffected and affected sides.

The *"finger abduction sign"* consists of abducing the fingers of the normal hand against resistance for 2 minutes in order to detect synkinetic movements (finger abduction) in the paretic hand. Surface electromyography (EMG) from first dorsal interossei and abductor digiti minimi corroborates with the data. The sign is dependent on uncrossed corticospinal tract pathways.

"Drift without pronation" of outstretched arms is another recently described test of upper limbs.

PSYCHOGENIC NONEPILEPTIC SEIZURES

About 15-30% of patients referred to an epilepsy clinic have nonepileptic events. Differentiating them from true epileptic seizures is challenging. While some of them may have nonepileptic physiological events like syncope, majority have functional seizures. 5-10% of patients may have both true and functional seizures. The various aspects of PNES are discussed elsewhere in this volume.

FUNCTIONAL TREMORS AND OTHER MOVEMENT DISORDERS

Functional tremors are characterized by variable frequency and a characteristic response to externally cued rhythmic movements (entrainment test).

Functional parkinsonism is characterized by excessive slowness without decrement and fatigue. There is variable resistance to passive movement. Concurrent functional tremors may coexist.

Functional dystonia manifests either in paroxysms or with fixed plantar flexion and inversion of the feet. The onset may be acute. Pain is common in functional dystonia, but rare in organic dystonia.

Newer Functional Disorders

Propriospinal myoclonus is characterized by flexor arrhythmic jerks of the trunk, hips, and knees. This is provoked when the patient is supine and may be stimulus sensitive. This was earlier considered an organic disorder. Recent studies have shown that majority of the patients are nonorganic. The diagnosis was based on acute onset, distractibility, and co-occurrence with functional somatic disorders. This was reinforced by the presence of a *bereitschaftspotential* (premovement potential in voluntary movement) on jerk-locked electroencephalogram (EEG) back averaging. Absence of *bereitschaftspotential* does not rule out FNDs.[9]

Functional facial movement disorder is a relatively common but underrecognized entity. It is characterized by unilateral facial contraction, usually of lower lip downward and ipsilateral jaw muscles. In addition, there may be ipsilateral tongue deviation. Depression of the eyebrow of the same side may occur due to contraction of the orbicularis oculi. In contrast, in patients with blepharospasm the contraction is shorter and the eyebrow is often elevated in an attempt to compensate.

Electrophysiological testing does not show *bereitschaftspotential*. It demonstrates the R2 blink reflex recovery cycle in patients with psychogenic blepharospasm.

Tic disorders can also be functional. These are adult onset, lack of premonitory symptoms, and are not voluntary suppressible. There is lack of echolalia, palilalia, or coprolalia. Other FNDs may coexist. Obsessive compulsive disorder and attention deficit hyperactive disorder, the usual accompaniments of organic tics are not seen in these patients.

Several studies have shown that a subset of patients presenting with lower leg weakness and urinary retention does not show any abnormality on imaging and other investigations. These "cauda equina syndrome" patients may be functional and overlap with Fowler's syndrome of chronic urinary retention.

Palatal myoclonus/tremor is usually ascribed to a lesion in the brainstem (triangle of Guillain and Mollaret). But a Queen Square group studied a series of patients and found the majority to be functional based on the principle of entrainment of tremor and distractibility with ballistic tasks.

FUNCTIONAL NEUROLOGICAL DISORDERS WITH SENSORY SYMPTOMS

There are some positive signs in FNDs with sensory symptoms. Precise midline splitting of vibration sense in patients with hemisensory symptoms (even in case of single bones such as the frontal bone and sternum) is a helpful clue. Sharply demarcated sensory loss at groin or shoulder not corresponding to any dermatomal distribution is characteristic.

In functional visual loss, tubular visual fields without any change in width with increasing the distance between the subject and the examiner may be present. Sometimes, there may be hemianopia with the "affected eye" or a bizarre field defect which cannot be explained by any lesion in the optic pathway or the eye itself.

Axial Functional Neurological Disorders

These include the disorders of gait and posture. Some common examples include excessive gait slowness, astasia-abasia, and knee buckling. Disproportionate demonstration of effort during ambulation (also referred to as huffing and puffing sign) has poor sensitivity but high specificity for functional gait disorders. Fixed forward flexion deformities of the spine (camptocormia) seen in Parkinson plus syndromes like multiple system atrophy can also be seen in FNDs.[10] Functional gait disorders including astasia-abasia are discussed in detail elsewhere in this volume.

Functional Neurological Disorders Involving Speech

Lack of fluency, visible demonstration of excessive effort, and change of prosody in different combinations are features of functional speech disorders. Aphonia or dysphonia may also occur without accompanying central nervous system (CNS) or laryngeal pathology. Functional aphonic/dysphonic subjects speak with a markedly husky voice but can cough loudly.

Functional Memory Disorder

Functional memory disorder (FMD) is a term used for persistent and credible, but presumably nonorganic deficits of memory in daily life. FMD can be associated with depression in various ways: (1) Both can be caused by third factors, (2) FMD can cause or promote depression, and (3) depression can cause cognitive deficits. However, most patients with FMDs are not clinically depressed. On formal neuropsychological testing, the results are usually normal. Psychogenic memory loss and its differentiation from transient global amnesia are discussed elsewhere in this volume.

Pitfalls in the Diagnosis of Functional Memory Disorders

- *Pitfall 1*: All bizarre phenomena may not be of functional origin
- *Pitfall 2*: Not all events triggered by an emotional disturbance may be a functional disorder
- *Pitfall 3*: Not all topographical incongruities are suggestive of functional disorders
- *Pitfall 4*: A subject may have both functional and organic symptoms at the same time; often encountered is association of epilepsy and PNES
- *Pitfall 5*: Psychiatric comorbid condition may not always be evident in the history of a patient with a functional disorder
- *Pitfall 6*: Lack of proper communication and inadequate elicitation of history at the time of diagnosis can compromise treatment and prognosis

MANAGEMENT PRINCIPLES

Treatment of FNDs is complex. There is an overlap between neurology and psychiatry. Sometimes, this dichotomy lands the patient in a no man's zone.

Stone has suggested that this problem can be overcome only when the neurologist takes up the responsibility for managing the patient. They should follow a model of care like in other neurological disorders. Treatment usually starts with the delivery of the diagnosis. However, Stone in his seminal works have gone one step beyond. He has suggested that treatment should start at the time of neurological history and assessment.[11]

Of utmost importance is to provide sufficient time to the patient. The first encounter should ideally last for an hour. The patient should be encouraged to enlist all his/her symptoms. Specific questions should be asked regarding fatigue and sleep. Questions pertaining to feeling of dissociation and depersonalization are more difficult to ask. The patient may not be able to find the appropriate words to describe these feelings or may not volunteer information in view of being stamped "crazy". That is where the neurologist can help by gradual description of the symptoms and reassurance. The neurologist's expectations should be tailored according to the needs of the patient. Often, the ability to bring out all the symptoms provides enormous relief to the patient. The patient should be allowed to vent out frustration with previous medical encounters. Intrusive personal questions about anxiety, mood disorders or past psychological trauma should not be asked in the first encounter, unless the patient volunteers.

During examination, a hands-on approach is of immense help. Demonstration of the positive signs (e.g., Hoover's sign and entrainment test) establishes that it is not a diagnosis of exclusion. It also demonstrates the potential for reversibility. Thirdly, it emphasizes on the role of focused attention in perpetuating the disorder. Lastly, it shows the benefits of distraction.[12]

Explanation of the disease process helps the patient understand and in turn improves adherence. A simple reassuring way is to tell the patient that based on history, examination, and investigations, a diagnosis has been reached. The primary fault is with the "software". The hardware is intact.

A Step Care Approach is Useful

Step 1 is the first encounter where the neurologist can start the treatment process on the basis of history and examination. Acceptance of the diagnosis goes a long way in improving adherence to therapy and improving outcome. Cognitive behavior therapy (CBT) is immensely useful. It may not always be very complex. Simple change of behavior based on cognitive changes (explanation provided to the patient) brought about by the treating neurologist is a positive first step of CBT. Self-help information and internet resources (such as www.neurosymptoms.org or www.nonepilepticattacks.info) and optimizing function are all important. A timely second visit should also be scheduled at this stage.

Step 2 involves additional help of a physiotherapist (if motor symptoms) or psychologist (if PNES) depending on the phenomenology of the FNDs.

Step 3 is more complex and involves a multidisciplinary team that accounts for a combination of factors: education, physiotherapy, occupational therapy, and of course psychotherapy (CBT).

There is growing evidence that has emerged in the last few years that supports the role of physiotherapy, especially in functional movement and gait disorders. The duration of the rehab programs has varied from 5 days to several weeks. The benefits were sustained even beyond the duration of the programs.

What if the Standard Approach Fails?

A detailed analysis is necessary to understand the reasons behind failure. The commonly encountered situations can be overcome by:
- An open dialogue with patients who are not accepting the diagnosis;
- Exploring the evolving complexity of predisposing, precipitating, and perpetuating factors;
- Encourage and accelerate psychotherapy treatment by collaboratively identifying unhelpful thoughts, maladaptive behaviors, negative emotions, and/or psychosocial stressors by additional exploration; and
- Enquiring about other treatment details and help educate the other caregivers.[13,14]

PROGNOSIS

The overall prognosis of FNDs is poor. This is because of three main factors. Firstly, there is under recognition of these disorders. Secondly, the diagnosis is delivered poorly. Thirdly, there is lack of skilled and knowledgeable therapists. Longer duration of symptoms before diagnosis and presence of preexisting personality disorders are negative prognostic markers. Younger age and early diagnosis are markers of good prognosis. Some patients continue to go downhill in spite of good acceptance of the diagnosis. Even in the unfavorable cases, treatment of the comorbidities and limitation of iatrogenic harm can be helpful.

CONCLUDING REMARKS

The concept of FMD helps in identification of a subset of patients who are not at risk of significant cognitive decline. Perceived distress, rather than clinically relevant distress may be important. Majority have psychological burden factors such as dysthymia, adjustment disorder, overwork, interpersonal conflicts, somatic disease, and fear of developing Alzheimer's disease.[11]

LEARNING POINTS

- FNDs are common and disabling but potentially reversible.
- A positive or inclusionary diagnosis can be made with a high level of certainty.
- Treatment includes psychological interventions, such as CBT, behavioral therapy, or psychodynamic therapy and, for functional motor disorder, rehabilitation strategies. The dose and duration of various approaches, the value of combination and multidisciplinary therapy, and the appropriate therapeutic modality for each patient should be determined carefully.
- Therapeutic success is dependent on diagnostic delivery that validates the patient's symptoms and disability and includes full understanding and acceptance of the diagnosis by the patient.

REFERENCES

1. Lehn A, Gelauff J, Hoeritzauer I, Ludwig L, McWhirter L, Williams S, et al. Functional neurological disorders: mechanisms and treatment. J Neurol. 2016;263(3):611-20.
2. Raynor G, Baslet G. A historical review of functional neurological disorder and comparison to contemporary models. Epilepsy Behav Rep. 2021;16:100489.
3. Veith IH. Hysteria: The History of a Disease. Chicago: University of Chicago Press; 1965.
4. Janet P. The Major Symptoms of Hysteria: Fifteen Lectures Given in the Medical School of Harvard University. New York: MacMillan & Co., Ltd.; 1907.

5. Goetz CG. Charcot, hysteria, and simulated disorders. Handb Clin Neurol. 2016:139:11-23.
6. Tremolizzo L, Susani E, Riva MA, Cesana G, Ferrarese C, Appollonio I. Positive signs of functional weakness. J Neurol Sci. 2014;340(1-2):13-8.
7. Espay AJ, Aybek S, Carson A, Edwards MJ, Goldstein LH, Hallett M, et al. Current Concepts in Diagnosis and Treatment of Functional Neurological Disorder. JAMA Neurol. 2018;75(9):1132-41.
8. Waddell G, McCulloch JA, Kummel E, Venner RM. Nonorganic Physical Signs in Low-Back Pain. Spine. 1980;5:117-25.
9. McWhirter L, Stone J, Sandercock P, Whiteley W. Hoover's sign for the diagnosis of functional weakness: a prospective unblinded cohort study in patients with suspected stroke. J Psychosom Res. 2011;71:384-6.
10. Van der Salm SMA, Erro R, Cordivari C, Edwards MJ, Koelman JHTM, van den Ende T, et al. Propriospinal myoclonus: clinical reappraisal and review of literature. Neurology. 2014;83:1862-70.
11. Schmidtke K, Polmann S, Metternich B. The syndrome of functional memory disorder: Definition, etiology and natural course. Am J Geriatr Psychiatry. 2008;16(12):981-8.
12. Stone J. Functional neurological disorders: The neurological assessment as treatment. Neurophysiol Clin. 2014;44(4):363-73.
13. Stone J, Edwards M. Trick or treat? Showing patients with functional (psychogenic) motor symptoms their physical signs. Neurology. 2012;79:282-4.
14. Adams C, Anderson J, Madva EN, LaFrance WC Jr, Perez DL. You've made the diagnosis of functional neurological disorder: now what? Pract Neurol. 2018;18(4):323-30.

CHAPTER 4

Systemic and Neurological Red Flags in the Diagnosis of Psychiatric Diseases

Sarosh M Katrak

■ INTRODUCTION

In psychiatry practice, there are many symptom complexes which fall in the border zone of neurology and psychiatry. Prominent among these are behavioural and cognitive dysfunction. Neuropsychiatry is the study and treatment of these disorders. The psychiatrist should be aware when a behavioral disorder has an "organic" (neurological basis), as there are many pitfalls in the diagnosis of such disorders.[1] The main symptom complexes considered here are acute confusional states (ACS), psychotic disorders, disorders of mood and affect, and cognitive dysfunction.

The focus of this chapter is to outline when ACS, delirium and psychosis, and to some extent mood disorders, form "red flags" in psychiatric practice and the common term "neuropsychiatric symptoms (NPS)" has been used. In the majority of cases, the NPS occur during the course of the illness and the diagnosis is evident. The problem arises when NPS are present at the onset of the disease! What are the red flags which help you to differentiate between a primary psychiatric disorder (PPD) and an organic one? As they say, "common things occur commonly". I will discuss conditions which are more frequently encountered and reserve the rare ones for a brief note.

■ NEUROPSYCHIATRIC ASPECTS OF CEREBROVASCULAR DISEASE

A variety of neuropsychiatric (NP) disturbances have been described in patients with strokes. These occur with infarcts in the anterior and posterior cerebral artery (PCA) territories. Infarcts in the dominant middle cerebral artery (MCA) territory usually produce language disorders, which at times, could be mistaken for acute psychosis.

Infarcts in the Anterior Cerebral Artery Territory

Usually bilateral infarcts in the anterior cerebral artery (ACA) territory cause akinetic mutism (AM). It is a syndrome of negatives—the patient seems awake but is silent and immobile. Eye movements and blinking are present. The best way to describe this condition is "seeming wakefulness without content".[2] The main differential diagnosis is major depressive disorders. AM is usually seen when the patient is recovering from an acute insult to the nervous system. Besides this, many clinical features of the ACA syndrome will be present. Grasping and sucking reflexes may be prominent. Although, there is a paucity of corticospinal tract deficits, there may be minor motor deficits in the foot and leg. A classic feature of bilateral ACA infarct is incontinence of urine. Although this is a classic sign, it is not very frequently seen.[3] Another form of AM occurs with infarcts in the PCA territory. This is said to be apathetic AM, as initially the patient is drowsy to stuporous because of the involvement of the ascending reticular activating system. A classic feature of this variety of AM is conjugate vertical gaze palsy due to involvement of the tectum of the midbrain.

Thalamic Infarcts

The thalamus has blood supply from four arteries, i.e., he polar, thalamic-subthalamic, thalamogeniculate, and the posterior choroidal arteries. The polar artery is a branch of the posterior communicating artery (PComA) and the rest are branches of the PCA. Thalamic infarcts usually produce hemisensory or sensorimotor strokes. NPS are characteristically found in polar artery infarcts.[4] Bilateral infarcts may have partial features of apathetic AM and anterograde amnesia. Occasionally, mild transient hemiparesis or hemisensory deficits may be noted and further help to differentiate from major depressive disorders. Unfortunately, AM from bilateral infarcts has a poor prognosis for meaningful recovery.

Wernicke's Aphasia

This results from a posteriorly placed infarct in the left MCA territory; hence there is hardly any paresis. The infarct involves the left posterior temporal gyrus. The speech is fluent with normal or even above normal output (logorrhea). However, the content is meaningless because of a lack of specific nouns, substitution of one word for another (semantic paraphasia, e.g., grass is blue) or a similar sounding but incorrect word (phonemic paraphasia, e.g., grass is green). In extreme cases, the speech is said to be jargon. This markedly reduces the ability of the patient to communicate. Compounding this is the main problem of Wernicke's aphasia (WA)—the inability to comprehend spoken speech. In some patients with WA there is paranoid behavior. A combination of paranoid behavior and abnormal speech could easily lead to a mistaken diagnosis of acute psychosis. The clinical differentiation lies in the fact that grossly abnormal speech is rarely a presenting symptom of acute psychosis.[5] The other differentiating points are the presence of risk factors for stroke in an elderly individual with a previously stable personality. Neuroimaging will confirm the infarct.

Transient Global Aphasia

The cause of transient global aphasia (TGA) is not known. Many hypotheses are have been offered. The abrupt onset and transient nature of TGA has raised the possibility of a vascular mechanism, and hence its inclusion in this section.

Transient global aphasia is a syndrome in which there is an abrupt onset of transient but complete anterograde amnesia together with retrograde amnesia going backward for several hours or days.[6] This usually occurs in a middle aged or elderly individual with preserved alertness and other cognitive functions. They appear to be in an ACS, as they repeatedly ask the same questions such as "Where am I?", "How did I get here?", and "When did you come?" However there is no clouding of consciousness, the individual is aware about self and can perform complex procedures during an attack. Neurological examination during or after the attack is normal as in brain imaging. These features make it easy to differentiate TGA from ACS. The attack ceases after several hours. Awareness of personal identity helps to differentiate from hysterical or malingering amnesia.

NEUROPSYCHIATRIC ASPECTS OF EPILEPSY

Psychosis is the main problem among the NPS in epilepsy. Psychosis in epilepsy is usually ictal, interictal, and postictal. Temporal lobe epilepsy (TLE) is the most common form of focal epilepsy. It is divided into a median TLE—mesial TLE (mTLE) and a lateral or neocortex TLE (nTLE). In mTLE, the hippocampus, entorhinal cortex, amygdala, and the parahippocampal gyrus are involved.[7] There is a greater prevalence of psychotic symptoms in mTLE, at times reaching up to 70%.

Ictal Psychosis

This form of psychosis occurs in a nonconvulsive seizure and in which the features are due to epileptic activity. It should be emphasized that this short-term psychosis has an abrupt onset with clouding of consciousness and accompanied by automatic behavior such as closing a window, running in circles, picking at clothes, and even micturition in public. These attacks typically last for minutes to an hour. If they last longer, they form a good example of partial complex status epilepticus.[8] Hallucinatory symptoms may be visual—metamorphopsia, micropsia or macropsia, auditory—ringing or buzzing sounds or a voice calling the patient's name, gustatory—metallic or foul taste in the mouth, or olfactory—odor of burning rubber, garbage or decaying or fecal odor. Memory flashbacks like experiences déjà vu are also described. These psychotic episodes (PEPs) are stereotypic in an individual patient and responsive to antiseizure medications (ASM). If these features are borne in mind, misdiagnosis with other forms of psychosis will be avoided.

Interictal Psychosis

A chronic interictal psychosis (IIP) with occasional exacerbation is frequently seen in patients with uncontrolled epilepsy. IIP and primary schizophrenia are closely related with a greater overlap of symptoms, risk factors, and etiologies. Although mTLE with IIP has been said to be indistinguishable from primary schizophrenia, many studies have noted subtle differences which help to differentiate one from the other. In IIP, hallucinations are characteristically visual or auditory and the delusions are more persecutory. There is a greater preservation of affect and fewer negative symptoms such as lack of interest and social interaction, lack of motivation, or being withdrawn. Patients with IIP have a greater insight in contrast to patients with primary schizophrenia. A family history of psychosis and premorbid personality disturbances are conspicuous by their absence in IIP. Lastly, it should be emphasized that IIP almost always develops when epilepsy is present for many years, usually a decade and the control has been poor.[9]

This differentiation will avoid stigmatization and pave the path for appropriate management. In most cases, antipsychotic medication (APM) is required. Unfortunately, all available APMs are mildly epileptogenic but if a patient is comedicated with ASMs, risk of increase in seizures is lower.[9]

An often under-recognized problem encountered in the intensive care unit (ICU) is sudden unresponsiveness due to nonconvulsive status epilepticus (NCSE). This needs a high index of suspicion as motor symptoms may be minimal or absent. The patient may present with an ACS. At times, positive symptoms like tonic eye deviation or nystagmoid jerking of the eyes may give a clue to the correct diagnosis. The common underlying etiologies are strokes, subarachnoid hemorrhage, infections, trauma, or metabolic/toxic encephalopathies. Multiagent chemotherapies and antibiotics, particularly cephalosporins, penicillin/tazobactam, and quinolones in conjunction with chronic kidney disease can precipitate NCSE. Thus the clinician must be aware of NCSE, when any patient in the ICU presents with an unexplained and abrupt alteration in behavior or consciousness. An electroencephalogram (EEG) will detect NCSE and prompt management is very gratifying.[2]

Another problem for the clinician in the ICU is psychogenic unresponsiveness (PUR). Its differentiation from stupor is essentially clinical and relatively easy if one knows what to look for. If the eyes are closed the eyelids may flicker spontaneously and any attempt to open the eyes is met with active resistance. When released, the upper eyelid closes rapidly. This is in sharp contrast to a patient in stupor where there is no spontaneous flickering of the eyelid, the eyes can be opened without any resistance and on releasing the upper eyelid, the eyes slowly close. Dropping a raised arm toward the face will elicit an avoiding movement to prevent self-injury and lastly tickling either nostril with a wisp of cotton may elicit a response on the face or may even restore "consciousness" in PUR.[2,10]

NEUROPSYCHIATRIC ASPECTS OF NEURODEGENERATIVE DISORDERS

Neuropsychiatric symptoms are common in neurodegenerative disorders. Hallucinations and delusions should be differentiated from primary psychosis of schizophrenia. Fortunately, these symptoms appear late in neurodegenerative disorders such as Alzheimer's and Parkinson's disease, by which time the diagnosis of the dementia is already established.[11,12] Dementia with Lewy body (DLB), behavioral variant of frontotemporal dementia (bvFTD), and corticobasal degeneration (CBD) are exceptions to the rule. In these disorders, behavioral abnormalities are seen early in the disease and could be the presenting feature. The onset is usually insidious, but at times they may present with acute psychosis.[1] Awareness of these entities may avoid a misinterpretation, thereby guiding the clinician to the right path, not only for the diagnosis but also for the management of these problems.

Dementia with Lewy Body

Dementia with Lewy body is applied to cases of parkinsonian syndrome in which cognitive impairment precedes or runs parallel with the parkinsonian features, usually within 1 year of each other. Early visual hallucinations occur in 60–80% of cases.[12,13] Another striking feature is the fluctuation in the visual hallucination and the parkinsonian features. Many of the care givers have said "he has good days and bad days. On a good day, he behaves normally and you would not say he has parkinsonism." Lastly, a point to remember is that patients with DLB have a marked neuroleptic sensitivity. This has a bearing on management of the psychosis. Neuroleptics produce a marked extrapyramidal syndrome and are best avoided in cases of DLB. Olanzapine and risperidone may be safer. Antiparkinsonian therapy should be started cautiously in small doses with very slow increments to avoid drug induced confusion.[12,13]

Frontotemporal Dementia

The frontotemporal dementias (FTDs) have three clinical variants based on the anatomical site of the initial involvement. If the pathology begins in the frontal lobes, the disorder is characterized by executive dysfunction, behavioural and social misconduct—the bvFTD. In the other two variants, semantic dementia and nonfluent progressive aphasia, the characteristic features involve disturbance of speech and language and will not be considered here.

In bvFTD, social skill impairment and personality changes occur early. The patient has difficulty at work and has disinhibited social behavior. Loss of empathy and personality are distressing to the family, particularly the spouse.[13] A particularly distressing feature of bvFTD is the Capgras' syndrome. The patient falsely believes that an identical duplicate has replaced someone significant to her, usually the spouse.[14] This results in a lot of aggressive and at times violent behavior. The main differentiation of bvFTD is from schizophrenia and schizoaffective disorders. The clinical pointers to remember are that the behavioral dysfunction runs parallel with deterioration in personality and social misconduct. Perception, visuospatial skills, praxis, and memory are relatively well preserved, particularly perception. As the disease progresses to involve the temporal lobes, the speech gets reduced—another clinical pointer. Other behavioral changes, peculiar to bvFTD, are a preference for sweet food and a ritualistic behavior for daily routine activity.[12,13] Lastly, delusions and hallucinations are rare symptoms in bvFTD.[15]

Corticobasal Degeneration

Corticobasal degeneration is characterized by a striking asymmetric, akinetic-rigid syndrome with cortical sensory loss, apraxia, and the alien limb phenomenon. Besides the parkinsonian features, other extrapyramidal signs are myoclonus and dystonia particularly of the affected limb.[16,17] The hallmark of CBD is the asymmetry, the alien limb in 50% of patients and a characteristic apraxia. The alien limb (a feeling that the limb does not belong to the patient's body) could be from a posteriorly placed lesion in which the patient has a parietal lobe type of hemineglect (the sensory type). In the anterior or motor type, the patient has an intermanual conflict, i.e., the affected hand interferes with the movements of the opposite hand in bimanual tasks. This clinical picture is fairly classical and does not pose any problem in the diagnosis.

NEUROPSYCHIATRIC ASPECTS OF AUTOIMMUNE ENCEPHALITIS

Autoimmune encephalitis (AIE) is a form of central nervous system (CNS) inflammation with a variety of clinical phenotypes. Most of these cases are associated with specific auto antibodies (Abs) to a number of structures. In recent years, cell surface or synaptic Ab-mediated AIE are increasingly recognized. These occur in children or younger patients and have a more favorable outcome if detected and treated early. Only a minority of these patients have an associated tumor. The practical challenge of diagnosing AIE is complicated by the fact that Ab testing is not universally available, maybe negative initially and newer Abs have been identified in atypical phenotypes such as a first presentation of psychosis.[1,18] Thus the clinician must make a diagnosis based on the clinical phenotype,[19] aided by cerebrospinal fluid (CSF) results and neuroimaging.

For the purpose of this chapter, the basic discussion will be on limbic encephalitis (LE). This is a clinical syndrome, which is subacute in onset (days to weeks) with evolving limbic symptoms and signs and evidence of structural and functional damage to the medial temporal lobe based on an autoimmune (AI) or paraneoplastic cause. The features common to all forms of LE are a triad of short-term memory loss, complex partial seizures and NPS of agitation, depression, and change in personality.

Anti-N-methyl-D-aspartate Receptor Encephalitis

Among the AIE, the most common disease associated with NPS, especially psychosis is N-methyl-D-aspartate receptor encephalitis (NMDARE). The median age is 21 years with a wide range from 1 to 93 years. Initially, there is a prodromal phase which resembles a viral infection—headache and fever. In the following days or weeks, there are behavioral changes marked by anxiety, agitation, insomnia, hallucinations, and persecutory delusions. In view of this presentation, it is not surprising that many patients are initially treated in the psychiatry ward. At this stage, the differentiation from PPD can be difficult. MRI and routine CSF cytochemistry are normal.[20] An important point to remember is that the EEG is usually abnormal from disease onset. In 30% of cases, it shows an "extreme delta brush" pattern—slow 1–3 Hz delta activity with superimposed fast 20–30 Hz beta activity. A normal EEG rules out an AIE.[18] In the next few days or weeks, most patients develop short-term memory deficits, confusion, cognitive and language deterioration, and catatonia. Complex partial seizures can occur at any stage of the illness although they are usually present in the early stages of the illness. Most patients younger than 18 years have orofacial dyskinesia and dyskinetic movements of the upper limbs. Autonomic disturbances, hypoventilation, and deterioration in the level of consciousness will require ICU management. At this stage, the CSF in approximately 90% of the patients will show a pleocytosis suggesting an AI inflammatory disorder.[20]

A detailed attention to clinical features, aided by investigations helps to differentiate NMDARE from a PPD. In NMDARE, the onset is subacute whereas in PPD the illness runs into months or years. A viral-like prodromal illness helps in favor of NMDARE. When the presentation is with acute psychosis, atypical features such as severe anxiety/agitation and catatonia favor an organic psychosis compared to a PPD. At this stage, EEG is very helpful in differentiating one from another. In children and young adults, it is prudent to consider NMDARE in cases of isolated psychosis as a presenting feature even in the absence of other neurological symptoms and an EEG should be done.[21] Lastly, in contrast to patients with schizophrenia, who lose insight, patients with NMDARE tend to retain some insight despite the psychosis.[18,20,21]

Psychosis as the presenting feature has been reported in a few patients with LE due to other neuronal cell surface or synaptic proteins. They are as follows:
- Anti-alpha-amino-3-hydroxy-5-methyl-4-isoxazolepropionic acid receptor (AMPAR)
- Leucine-rich glioma-inactivated protein 1 (LGI1)
- Dipeptidyl-peptidase-like protein 6 (DPPX)
- Contactin-associated protein-like 2 (CASPR2)

Limbic encephalitis due to anti-AMPAR Ab presents with confusion, disorientation, and memory loss evolving subacutely over 8 weeks. Over 40% have seizures and most patients have CSF pleocytosis. MRI will show fluid-attenuated inversion recovery (FLAIR) hyperintense signals in the medial temporal lobe. In 70%, cancer is usually seen in the lungs or thymus. Blood AMPAR-positive serology is seen in almost all and in 67% it is positive both in the blood and CSF. Patients show a partial short-term therapeutic response to immunosuppressant oncotherapy but overall the prognosis is unsatisfactory.[22,23]

Patients with LGI1 encephalitis also show typical features of LE. Two features help to differentiate it from PPD. The first is hyponatremia due to syndrome of inappropriate antidiuretic hormone (SIADH) and the second is faciobrachial dystonic seizures (FBDS). The latter involves a dystonic unilateral posturing of the upper limb and face. In the majority of patients, FBDS precedes the onset of LE by a few weeks, when other symptoms follow. Awareness of FBDS as a prodromal feature of anti LGI1 encephalitis might enable early treatment.[23]

Patients with DPPX encephalitis show cognitive dysfunction associated with symptoms of CNS hyperexcitability—exaggerated startle response to sound or touch, myoclonus, and/or tremors. In the majority of patients this is preceded by gastrointestinal symptoms such as diarrhea and significant weight loss.[20,23]

CASPR2 Abs are predominantly associated with peripheral nerve hyperexcitability and a combination of central and peripheral nervous system involvement. CASPR2 associated LE is very rare.

NEUROPSYCHIATRIC ASPECTS OF CENTRAL NERVOUS SYSTEM INFECTIONS

The CNS is affected by hematogenous spread of any infectious agents. These include viral, bacterial, spirochetal, fungal, and parasitic agents. In this chapter, only those infections which produce significant NPS and are endemic to India will be considered.

Viral Encephalitis

The classical clinical presentation of viral encephalitis (VE) is with fever, headache, and altered sensorium. The other symptoms and signs maybe acute memory disturbances, confusion, agitation, hallucinations, psychosis, focal neurological deficits, and seizures. The geographical location or travel history may provide clues to certain causative viruses which are prevalent in that geographical area. Seasonal peaks are also known as post monsoon peak of cases of Japanese encephalitis (JE) or dengue. Investigations including EEG, neuroimaging, and virological tests are necessary to establish the exact diagnosis. In general, with the earlier mentioned presentation the NPS are part of the symptoms and signs and do not pose any "red flags" for the clinician.[24]

Herpes simplex encephalitis (HSE) is the most common sporadic VE. It has a predilection to involve the orbitofrontal and temporal lobes. The onset is with fever and headaches followed by symptoms of frontotemporal lobe involvement—agitation, fear, and hallucinations. Seizures occur in 70% and focal neurological deficits like hemiplegia or aphasia in 75%. In atypical cases, fever, headache, and NPS occur in the absence of seizures and focal deficits. This may raise the possibility of an "organic" psychosis because of the fever and the headache. As herpes simplex virus (HSV) spreads to the CNS via the olfactory pathways, there may be associated anosmia—a clue to the diagnosis. Neuroimaging is a very useful test. If the MRI shows a frontotemporal lesion, it is practically pathognomonic of HSE and initiation of acyclovir therapy pending virological confirmation is warranted.[24]

Japanese encephalitis is one of the three purely neurotropic viruses. Behavioral abnormalities are part of the encephalitic stage which usually follows a prodromal stage of fever, headache, nausea, vomiting, and anorexia. JE usually occurs in a rural setting in the lower socioeconomic group and in India, is more prevalent in the Northeastern states. MRI will show characteristic lesions in the thalamus and basal ganglia. Hence, the NPS hardly pose a problem for diagnosis in such patients.

Human Immunodeficiency Virus Infection

Neuropsychiatric disorders are an important problem in people living with human immunodeficiency virus (HIV). The main risk factors for such symptoms are pre-existing psychosocial problems and substance abuse. One must remember that besides HIV itself, associated opportunistic infections (OIs) and adverse effects (AEs) of antiretroviral therapy (ART) can produce NPS. This section deals with NPS due to primary HIV infection.

Neuropsychiatric symptoms occur in HIV infection in two stages of the disease. Chronic aseptic meningitis is a seroconversion illness which begins 2–4 weeks after exposure. There is an insidious onset of afebrile headaches, without meningeal signs. Some patients may have seizures and confusion independent of seizures.

There is a predilection to develop a lower motor neuron (LMN) facial palsy, a good biomarker for this illness. The symptoms and signs spontaneously resolve in 4 weeks. At this stage of the disease, HIV serology is usually negative. Therefore, a high index of suspicion should be aroused in a young patient with a history of high-risk behavior, who presents with confusion, associated with or without seizures, and perhaps a LMN facial palsy. Leukopenia and thrombocytopenia are useful laboratory markers. HIV ribonucleic acid (RNA) levels and p24 antigen are more sensitive than HIV serology.[25]

HIV-associated Neurocognitive Disorders or AIDS Dementia Complex

This is a late manifestation of HIV infection and is an acquired immunodeficiency syndrome (AIDS) defining entity. Therefore, the diagnosis is obvious. There is an insidious onset of forgetfulness, lack of concentration, apathy, waning interest at work, and social withdrawal—features simulating depression.[25,26]

Progressive Multifocal Leukoencephalopathy

This form of leukoencephalopathy is caused by the JC virus and is due to the reactivation of the virus due to the immunosuppression by disease, including HIV infection or immunosuppressant therapy. Fortunately progressive multifocal leukoencephalopathy (PML) has decreased with ART. The onset in insidious and occurs in the evolution of an established predisposing disease and therefore does not raise any red flags. Rarely, PML may be the presenting manifestation of a previously undiagnosed illness which causes immunosuppression. Clinical features are based on the location of the demyelinating plaques and range from aphasia, apraxia, agnosia, visual field defects, hemiplegia, hemisensory deficits, ataxia, and movement disorders. NP features are catatonia, emotional lability, or AM but usually in association with other neurological deficits. The MRI shows one or more large demyelinating lesions—a finding characteristic for a diagnosis of PML. Thus, PML is also unlikely to pose any "red flags" apart from the rare situation in which NPS are the presenting manifestation.

Bacterial Infections

Bacterial/pyogenic meningitis is an acute fulminant infection with a classic triad of high fever, neck stiffness, and altered level of consciousness. Therefore, it is not within the purview of this chapter.

Tuberculous meningitis (TBM) is a medical emergency and requires a prompt diagnosis and initiation of antituberculous therapy (ATT). Complications of TBM occur when there is a delay between onset of symptoms and initiation of therapy. The clinical manifestations of TBM can be varied. Atypical presentations can be progressive dementia, psychosis, movement disorders, and rarely status epilepticus.[27]

Strokes in TBM occur in 13–57% of patients based on the methods of evaluation. The resultant focal neurological deficit usually occurs acutely and involves the internal capsule and basal ganglia. Rarely, patients with thalamic involvement may have NPS.[28] This is already discussed. If the focal deficit occurs insidiously, a tuberculoma should be suspected. If this is in the frontal region, there may be no motor deficits and only NPS. Lastly communicating hydrocephalus may produce subcortical cognitive impairment. All these complications occur during the course of the illness, when the diagnosis is already established and the patient is monitored for any complications.

Hyponatremia is an often overlooked complication of TBM. Specifically looked for, it occurs in 40–50% of patients. It may be due to cerebral salt wasting (CSW) syndrome or SIADH. During the course of the illness, symptoms appear insidiously—nausea, confusion, and seizures. Awareness of hyponatremia is the key to the diagnosis. However, for the management of this complication, it is important to distinguish between CSW and SIADH as the former is managed by fluid administration and the latter by fluid restriction.[28]

Lastly, in our study comparing patients of TBM with and without HIV infection, we found that patients coinfected with HIV had significantly more cognitive deficits at the time of diagnosis. Such patients had a shortened prodromal phase with significant weight loss. Fever and headache were present in 80%, but neck rigidity was evident in only 59%. These patients had a more fulminant illness and the mortality was significantly higher.[29]

Parasitic and Fungal Infections

Neurocysticercosis

The most common presentation of neurocysticercosis (NCC) is focal with secondary generalized seizures. In "miliary" NCC, when hundreds of cysts are lodged in the cerebral parenchyma, dementia and cognitive impairment are associated with signs of increased intracranial pressure. Hence, focal epilepsy of late onset with NPS should draw attention to NCC. The associated features of headache and papilledema, when present make the appropriate diagnosis easy. The MRI is very useful in confirming the diagnosis.[30]

Toxoplasmosis

Toxoplasma gondii is an obligatory intracellular protozoan, commonly found throughout the world. Immunosuppression activates the latent bradyzoites, leading to clinical disease. Common presentations are fever, headache, and focal neurological deficits in the majority of patients. Confusion and altered sensorium can occur in 30-40% but usually with other neurological deficits.[25]

Malaria

In malaria, NPS occur at three stages of the illness:
1. *Cerebral malaria*: The usual presentation is that of a hyper febrile patient with rapidly deteriorating level of consciousness, with or without seizures, which occur in 50-66% of patients. Children are more prone to seizures which are largely generalized. Most patients will also have other systemic manifestations of severe malaria—renal failure, jaundice, severe anemia, and adult respiratory distress syndrome. The mortality in such cases can be very high.
2. *Postmalaria syndrome*: The patient may have aphasia, tremors, myoclonus, and NPS, weeks or months after recovery. A delayed cerebellar ataxia is also known and is believed to be a postinfective immune-mediated disorder.[31]
3. *Mefloquine induced*: In 28% of patients, mefloquine may produce severe depression, bizarre behavior, and psychotic hallucinations.[32]

As one can see, the diagnosis of malaria is well established in all the three clinical situations.

Cryptococcal Meningitis

Cryptococcal meningitis (CrM) is one of the most common OI in HIV affected patients. This usually presents with fever and headache in approximately 80%. Unbearable headaches have been stressed by one center in India.[25] These symptoms may be followed by altered sensorium and are associated with a poor prognosis. Thus, in CrM, NPS are known but never in isolation and therefore do not pose any "red flag" situation.

Neurosyphilis

In this section, only general paralysis (GP) will be discussed. GP occurs 10-20 years after the infection and is considered a late/tertiary manifestation of syphilis. It combines neurological and psychiatric features. Classic neurological abnormalities are a mask-like face, tremors of the tongue (also called trombone tongue), dysarthria, hyperreflexia, and the Argyll Robertson pupil—small pupils which do not react to light but accommodate normally (light-near dissociation). The psychiatric manifestations are mainly delusions of grandeur but hallucinations, agitation, and emotional lability can also occur. The problem arises when the history of syphilis is hidden for obvious reasons. Nevertheless GP should be suspected when the earlier mentioned combination of classic findings are present.[33]

Prion Diseases

Sporadic Creutzfeldt–Jakob disease (sCJD) accounts for 85-90% of all cases of prion disease. The onset is usually in the late 50s or early 60s. sCJD should be considered in any patient in the above age group with a rapidly progressive dementia and myoclonus. Hence, "red flags" may be raised only in the initial phase of the illness when the patient has apathy, depression, hypersomnia, or insomnia. Soon, rapid deterioration of cognitive functions and myoclonus become the dominant feature in most cases, clarifying the diagnosis. The MRI is highly sensitive (91%) and specific (96%). It shows the characteristic hyperintense cortical-ribboning pattern on the diffusion-weighted imaging (DWI) and FLAIR sequences clarifying the diagnosis.[34]

Familial Creutzfeldt–Jakob Disease

About 5-15% of all cases of CJD are familial. The inheritance is autosomal dominant and hence the family history is positive. Patients with familial Creutzfeldt–Jakob disease (fCJD) have an earlier age of onset (mean 46 years) and a more protracted course (mean 23 months). Hence, the problem may be with the index case in a family. Working memory loss, behavioral and personality changes, and depression with social withdrawal and mood swings can last for several months as was the problem with the index case of our family with fCJD.[35] Dementia is an invariable feature, though appearing late in the clinical course. In such a clinical scenario with NPS, a positive family history of a similar problem, together with the MRI findings, helps to clinch the diagnosis.

Variant Creutzfeldt–Jakob Disease or Mad Cow Disease

In variant Creutzfeldt–Jakob disease (vCJD), the age at onset is much younger (16-48 years), the clinical course is more protracted, and the presentation is with prominent sensory disturbance—paresthesia/dysesthesia over the face or body—and psychiatric disorders. The latter may include apathy, depression, anxiety, irritability, and uncommonly frank psychosis with hallucinations. As the disease progresses, ataxia and dysarthria become obvious. Dementia, immobility, and mutism are late features and practically herald the patient's demise. A high index of suspicion is required in such cases as Hashimoto's encephalopathy maybe a close differential diagnosis.

A history of eating beef in the UK between 1996 and 2014 is a useful clinical pointer for the diagnosis. Besides the psychosis there is working memory loss pointing to an organic psychosis. The MRI may show hyperintense lesion in the pulvinar of the thalamus (pulvinar sign) and in both, the pulvinar and dorsomedial thalamus (the hockey stick sign). Tonsillar biopsy tissue analysis for prion protein appears to be a sensitive and specific method for diagnosis of vCJD in the appropriate clinical setting.[34]

NEUROPSYCHIATRIC ASPECTS OF SYSTEMIC DISORDERS

In most of the systemic disorders, NPS occur when the disease is well established. Here, I would like to discuss only those systemic disorders in which NPS are a prominent part of the clinical profile or at times when they may be the presenting feature.

Gastrointestinal and Nutritional Disorders

Essential micronutrients cannot be synthesized by our bodies but are essential for normal functioning. They include water- and fat-soluble vitamins and trace minerals that are obtained through out diet. Deficiencies of these vitamins occur in individuals with a poor nutritional intake or malabsorption.

Vitamin B12 Deficiency

The clinical approach to patients at risk is to look for a clinical syndrome rather than a specific deficiency. For vitamin B12 deficiency, "at risk" individuals are vegetarian/vegans, diabetic patients on metformin, elderly patients with poor intake and on H2 blockers or proton pump inhibitors (PPIs) and alcohol abuse. The B12 deficiency syndrome consists of a predominantly large fiber sensory neuropathy, subacute combined degeneration (SCD), and subacute to chronic cognitive NPS. One must remember that peripheral neuropathy is the most common neurological manifestation. NPS are uncommon and although they maybe the presenting symptoms, they are invariably associated with some features of a peripheral neuropathy like absent ankle jerks. The earliest effect of B12 deficiency is on the bone marrow, i.e., a megaloblastic anemia. A mean corpuscular volume of over 100 μm^3 is a good pointer to the etiology.[36]

Wernicke–Korsakoff Syndrome

Wernicke's encephalopathy (WE) consists of a triad of ophthalmoplegia, ataxia, and mental confusion which occur acutely or subacutely following a more abrupt deficiency of vitamin B1 (thiamine). Patients at risk are mainly alcoholics but it can also occur in women with hyperemesis gravidarum. Although the triad is seen in only 33% of patients, the disease often begins with two of the three features. A global confusional state occurs at some stage in approximately 90% of cases. Drowsiness commonly occurs in such patients. The diagnosis of WE should be suspected when a patient at risk has an acute to subacute onset of one or two components of the syndrome. In an acute confusional presentation, examination of the eyes may reveal nystagmus, gaze paresis, or abducens nerve palsy—features pointing to the right diagnosis. It is prudent to give thiamine at this stage without waiting for confirmation of the diagnosis. The benefits are two-fold. Firstly, all the clinical features clear up rapidly and secondly treatment with thiamine prevents the permanent Korsakoff syndrome which follows in 75% of survivors of WE. The main features of Korsakoff syndrome is an anterograde amnesia and prominent confabulations. Apart from memory deficits the other cognitive domains are relatively well preserved.[36]

Rheumatologic Disorders

Rheumatologic disorders are multisystemic disorders with a wide range of clinical and radiologic syndromes. They can affect the central as well as the peripheral nervous system. In this section of this chapter, I will only discuss neuropsychiatric systemic lupus erythematosus (NP-SLE).

Systemic lupus erythematosus (SLE) is a chronic multiorgan AI inflammatory disorder that mainly affects women. NP-SLE encompasses various NP syndromes and occurs in about 20–30% of patients with SLE. But NPS can also occur from complications of SLE such as OI, metabolic derangements, or medication toxicity. Acute psychosis is rare but well described.[37] Objective cognitive impairment is associated with detection of anticardiolipin Ab and lupus anticoagulants which in turn are associated with strokes in SLE. At times NPS appear first in a patient without a preexisting diagnosis of SLE. The clinical situation is usually in a young female with a stable background personality who abruptly develops a NP syndrome. The presence of multisystemic involvement, an obstetric history of multiple miscarriages due to the antiphospholipid Ab syndrome, and detection of auto-Abs associated with SLE should be suggestive of the diagnosis.[37]

Endocrine Disorders

Adrenal Disorders

The most relevant adrenal hormone is cortisol. From a practical point of view, Cushing syndrome is due to prolonged prescription of corticosteroids for presumed or confirmed AI disorders. The main AEs are proximal limb girdle myopathy and NP manifestations. Proximal myopathy is by far the most common AE of prolonged glucocorticoid administration and is detected by the patient as difficulty in arising from the squatting position. The concomitant steroid-induced hypokalemia further potentiates the weakness. However, depression is the most common NPS and is seen in 70-80% of patients.[38] Acute psychosis is rare and is usually seen when methylprednisolone is given intravenously in high doses as pulse therapy. Besides the NPS there is general and systemic evidence of excess glucocorticoid levels. For these reasons there is no difficulty in making a confident diagnosis in such cases.

Thyroid Disorders

Hypothyroidism

Symptoms of hypothyroidism may develop insidiously and many patients may have a history of being treated earlier for hyperthyroidism. The most salient NPS are confusion, psychosis, and seizures. With a greater degree of hypothyroidism, drowsiness, stupor, and life-threatening coma can ensue. Delayed relaxation of the deep tendon reflexes may be a significant clue to the diagnosis. Other clinical features are hypothermia, bradycardia, and hypoventilation. Hypoglycemia and hyponatremia are useful laboratory clues. With supportive care and thyroid replacement therapy, the patient can make a full recovery. Considering the frequency with which thyroid function tests are ordered, severe hypothyroidism or coma is a rarity.[38]

Hyperthyroidism

This produces a more hyperkinetic and excitable syndrome. NPS include anxiety, irritability, emotional lability, insomnia, inattention, headaches, and weakness. Rarely, executive dysfunction is also reported. The hyperkinetic neurological features are a fine postural tremor, chorea, and myoclonus. Weakness is a common feature and occurs in nearly 60% of patients with an acute or subacute onset. It may be due to a combination of myopathy, neuropathy, myasthenia gravis, or hypokalemic periodic paralysis. Replacement therapy to achieve a euthyroid state and beta-blockers often leads to a good or full recovery.[38]

Hashimoto Encephalopathy

Autoimmune thyroiditis (hashimoto thyroiditis) produces a goiter and varying degree of thyroid dysfunction. Approximately 2 out of 100,000 patients with AI thyroiditis develop a steroid-responsive encephalopathy associated with autoimmune thyroiditis (SREAT) or hashimoto encephalopathy (HE). This is a rare entity, which occurs predominantly in females. The pathogenesis is not well understood. High titers of Ab against thyroglobulin and/or thyroid peroxidase are necessary for the diagnosis, though they may be in low titers or even normal. The NPS include stroke-like focal deficits, a progressive cerebellar ataxia, seizures, myoclonus, and psychosis with hallucinations. CSF shows high proteins but is acellular. This rare disorder is associated with other concurrent AI disorders. A classic example is HE and myasthenia gravis occurring together. The diagnosis is suspected when a middle-aged female with goiter and thyroid dysfunction develops the earlier mentioned symptoms. The EEG is practically always abnormal but shows nonspecific slowing. This helps to differentiate between HE and PPD. In general, the patients respond well to steroids.[38,39]

NEUROPSYCHIATRIC ASPECTS OF SUBSTANCE USE, ALCOHOL, DRUGS, AND TOXINS

Substance Use

Toxic insult to the CNS due to illicit drugs can range from mild to fatal **(Box 1)**. Severe intoxication always appears acutely and "comedown" or withdrawal symptoms may be acute or subacute based on the degree of addiction and the illicit drug. Multiple exposures to illicit drugs have a strong tendency to addiction with chronic symptoms. The pattern of injury to the CNS is also important for the clinician when it comes to identifying the incriminating agent, as a history of exposure may not be forthcoming because of the stigma or the patient's unwillingness to disclose illicit activity.[40]

Most of these produce hyperactive AEs except opioids and sedative/hypnotics. The main AEs are neurological—seizures and encephalopathy—and are associated with systemic and autonomic AEs such as respiratory depression, pupillary abnormalities (meiosis or mydriasis), tachycardia, and sweating. Those that predominantly produce NPS will be discussed here.

BOX 1: Classes of illicit drugs.

- Opioids and derivatives:
  - Nonsynthetic: Morphine and heroin
  - Synthetic: Fentanyl
- *Psychostimulants*: Cocaine and derivatives
- Sedatives and hypnotics
- Marijuana and synthetic derivatives
- *Hallucinogens*: Lysergic acid diethylamide (LSD)
- *Dissociative agents*: Phencyclidine and ketamine
- Inhalants and E-cigarettes

Psychostimulants

These illicit drugs promote neurotransmission of dopamine, serotonin, and norepinephrine producing an enjoyable "high". Overdosage produces a hyperactive encephalopathy complicated by psychosis, seizures, cardiac arrhythmia, dilated pupils, and hyperthermia/muscle stiffness. Rhabdomyolysis is a known complication of the latter.

Marijuana and Synthetic Derivatives

Marijuana or *Bhang* as it is known in India, produces an euphoric state with jocularity and relaxation. It also produces increased appetite and an altered sense of perception and passage of time. Synthetic cannabinoids are more likely to produce NP effects—agitation, paranoia, delusions, and psychosis. They also increase the risk of seizures. Marijuana is a risk factor not only for ischemic or hemorrhagic strokes but also for reversible cerebral vasoconstriction syndrome. Finally, the clinician should be aware that chronic cannabis exposure produces centrally induced intractable nausea and vomiting. Cannabis hyperemesis uniquely responds to hot water bathing—a near pathognomonic feature.[40]

Dissociative Agents

Phencyclidine (PCD) and ketamine cause significant blockade of NMDA receptors. Acute intoxication can present with acute psychosis. These agents should be considered as chemical precipitants of any new-onset undifferentiated schizophrenia.[40]

Alcohol

Chronic alcohol use can produce primary or secondary damage to the nervous system. Cerebellar degeneration or peripheral neuropathy are classic examples of the former whereas hepatic encephalopathy following alcoholic cirrhosis, the latter. Withdrawal symptoms are known as delirium tremens. This begins 48–72 hours after abstinence and is marked by tachycardia, agitation, hyperthermia, hallucinations, and generalized seizures. Hallucinations, which start within the first day of abstinence and resolve within 48 hours is a separate entity.[40]

ADVERSE EFFECTS OF COMMONLY PRESCRIBED DRUGS

One of the most common causes of confusion, delirium, or psychosis in clinical practice is drug intoxication due to commonly prescribed drugs. The associated risk factors are old age, chronic kidney disease, and prior CNS disease. The most distinctive syndrome is with anticholinergic drugs. This is usually accompanied by peripheral cholinergic effects—dry skin and mouth, constipation, and urinary hesitancy or frank retention. By contrast, serotonergic agents used to treat depression, can also produce delirium but with normal salivation, excessive sweating, and a hyperactive gut with diarrhea. In addition, the deep tendon reflexes are exaggerated with clonus.[41]

Dopaminergic drugs, including agonist and amantadine hydrochloride, are notorious for inducing confusion and delirium in patients of PD. This is more frequent in the akinetic-rigid variant compared to the tremorgenic one. In this context, one should mention the neuroleptic malignant syndrome (NMS)—an agitated confusional state which may be followed by stupor. However, the most characteristic feature of NMS is progressive muscle rigidity resulting in hyperthermia which may be confused for VE. The muscle rigidity is the cause of hyperthermia and markedly elevated serum creatine kinase. This responds to cooling and dantrolene sodium. Thus, a thorough history and differences in the peripheral AEs help to determine which class of drug is involved.

Efavirenz is a non-nucleoside reverse transcriptase inhibitor (NNRTI) class of drug used in highly active antiretroviral therapy (HAART). NP side effects include mania, depression with suicidal thoughts, aggression, and psychosis. These AEs usually begin in the first few weeks of therapy and accommodation to them may take over 6 months. Delirium usually is an idiosyncratic reaction to ART.[26]

Heavy Metals

Many heavy metals are also toxic to the nervous system. Most of them produce a peripheral neuropathy (arsenic, thallium, lead, and gold). Mercury produces an ataxia, intention tremors, and dysarthria. Some patients, in addition, may have mental confusion. Lead, in adults, produces abdominal colic, anemia, and a peripheral neuropathy. Lead encephalopathy is decidedly rare. In the Indian context, it should be mentioned that heavy metals, known as *Bhasmas*, are a component of many *Ayurvedic* medicines given for conditions such as diabetes and arthritis. In a patient with such symptoms and a new-onset encephalopathy, a detailed history of medication, especially *Ayurvedic* should be obtained.[42]

Neoplasms and structural lesions do produce NPS but as part of the disease progression and do not create a problem with diagnosis.

CONCLUDING REMARKS

There are a host of neurological and systemic disorders which can produce NPS. In this chapter, those conditions in which, NPS are a predominant part of the clinical profile or can be a presenting feature are discussed. Careful attention to history and clinical findings often differentiates organic psychosis from PPDs. The focus has been mainly on clinical features and the value of investigations such as laboratory parameters, EEG, and neuroimaging have been highlighted when relevant.

LEARNING POINTS

- Many general medical conditions may first manifest as isolated psychotic symptoms, and a significant proportion of them are eligible for specific and/or potentially curative treatment.
- The question of somatic differential diagnosis in the face of a first PEP is therefore essential. Regarding the various possible causes, we have retained the psychotic symptoms linked to toxic substances, drugs, pathologies of the CNS, autoimmune or inflammatory systemic pathologies, of infectious origin, of genetic and nongenetic metabolic origin.
- A detailed anamnesis and a careful clinical examination must be carried out in the event of any first psychiatric episode, as well as a biological check-up.[4] Cerebral imaging and complementary tests (targeted according to the context) are desirable during psychotic-like manifestations, and careful attention should be paid to seeking a general medical condition whenever there are signs of alert.
- A large number of nonpsychiatric pathologies can induce psychotic symptoms such as drug or drug intake, pathologies of the CNS, AI or inflammatory or infectious systemic diseases, metabolic, and genetic or nongenetic diseases.
- A big many of them depend on specific treatments, and even in the case of genetic pathology without known treatment, given the family impact, it is important to seek one of these causes by a careful and early anamnestic and clinical evaluation, supplemented by a basic biological assessment.
- At the slightest sign suggestive of psychotic symptoms of secondary origin, it is essential to refer the patient for further targeted investigations depending on the context.

REFERENCES

1. Gout J, Killian MR, Antoine JC, Massoubre C, Fakra E, Cathébras P. First-episode psychosis as primary manifestation of medical disease: An update. Rev Med Interne. 2019;40(11):742-9.
2. Katrak SM. Approach to coma. In: Khadilkar SV, Singh G (Eds). IAN Textbook of Neurology, 2nd edition. New Delhi: Jaypee Brothers Medical Publishers (P) Ltd.; 2024. pp. 248-52.
3. Miller-Fischer C. Abulia. In: Bougousslavsky L, Caplan L (Eds). Strokes Syndromes. New York, USA: Cambridge University Press; 1995. pp. 182-7.
4. Barth A, Bogousslavsky, Caplan L. Thalamic infarcts and hemorrhages. In: Bougousslavsky J, Caplan L (Eds). Strokes Syndromes. New York, USA: Cambridge University Press; 1995. pp. 276-83.
5. Benson FD, Gershwind N. Aphasias and related disorders: a clinical approach. In: Mesulam MM (Ed). Principles of Behavioural Neurology. Philadelphia, USA: F.A. Davis Company; 1985. pp. 201-14.
6. Ropper AH. Transient Global Amnesia. N Engl J Med. 2023; 388:635-40.
7. Vinti V, Dell'Isola GB, Tascini G, Mencaroni E, Cara GD, Striano P, et al. Temporal Lobe Epilepsy and Psychiatric Comorbidity. Front Neurol. 2021;12:775781.
8. Spier PA, Schomer DL, Blume HW, Mesulam M-M. Temporolimbic epilepsy and behaviour. In: Mesulam MM (Ed). Principles of Behavioural Neurology. Philadelphia, USA: F.A. Davis Company; 1985. pp. 289-326.
9. Shorvon S. Principles of treatment. In: Shorvon S (Ed). Handbook of Epilepsy Treatment, 3rd edition. New Delhi, India: Wiley-Blackwell Publication, Wiley India Pvt. Ltd; 2011. pp. 75-126.
10. Ridley A. Persistent states of altered consciousness. In: Swash M, Oxbury J (Eds). Clinical Neurology. New York, USA: Churchill Livingstone; 1991. pp. 203-9.
11. Tariot PN, Mack JL, Patterson MB, Edland SD, Weiner MF, Fillenbaum G, et al. The Behavior Rating Scale for Dementia of the Consortium to Establish a Registry for Alzheimer's disease. The Behavioral Pathology Committee of the Consortium to Establish a Registry for Alzheimer's disease. Am J Psychiatry. 1995;152:1349-57.
12. Burghaus L, Eggers C, Timmermann L, Fink GR, Diederich NJ. Hallucinations in Neurodegenerative Diseases. CNS Neurosci Ther. 2012;18:149-59.
13. Rossor M. The dementias. In: Donaghy M (Ed). Brain's Diseases of the Nervous System, 12th edition. Oxford: Oxford University Press; 2009. pp. 978-90.
14. Berson RJ. Capgras' Syndrome. Am J Psychiatry. 1983;140:969-78.
15. Mendez MF, Shapira JS, Woods RJ, Licht EA, Saul RE. Psychotic Symptoms in Frontotemporal Dementia: Prevalence and Review. Dement Geriatr Cogn Disord. 2008;25:206-11.
16. Fletcher N. The akinetic-rigid disorders. In: Donaghy M (Ed). Brain's Diseases of the Nervous System, 12th edition. Oxford: Oxford University Press; 2009. pp. 1240-67.
17. Garg D, Goyal V. Parkinson plus syndrome. In: Khadilkar SV, Singh G (Eds). IAN Textbook of Neurology, 2nd edition. New Delhi: Jaypee Brothers Medical Publishers (P) Ltd.; 2024. pp. 783-90.
18. Ganesh A, Wesley SF. Practice Current: When do you suspect autoimmune encephalitis and what is the role of antibody testing? Neurol Clin Pract. 2018;8:67-73.

19. Gaus F, Titulaer MJ, Balu R, Benselar S, Bien CG, Cellucci T, et al. A Clinical Approach to the Diagnosis of Autoimmune Encephalitis. Lancet Neurol. 2016;15:391-404.
20. Dalmau J. Neuropsychiatry and encephalitis. In: Dalmau J (Ed). Autoimmune Neurology-II Advanced, C-182 Teaching Course. Boston USA: Frontiers of Neurosciences, AAN Annual Meeting; 2017.
21. Subeh GK, Lajber M, Patel T, Mostafa JA. Anti-N-Methyl-D-Aspartate Receptor Encephalitis: A Detailed Review of the Different Psychiatric Presentations and Red Flags to Look for in Suspected Cases. Cureus. 2021;13(5):e15188.
22. Rosenfeld MR, Titulaer MJ, Dalmau J. Paraneoplastic syndromes and autoimmune encephalitis. Neurol Clin Pract. 2012;2: 215-22.
23. van Sonderen A, Titulaer MJ. Autoimmune encephalitis. In: Deisenhammer F, Sellebjerg F, Teunissen CE, Tumani H (Eds). Cerebrospinal Fluid in Clinical Neurology. Switzerland: Springer International Publishing; 2015. pp. 247-76.
24. Misra UK, Kalita J. Acute viral encephalitis. In: Khadilkar SV, Singh G (Eds). IAN Textbook of Neurology, 2nd edition. New Delhi: Jaypee Brothers Medical Publishers (P) Ltd.; 2024. pp. 614-27.
25. Katrak SM. Neurological manifestations of acquired immuno-deficiency syndrome. In: Wadia NH (Ed) Neurological Practice: An Indian Perspective. New Delhi, India: Elsevier India Pvt. Ltd.; 2005. pp. 52-73.
26. Singer EJ, Thames AD. Neurobehavioral Manifestations of HIV/AIDS: Diagnosis and Treatment. Neurol Clin. 2016;34:33-53.
27. Radhakrishnan VV, Ashalatha R. Clinicopathological spectrum of chronic meningitis. In: Radhakrishnan VV, Ashalatha R (Eds). Reviews in Neurology. New Delhi, India: Wolters Kluwer Medknow; 2003. pp. 49-70.
28. Katrak SM. Central Nervous System Tuberculosis. J Neurol Sci. 2021;421:117278.
29. Katrak SM, Shembalkar PK, Bijwe SR, Bhandarkar LD. The Clinical, Radiological and Pathological Profile of Tuberculous Meningitis in patients with and without Human Immunodeficiency Virus Infection. J Neurol Sci. 2000;181:118-26.
30. Singh G. Neurocycticercosis. In: Khadilkar SV, Singh G (Eds). IAN Textbook of Neurology, 2nd edition. New Delhi: Jaypee Brothers Medical Publishers (P) Ltd.; 2024. pp. 607-13.
31. Sorabjee J. Cerebral malaria. In: Wadia NH (Ed). Neurological Practice: An Indian Perspective. New Delhi, India: Elsevier India Pvt. Ltd.; 2005. pp. 252-63.
32. Goyal G, Kaur U, Sharma M, Sehgal R. Neuropsychiatric Aspects of Parasitic Infections—A Review. Neurol India. 2023;71:228-32.
33. Tramont EC. Syphilis of the central nervous system. In: Lambert HL (Ed). Infections of the Central Nervous System. London, UK: Edward Arnold; 1991. pp. 207-17.
34. Katrak SM, Irani AM. Prion diseases. In: Bhattacharyya KB, Lalkaka JA, Sankhla CS, Wadia PM (Eds). Parkinson's Disease and Movement Disorders. New Delhi: Jaypee Brothers Medical Publishers (P) Ltd.; 2024. pp. 447-53.
35. Katrak SM, Pauranik A, Desai SB, Mead S, Beck J, Brandner S, et al. Familial Creutzfeldt-Jakob Disease in an Indian Kindred. Ann Indian Acad Neurol. 2019;22:458-61.
36. Diesing TS. Neurologic Manifestations of Gastrointestinal and Nutritional Disorders. Continuum. 2023;29:708-33.
37. Toledano M. Neurologic Manifestations of Rheumatologic Disease. Continuum. 2023;29:734-62.
38. Reda H. Neurologic Complications of Endocrine Disorders. Continuum. 2023;29:887-902.
39. Chong JY. Hashimoto encephalopathy. In: Rowlands LP, Pedley TA (eds). Merritt's Neurology, 12th Edition. Philadelphia USA: Lippincott Williams & Wilkins; 2010. pp. 1051-2.
40. Still D. Substance Use and the Nervous System. Continuum (Minneap Minn). 2023;29:923-45.
41. Ropper AH, Samuels MA, Klein JP. Delirium and other confusional states. In: Ropper AH, Samuels MA, Klein JP (Eds). Adams and Victor's Principles of Neurology, 10th edition. New York, USA: McGraw Hill Education Medical; 2014. pp. 421-33.
42. Ropper AH, Samuels MA, Klein JP. Disorders of the nervous system caused by drugs, toxins and chemical agents. In: Ropper AH, Samuels MA, Klein JP (eds). Adams and Victor's Principles of Neurology, 10th edition. New York, USA: McGraw Hill Education Medical; 2014. pp. 1200-33.

A Truly Neuropsychiatric Problem!

Ambar Chakravarty

CASE VIGNETTE

A 24-year-old lady was referred to the present author while being admitted in a psychiatric nursing home when she developed a febrile encephalopathy with an abnormal cerebrospinal fluid (CSF) study and an abnormal magnetic resonance (MR) scan of brain. She was admitted under care of a psychiatrist with a history of personality change and bizarre behavior. Her symptoms started with increased irritability about 3 weeks before admission. 1 week before admission she began having confusion, memory lapses, and had been sleeping only for a couple of hours at night. A few days before admission she was unable to identify family members and expressed nihilistic delusions. Episodes of dancing, chanting, pressured speech, and flight of ideas followed. She was also hypersexual, confused, and fatigued. The patient had no prior psychiatric illness or exposure to neuroleptics. There was no history of drug or alcohol abuse. The family history was significant for a brother with alcohol abuse. An aunt was reported to have had an unspecified psychiatric illness. There was no family history of suicide. Her physical and neurologic examinations were within normal limits, as reported to the author by the resident doctor. Shortly after admission she developed catatonic excitement, with chanting, fondling, and choreiform movements. These alternated with episodes of stupor. Urine drug screen was negative for phenothiazines and drugs of abuse. Creatinine phosphokinase was elevated at 519 U/L (normal up to 180 U/L). Complete blood count (CBC) revealed 12,000 white blood cells with 77% neutrophils with a platelet count of 90,000/mm³. Liver enzymes were marginally raised and rest of the biochemical profile was normal.

Two days after admission she developed fever of 102°F, diaphoresis, and fluctuating blood pressure. She had periods of fluctuating sensorium with auditory and visual hallucinations. She had staring, mutism, refusal to eat or drink, negativism, stereotypies, choreiform movements,

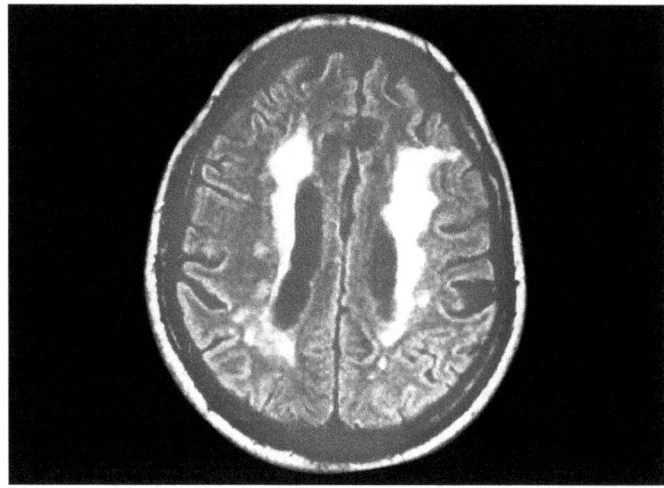

FIG. 1: MRI brain [fluid-attenuated inversion recovery (FLAIR)] of the patient.

and cogwheel rigidity. An electroencephalogram (EEG) showed mild diffuse slowing without any epileptiform features. A CSF was done and that revealed a protein of 90 mg%, normal glucose, and 20 cells/mm³ (all lymphocytes). CSF adenosine deaminase (ADA) and GeneXpert for *Mycobacterium* were negative. A MRI of brain was done and shown in **Figure 1**.

DISCUSSION

- The initial psychiatric diagnosis had been catatonia associated with schizophrenic features such as visual and auditory hallucinations. According to Diagnostic and Statistical Manual of Mental Disorders, Fifth Edition (DSM-5), catatonia is associated with a mental disorder and is diagnosed when the clinical picture is dominated by at least three of the following: Stupor; catalepsy; waxy flexibility; agitation; mutism; negativism; posturing; mannerisms; stereotypy;

grimacing; echolalia; and echopraxia. The present case had altered sensorium, negativism, mutism, echopraxia, and muscle rigidity. The choreiform movements described in the psychiatric record was in fact stereotypic movements. Catalepsy is defined as a state of marked loss of voluntary motion in which the limbs remain in whatever position they are placed. This was demonstrable when examined by the author. Waxy flexibility is closely similar. Gegenhalten is reverse of waxy flexibility where patient's resistance to passive movements increases as the examiner continues to move that part of the body of the subject passively. Gegenhalten can be elicited in patients with catatonia as well as in several neurodegenerative conditions in their advanced stages.

- The differential diagnosis of catatonic stupor include neuroleptic malignant syndrome (NMS); akinetic mutism; nonconvulsive status epilepticus (NCSE); stroke; delirium; dementia; and elective mutism.
- Although serum creatine phosphokinase (CPK) was raised in the present case along with some degree of muscle rigidity, the diagnosis of NMS was not considered as the rise of CPK was small, there was no history of intake of any neuroleptic drugs and lastly the behavioral pattern had been highly suggestive of catatonic stupor. Absence of any focal signs would exclude a stroke-like illness and absence of any epileptiform discharges in the ictal state, would exclude the possibility of NCSE.
- Features noted in the initial evaluation which could have been suggestive of an underlying systemic illness were the leukocytosis along with thrombocytopenia. In the subject, these hematological features along with the clinical features of a stuporous state would have raised the possibility of an encephalopathy with sepsis. Patient was afebrile at that time but that itself would not exclude sepsis totally. However, considering that the subject was young and female, more likely possibilities would have been an early central nervous system (CNS) infection and CNS affection from a systemic connective tissue disease.
- When the patient became febrile and the CSF was abnormal, the possibility of a CNS infection was a very distinct possibility. A bacterial infection (including tuberculosis) was unlikely because of the leukocytosis (rather than leukopenia), thrombocytopenia, normal CSF glucose, CSF lymphocytic pleocytosis, and a negative GeneXpert test. The remaining possibilities would include a viral encephalitis/encephalopathy, an autoimmune encephalitis (AIE), and CNS involvement from a systemic connective tissue disease, especially in a young female.
- The MRI brain revealed extensive periventricular white matter hyperintensities in the T2-weighted and fluid-attenuated inversion recovery (FLAIR) sequences. Such changes could have been caused by small vessel disease resulting from long-standing hypertension, cerebral autosomal dominant arteriopathy with subcortical infarcts and leukoencephalopathy (CADASIL) and demyelinating diseases such as multiple sclerosis (MS) or acute demyelinating encephalomyelitis (ADEM). Similar changes could have been caused by demyelination secondary to CNS involvement of systemic connective tissue diseases. In current time, CNS manifestation of coronavirus disease-2019 (COVID-19) would have been a distinct possibility; but this patient was seen a few years earlier. The causes of signal alterations in white matter in T2-weighted image are detailed in **Box 1**.

BOX 1: Differential diagnosis of white matter diseases of the central nervous system.[1]

- *Infectious*: Human immunodeficiency virus and associated infections; human T-lymphotropic virus (HTLV), tuberculosis, syphilis, viral encephalitis, cystic inflammatory diseases—neurocysticercosis, subacute sclerosing panencephalitis (SSPE) and other slow viral diseases, Lyme disease, and Whipple's disease
- *Inflammatory*: Acute disseminated encephalomyelitis, postinfectious/postvaccinal; site-specific demyelinating disorders, transverse myelitis, neuromyelitis optica, brainstem encephalitis, multiple sclerosis, Hashimoto's encephalopathy, Behçet syndrome, and neurosarcoidosis
- *Metabolic/nutritional*: Wernicke's encephalopathy, osmotic demyelination syndrome, and subacute combined degeneration (vitamin B12 deficiency)
- *Mitochondrial disorders*: Mitochondrial encephalopathy with stroke-like episodes (MELAS), Leigh's syndrome, and Leber's optic atrophy
- *Vascular*: Vasculitis—systemic lupus erythematosus, antiphospholipid antibody syndrome, isolated angiitis of the central nervous system (CNS); vasculopathy—moyamoya disease, retinocochleocerebral vasculopathy of Susac, cerebral autosomal dominant arteriopathy with subcortical infarcts and leukoencephalopathy (CADASIL); and cerebral venous thrombosis
- *Neoplastic*: Gliomatosis cerebri, primary CNS lymphoma, and paraneoplastic syndrome
- *Other degenerative disorders*: Spinocerebellar ataxia, leukodystrophies, radiation; toxic—carbon monoxide clioquinol, chemotherapy (methotrexate and 5-fluorouracil); reversible posterior leukoencephalopathy

- In the present case, in view of the profound psychiatric manifestations, the possibility of an underlying systemic connective tissue disease was first probed.
- Her erythrocyte sedimentation rate (ESR) was raised to 110 mm; C-reactive protein (CRP) 84 mg; antinuclear antibody (ANA), anti-double-stranded deoxyribonucleic acid (dsDNA) antibody, antiribonucleoprotein antibody, and lupus anticoagulant were all strongly positive. A final diagnosis of neuropsychiatric systemic lupus erythematosus (NPSLE) was made. A course of high-dose methylprednisolone (1 g/day by intravenous infusion) was given. She improved significantly at the completion of the course. Her subsequent management was done under care of a rheumatologist in joint consultation with the psychiatrist.
- The American College of Rheumatology (ACR) defines 19 distinct clinical central and peripheral neuropsychiatric (NP) syndromes that can occur in systemic lupus erythematosus (SLE), 12 of which are due to CNS involvement. These syndromes may be the presenting symptom of lupus or may develop later in the course.

The major CNS features include:[2-7]
- *Seizures*: Both focal and generalized seizures may occur in some 20% of SLE patients. The underlying pathology may be a focal vasculitis or a localized immune-mediated encephalopathy.
- *Cerebrovascular disease*: Both arterial and venous strokes may occur commonly in around 20% of cases. The stroke subtype may be vaso-occlusive with infarction or hemorrhagic. In SLE, several factors might predispose to stroke and these include antiphospholipid antibodies (present in up to 55% of SLE patients), vasculitis (lupus angiitis), hypertension, accelerated atherosclerosis (e.g., related to long-term steroid use), carditis (e.g., Libman–Sacks endocarditis), thrombocytopenia, and age. Lupus cerebral vasculitis presents with a distinct clinical syndrome of headache, fever, and psychiatric symptoms in addition to those of the stroke.
- *Demyelinating syndrome*: MRI brain features closely akin to MS/ADEM may be encountered in SLE with neurological, psychiatric or mixed neurological and psychiatric presentation. A few cases of SLE presenting with catatonic stupor, like the present case, had been reported earlier.
- *Myelopathy*: Transverse myelitis-like presentation of lupus is rare. When it does occur, rather rarely, the pathogenetic mechanism is vascular rather than demyelination.
- *Headache*: It is doubted what role SLE plays in the genesis of migraine headaches as also in idiopathic intracranial hypertension. However, headaches, migrainous or not, are common in patients with SLE.
- *Movement disorder*: Movement disorders occur uncommonly in patients with lupus. The most well recognized one is chorea occurring in 1% of cases. It is possible that vascular or neuronal antibodies may have a role in its genesis.
- *Aseptic meningitis*: This is a rare manifestation. The diagnosis can only be made when an infectious etiology can be carefully excluded in view of the immunocompromised state.

PSYCHIATRIC MANIFESTATIONS

- *Psychosis*: Delusions and hallucinations occur in about 5% cases. It may be immune mediated or related to vasculitis. An association with antiribosomal P and anti-NMDA receptor antibodies has been noted.
- *Acute confusional state*: This may manifest as either a hypoaroused state or a hyperaroused state, alternatively called delirium. The former refers to varying disturbances of consciousness ultimately leading to coma. The underlying pathophysiology may be multifactorial from immune mediated one to vasculitis.
- *Cognitive dysfunction*: This may occur in as high as 80% of patients. The clinical picture may vary from one with short-term memory loss to frank dementia in advanced cases.
- *Mood disorder*: Depression is common. Mostly this is related to coping with a chronic illness and is nonmelancholic. However, complex mechanisms may be involved in its genesis.
- *Anxiety disorder*: Similar to mood disorders, this may be a reaction to coping with a chronic illness but again it may also have an immunological basis.

Lastly, the peripheral nervous system involving conditions in the ACR criteria include acute inflammatory demyelinating polyradiculoneuropathy; autonomic disorders; cranial neuropathy; mononeuropathy; myasthenia gravis; plexopathy, and polyneuropathy.

KEY POINTS

- In a young female, new onset of a psychiatric illness or a movement disorder should always raise suspicion of NPSLE.
- MRI features in NPSLE are extremely variable, ranging from normal appearance to pictures simulating

MS/ADEM to features of posterior reversible encephalopathy syndrome (PRES).
- Confirmatory methods for diagnosis of NPSLE are controversial. Use of CSF level of cytokines [interleukin-6 (IL-6) in particular] and presence of antineuronal antibodies have been highlighted. However, advanced neuroimaging methods would probably score over immunological methods

REFERENCES

1. Sibbitt WL Jr, Sibbitt RR, Brooks WM. Neuroimaging in neuropsychiatric systemic lupus erythematosus. Arthritis Rheum. 1999;42(10):2026-38.
2. Rogers JP, Pollak TA, Blackman G, David AS. Catatonia and the immune system: a review. Lancet Psychiatry. 2019;6:620-30.
3. Carroll BT, Anfinson TJ, Kennedy JC, Yendrek R, Boutros M, Bilon A. Catatonic Disorder Due to General Medical Conditions. J Neuropsychiatry Clin Neurosci. 1994;6:122-33.
4. Ali A, Taj A, Zehra M. Lupus catatonia in a young girl who presented with fever and altered sensorium. Pak J Med Sci. 2014;30(2):446-8.
5. Grover S, Singh A, Sarkar S, Bhalla A. SLE presenting with catatonia in an adolescent girl. J Pediatr Neurosci. 2013;8(3): 262-3.
6. Grover S, Parakh P, Sharma A, Rao P, Modi M, Kumar A. Catatonia in systemic lupus erythematosus: a case report and review of literature. Lupus. 2013;22:634-8.
7. Sommerlad A, Duncan J, Lunn MPT, Foong J. Neuropsychiatric systemic lupus erythematosus: a diagnostic challenge. BMJ Case Rep. 2015; 2015:bcr2014208215.

CHAPTER 5

Cognition Testing at the Bedside

Amit Halder, Ambar Chakravarty

INTRODUCTION: TESTING COGNITION THROUGH THE AGES

Physicians in the 17th and 18th centuries first observed the notable dissociations of mental faculties that were impaired while others remained intact in various brain disorders, Carl Wernicke (1848-1905), a German physician, anatomist, psychiatrist, and neuropathologist, first began to develop procedures for assessing more specific components of mental functioning in the mid-19th century. Konrad Rieger (1855-1939) and Theodor Ziehen (1862-1950), both German, a neurologist and the other, a psychiatrist, developed the first neuropsychological test batteries. Kurt Goldstein (1878-1965), a student of Wernicke and Edinger, laid more importance on the way patients performed with the test batteries rather than how much they scored. Alexander Luria (1902-1977) the Soviet neuropsychologist considered the father of modern clinical neuropsychology, developed an extensive and original battery of neuropsychological tests during his clinical work with brain-injured victims of World War II. Soon thereafter, Alfred Binet (1857-1911), a French psychologist and a pupil of Charcot, along with another psychologist Théodore Simon (1873-1971), developed the intelligence testing battery. Later this was transformed into the Army Alpha and Army Beta tests for selecting soldiers. However, the basics of this battery of tests are still being used by modern-day neuropsychologists for assessing intelligence. The 20th century witnessed the contributions of two great neuropsychologists, Shepherd Ivory Franz (1874-1933) an American psychologist, favoring a clinical approach, and Ward Halstead (1908-1968) another American, who stimulated a strongly psychometric-based approach. Henry Charlton Bastian (1837-1915), a Queen Square neurologist, formulated the first comprehensive language battery tests. While in the 19th and the first half of the 20th century, neurologists and psychiatrists had to depend solely on autopsy studies for clinicoanatomical correlation of different domains of cognition, advancements in neuroimaging techniques in the latter part of the 20th century and early 21st century greatly enriched our knowledge in regard to structure-function correlation.

The myth has been propagated through generations of medical practitioners that the mental status of an individual cannot be evaluated at the bedside and need extensive standardized neuropsychological testing. This notion is impractical as in the hospital ward or intensive care unit, the real-life situation is entirely different. The clinician is often faced with the challenging job of evaluating a patient who has suddenly become confused and/or agitated. Time is of the essence and bedside testing is the only way forward. The clinician is faced with a plethora of questions. Is it delirium? Or, is it preexisting cognitive impairment that has got unmasked? Or, is it some new-onset neurological disease that is manifesting with altered mentation?

"Bedside cognitive testing" denotes a flexible, goal-oriented evaluation of mental function by the clinician that uses prepared test material or ad hoc devised tests (depending on the clinical situation).[1-3] Impaired cognition generally denotes a deficiency in knowledge, thought process, or judgment. Bedside cognitive testing can diagnose major cognitive impairment (i.e., dementia) mild cognitive impairment (MCI), evaluate overall brain functions in traumatic brain injuries, and help determine the decision-making capacity of an individual (needed for assessment for fitness to continue in a responsible job), and make an approximation of any significant intellectual dysfunction.[4-7]

According to the Diagnostic and Statistical Manual of Mental Disorders, 5th edition (2014 updated 2018),[8] major neurocognitive disorder requires demonstration of significant cognitive decline in at least one of the following cognitive domains: Complex attention, executive function, language, learning and memory, perceptual-motor, and social cognition. Recognition of minor neurocognitive disorder requires only modest cognitive decline that does not interfere with instrumental activities of daily living. Most of the features mentioned above can be assessed with reasonable accuracy at the bedside using well-standardized methods and only cases with doubtful and difficult to make decisions can be the candidates for detailed neuropsychological testing.

ANATOMICAL BASIS OF COGNITIVE DEFICITS

Localization is the key to the diagnosis of neurological disorders. In the field of cognition, there is a dichotomy. Some cognitive functions can be localized. Others cannot be. The term "distributed" is used to describe brain functions that cannot be strictly localized to one lateralized brain region (**Table 1**). The three main domains of cognition that are distributed include: (1) Arousal/attention, (2) memory, and (3) executive functions. Abnormalities of distributed brain function thus arise only in bilateral extensive lesions. A localized thalamic lesion may be an exception. Localized functions on the other hand can be divided into those associated with the dominant (usually, left) or nondominant hemisphere.[3] This is summarized in **Table 1**. Brain regions affected by different forms of cognitive dysfunctions are schematically shown in **Figures 1 and 2**. Some detailing of the anatomical basis of the different domains of cognition will be made later in this chapter.

TABLE 1: Localizations of cognitive functions.[3]

Cognitive functions	Probable localizations
Arousal/attention/concentration	Reticular activating system and the thalamic projections along with multimodal association areas (prefrontal and parietal) with right hemispheric bias
Memory	The limbic system (hippocampus and diencephalon)
Complex executive functions	Frontal Lobes

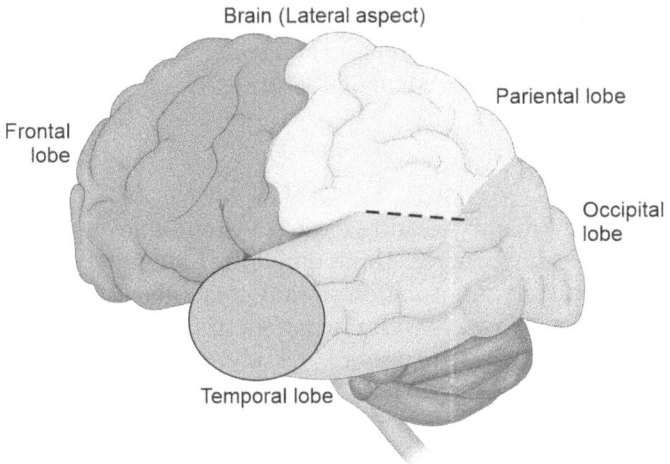

FIG. 2: Lobes of the brain (to be correlated with the Index in Fig. 1).

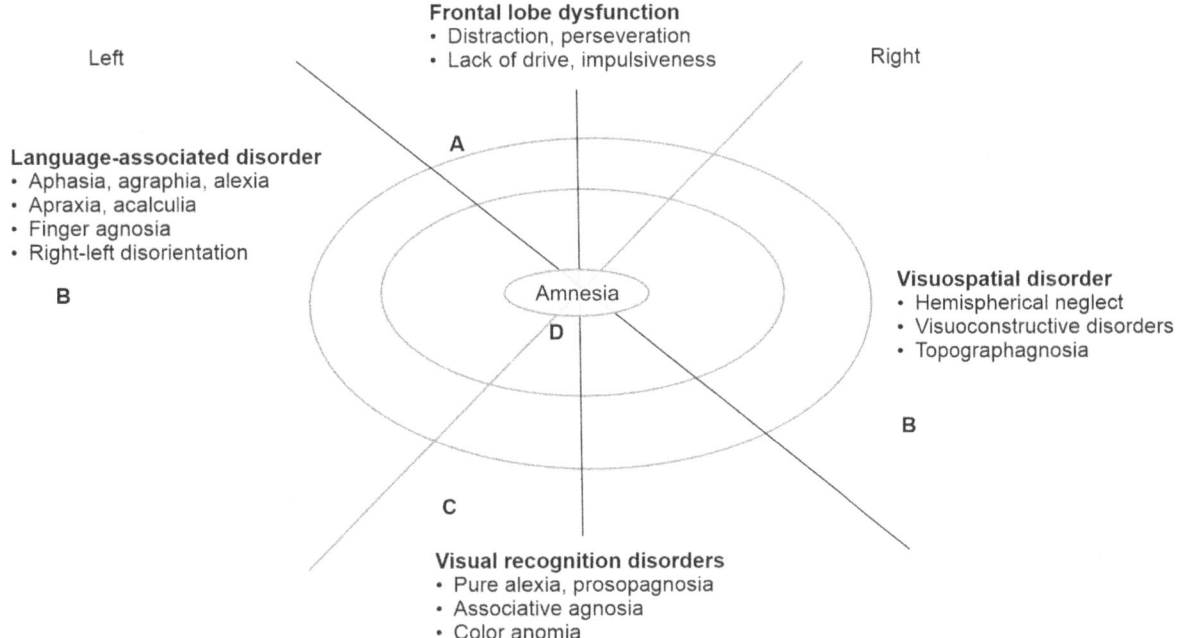

FIG. 1: Schematic representations of brain regions affected by different cognitive dysfunctions. Index A—frontal Lobe; B—parietal lobe and posterior temporal lobe; C—Occipital Lobe; D—anterior temporal lobe.

THE TESTING PROCESS

The classical scheme of history, observation, and examination is the key. The purpose of the clinical evaluation needs to be chalked out at the outset. Firstly, the presence or absence of well-defined behavioral/cognitive changes indicative of organic brain disease needs to be established. This has to be correlated with the patient's preexisting level of functioning. Knowing the educational and occupational status of the individual helps in this process. The possibility of adjustment disorder or functional psychiatric disorder needs to be looked into. The patient's general medical condition needs to be carefully ascertained. Endocrine diseases, hepatic or renal failure, alcohol or drug abuse, and systemic infection can all present with altered mental status.[2]

HISTORY

A detailed history relating to the presenting problem is of utmost importance. If the patient is unable to give a proper history, information should be obtained from an informant who stays with the patient. If both the patient and the informant are present, it is advisable to talk to the patient alone for some time. This may help the patient to reveal confidential information relevant to the illness to the examiner.

History taking is important as it helps out in finding the precise complaints of the patient. Secondly, it helps in assessing the severity of the disorder and its impact on the patient's life. A person coming with a "memory complaint" and having difficulty in remembering names does not have the same severity of the illness as someone who has lost his way home. Thirdly, the premorbid cognitive abilities can be assessed from history. Lastly, the ease and precision of the patient's response can give the examiner an idea about the patient's language and memory functions. Behavioral abnormalities are sometimes more evident during history taking. A common but often overlooked entity is the "head-turning sign". Here, the patient looks to his accomplice for help when asked questions; this may be a useful sign in identifying a patient with major cognitive dysfunction.[3] The examiner must be capable of adjusting the examination process based on observations made during the elicitation of history.

The following pieces of information need to be obtained—(1) onset of the condition (insidious or acute), (2) presenting symptom, (3) course of the condition (gradually progressive, stepwise, fluctuating, or improving), and (4) duration of the symptoms.[2,3]

The establishment of rapport with the patient is the initial step. A few nonconfrontational questions about the patient's background including his/her hobbies and interests may go a long way in putting the patient at ease. If the patient is unable to engage in sensible conversation to answer coherently, the role of the informant becomes more important. The reason for referral to the clinic or admission to the hospital needs to be ascertained. Often, a cognitively impaired patient may not be able to provide correct answers.

Open-ended questions are preferred to obtain an unbiased narrative reply. The colloquial "phrases" used by the patient to describe his/her problems should be noted *ad verbatim* rather than using medical terms. A description of the principal symptoms along with their duration and progression is obtained. Alongside, questions need to be asked about any alteration or disturbance (unusual/inappropriate behavioral pattern). One should specifically ask for any history of poor judgment, difficulty in concentration, or language functions (not articulatory but inappropriate). Memory problems, history of losing way (even indoors) or trouble carrying out activities of daily living (e.g., cooking or driving) may give important clues about the underlying domains affected.

The term "memory difficulty" used by the patient or the relatives may have various connotations—it may be the inability to concentrate while reading a book; it may be the inability to follow the conversation; there may be the inability to remember why they entered a room or also, remembering the proper sequence of mixing up ingredients during cooking. These are all examples of the inability to learn/retain new information.

Specific history for any psychiatric disorder such as depression, anxiety, or schizophrenia needs to be obtained. Any symptoms of delusion or hallucination must be recorded. Past medical history including any history of infection, head injury, stroke, or epilepsy may point to a possible underlying etiology for the cognitive decline. A history of intake of drugs or alcohol or exposure to toxins should not be missed (e.g., lead poisoning). A detailed birth and developmental history should be taken to account for any preexisting cognitive deficits. Educational history and academic records may corroborate this.

History is not complete without a detailed family history of neurological disorders or mental illness. For example, a family history of suicide may point to underlying Huntington's disease. Lastly, the dietetic history and sexual behavior need exploration (vitamin B12 deficiency and sexually transmitted diseases causing neurocognitive problems are not very uncommon).

OBSERVING THE BEHAVIOR

During the process of history taking, the general behavior of the patient should be observed. This can provide important clues regarding an organic or functional disorder. Several neurobehavioral syndromes (e.g., delirium and frontal lobe syndrome) can be diagnosed primarily based on their behavioral manifestations. Frontal lobe disinhibition may lead to a person being inappropriately jocular or making obscene comments. A delirious patient, on the other hand, can be noisy, restless, and easily distractible. This problem may also interfere with subsequent formal testing of specific domains like memory.[4] Delirium (as defined in the DSM5) is an acute and fluctuating neurological disorder that reflects a change from baseline cognition and is characterized by the cardinal features of inattention and disorganized thinking.[8] Several factors may predispose an elderly subject to develop this state. These include acute medical comorbidities (e.g., heart failure), disturbed sleep, sensory impairment, hospital isolation, lack of exposure to daylight, infections, drug/alcohol withdrawal, dehydration, blood loss, dyselectrolytemia, acid-base abnormalities, desaturation/hypoxemia, pyrexia, seizures, and endocrinologic dysfunction. A close lookout for these would be warranted. Observation of the general physical appearance of the subject is equally important. Unilateral neglect, both for body part and visual field, can be ascertained with ease at the bedside and this can be confirmed later during physical examination. This would be of significant localizing value. Improper attire and lack of cleanliness suggest a lack of self-care may be observed in both demented as well as severely depressed subjects.

The observed behavior of a subject in a specified situation is closely linked to the underlying emotion generated internally. While emotional responses are mostly generated in deep cortical and subcortical structures (hippocampus, amygdala, hypothalamus, and multiple regions in the brainstem), the final expression of the emotional response is largely modified by the prefrontal cortices. And here comes the role of the inhibitory functions of the frontal lobes.

ANATOMICAL BASIS OF MEMORY AND EMOTION

There exists an extensive network of regions in the frontal and temporal lobes involved in emotional and social processing. The well-known Papez circuit **(Fig. 3)** plays an important role.[9] The circuit involves such structures as—the hippocampus, its efferent pathway through the fimbriae, posterior columns of the fornix, body of the fornix, and finally the anterior columns of the fornix, terminating in the mammillary bodies. The latter structures are connected to the anterior nucleus of the thalamus which in turn project to the prefrontal and anterior cingulate cortices. Apart from generating emotional responses, many of the aforementioned structures are involved in the preservation of memory as well. Emotional responses to specified situations are indeed often governed by the memory of past experiences.

The inhibitory functions of the frontal lobes are often needed in the proper execution of our day-to-day activities as well as in determining our social responses. In daily life, it is sometimes necessary to suppress the impulse to perform certain tasks to reach our goals. The terms

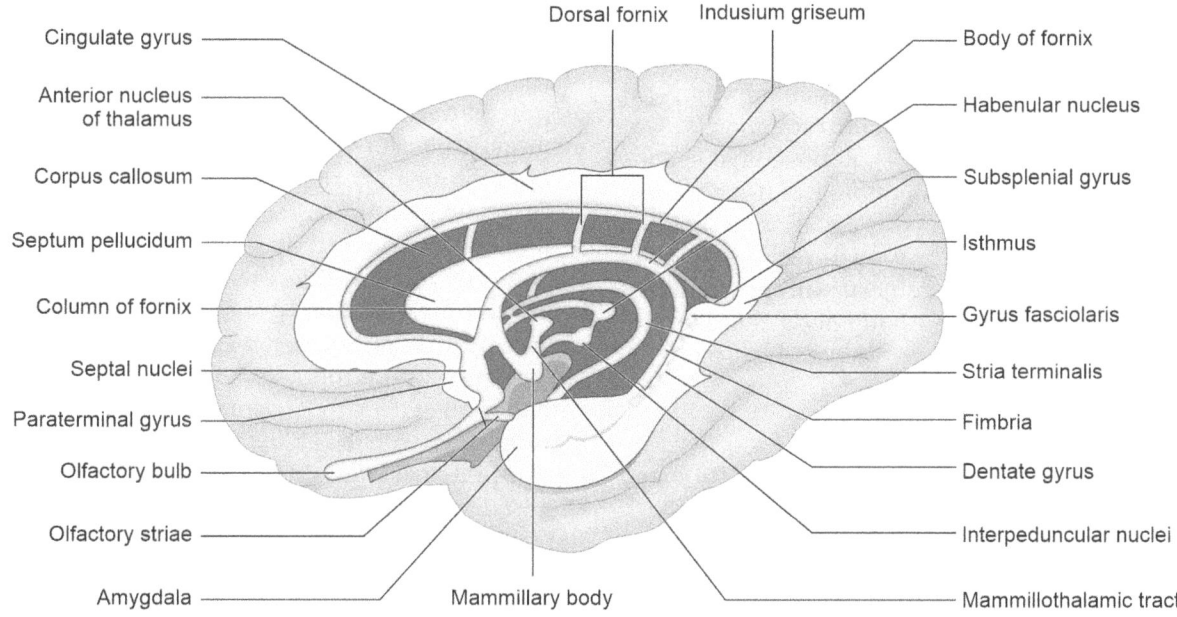

FIG. 3: The components of the Papez circuit and the limbic system.

"utilization behavior" and "environmental dependency" were used by Lhermitte to describe the impaired inhibition seen in the daily activities of patients with frontal lobe injury.[10] Such patients lose the ability to inhibit motor programs (e.g., when given an empty cup, starts drinking from it), as the drive/desire to use an object overrides any logic whether such action is appropriate or not. Environmental dependency, on the other hand, relates to the tendency to passively follow the cues and gestures of others, even though that would not be socially appropriate (e.g., holding and shaking a guest's hand when the latter had only moved his hand to scratch his/her face). All these can be detected at the bedside in patients with frontal lobar lesions, with close observation, and also can be noted during detailed history elicitation.

PHYSICAL EXAMINATION

Examination usually begins by testing the patient's alertness. Descriptive common-sense terms such as wakeful and cooperative are preferred to vague medical jargon like stupor. A summary of the key deficits that can be elicited by testing the brain functions along with their localization are summarized in **Figures 1 and 2**.

Testing Attention

These include digit span, serial subtraction of 7s, and spelling familiar words backward. The problem with serial 7s is that the elderly and patients with left hemispheric dysfunction, may not be able to perform the test even with intact attention.[11] The Mini-Mental State Examination (MMSE) and the Addenbrooke Cognitive Examination (ACE3)[12] have thus used spelling the word "WORLD" backward for those who are unable to perform the serial seven subtraction.[11] Ability to recite the months in a year backward is also a good test of sustained attention.

The normal digit span is 6 (±1). Reverse digit span is also an accurate measure of attention. It is usually 1 less than the forward digit span.[2,3] This depends on working memory which is determined by frontal executive function and phonological processes. Subjects with predominant amnesic disorders such as Alzheimer's disease and Korsakoff's syndrome may have preserved digit span.

Orientation

Orientation is usually described in relation to time and place. This can be done practically as shown in **Table 2**. Date orientation is the least reliable test. Some clinicians would consider a date range of (±) 2 of the actual date to be a normal response. Hospital-admitted patients, often do not have any clue as to the date (and often the time

TABLE 2: Testing orientation.

Orientation	Time	Day of the week
		Date
		Month
		Season
		Year
	Place	Building
		Floor
		Town
		Country/State (as applicable)
		Country

of the day); one needs to specifically ask for how long the patient has been admitted and whether it is daytime or night. The latter may be impossible for some staying in an intensive care ward with continuous artificial lighting. Disorientation in time is more prominent in acute confusional states (e.g., delirium) due to metabolic causes or diffuse brain injury. This may not be prominent in subjects with early dementia. Orientation to place is a less sensitive test of cognition than orientation to time.[13]

Even subjects with advanced dementia or with acute confusional state, are usually able to tell his or her name correctly. If a patient is unable to do that, the possibility of psychogenic amnesia needs to be considered. Subjects with motor aphasia may also be unable to utter their names, but can choose the right name if given options. Comprehension needs to be reasonably intact to understand the meaning of the question asked.

Memory

Memory can be divided into two main types—(1) implicit or procedural memory and (2) explicit or declarative memory. Explicit memory is again divided into two parts—(1) episodic memory and (2) semantic memory.[1]

Episodic memory is responsible for laying down of personally experienced and temporally specific events. Semantic memory on the other hand acts as a storehouse of facts and meanings about objects, concepts, and people.

Episodic memory can again be subdivided into anterograde and retrograde. Anterograde memory deals with the ability to learn new information while retrograde memory deals with the ability to recall old information.

The principal brain structures needed for the retention of episodic memory include the hippocampus (along with the subiculum), the entorhinal cortex part of the para-hippocampal gyrus, the mammillary bodies and the thalamus.[14] Two major neural tracts, namely: (1) The septohippocampal and (2) the mammillothalamic tracts, are needed for the maintenance of episodic memory. The former, a major cholinergic projection arising from the septal nuclei in the septum pellucidum, travels through the fornix and reaches the hippocampus and the entorhinal cortex in the parahippocampal cortex. The mammillothalamic tract is a part of the Papez circuit and its course and projections have been discussed earlier in this chapter. The anterior cingulum, receiving the projection from the mammillothalamic tract, projects back to the hippocampus through anatomical continuity. Thus the mammillothalamic system is connected to the septohippocampal tract. This intricate interconnecting pathway is needed for spatial processing controlled by the hippocampus. This organ can thus associate "what", "when", and "where" together.[15] Also the Limbic system links the pathways controlling memory functions and emotional expressions, which thus are interdependent.

A lesion anywhere along the septohippocampal pathway would lead to a severe loss of episodic memory. Such subjects would have anterograde amnesia with the inability to retain/memorize any new information. Memories that were established before, (remote memories), would be relatively preserved. However, retrograde amnesia, going as far back as years, may be present. The extent of this retrograde memory loss would be dependent on the size of the lesion; with the healing of the lesion, the degree of memory loss tends to lessen. The most common cause of entorhinal cortical dysfunction is Alzheimer's disease; the entorhinal pathology subsequently involves the hippocampus. Hippocampal injury can also be caused by trauma, stroke, and encephalitis, commonly herpes simplex infection. Classical injury to the mammillary bodies leads to Korsakoff's syndrome and a stroke involving the dorsomedial nucleus of the thalamus can cause severe amnesia.

TESTING ANTEROGRADE MEMORY

Anterograde memory can be verbal or nonverbal.

There are formal and nonformal tests of anterograde verbal memory. Nonformal tests include asking the patient how he came to the hospital or what he had seen on television the previous weekend.

In ACE3, the patient is asked to repeat seven part name and address. This is repeated thrice, even if the response is correct on the first occasion. After a gap of about 10 minutes, when the rest of the test is completed, the patient is asked to recall the same name and address. A completely correct response virtually rules out a major amnesic deficit. Intermediate results are more difficult to judge. Recognition of the components that they have failed to recall will indicate anxiety, depression, or frontal lobe retrieval problems.[12]

Story recall and word list learning tasks can be employed for formal assessment. These are usually derived from the Wechsler Memory Scale.[16] The 15-item Rey Auditory Verbal Learning Test is frequently employed.[17] It consists of five learning trials of list A followed by an interfering list B. This is followed by a recall of list A and again after 20 minutes a delayed recall of list A.

Verbal memory, relies disproportionately on the left (or dominant) hippocampus. With dominant side hippocampal lesions, the ability to learn new vocabulary is lost. Additionally as much of day-to-day new learning requires intact verbal memory, it is not uncommon for such subjects to forget the time or place of appointments, the names of friends, or the content of the previous conversation. Dominant (mostly left) hippocampal lesions and dorsomedial thalamic lesions lead to more severe amnesia than damage to the other side.[18] Interestingly, damage to the right hippocampus seems to have a greater impact on memory for visual and spatial information than for verbal ones.

Anterograde Nonverbal Memory

The decline in nonverbal memory usually parallels the decline in verbal memory except in cases where there is selective damage to the nondominant medial temporal lobe. Unfortunately, there are no good bedside tests for nonverbal memory. Spatial learning can be tested by walking a route around the ward or clinic with the patient and then asking him/her to retrace the part. Tests of face memory using nonfamous face photographs from various magazines can also be employed.

A formal Paired Associate learning (PAL) from a computerized Cambridge Neuropsychological Test Automated Battery (CANTAB) battery and recognition memory test can be used.[19,20]

Retrograde Memory

Systematic questioning about past events from the preceding months, years, or decades can give a holistic picture. It must be correlated according to the patient's baseline performance. It is better to start with open-ended questions and then go to the details. A temporal gradient for retrograde memory loss may be present. They may be better for events of the distant past than for those of the recent past. This is known as Ribot's law of retrograde amnesia.[21,22] In Alzheimer's disease or Korsakoff''s syndrome, memory loss is more extensive than in pure hippocampal damage.

Autobiographical or personal memory can be tested by asking the patient to correctly chronologically sequence some specific events of his/her personal life, e.g., educational career or professional career.[23]

Semantic Memory

This involves multiple domains of cognition. Hence, there is no single test. It may be both verbal and nonverbal. The common examples include:
- Category fluency (e.g., animals and fruits) is very sensitive, but is affected by executive functions.
- Naming pictures
- Tests of verbal knowledge
- Picture pointing in response to spoken name

Confrontation naming detects/semantic defects, word finding capacity and visual processing, need to be intact for reliable testing.[24]

With semantic memory loss, the individual usually has no recollection of when or where the information was acquired. For example, when a subject is asked how many days are present in a month, most people would respond spontaneously with the answer "30 or 31". Retaining the knowledge that "30/31" days are present in a month is possible because the brain holds a complex set of constructs that include an abstract awareness of what a day represents, and how many of these abstract units of time are present in another abstract time concept, namely the month. The semantic memory system is capable of holding these ideas together. This system works independently of the septohippocampal and mammillothalamic memory systems and likely involves the anterior and lateral temporal lobes. Patients with MTL injury, usually maintain their access to semantic knowledge, while patients with primarily anterior and lateral temporal lobe damage show intact episodic memory but impaired semantic memory.[25-27] In semantic dementia (a subtype of frontotemporal dementia), both simply naming an object and later knowledge about the identity of people and objects are lost. Such patients would tend to classify objects into increasingly superordinate categories (e.g., calling a "parrot" as just a "bird" and later with disease progression that "bird" becomes just an animal). It has been suggested that the hippocampus can store semantic memories for approximately 2 years and after that, these memories are transferred to the left temporal neocortex.[28] Hence, patients with semantic dementia can often remember current events as their hippocampi are spared, but they would reveal profound loss of remote memory, as their temporal neocortices are degenerated and dysfunctional. While bilateral (though at times asymmetrically), temporal lobar degeneration is a characteristic feature of semantic dementia, such a situation can also occur following herpes zoster encephalitis.

Working Memory

This may be considered a form of episodic memory "that allowed the individual to hold and manipulate information for short periods: from seconds to minutes".[29] A simple way to test this would be to call an operator and ask for a telephone number.

Working memory is needed to remember these numbers while they are being dialed into the telephone. Functional magnetic resonance imaging (fMRI) studies have shown that the dorsolateral frontal lobes, particularly Brodmann area 46, are critical for working memory. Working memory deficit may hamper the learning process in a subject and may affect daily life activities. Subjects with classic amnesic syndrome possess intact working memory but are unable to transfer information from working memory into a long-term store.[30,31]

FRONTAL EXECUTIVE FUNCTIONS

The frontal lobe is subdivided into several structurally and functionally specific regions for carrying out several important functions. These include motor planning, language, intelligence, working memory, generation/initiation of movements, inhibition of inappropriate social behavior, attention, abstraction, sequencing alternate tasks, drive, emotional expression, self-awareness, insight, and personality. All these functions (often grouped as frontal executive functions) are of higher order or executive processes that involve the organization of more basic cerebral processes to promote efficient and flawless task performance.[32,33] Current research casts some doubt about the sole role of the frontal cortex in executive memory functions as: (1) executive processes involve links between different brain areas, not exclusively with the frontal cortex, and (2) patients with no evidence of frontal damage present with executive deficits, and (3) patients with frontal lesions do not always show executive deficits. It is felt that it is time for a more dynamic and flexible view of the neural substrate of executive processes to be considered.[34]

History and observance of the patient's behavior may be more important than formal testing in assessing the executive functions. Nevertheless, there are several tests that can be useful for confirming the clinical impression. These include:
- Initiation
- Abstraction
- Problem-solving and decision making
- Response inhibition and set-shifting

Initiation

Verbal fluency tests can range from words beginning with a particular letter (e.g., F, A, and S) to those from a common semantic category (e.g., fruits and animals). They depend on the coordinated functions of the frontal and temporal lobes. The patient is asked to generate as many words as possible in 1 minute excluding proper nouns starting with the letters FAS. Normal young subjects should produce at least 15 words for each letter. A total of FAS of <30 words is abnormal. Patients with frontal lobe dysfunction, e.g., due to frontotemporal degeneration, produce few words and make rule breaks. Amnesic patients tend to repeat the same words several times in category fluency tests. The test is also a sensitive test for detecting speech disorders.[35,36]

In the category fluency test, subjects are asked to generate as many words as possible from semantic categories such as animals, fruits, and vegetables. Ten or below is usually considered abnormal.

It should be borne in mind that these tests are dependent on the age and the baseline intellect of the subject.

Nonverbal drive and flexibility can be explored with the five-point test[37] in which subjects are asked to produce within 3 minutes, simple designs by combining two to five points in a fixed array of five points. Normal subjects can produce at least 20 designs in 3 minutes. This is a sensitive test of right frontal dysfunction.

Abstraction: Proverbs, Similarities and Cognitive Estimates

An idea about abstraction can be gained by proverb interpretation and similarities test. Subjects who lose this ability often have acquired frontal lobe lesions. Participation of multiple brain regions is needed in the process of abstraction, but the final pathway probably requires the proper functioning of the frontal lobes.

Test of Proverb Interpretation

While interpreting such common proverbs as *"A rolling stone gathers no moss"*, concrete interpretation with an inability to use analogies is a salient feature of patients with frontal lobe dysfunction. Again, this test is dependent on the educational and cultural background of the patient and is often language specific. Alternatives in regional languages need to be formulated beforehand.

Test of Similarities

Here subjects are asked in which way conceptually linked items are alike. For example, table and chair; apple and banana and like that. Patients with frontal lobe dysfunction and dementia often fail to make proper associations or make wrong associations.

Cognitive Estimates Test

Here a subject is asked a range of questions that require common sense judgment to answer correctly. For example, *"what is the average height of a man"*? This would assess the subject's ability to conceptualize.

Response Inhibition and Set-shifting

These tests are designed to check a subject's ability to shift from one cognitive set to another and his/her ability to inhibit/suppress inappropriate responses.

Wisconsin Card Sorting Test

It is a formal test of set-shifting and also involves problem-solving and hypothesis testing.[38] The test involves sorting out cards containing geometric forms which differ in number, shape, and color. After the correct sorting dimension, asked for, is made, subjects are required to shift to another dimension. Patients with frontal lobe impairment are unable to shift from one dimension to another. They make errors in way of repetitions. This phenomenon is called perseveration.

Go-no-go Test

This is also a test of response inhibition (impulsivity) and may be impaired in subjects with frontal lobe dysfunction.[39] Subjects respond to certain stimuli ("go" stimuli) and make no response for others ("no-go" stimuli). The examiner assesses the commission error rate (making a "go" response wrongly on a "no-go" task stimulus); fewer errors signify better response inhibition, signifying intact frontal inhibitory functions.

Trail-making Test

This is a good measure of mental speed, attention shifting, and response inhibition.[40] Age and education can influence performance. There are two parts. In the first part, the patient is asked to draw a line connecting randomly arranged numbers in numerical sequence. In the second part, the numbers are intermixed with letters and the subject is asked to connect the numbers and alphabets in an alternating sequence.

Motor Sequencing: The Luria Three-step Test and the Alternating Hand Movements Test

In Luria's three-step test, the examiner demonstrates a series of hand movements—fist, edge, palm, in sequence, five times without any verbal clues.[41] The subject is then asked to repeat the same series. Patients with frontal lobe dysfunction are unable to do the sequence correctly (even with verbal clues).[42] In the alternating hand movements test, the examiner again demonstrates a series of hand movements and asks the subject to repeat them.

SOCIAL DISINHIBITION AND CHANGES IN EMOTIONAL REACTIVITY

Good social behavior includes maintaining good judgment, and honesty, understanding one's appropriate place in society, and shaping and modifying one's behavior and manners as required from time to time in response to social cues/needs.

Subjects with lesions in the orbitofrontal cortex (resulting from tumors, head trauma, anterior communicating artery aneurysms, and frontotemporal dementia) often present with selective deficits in social behavior (inappropriate behavior) but have relative sparing of drive and other neuropsychological functions.[43] The term "pseudopsychopathic personality disorder" had been used to describe such behavioral changes.[44] While these patients are socially disinhibited, inappropriately friendly, unreliable, and in constant trouble, they would rarely exhibit the systematic cruelty, or the careful planning of crimes, as noted in true psychopaths. These subjects have been noted to exhibit remorse, on occasions, after exhibiting some inappropriate social behavior.

Mood disorders such as depression and mania are often noted in subjects with lesions of the prefrontal cortex. Depression may be more common with left rather than right frontal lobe lesions.[45] Manic syndromes, on the other hand, are more likely to occur with right frontal pathologies. Frontal lobar dysfunction may lead to a lower threshold for crying, and occasionally for laughing (pseudobulbar affect).

The right hemisphere plays an important role in emotional processing and hence subjects with right hemispheric pathology are at times emotionally flat, and exhibit difficulty in expressing the normal emotional signals in the voice with variations in pitch, speed, and loudness—designated as a prosody and a melody.[46] Although such subjects are emotionally flat, they would rarely complain of feeling depressed, the emotional blunting may make a true assessment of the affective disorder in these patients.

There cannot be any specific test to quantify the disinhibitory and emotional aberrations in patients with frontal lobar lesions; careful observation of patients' behavior during history elucidation and physical examination, is essential to gauge the patient's mental and emotional status.

Localization-related Cerebral Functions

The second part of cognitive assessment addresses the localizable functions of the cerebral cortex. Specific cognitive functions are divided by their localization in the dominant (usually left) and the nondominant hemisphere (usually right). In almost 90% of people, the left hemisphere is the dominant hemisphere and houses the language functions.

DOMINANT HEMISPHERE FUNCTIONS

The dominant hemisphere functions that are tested include speech and language, calculation, and praxis.

Language

Aphasia/dysphasia is defined as an impairment of language function caused by brain damage. This needs to be differentiated from dysarthria or anarthria, which are articulatory disorders without any affection of language. Since speech/language disorders would be discussed separately in this volume, only brief mention would be made of the neuroanatomical basis, classification, and bedside testing modalities.

Since the times of Paul Broca and Carl Wernicke,[47,48] it has been recognized that most aphasias occur with left hemispheric, particularly perisylvian, lesions. Broca's aphasia is characterized by the presence of nonfluent speech, phonemic paraphasias, and relatively intact language comprehension. Classically, this syndrome is associated with a lesion in the posterior portion of the left inferior frontal gyrus. On the other hand, lesions affecting the left parietal/posterior temporal region are associated with fluent, "gibberish" speech, comprehension difficulties, and semantic paraphasias. These are constituents of Wernicke's aphasia. A milder syndrome of relatively isolated anomia can occur as a result of any left-hemisphere lesion. Many aphasic patients evolve from a severe aphasic syndrome developing soon after the onset of the brain lesion to anomic aphasia on recovery. Global aphasia, where there is a complete inability to understand or produce language, results from large perisylvian lesions in the dominant hemisphere. In classical Broca's or Wernicke's aphasias, the ability to repeat words is impaired as much as the inability to speak spontaneously. A combination of features, like speech pattern (fluent or non-fluent), word usage, comprehension, and repetition abilities have been used to describe different aphasic syndromes with specific anatomical localizations.

The following language functions are commonly performed at the bedside—spontaneous speech; naming;

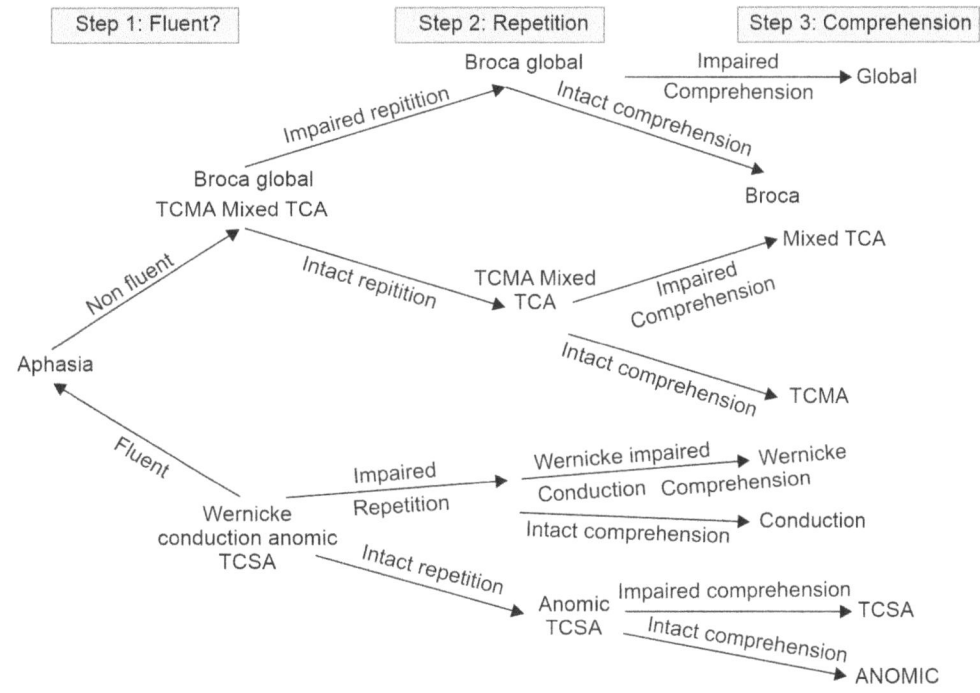

FLOWCHART 1: A stepwise approach to speech disorders.
(TCA: transcortical aphasia; TCMA: transcortical motor aphasia; TCSA: transcortical sensory aphasia)

comprehension; repetition; and reading and writing. While detailed testing procedures would be discussed elsewhere in this volume, based on the results obtained, speech disorders can be classified as follows:

- *Broca's aphasia*: Nonfluent speech; impaired naming; impaired repetition; and intact comprehension
- *Wernicke's aphasia*: Fluent aphasia; intact naming; impaired repetition; and impaired comprehension
- *Conduction aphasia*: Fluent speech; intact naming; impaired repetition; and intact comprehension
- *Transcortical motor aphasia*: Nonfluent speech; impaired naming; intact repetition; and intact comprehension
- *Transcortical sensory aphasia*: Fluent speech; intact naming; intact repetition; and impaired comprehension (except auditory)
- *Global aphasia*: Nonfluent speech/mute: Impaired naming; impaired repetition; and impaired comprehension

Lesion localization of conduction aphasia is in the superior temporal lobe but without any significant damage to Wernicke's area or it may involve the inferior parietal region. Conduction aphasia may be considered to be a form of "disconnection syndrome" wherein a lesion interrupting the arcuate fasciculus, connecting the anterior temporal lobe to the inferior frontal region, occurs. The site of lesion in transcortical motor aphasia may be anterior to Broca's area buried deep in the white matter; localization of transcortical sensory aphasia may also be close to Wernicke's area.[49] The following **Flowchart 1** may be helpful in the diagnosis of the classical eight aphasia syndromes.

Calculation

Calculation is tested if there are suggestions from the history of a suspected dementing illness or if the patient is aphasic. The following sequence may be followed:

- *Number reading and writing:*
  - The subject is asked to read and write from a series of simple and complex numbers written by the examiner.
  - Then the subject is asked to write numbers to dictation.
  - If there are errors in the first two steps, copying the numbers and pointing to the numbers on command can also be done.
- *Arithmetic operations:* After the basic reading and writing of numbers, the subject should be tested for basic arithmetic operations—addition, subtraction, multiplication, and division. This is followed by written calculations. At the bedside, often the serial subtraction ("100-7") test usually suffices and this also tests the patient's ability for sustained attention.

Disorders of Calculation

Acalculia is a disturbance in the ability to comprehend or write numbers properly. It is common in patients with aphasia. Lesion localization is usually in the angular gyrus of the left hemisphere.[49] Some aphasic patients can perform calculations mentally and perform well with multiple choice answers.

Anarithmetria is characterized by the inability to perform numerical manipulations. These individuals can recognize and correctly reproduce numbers, but cannot perform simple arithmetic calculations (mental arithmetic).[50] This is common in patients with dementia such as Alzheimer's disease. An occasional patient with an isolated left parietal lesion may have impaired calculating skills without producing any language disorder. This is the true syndrome of anarithmetria or loss of the concept of numbers. On the other hand, some patients with severe aphasia can play cards and look at business ledgers and accounting sheets.[50,51]

Spatial dyscalculia is a disorder of performing written calculations. These patients have difficulty aligning columns of figures and performing carrying tasks. They usually have right hemispherical damage and exhibit the phenomenon of neglect.

Gerstmann's syndrome is characterized by a constellation of clinical features that include:
- Agraphia
- Acalculia
- Right-left disorientation (disorder in demonstrating the correct hand or body part on command)
- *Finger agnosia*: Inability to name the fingers or point to/move a finger when its name is given.

The anatomical localization for this syndrome is in the angular gyrus. It is also known as the *angular gyrus syndrome*. In practice, often the full tetrad of Gerstmann's syndrome may not be obvious.[52,53] While the presence of at least three of the four features may suffice for an eponymous diagnosis, it is not uncommon to find additional features such as anomia, alexia, constructional apraxia, mild fluent dysphasia, and visual field defects. Some authorities would call the association of additional features the "angular gyrus syndrome" making a difference from classical Gerstmann's syndrome. The angular gyrus region, now designated as "heteromodal association cortices" coordinates information transfers among different sensory modalities.[49]

Apraxias

Apraxia is defined as "the inability to perform a skilled motor activity that is not explicable based on problems with basic motor function due to weakness, sensory loss, tremor, chorea or other movement disorders, or to deficits in attention, memory, or motivation".[54] The most common form is "ideomotor apraxia", where patients fail to perform skilled movements such as the use of a knife, toothbrush, or scissors, or learned limb movements not requiring the use of an object, such as waving goodbye or making the "OK", or "victory" sign, though it may be observed that they can perform these actions spontaneously. The other types of apraxia include limb kinetic apraxia, ideational apraxia (which needs differentiation from ideomotor apraxia; in the former patients lack the very concept of using an object), and constructional apraxia, dressing apraxia, and orobuccal apraxia.

Apraxia almost always results from a left hemispheric lesion especially involving the left frontal or parietal lobe.[55,56] Corpus callosum lesions may cause apraxia limited to the left arm only. Loss of communication between the two hemispheres may be a cause.[57] It is possible that lesioning anywhere in the motor system in the dominant hemisphere may cause problems with skillful activities. Apraxia with the use of either limb can occur with lesions in the frontal lobar dorsomedial part, where complex motor movements are coordinated.[58]

DETECTION OF RIGHT (NONDOMINANT) HEMISPHERIC LESIONS

The deficits produced by damage to the right hemisphere are more subtle and hence tougher to detect at the bedside. Close observation of the patient's behavior and movements are needed during elicitation of history and general physical examination. The following features may be noted.

Neglect

It is a term used to describe deficits in spatially designed attention. It can again be of various types:
- Personal neglect
- Motor and sensory neglect
- Extrapersonal neglect

Personal Neglect

Some patients with left hemiplegia (right or nondominant hemispherical lesion) may not realize that they are paralyzed on one side and deny their deficit.

Firstly, they may deny the existence of one side (the paretic side), along with somatic delusions.

Secondly, they accept the existence of the paretic side but refute the presence of hemiparesis. This is defined by the term *anosognosia*.

Thirdly, they accept they are hemiparetic, but underplay its severity and resultant disability *(anosodiaphoria)*.

Personal neglect may be evident in appearance when the patient fails to groom or shave one side.

Sensory Neglect

Persons with sensory neglect consistently ignore sensory inputs from the side contralateral to the side of their brain lesion. Commonly there is left hemineglect as the causative lesion is generally on the nondominant right side. Neglect is particularly evident about the visual field; the subject ignores a person standing on the left side or fails to eat food lying on the left side of the plate. While drawing a clock face, the patient fails to put the numbers on the left side—and puts all numbers on the right **(Fig. 4)**. It is sometimes difficult to distinguish between visual hemineglect and hemianopic visual field loss. The line bisection test may be helpful in some such cases.

Sensory extinction or perceptual rivalry is seen when patients respond to stimuli presented to each side, but fail to respond on the neglected if the stimuli are presented on both sides simultaneously.[59] This, again, becomes more evident while testing visual field by confrontation.

Extrapersonal Neglect

This is tested by asking the patient to bisect lines of varying lengths, cancellation tasks, and drawing and copying figures.

A patient with a right hemispherical stroke is asked to copy a figure of a clock face. He draws the right half of the clock face, but misses out to copy the left half. This is an example of object-centered neglect. However, this could have resulted from a left homonymous hemianopia as well as he would be unable to see the left half of his visual field. How to distinguish between the two—(1) hemianopia or (2) hemineglect? The line bisection test may help to differentiate between hemianopia on one side and a hemineglect on the same side due to a lesion in the contralateral parieto-occipital region.[60] Hemianopic patients tend to put the bisecting mark much beyond the actual central point; whereas patients with visual hemineglect on the same side, would tend to put the bisecting mark much proximal to the actual midpoint. Visual hemineglect is usually more persistent in right hemispherical disorders, but can occur with lesions of either hemisphere. Lesions causing visual hemineglect need not necessarily be only in the visual association areas, but may be located much anteriorly in the nondominant hemisphere **(Fig. 5)**.

Dressing Apraxia

The term "apraxia" is a misnomer about dressing. The disturbance inability to dress is not a motor disorder. It is a deficit in the orientation of body parts about garments due to a disorder of the visuospatial mechanism. The site of the lesion is usually in the right posterior parietal area. Dressing apraxia may be evident when a subject is asked to wear a shirt or blouse after turning it inside out.

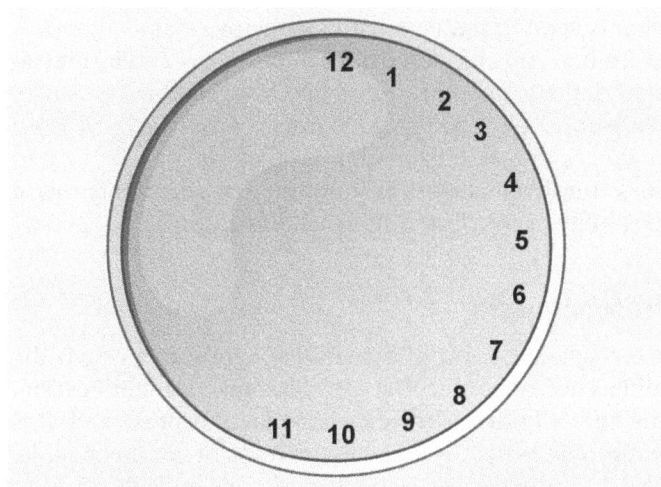

FIG. 4: Clock-face drawing in a patient with left visual hemineglect. All numbers are put on the right side leaving the left side blank.

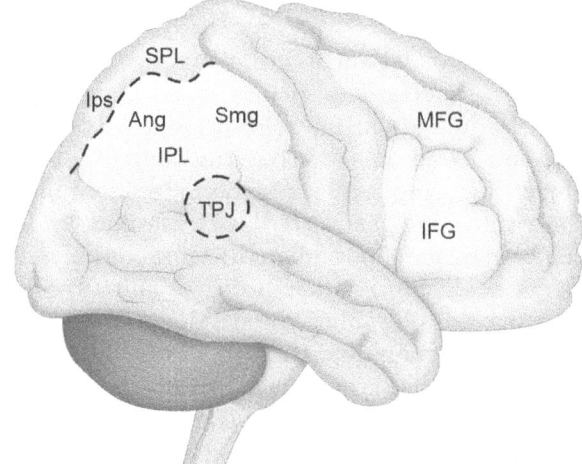

FIG. 5: Cortical areas in the nondominant hemisphere where lesions may produce visual hemineglect on the contralateral side.

(MFG: middle frontal gyrus; IFG: inferior frontal gyrus; SPL: superior parietal lobule; IPL: inferior parietal lobule; Ang: angular gyrus; Smg: supramarginal gyrus; TP3: temporoparietal association area)

Testing Visuospatial and Constructional Ability

Disorders of constructional ability can be tested by asking the subject to draw 3D drawings or a complex 2D shape like the intersecting pentagons. For a more objective assessment, Rey–Osterrieth Complex Figure Test is recommended.[61,62]

The clock setting/drawing test is not only a useful test of constructional ability but it also tests the conceptualization of time and its abstract relation to the placement of hands. Patients with early dementia can usually draw the clock correctly, but have problems with placement of hands when asked to set a time. Some authorities have suggested that the patient should be asked to set a time when one arm of the clock should be placed on the right side and the other on the left (e.g., 10 minutes past 10 o'clock). This is useful in detecting unilateral neglect as discussed earlier.[63]

AGNOSIAS

Agnosias are disorders of recognition that cannot be attributed to general intellectual impairment, aphasia, or basic sensory dysfunction. Agnosias can be visual, tactile, or sensory.

A person with visual agnosia sees an object but is unable to recognize them. This can be again for different categories of stimuli such as colors, objects, and faces.

The object recognition disorder can be categorized into two main types depending on the stage at which visual perception breaks down.

Apperceptive Visual Agnosia

In this type of visual agnosia, patients have preserved elementary visual faculties such as acuity, simple shape, contour discrimination, and color perception, but fail to identify and name objects. They can sometimes name the objects by using tactile palpation. Common objects such as watches and pen can be used for testing. This may happen with bilateral posterior cortical lesions involving the visual association cortex (areas 18 and 19) and in carbon monoxide poisoning. When a person fails to name or identify a common object, differentiation needs to be made between anomia, and visual agnosia. In the former case, the person would be able to choose the right name when given options and would explain the use of the object through gestures/pantomime. None of these would be possible for a person having apperceptive visual agnosia.

Associative Visual Agnosia

In this type of agnosia, a patient can demonstrate the use of an object, but is unable to recognize and name the object. It is believed to be caused by the disconnection of the visual area from the language area and the visual memory stores. The site of the lesion is usually in the bilateral inferior temporo-occipital junction or a lesion in the left occipital lobe and adjacent posterior corpus callosum. The same lesion can also cause alexia without agraphia.

Visual agnosias can be tested by:
- Visual object identification by inspecting shape, color, etc., but not feeling with hands.
- Copying line drawings of common articles such as a house and bicycle.

Visual matching tasks the ability to match pictures to objects. Some additional tests such as object knowledge (that is the ability to generate accurate verbal descriptions when given the name of objects) and *tactile naming*—the ability to name objects by touch, may help in detailed lesion localization. In cross-modal associative agnosia, there is generalized semantic memory impairment. These patients are unable to identify objects by any modality (visual, verbal, and touch). They can identify the picture of an animal, but are unable to name the animal or describe its size or habitat. The site of the lesion is in the left anterior temporal lobe. This may be present in advanced Alzheimer's disease or patients with semantic dementia.[64]

Optic Aphasia

Optic aphasic subjects have a modality-specific (visual) recognition deficit but can recognize objects through both auditory and tactile modalities. This is similar to what is seen in patients with associative visual agnosias. As both groups of patients tend to display similarities in their deficits, one may argue for classification as a single syndrome, with varying degrees of severity. In both instances, lesion localization is suggestive of damage to the ventral visual stream.[65] Both types of patients retain the ability to copy presented line drawings.

Prosopagnosia

It is a specific form of associative agnosia in which the subject has a disorder of face recognition and identification. The ability to describe and match faces is preserved. It is commonly tested by showing pictures of famous people, friends, and relatives. The site of the lesion is in the right posterior temporal lobe (fusiform gyrus) usually due to a stroke.

In semantic dementia, there is progressive atrophy of the right temporal lobe. These patients not only lose the ability to recognize people, but are also unable to provide knowledge about the faces.[66]

LIMITATIONS OF BEDSIDE COGNITIVE TESTING

Bedside cognitive testing has got multiple limitations. Some of these, but not all, can be overcome by elaborate neuropsychological testing batteries.

First of all, most of these tools and test batteries have evolved in Western countries. Consequently, in non-English speaking populations like ours, these scales may lack reliability. Efforts are being made to develop reliable diagnostic tools and instruments that are culturally and linguistically valid for making an accurate diagnosis in the Indian population. The NIMHANS neuropsychological battery[67] for the elderly and the Kolkata Cognitive Battery[68] are examples of this. But in a country like India, where there is so much linguistic and cultural diversity, the same scale may not have uniform utility everywhere. Another important limitation is the lack of normative data for different communities.

Secondly, it is tough to follow the hierarchy of assessment in bedside testing or a busy clinic. The clinician tries to use one or two tests to come to a quick diagnosis. The clock drawing test described above is one such example. It is a test for visuospatial (agnosia) and visual constructional (apraxia) abilities. Visual or hearing defects or lack of basic education can all impair the test results.

Thirdly, high-functioning individuals may perform well in the standard cognitive tests, even if they may be having major cognitive defects.

Last, of all, abnormality of a single test does not signify impairment of a particular cognitive domain. For example, the serial subtraction seven test may be an attention test. But, it can be impaired in patients with impaired calculative skills.

It should be remembered at the bedside that the way a subject performs a test may be more important than the absolute scores.

INDIVIDUALIZED TESTING VERSUS STANDARDIZED MENTAL TESTS

In this chapter, we have described a bedside testing scheme for cognition excepting those used for language and praxis assessment (discussed elsewhere in the volume). But time constraints often may prevent the examiner from utilizing all these tests. Standardized mental tests have evolved. Some of these are elaborate like the Dementia Rating Scale. Shorter scales like the MMSE, Montreal Cognitive Assessment (MoCA),[69] and Addenbrooke's Cognitive Examination have been developed for use in the clinic or bedside.

The MMSE, devised by Folstein and colleagues in 1975,[70] had been the most popular bedside testing scale till a few years back. It was easy and standardized for testing the important domains of attention, language, memory, and visuospatial abilities. A person is scored out of 30. A score below 24 was considered abnormal. But it was not sensitive for detecting MCI, frontal lobe dysfunction, and focal cognitive deficits. Recently, it has been copyrighted (making it expensive) and this has contributed to its loss of popularity and usage. This is very disheartening.

The decline in usage of MMSE has led to the rise in popularity of the MoCA. This is 30-point test that can be administered in 10 minutes. The test is free and can be accessed by clinicians at http://www.mocatest.org. It has shown promise in detecting MCI and early Alzheimer's disease.[69]

The ACE has been modified to ACE3 (Indian English version).[12] It is more elaborate and time-consuming, but can help in separating frontotemporal dementia from Alzheimer's disease. The test toolkit can be accessed free at https://doi.org/10.1093/occmed/kqv041.

CONCLUDING REMARKS

Cognitive neurology is a fascinating subject. It had been made more interesting and intriguing with the introduction of advanced functional neuroimaging modalities which have made clinicoanatomical localizations more challenging. Accuracy of bedside lesion localization, in essence, depends on a very thorough knowledge of the clinical anatomy of the cerebral cortex. Testing without any attempt at lesion localization, would have no value. Furthermore, as already stated, at the bedside, the way a subject performs a test may be more important than the absolute scores.

LEARNING POINTS

- Testing higher mental functions at the bedside is an exhaustive process. However, an astute clinician can, with appropriate questions, test various facets of cognition such as memory, orientation, behavior, emotion, speech, calculation, and praxis, during the process of elicitation of the clinical history from conscious co-operative patients and/or their relatives.
- Trainees should strive hard to master the art of good history taking.

- In neurological practice, diagnoses are generally made at the end of history taking; clinical examination and investigations only help in fine tuning the historical diagnosis.

ACKNOWLEDGMENT

Authors would like to thank the Editors of IAN Textbook of Neurology, Second Edition 2023 and the Publisher Jaypee Brothers for their kind permission to reproduce this Chapter with modifications.

REFERENCES

1. Schnidner A. Neuropsychologic testing: Bedside approaches. In: Goldenberg G, Miller BL (eds). Neuropsychology and Behavioral Neurology: Volume 3 (Handbook of Clinical Neurology). Philadelphia: Elsevier; 2008. pp. 137-54.
2. Strub RL, Black FW. The Mental State Examination in Neurology, 4th edition. New Delhi: Jaypee Brothers Medical Publishers (P) Ltd.; 2003.
3. Hodges RJ. Cognitive assessment for Clinicians, 3rd edition. Oxford, United Kingdom: Oxford University Press; 2018.
4. Sanford AM. Mild Cognitive Impairment. Clin Geriatr Med. 2017;33(3):325-37.
5. Petersen RC. Mild Cognitive Impairment. Continuum (Minneap Minn). 2016;22(2 Dementia):404-18.
6. Harmon KG, Drezner JA, Gammons M, Guskiewicz KM, Halstead M, Herring SA, et al. American Medical Society for Sports Medicine position statement: concussion in sport. Br J Sports Med. 2013;47(1):15-26.
7. Snyderman D, Rovner B. Mental status exam in primary care: A review. Am Fam Physician. 2009;80(8):809-14.
8. American Psychiatric Association. Diagnostic and Statistical Manual of Mental Disorders, 5th ed. Washington, DC: American Psychiatric Association; 2014 (updated 2018).
9. Papez JW. A proposed mechanism of emotion. Arch Neurol Psychiatry 1937;387:25-38.
10. Lhermitte F. Human autonomy and the frontal lobes. Part II: Patient behavior in complex and social situations: the 'environmental dependency syndrome'. Ann Neurol. 1986;19:335-43
11. Smith A: The series sevens subtraction test. Arch Neurol. 1976; 17:18.
12. Noone P. Addenbrook's Cognitive Examination-III. Occup Med. 2015;65(5):418-420.
13. Ettlin TM, Kischka U, Beckson M, Gaggiotti M, Rauchfleisch U, Benson DF. A frontal lobe score. I: Construction of a mental status of frontal systems. Clin Rehabil. 2000;14:260-71.
14. Zola-Morgan S, Squire LR, Amaral DG. Human amnesia and the medial temporal region: Enduring memory impairment following a bilateral lesion limited to the CA1 field of the hippocampus. J Neurosci. 1986;6:2950-67.
15. Rolls E. A theory of hippocampal function in memory. Hippocampus 1996;6:601.
16. Wechsler D. Wechsler memory scale. USA: Psychological Corporation.1945.
17. Schoenberg MR, Dawson KA, Duff K, Patton D, Scott JG, Adams RL. Test performance and classification statistics for the Rey Auditory Verbal Learning Test in selected clinical samples. Arch Clin Neuropsychol. 2006;21(7):693-703.
18. Abrahams S, Pickering A, Polkey CE, Morris RG. Spatial memory deficits in patients with unilateral damage to the right hippocampal formation. Neuropsychologia. 1997;35:11-24.
19. Eling P. History of Neuropsychological Assessment. Front Neurol Neurosci. 2019;44:164-78.
20. Lenehan ME, Summers MJ, Saunders NL, Summers JJ, Vickers JC. Does the Cambridge Automated Neuropsychological Test Battery (CANTAB) Distinguish Between Cognitive Domains in Healthy Older Adults? Assessment. 2016;23(2):163-72.
21. Wixted JT. On Common Ground: Jost's (1897) law of forgetting and Ribot's (1881) law of retrograde amnesia. Psychol Rev. 2004;111(4):864-79.
22. Pearce JM. A note on aphasia in bilingual patients: Pitres' and Ribot's laws. Eur Neurol. 2005;54(3):127-31.
23. Piolino P. Autobiographical memory in aging. Psychol Neuropsychiatr Vieil. 2003;1(1):25-35.
24. Hodges JR, Salmon DP, Butters N. Semantic memory impairment in Alzheimer's disease: Failure of access or degraded knowledge? Neuropsychologia. 1992;30:301-4.
25. Hodges JR, Graham KS. A reversal of the temporal gradient for famous person knowledge in semantic dementia: implications for the neural organisation of long-term memory. Neuropsychologia. 1998;36(8):803-25.
26. Viskontas IV, McAndrews MP, Moscovitch M. Remote episodic memory deficits in patients with unilateral temporal lobe epilepsy and excisions. J Neurosci. 2000;20(15):5853-7.
27. Estmacott RW, Moscovitch M. Temporally graded semantic memory loss in amnesia and semantic dementia: Further evidence for opposite gradients. Cogn Neuropsychol. 2002;19(2):135-63.
28. Simons JS, Verfaellie M, Galton CJ, Miller BL, Hodges JR, Graham KS. Recollection-based memory in frontotemporal dementia: implications for theories of long-term memory. Brain. 2002;125 (Pt 11):2523-36.
29. Baddeley A, Della Sala S. Working memory and executive control. Philos Trans R Soc Lond B Biol Sci. 1996;351(1346):1397-403.
30. Moscovitch M. Multiple dissociations of function in amnesia. In: Cermak LS (Ed). Human Memory and Amnesia. United States: Erlbaum, Hillsdale, NJ; 1982. pp. 337-70.
31. Milner B, Petrides M, Smith ML. Frontal lobes and the temporal organization of memory. Hum Neurobiol. 1985;4(3):137-42.
32. Luria AR. Human Brain and Psychological Processes. New York: Harper Row; 1966.
33. Fuster J. The Prefrontal Cortex. New York: Raven Press; 1997.
34. Andrés P. Frontal cortex as the central executive of working memory: Time to revise our view. Cortex. 2003;39(4-5):871-95.
35. Strauss E, Sherman EMS, Spreen O, Spreen O. A Compendium of Neuropsychological Tests: Administration, Norms, and Commentary, 3rd edition. New York, NY: Oxford University Press; 2006.
36. Thurstone LL, Thurstone TG. Primary Mental Abilities (rev). Chicago: Science Research Associates; 1962.
37. Regard M, Strauss E, Knapp P. Children's production on verbal and nonverbal fluency tasks. Percept Mot Skills.1982;55(3):839-44.

38. Miles S, Howlett CA, Berryman C, Nedeljkovic M, Moseley GL, Phillipou A. Considerations for using the Wisconsin Card Sorting Test to assess cognitive flexibility. Behav Res Methods. 2021;53(5):2083-91.
39. Wessels AM, Edgar CJ, Nathan PJ, Siemers ER, Maruff P, Harrison J. Cognitive Go/No-Go decision-making criteria in Alzheimer's disease drug development. Drug Discov Today. 2021;26(5):1330-6.
40. Llinàs-Reglà J, Vilalta-Franch J, López-Pousa S, Calvó-Perxas L, Torrents Rodas D, Garre-Olmo J. The Trail Making Test. Assessment. 2017;24(2):183-96.
41. Weiner MF, Hynan LS, Rossetti H, Falkowski. Luria's three-step test: what is it and what does it tell us?. J Int Psychogeriatr. 2011;23(10):1602-6.
42. Luria AR. Higher Cortical Functions in Man, 2nd edition. New York: Basic Books; 1980.
43. Damasio AR, Graff-Radford NR, Damasio H. Transient partial amnesia. Arch Neurol. 1983;40:656-7.
44. Blumer D, Benson DF. Personality changes with frontal and temporal lobe lesions. In: Benson DF, Blumer D (eds). Psychiatric Aspects of Neurologic Disease. New York: Grune & Stratton; 1975. pp. 151-69.
45. Robinson RG, Kubos KL, Starr LB, Rao K, Price TR. Mood disorders in stroke patients: Importance of lesion location. Brain. 1984;107:81-93.
46. Ross ED. The Aprosodias. In: TE Feinberg, MJ Farah (eds). Behavioral Neurology and Neuropsychology. New York: McGraw-Hill; 1997.
47. Broca P. Remarques sur le siége de la faculté du langage articulé, suivies d'une observation daphémie. Bull Assoc Anat (Nancy). 1861;2:330-57.
48. Wernicke K. Der Aphasische Symtomencomplex. Breslau: Cohn & Weigert; 1874.
49. Kirshner HS. Speech and Language Disorders. Behavioral Neurology, Second edition. Butterworth: Heinemann; 2002.
50. Mayer E, Reicherts M, Deloche G, Willadino-Braga L, Taussik I, Dordain M, et al. Number processing after stroke: Anatomoclinical correlations in oral and written codes. J Int Neuropsychol Soc. 2003;9:899-912.
51. Pavlović D. Acalculia. Srp Arh Celok Lek. 1997;125(11-12):353-5.
52. Ardila A. Gerstmann Syndrome. Curr Neurol Neurosci Rep. 2020;20(11):48.
53. Rusconi E. Gerstmann syndrome: Historic and current perspectives. Handb Clin Neurol. 2018;151:395-411.
54. Rosen HJ, Viskontas IV. Cortical Neuroanatomy and Cognition. Neuropsychology and behavioral neurology: Volume 88 (3rd series) (Handbook of Clinical Neurology). In: Goldenberg G, Miller BL. Philadelphia: Elsevier: 2008; pp. 41-60.
55. Heilman KR, Valenstein E. Two forms of ideomotor apraxia. Neurology. 1982;32:342-6.
56. Rothi L, Heilman KM, Watson RT. Pantomime comprehension and ideomotor apraxia. J Neurol Neurosurg Psychiatry. 1985;48:207-10.
57. Watson RT, Heilman KM. Callosal apraxia. Brain. 1983;106: 391-403.
58. Watson RT, Fleet WS, Rothi LJG, Heilman KM. Apraxia and the supplementary motor area. Arch Neurol. 1986;43:787-92.
59. Heilman KM, Watson RT, Valenstein E. Neglect and related disorders. In KM Heilman, E Valenstein (Eds). Clinical Neuropsychology, 4th edition. New York: Oxford University Press; pp. 296-346.
60. Barton JJS, Black SE. Line bisection in hemianopia. J Neurol, Neurosurg Psychiatry. 1998;64:660-2.
61. Spreen O, Strauss E. A Compendium of Neuropsychological Tests. Administration, Norms, and Commentary, 2nd edition. New York: Oxford University Press; 1998.
62. Zhang X, Lv L, Min G, Wang Q, Zhao Y, Li Y. Overview of the Complex Figure Test and Its Clinical Application in Neuropsychiatric Disorders, Including Copying and Recall. Front. Neurol. 2021;12:680474.
63. Freedman M, Leach L, Kaplan E, Winocur G, Shulman K I, Delis C. Clock drawing: A neuropsychological analysis. Oxford: Oxford University Press;1994.
64. Grusser OJ, Landis T. Visual Agnosias and Other Disturbances of Visual Perception and Cognition. London: MacMillan; 1991.
65. Schnider A, Benson DF, Scharre. DW. Visual agnosia and optic aphasia: are they anatomically distinct? Cortex. 1994;30(3): 445-57.
66. 64. Meadows J. The anatomical basis of prospognosia. J Neurol Neurosurg Psychiatry. 1974;37:48.
67. Tripathi R, Kumar JK, Bharath S, Marimuthu P, Varghese M. Clinical validity of NIMHANS neuropsychological battery for elderly: A preliminary report. Indian J Psychiatry. 2013;55(3):279-82.
68. Das SK, Bose P, Biswas A, Dutt A, Banerjee TK, Hazra AM, et al. An epidemiologic study of mild cognitive impairment in Kolkata, India. Neurology. 2007;68(23):2019-26.
69. Nasreddine ZS, Phillips NA, Bédirian V, Charbonneau S, Whitehead V, Collin I, et al. The Montreal Cognitive Assessment, MoCA: A brief screening tool for mild cognitive impairment. J Am Geriatr Soc. 2005;53(4):695-9.
70. Folstein MF, Folstein SE, McHugh PR. "Mini-mental state". A practical method for grading the cognitive state of patients for the clinician. J Psychiatr Res. 1975;12(3):189-98.

A Relook at Acute Onset Amnesia Syndromes

Ambar Chakravarty

INTRODUCTION

Acute-onset amnesia is an emergency neurological presentation that can lead to considerable concern to both patient and clinician. The patient classically presents with being not only to retain new memories but also access those previously acquired, suggesting disturbance of hippocampal function.[1] Transient global amnesia (TGA) is the most common cause of acute-onset amnesia and is characterized by a profound anterograde and retrograde amnesia that classically resolves within 24 hours.

This commentary will not consider acute amnesia associated with impairment of conscious level (e.g., encephalopathy), broader cognitive and behavioral dysfunction (e.g., delirium), or additional neurological features such as seizures (e.g., autoimmune or paraneoplastic encephalitis). As TGA has been discussed in some details elsewhere in this volume, only the salient features would be mentioned including its diagnostic criteria and its differentiation from functional/psychogenic amnesia. Instead important differential diagnoses discussed within this commentary would include posterior circulation strokes, transient epileptic amnesia (TEA), psychogenic amnesia, post-traumatic amnesia (PTA), and toxic/drug-related amnesia. The neurologist would generally see the patient after the amnesic episode has resolved. Therefore, as with most patients in acute neurology, and especially when cognitive function is altered, a witness account of the episode is key to making an accurate diagnosis.

TYPES OF MEMORY

There are different forms of memory. Declarative memories are, basically, those memories than can be communicated to others. This type of memory contrasts with various forms of "nondeclarative memory", including motor skills, priming, and conditioned "Pavlovian" responses. Declarative memory can be subdivided into two major forms, or systems: (1) episodic memory and (2) semantic memory. Episodic memories—which in day-to-day life are often autobiographical in nature—are typically complex memories of temporally unfolding events, allowing us to re-experience specific "episodes" of our lived past (like remembering a birthday day).[2] Whilst the neuroanatomical basis of episodic memory is controversial[3-6] and to a degree diffuse,[7-10] from a clinical perspective episodic memory loss should prompt the clinician to suspect pathology in or around the hippocampus. The hippocampus sits above a hierarchy of multimodal processing streams[10] and is thought to create associations between distinct elements of a memory (e.g., people and objects) within a specific spatial context.[2] Episodic autobiographical memories also contain first person emotional and thought content pertaining to these specific events. In contrast to episodic memories, semantic memories do not have re-experiential content and do not rely upon the binding together of multiple features into a single episode. They are instead fact-like and reflect our knowledge of the world. Two forms of semantic memory exist, distinguished by their relation to the self—(1) public semantic memory (e.g., knowing that New Delhi is the capital of India) and (2) personal semantic memory (such as knowing the names of the schools we attended in our childhood days).

These types of declarative memory are highly-interdependent[11] and can be hard to fractionate without specific neuropsychological tools. The principal neuropsychological deficits in TGA are centered around episodic memory, whilst semantic memory remains largely intact.

THE TEMPORAL PERIOD OF AMNESIA

It is very important to identify the period of time for which the patient is amnesic. If the memory loss predominantly reflects information acquired in the period *before* the onset of amnesia, this is termed *retrograde* amnesia. If the memory loss is primarily for events in the period *after* the onset of amnesia, this is called *anterograde* amnesia. Acute amnesia may affect both time periods, but one will usually predominate.

In TGA, there is usually a dense anterograde amnesia and a variable degree of retrograde amnesia (which can vary from a few hours up to several years before to the onset of the amnesic episode).[12] The retrograde amnesia tends to spare very remote (>10 years) memories intact—or at least rough impressions of them[13]—and as the amnesia resolves memories tend to return sequentially, with the oldest lost memory coming back first.[1]

ANATOMICAL LOCALIZATION

The hippocampus and medial temporal lobes are critical for declarative memories. The hippocampus and its subfields **(Fig. 1)** are considered to provide the neuroanatomical basis for this associative process to occur.[14] Episodic recall depends on a well-defined neural circuit beginning in the entorhinal cortex (ERC), continuing, via the "trisynaptic circuit" through the hippocampal subfields [dentate gyrus, DG (which is often collocated with cornu ammonis (CA)], CA3, CA2, and CA1 (direct ERC-CA1 projections also exist), then via the subiculum (and its components) back into the ERC.[15] Experimental damage to DG[16] and CA3[16,17] has been shown to impair episodic memories and autobiographical memories respectively. In TGA, lesions to CA1—a critical area of output from the hippocampus—have been shown to cause episodic amnesia.[16]

Widely distributed areas in the brain are involved with personal and public semantic memory but specific representation of abstract information concerning event knowledge seems to rely particularly on anterior and lateral temporal and inferior parietal cortex.[17] Disruption to personal and public semantic memories should alert the clinician to consider dysfunction in these regions.[1,17]

Transient Global Amnesia

Transient global amnesia is the most widely recognized acute amnesic syndrome[18,19] and was first described in the 1950s. The diagnostic criteria are shown in **Box 1**.[18]

Neuroimaging has an important role in diagnosis of TGA. Diffusion-weighted imaging (DWI) is most useful during the postamnesic phase, as TGA can be associated with punctate DWI changes within the hippocampus after the amnesic period has resolved. These lesions generally appear 12–48 hours[20,21] following symptom resolution and can then persist for up to 6 days.[12]

BOX 1: Diagnostic criteria for TGA.[19]

- Attacks must be witnessed
- There must be anterograde amnesia during the attack (usually evidence with repetitive questioning)
- Cognitive impairment must be limited to amnesia
- No clouding of consciousness or loss of personal identity
- No focal neurological signs or symptoms
- No epileptic features
- Attacks must resolve within 24-hour
- No recent head injury or active epilepsy

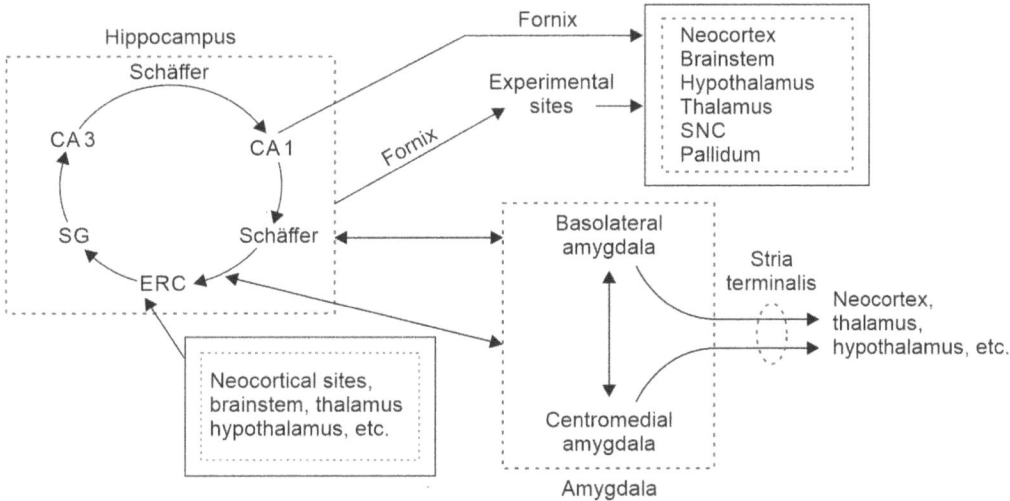

FIG. 1: Limbic circuitry.

The lesion detection time is maximal 2 days after symptom onset.[20] DWI lesions are well seen in the CA1 region of the hippocampus,[12,20,21] which is the principal area of information outflow from the hippocampus.[12] From a practical perspective, the appearance of lesions only after cognitive normalization is to be expected. A normal magnetic resonance imaging (MRI) at the time of acute presentation of amnesia should not go against diagnosing TGA, nor should the presence of isolated intrahippocampal DWI lesions after the resolution of symptoms would go against making the diagnosis of TGA. Moreover, in a proportion of cases, the MRI never becomes abnormal.[1]

Differentiating TGA from Hippocampal Ischemia

How might the neurologist practically distinguish between hippocampal/posterior cerebral artery ischemia and TGA? The initial step is to define the clinical syndrome. Ischemia within the hippocampal artery territory (a rare presentation of stroke) appears to be associated with five different presentations—(1) anterior hippocampal infarcts, with changes in sensorium, visual hallucinations, and anterograde memory deficits; (2) posterior hippocampal infarcts with vertigo/dizziness, a confused state, anterograde memory deficits; (3) unilateral complete hippocampal infarcts with confusional state, visual hallucinations, mood alterations including depression, and impulsivity; (4) bilateral hippocampal infarcts (typically due to embolic stroke) with a dense anterograde amnesia; and, (5) punctiform lesions in unilateral or bilateral hippocampi associated with anterograde amnesia and dysphasia.[21]

Despite these, it is not possible with 100% certainty to rule out using solely bedside evaluation the unlikely but important possibility of stroke in patients presenting with acute amnesia. The present author's recommendation is therefore that, where possible, all patients should have an MRI scan on presentation.

Neuroradiologically, DWI lesions associated with strokes tend to show larger restricting lesions compared to TGA. Punctate ischemic lesions also tend to be associated with dysphasia and vertigo, rather than pure amnesia.[21] As mentioned above, the timing of DWI lesions is also important—lesions visible during the amnesic period would suggest to the clinician to consider hippocampal ischemia. The absence of DWI lesions during amnesia is generally noted in cases of TGA, since these lesions typically appear once the amnesia has passed off.

Amnesic Seizure

Transient epileptic amnesia is a mesial temporal epileptic syndrome and the diagnostic criteria[22] are—(1) A history of recurrent witnessed episodes of transient amnesia; (2) cognitive functions other than memory judged to be intact during typical episodes by a reliable witness; (3) evidence for a diagnosis of epilepsy based on one or more of the following—(i) epileptiform abnormalities on electroencephalography; (ii) The concurrent onset of other clinical features of epilepsy (e.g., lip-smacking and olfactory hallucinations); and (iii) a clear-cut response to anticonvulsant therapy.

The TEA is a distinct form of late-onset epilepsy of limbic origin. Patients have recurrent episodes of transient amnesia, generally lasting for around 30 minutes, mostly when awake, occurring mostly at intervals of around 1 month. Other reported symptoms happening concurrently include olfactory hallucinations, repetitive questioning, or motor automatisms.[23] Patients can carry on a conversation and act appropriately[24] during the amnesic attacks, suggesting the preservation of other cognitive functions (other like the attention, perception, language, and executive functions). The condition of TEA syndrome is most often of idiopathic etiology and has a benign prognosis.

The exact time relationship between onset of seizure and termination and the associated amnesia is, often uncertain in the majority of cases of TEA.[24] Epileptiform abnormalities on the EEG are rarely seen on a standard waking EEG but often on a nocturnal prolonged sleep EEG.[24] It may be suggested that rapidly developing short-term memory loss and impaired autobiographical memory are the result of inadequately controlled epileptic activity. The acute amnestic attacks of TEA can be controlled with low dose of a single anticonvulsant, although the interictal memory deficits often tend to persist despite treatment. There is no evidence of progression of these deficits over time or of an increased risk of dementia. A summary of the differences between TGA and TEA are shown in **Table 1**.

Psychogenic Amnesia

Psychogenic amnesia which is rare, can be subdivided into four different types[25]—(1) a fugue state, with an abrupt loss of autobiographical memory (resolving within 4 weeks) with a loss of personal identity and/or wandering; (2) fugue-to-focal retrograde amnesia, which is a prolonged period of retrograde amnesia after an initial fugue state; (3) focal retrograde amnesia, a loss of retrograde autobiographical memory but no wandering and usually staying for more than 4 weeks often associated with loss of personal identity; and, (4) patchy memory, where patients have discrete memory loss that may be associated with psychosocial stress, but without any loss of personal identity.[26] There is an association with severe psychological or physiological stress in most cases, though such triggers

TABLE 1: Distinguishing between transient global amnesia and transient epileptic amnesia.

	Transient global amnesia	Transient epileptic amnesia
Typical number of attacks	Usually one, rarely two, in an entire lifetime	Approximately 14–15 attacks per year
Typical duration of attacks	4–6 hours (range: 30 min–24 hours)	Usually less than an hour
Typical time of day of attacks	Any time of day	On waking
Triggers	Emotional or physical stress	
Associated features	Generally no memory for ictal period returns. Possible migrainous symptoms on direct questioning	• Other features of temporal lobe epilepsy: Olfactory/gustatory hallucinations, orofacial automatisms, behavioral arrest, and hand stereotypies • Some memory of event may return • May have retrograde episodic amnesia for memories outside of the acute attacks

TABLE 2: Differentiation of organic amnesic syndromes from functional/psychogenic amnesia.

	Organic amnesic syndrome	Functional/Psychogenic amnesia
Stressful precipitant	Usually absent	Typically present
Typical precipitants	Cerebrovascular disease; viral encephalitis; neurosurgical lesions; hypoxia; and early AD	Mild head trauma; legal witness
Autobiographical memory	Mildly impaired	Severely impaired
Personal identity	Preserved	Often lost
New learning ability	Severely impaired	Typically normal
Everyday functioning	Impaired	Typically normal
Premorbid psychopathology	Not significant	More frequent (major depression)
Premorbid personality	Unremarkable	High prevalence
Legal involvement	Rare	Frequent

are not always elicitable.[27] A minor head injury (without loss of consciousness) may be a precipitating cause of psychogenic amnesia, especially in patients with a history of psychiatric illness. Psychogenic amnesia varies from patient to patient and so makes it difficult to describe a single, well definable neuropsychological profile. Often, retrograde amnesia is predominant. Extensive remote memory loss can be seen in such conditions, as LGI1-limbic encephalitis and Korsakoff's syndrome, but patients with psychogenic amnesia usually demonstrate a preserved ability to acquire new memories. This is very different from the dense anterograde amnesia encountered in TGA.

Psychogenic amnesia is highly likely if the patient is unable to remember personal semantic information, such as their own name, address, and date of birth. Patients may also be unable to recognize family members or photographs of themselves.[28] Such forms of memory are generally intact in all but the most severe organic brain syndromes. Knowledge for public semantic information is often comparatively intact, except when patients may show loss of such information if it pertains to a traumatic personal event.[28]

Table 2 highlights the differentiation of organic amnesic syndromes from psychogenic ones.

The diagnosis and management of psychogenic amnesia are complex and should involve a multidisciplinary team.

Neuropsychometry is essential to assess measures of "effort" (or exertion) to exclude malingering, alongside measure of autobiographical episodic memory, and personal and public semantic memory.[28] Psychogenic amnesia is very different from malingering and the two should not be confused. Psychogenic amnesia is often associated with high scores on depression scales.[28] Overall prognosis for psychogenic amnesia is favorable specially in fugue patients who exhibit improvements in in both personal semantic memory and autobiographical memory.[28]

Patients with focal retrograde amnesia also show improvements but not as marked as patients with fugue. Whilst the pathophysiology of psychogenic amnesia is unclear, it is possible that it arises from psychologically mediated changes in the functional connectivity between the prefrontal and temporal cortices.[28]

Post-traumatic Amnesia

A period of PTA commonly follows many a traumatic brain injuries. amnesia. PTA includes anterograde amnesia, retrograde amnesia (for episodic but also sometimes for semantic information), and impairment in additional cognitive domains, like difficulty in sustained attention or concentration.[29] The history of head injury is commonly used to distinguish PTA from TGA (although mild head injury can trigger a "classical" TGA presentation).[30] Other suggestive features in clinical history often include headaches, anxiety, irritability, emotional lability, vertigo, phono-/photophobia, and fatigue.[31] The duration of PTA correlates with the severity of the brain injury. PTA is associated with disrupted functional connectivity within the default mode network,[32,33] a collection of cortical regions central to autobiographical memory that includes the hippocampus.[34-36] Specifically, there appears to be diminished functional connectivity between the parahippocampal gyrus and the posterior cingulate cortex, associated with diminished white matter integrity within the parahippocampal gyrus. These functional connectivity changes settle down as the PTA improves.

Toxic/Drug-related Amnesia

A final important differential diagnosis to consider for acute amnesia is toxic/alcohol or drug-related encephalopathy. One of the hallmarks of TGA is the dense anterograde episodic amnesia alongside the preservation of other cognitive processes. The patient presenting with acute amnesia due to alcohol or other toxic encephalopathies will often present with other features of encephalopathy such as a fluctuating conscious level. Patients under the influence of various psychoactive substances may also present with other neuropsychiatric features such as distractibility, pressure of speech, delusional or paranoid ideas, or dysphasia. There may also be clinical signs of drug ingestion such as hyper- or hypotension, tachy- or bradycardia, and pupillary changes. It is worth exploring a previous history of alcohol excess alongside a psychiatric history. A drug history might reveal possible sources of overdose (such as antidepressants, neuroleptics, anxiolytics, or hypnotics). Finally, there may also be biochemical evidence of drug ingestion such as a positive toxicology screen, acid-base imbalance on arterial blood gas, or changes in sodium balance.

Acute-onset amnesia is a striking neurological presentation that often causes concern to both patients and clinicians. Whilst memory is a complex area of cognitive neuroscience and the pathophysiology underlying acute memory impairment is poorly understood, the main clinical syndromes that cause acute memory loss are comparatively straightforward. Care should be taken to obtain a careful history and examination alongside a few, occasionally well-timed, investigations to define the clinical syndrome.

REFERENCES

1. Bartsch T, Butler C. Transient amnesic syndromes. Nature Rev Neurol. 2013;9:86-97.
2. Tulving E. Episodic memory: From mind to brain. Ann Rev Psychol. 2002;53:1-25.
3. Squire LR, Alvarez P. Retrograde amnesia and memory consolidation: A neurobiological perspective. Curr Opin Neurobiol. 1995;5(2):169-77.
4. Squire LR, Bayley PJ. The neuroscience of remote memory. Curr Opin Neurobiol. 2007;17:185-96.
5. Moscovitch M, Nadel L. Multiple-trace theory and semantic dementia: Response to K.S. Graham (1999). Trends Cogn Sci.1999;3:87-9.
6. Moscovitch M, Nadel L, Winocur G, Gilboa A, Rosenbaum RS. The cognitive neuroscience of remote episodic, semantic and spatial memory. Curr Opin Neurobiol. 2006;16:179-90.
7. Bonnici HM, Chadwick MJ, Lutti A, Hassabis D, Weiskopf N, Maguire EA. Detecting representations of recent and remote autobiographical memories in vmPFC and hippocampus. J Neurosci. 2012;32:16982-91.
8. Bonnici HM, Chadwick MJ, Maguire EA. Representations of recent and remote autobiographical memories in hippocampal subfields. Hippocampus. 2013;23:849-54.
9. Maguire EA. The retrosplenial contribution to human navigation: a review of lesion and neuroimaging findings. Scand J Psychol. 2001;42:225-38.
10. Turk-Browne NB. The hippocampus as a visual area organized by space and time: A spatiotemporal similarity hypothesis. Vision Res. 2019;165:123-30.
11. Greenberg DL, Verfaellie M. Interdependence of episodic and semantic memory: Evidence from neuropsychology. J Int Neuropsychol Soc. 2010;16:748-53.
12. Bartsch T, Dohring J, Rohr A, Jansen O, Deuschl G. CA1 neurons in the human hippocampus are critical for autobiographical memory, mental time travel, and autonoetic consciousness. Proc Natl Acad Sci USA. 2011;108:17562-7.
13. Moscovitch M, Cabeza R, Winocur G, Nadel L. Episodic memory and beyond: The hippocampus and neocortex in transformation. Ann Rev Psych. 2016;67:105-34.
14. Ranganath C. A unified framework for the functional organization of the medial temporal lobes and the phenomenology of episodic memory. Hippocampus. 2010;20:1263-90.
15. Bartsch T, Schonfeld R, Muller FJ, et al. Focal lesions of human hippocampal CA1 neurons in transient global amnesia impair place memory. Science. 2010;328:1412-5.
16. Binder JR, Desai RH. The neurobiology of semantic memory. Trends Cogn Sci. 2011;15:527-36.
17. Bender MB. Syndrome of isolated episode of confusion with amnesia. J Hillside Hospital. 1956;5:212-5.
18. Fisher CM, Adams RD. Transient global amnesia. Acta Neurol Scand. 1964;40:1-83.
19. Hodges JR, Warlow CP. Syndromes of transient amnesia: Towards a classification. A study of 153 cases. J Neurol Neurosurg Psychiatry. 1990;53:834-43.
20. Kumral E, Deveci EE, Erdogan CE, Enüstün C. Isolated hippocampal infarcts: Vascular and neuropsychological findings. J Neurol Sci. 2015;356:83-9.

21. Förster A, Al-Zghloul M, Wenz H, Böhme J, Groden C, Neumaier-Probst E. Isolated punctate hippocampal infarction and transient global amnesia are indistinguishable by means of MRI. Int J Stroke. 2016;12:292-6.
22. Zeman AZJ, Boniface SJ, Hodges JR. Transient epileptic amnesia: A description of the clinical and neuropsychological features in 10 cases and a review of the literature. J Neurol Neurosurg Psychiatry. 1998;64:435-43.
23. Baker J, Savage S, Milton F, Butler C, Kapur N, Hodges J, et al. The syndrome of transient epileptic amnesia: a combined series of 115 cases and literature review. Brain Commun. 2021;3:fcab038.
24. Butler C, Zeman A. Syndromes of Transient Amnesia. In: Laureys S, Gosseries O, Tononi G (Eds). The Neurology of Consciousness: Cognitive Neuroscience and Neuropathology. Amsterdam, Netherlands: Elsevier; 2016. pp. 365-78
25. Harrison NA, Johnston K, Corno F, Casey SJ, Friedner K, Humphreys K, et al. Psychogenic amnesia: syndromes, outcome, and patterns of retrograde amnesia. Brain. 2017;140:2498-510.
26. Markowitsch HJ, Staniloiu A. Functional (dissociative) retrograde amnesia. Handb Clin Neurol. 2016;139:419-45.
27. Staniloiu A, Markowitsch HJ. Dissociative amnesia. Lancet Psychiatry 2014;1:226-41.
28. De Simoni S, Grover PJ, Jenkins PO, Honeyfield L, Quest RA, Ross E, et al. Disconnection between the default mode network and medial temporal lobes in post-traumatic amnesia. Brain. 2016;139:3137-50.
29. Haas DC, Ross GS. Transient global amnesia triggered by mild head trauma. Brain. 1986;109:251-57.
30. Dwyer B, Katz DI. Postconcussion syndrome. Handb Clin Neurol 2018; 158: 163-78.
31. Fox MD, Raichle ME. Spontaneous fluctuations in brain activity observed with functional magnetic resonance imaging. Nat Rev Neurosci. 2007;8(9):700-11.
32. Raichle ME. The brain's default mode network. Ann Rev Neurosci. 2015;38:433-47.
33. Spreng RN, Mar RA, Kim AS. The common neural basis of autobiographical memory, prospection, navigation, theory of mind, and the default mode: a quantitative meta-analysis. J Cogn Neurosci. 2009;21(3):489-510.
34. Andrews-Hanna JR, Reidler JS, Sepulcre J, Poulin R, Buckner RL. Functionalanatomic fractionation of the brain's default network. Neuron 2010;65:550-62.
35. Andrews-Hanna JR, Saxe R, Yarkoni T. Contributions of episodic retrieval and mentalizing to autobiographical thought: Evidence from functional neuroimaging, resting-state connectivity, and fMRI meta-analyses. NeuroImage. 2014;91:324-35.
36. Parker TD, Rees R, Rajagopal A, Griffin C, Goodliffe L, Dilley M, et al. Post-traumatic amnesia. Pract Neurol. 2022;22(2):129-37.

CHAPTER 6

Pitfalls in Neuropsychological Testing in Adults with Suspected Dementias

Atanu Biswas

INTRODUCTION

Diagnosis of dementia or major neurocognitive disorder requires a good clinical assessment. A detailed history of the illness and careful clinical examination are important first step for the diagnosis. Neuropsychological assessment (NPA) is a very important next investigation for making a clinical diagnosis. NPA is also important for monitoring disease progression, and determining treatment efficacy of neurocognitive impairment. Although basic assessment of cognitive function is performed by most of the clinicians, patients are often referred to clinical psychologists for a detailed study, as NPA is time consuming and beyond the scope of a neurologist, psychiatrist, or geriatrician. NPA helps to differentiate normal ageing from minor and from minor to major neurocognitive disorders. It also helps to make a clinical diagnosis of a type of neurocognitive disorder. However, there are many difficulties in undertaking NPA and interpreting their results. In this chapter, an attempt is made to enumerate various difficulties encountered during NPA and while interpreting them.

NONAVAILABILITY OF PROPER VALIDATED TOOL FOR ASSESSMENT

Most of the available neuropsychological tools have been developed in Western countries. Getting a culturally validated tool is difficult for non-English speaking countries like India. Using tools developed for Western countries might result in underdetection as well as overdiagnosis of dementia in our country. Efforts have been made to develop reliable diagnostic tools and instruments that are culturally and linguistically valid for making an accurate diagnosis in Indian population. Some of these include 10/66 global dementia studies,[1] PGI battery for brain dysfunctions,[2] the National Institute of Mental Health and Neurosciences (NIMHANS) neuropsychological battery for the elderly,[3] Kolkata Cognitive Battery,[4] etc.

Unfortunately, these locally adapted and validated tools are not available in all Indian languages and India being culturally and linguistically diverse nation, some of them may not be useful in all parts of the country. For example, in picture naming test (PNT), animal pictures of tiger, elephant, rhinoceros, etc., may not be appropriate for a large part of the population due to nonexposure. Similarly, fruits like jackfruit or mango may not be useful for pan-India usage forcing researchers to settle to a common animal such as cow, cat, or dog and common fruit such as banana and guava. The idea of the test gets compromised as a relatively uncommon item is needed for the test. Researchers have tried to use the images of god and goddesses to test for semantic memory. India's religious diversity also makes this attempt difficult.

Another important limitation is the lack of normative data for the community. To make a diagnosis on the basis of performance, one need to know the cutoff score for the age, gender, and education matched control subjects of the community. Unfortunately, there is lack of cutoff for most of these tools for various ethnic and linguistic groups of this country. Community level cutoff scores are available for few languages with some tests.[4,5]

Illiteracy in India is another problem, and as most of the tools used for NPAs require subject to read and write, these are difficult to use in illiterate or low literate individuals. Difficulties in assessing a large population with no or very low education is a challenge for clinicians and neuropsychologists in this country.

The Indian Council of Medical Research (ICMR) Neurocognitive Tool Box was an attempt for developing a tool specifically for Indian cultural context and in various Indian languages.[6] This is a comprehensive instrument for diagnosis of neurocognitive dysfunction. Attempt is also made for developing the instrument for illiterate subjects as well.

CROSS-SECTIONAL VERSUS LONGITUDINAL ASSESSMENT

The primary requisite for making a diagnosis of neurocognitive dysfunction is to know the change of cognitive function over time. This is commonly judged from the history of change from previous level of functioning. Ideally, a repeat assessment gives more objective evidence of deterioration over time. This also helps in overcoming the problem of nonavailability of normative data in the community. The performance of repeat NPA helps in making comparison with the previous assessment.

In absence of longitudinal data of a subject, one needs to rely on the history. For this a reliable caregiver is essential to provide details account of change of cognition and behavior over time. Unfortunately, many old persons are now living alone and looking after by professional carer, and getting a good history is often difficult. Sometime the spouse is also not in a position to provide the history as he/she also is inflicted with amnesia.

FOLLOWING HIERARCHY OF ASSESSMENT IS ESSENTIAL

It is essential to follow a proper sequence of assessment while performing NPA. In a busy clinic, physician often tries to make a tentative diagnosis with only few tests. Clock-drawing test is popular as it provides much information about cognition. However, inability to properly draw the face of a clock can be accounted for multiple reasons. Essentially it tests the visuoconstructional and visuospatial functions. However, before undertaking this test, it is important to check for the vision and hearing. The subject must be attentive, and must have the ability to comprehend the instruction and must have certain level of education to complete the task. If all these are relatively well preserved, a defect in the drawing can be attributed to the defect in constructional ability, spatial defect, defect in concept about the clock, etc. If, however, a decision is drawn that the patient in having major neurocognitive dysfunction or dementia, it may be an overdiagnosis, unless all initial steps are followed.

Reasonably preserved vision and hearing is important for undertaking NPA. The arousal is important to carry forward further testing. Then the subject's attention needs to be assessed. Lack of attention results in false interpretation of other test performances. Subject in delirium exhibit derangement in arousal and attention and further testing would be useless. Once it is found that the person has relatively intact attention, the next step is to test for his language function. Preserved comprehension

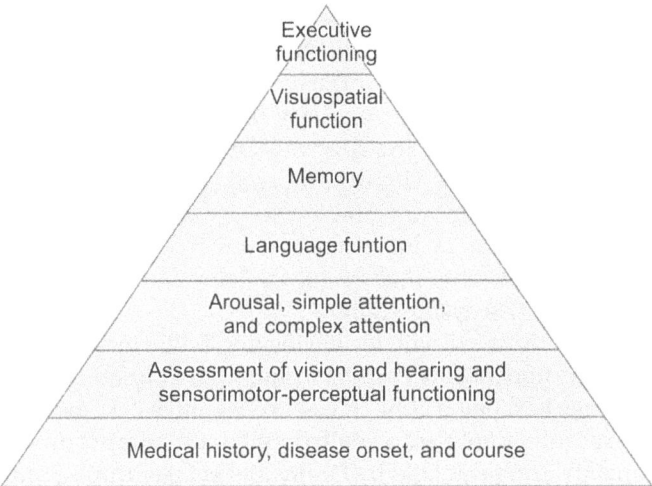

FIG. 1: Hierarchy of neuropsychological assessment.

and ability to communicate are vital prerequisites for additional tests. All other tests, namely recent memory, visuospatial ability, praxis, gnosis, and executive function are to be tested only if attention and language functions are relatively preserved **(Fig. 1)**.

HIGH FUNCTIONING INDIVIDUALS MAY SCORE NORMAL DESPITE HAVING NEUROCOGNITIVE IMPAIRMENT

Case Vignette

A 65-year-old right-handed individual with 15 years of education, editor of the mouthpiece of political party came with complaints of difficulties in remembering names of well-known and famous persons, places, or objects, as well as difficulty in finding appropriate words while writing articles, which he described, was very disturbing and embarrassing for him. His wife also complaints of loss of his memory of recent events that she noticed for last 6 months. He did not have any vascular risk factor; his mother had dementia after her 75 years of age. He scored 30/30 in mini–mental state examination (MMSE), 96/100 in Addenbrooke's Cognitive Examination (ACE), and his Clinical Dementia Rating (CDR) was 0. In Verbal Learning Test, he scored 6/10, 7/10, and 8/10 in three trials of immediate recall and 7/10 in delayed recall. In object naming test, he scored 100%. As he performed well in his tests, he told those were too easy for him. Asking to name the prime minister of Bangladesh assassinated in 1970s or to name the women prime minister of India were too simple for him. He expected much tougher questions like to name the US presidents chronologically, which would have been suitable for him.

Neuropsychological tools are developed to make them useful for all individuals in the community. Although, these tools are suitable for the majority, some individuals may find them either very easy or very difficult. They belong to the end of the spectrum of normal individuals in the community. Highly educated persons with high cognitive function may find a test very easy and scoring below the cutoff for impairment requires longer time for deterioration. This may result in delay in diagnosis of neurocognitive dysfunction.

Similarly, those who are having borderline intelligence, they may find these tests difficult and score below the cutoff and may be labeled as having neurocognitive dysfunction. These individuals are usually living with compromised capacity and protected by family and society throughout their life. In the modern educational system in India, they even may cross the secondary school level. The intellectual disability remains undetected due to the lack of systematic assessment as well as lack of resources for assessment and tolerance for "poor learners" in the different Indian schooling systems.[7] This results in a heterogeneous population even when the level of educational attainment is controlled, and so, education stratified normative data for cognitive tests may not be accurately available.[8] In cross-sectional community-based studies, these subjects often create difficulties in diagnostic labeling. However, a detailed history of lack of deterioration over time or follow-up assessment would help resolving the issue.

BORDER-ZONE BETWEEN NORMALCY AND MILD AND BETWEEN MILD AND MAJOR NEUROCOGNITIVE DYSFUNCTION ALSO REQUIRE USE OF ADDITIONAL INFORMATION FORM HISTORY AND FUNCTIONAL STATUS OF THE INDIVIDUAL

Normal aging process generally affects our cognition. The fluid intelligence deteriorates and the processing speed becomes slower. Despite these changes, old persons perform well in neuropsychological testing if sufficient time is given. Although aged person's performance is different from that of a young individual, their performance match with the age, gender, and education-matched individuals in the community.

When the performance deteriorates in respect to what is normal for the age, gender and education-matched individuals in the community, and the person remains functionally independent, it is called mild cognitive impairment (MCI) of mild neurocognitive dysfunction. If subject fails to perform his normal activities with this level of cognitive impairment, an early dementia or major neurocognitive dysfunction is considered. The thin line between MCI and early dementia is the preservation or disturbance of instrumental activities of daily life (IADL). Thus, CDR score 0.5 makes a person MCI, if his/her IADL is preserved, and dementia if IADL is affected.

Detailed NPA is needed to find out the domains of cognitive functions affected, but a thorough assessment of IADL with culturally valid tool is crucial for making a clinical differentiation. This requires an understanding of what is normal functioning for the subject, and a culturally valid scale for instrumental activities of daily living. In India, old persons are usually not challenged due to the protection from the family. This is more common in rural areas and in joint families, where, old persons are not allowed to go for shopping, do financial transactions, travel alone, or drive. This makes delay in making a diagnosis.

ABNORMALITY IN A SINGLE TEST DOES NOT SIGNIFY IMPAIRMENT OF A PARTICULAR COGNITIVE DOMAIN

As described earlier about clock drawing test, it is very important to analyze each test result with all probable causes of poor performance. Serial subtraction of 7 from 100 is a very common test used by clinicians. It tests the ability of doing mental arithmetic to subtract 7 from a number, thus testing the ability to calculate. However, it requires complex attention for subtraction or backward counting. The subject needs to hold on in his/her memory that he/she needs to subtract 7 from the number he just got from previous subtraction. Thus, the test may be abnormal, if the subject has defect in attention as well as in calculation. Another important test commonly used by clinicians is category fluency test. It is commonly used as a test of fluency to categorize the type of aphasia. It, however, also a test of frontal lobe function. The subject is supposed to generate words of a particular category and inhibiting names of other similar names. For example, when generating name of animals, one needs to say the name of animals only, not the birds or reptiles or fish. The subject also needs to control his/her desire to repeat the same word again and again. If that becomes evident, it suggests perseveration or inflexibility or features of obsession, suggesting frontal lobar dysfunction.

NEUROPSYCHOLOGICAL TESTS ARE TO BE INTERPRETED CAREFULLY, RELYING ON SCORE MAY BE MISLEADING

Case Vignette

A 70-year-old gentleman, a retired engineer, with 16 years of education, presented with slowness of all activities for 1 year with history of dream enactment. He was treated with levodopa by his primary care physician without much improvement. For last 4 months he also developed forgetfulness and seeing people around him when no one was there. He scored 95 of 100 in ACE III and 30 out of 30 in MMSE and a diagnosis of Parkinson's disease with drug-induced hallucination was made. In his next visit after 3 months, he was again tested and scored 78 in ACE III and 22 in MMSE. A history of fluctuation of cognition was obtained from his wife, who also gave history of two falls with transient loss of consciousness. Detailed assessment revealed deficits in attention, visuospatial, executive function, and recent memory. This helps in making a diagnosis of Lewy body dementia.

The case exemplifies the fallacy of relying on scores in NPA. Unless the clinical context is analyzed properly, scores may be misleading. Fluctuation of cognition is also common in delirium. Many-a-time a diagnosis may be missed if a single assessment is done. Thus, test scores are to be interpreted carefully and clinician must analyze history properly to make a clinical diagnosis.

QUALITATIVE ASSESSMENT OF HOW THE SUBJECT PERFORMS A TEST RATHER THAN WHAT IS PERFORMED IS IMPORTANT FOR MAKING A DIAGNOSIS

It is essential to look for the scores in many cognitive tests, e.g., in verbal learning test subject is asked to repeat a list of unrelated words and this is usually repeated for three times to make him/her learn. After a gap of 30 minutes he/she is asked to recall those words, and if unable then, cues or choices are given. The test is interpreted by the number of words subject could reproduce in initial three trials and after a delay of 30 minutes. This helps to know the subject's recent verbal memory. However, a qualitative assessment is also important. Subject may not be attentive and easily distractible, that can only be observed by the tester. Similarly, the intrusion of other words, repeating the same word or perseveration suggests frontal lobe dysfunction. A qualitative assessment of each test performance also gives important clue to differentiate dementia from pseudodementia.

LACK OF EXPOSURE TO NEUROPSYCHOLOGICAL TEST AND PRESSURE OF PERFORMING WELL

Elderly Indians not exposed to NPA often perform poorly due multiple other issues. The tests of cognition are treated akin to testing in schools and this leads to test anxiety which in turn affects test performance.[8] Another factor is the innate societal pressure of "scoring the highest" and "being the best". The elderly Indian population and their families are defensive about their cognitive abilities and frequently are not motivated enough to complete the testing, often giving up during testing.[9] Thus, determining the best level of cognitive functioning is challenging even in cognitively normal people, and often, the poor test performance may be due to the lack of test sophistication and not cognitive dysfunction. Many clinicians and neuropsychologists think that there is a need to repeat test instructions and give lengthy explanations to subjects and verbatim test instructions alone are not sufficient in many cases.[9,10]

NEUROPSYCHOLOGICAL TESTS ARE NOT ALWAYS TESTING REAL-LIFE DIFFICULTIES

Neuropsychological tests are developed to document the disability of cognitive functions of an individual. Ideally these instruments must simulate real-life situation faced in our day-to-day life. However, many real-life situations are difficult to simulate in a laboratory. For example, the problem of navigation is common visuospatial problem encountered in patients of neurocognitive dysfunction. Commonly used tests for visuospatial dysfunction are clock drawing, drawing of three-dimensional cube and complex figures, line bisection test, etc. They do not properly assess the ability of a person to navigate in a known environment. This requires improvisation of test instruments. Some computer-based tests simulating the real-life complexities developed to address this problem are developed. "The 4 Mountain Test" is one such example.[11] Use of digital platform and artificial intelligence would definitely improve the assessment of cognitive function is coming days.

MULTIPLE TESTS OF A COGNITIVE DOMAIN ARE NEEDED TO DETERMINE TRUE DEFICIT

Although neuropsychological tests are meant to elicit cognitive dysfunction, a singe test may not provide an accurate understanding about the domain it is supposed to assess. This means, we need to use more than one test for one particular domain to decide on impairment. This idea is used to build up the Movement Disorder Society (MDS) task force criteria for mild cognitive impairment in Parkinson's disease (PD-MCI). The level II guideline of this criterion mandates presence of impairment on at least two neuropsychological tests, represented by either two impaired tests in one cognitive domain or one impaired test in two different cognitive domains.[12]

CONVENTIONAL TESTS MAY NOT ALWAYS BE SUFFICIENT TO DETECT COGNITIVE IMPAIRMENT

Neuropsychological tests routinely used are not always sufficient to detect every aspect of cognition. For routine clinical use a set of tests are used to pick up major domains of cognition. Whenever there is a suspicion about higher order visual dysfunction, one need to expand the test protocol. This is also true for higher order language function. Conventionally, for assessment of language function, following aspects are tested: Comprehension, fluency, naming, repetition, reading, and writing. It is now established that higher level of language function like pragmatics which we acquire late in our development gets affected early in the course of neurodegeneration. Figurative language tests like metaphor comprehension have been found to be useful in detecting early neurocognitive dysfunction.[13]

TESTS ARE DONE IN ARTIFICIAL ENVIRONMENT AND THEY DO NOT ALWAYS REFLECT THE PROBLEM SEEN IN REAL LIFE

Neuropsychological tests are built to tests various aspects of cognition, to pick up difficulties faced in daily life. However, these are artificial methods and can never match the real-life difficulties. For example, tests of visuospatial deficit are too difficult in a laboratory. Navigational problem, heading difficulty, and landmark agnosia are difficult to simulate even in virtual platform.

Attempts to test a person's cognition in real-life situation are also gaining popularity. The "performance-based assessment of cognition" and the concept of "dementia studio" are thought to help overcome these problems.

CONCLUDING REMARKS

Although, many advancements are happening in the field of NPA, they may not be useful in India due to various reasons including illiteracy, cultural, and linguistic diversity and the so-called "digital divide" prevailing in the country. The COVID-19 pandemic has resulted in significant change in our life. Face-to-face NPA becomes difficult and clinicians and neuropsychologists are contemplating online assessment. This requires a paradigm-shift in the assessment procedure and new methods and newer test modules are to be developed to accomplish the goal. Despite all the challenges, a detailed history from a reliable caregiver and careful NPA with appropriate tools would help clinician making a diagnosis of neurocognitive disorders.

LEARNING POINTS

The major pitfalls in conduction of neuropsychological tests in the diagnosis of dementias include:
- Nonavailability of proper validated tool for assessment.
- Following hierarchy of assessment is essential.
- High functioning individuals may score normal despite having neurocognitive impairment.
- Border-zone between normalcy and mild and between mild and major neurocognitive dysfunction also require use of additional information form history and functional status of the individual.
- Neuropsychological tests are to be interpreted carefully, relying on score may be misleading.
- Qualitative assessment of how the subject performs a test rather than what is performed is important for making a diagnosis.
- Neuropsychological tests are not always testing real-life difficulties.
- Multiple tests of a cognitive domain are needed to determine true deficit.
- Conventional tests may not always be sufficient to detect cognitive impairment.

REFERENCES

1. Prince M, Acosta D, Chiu H, Scazufca M, Varghese M, Group DR. Dementia diagnosis in developing countries: A cross-cultural validation study. Lancet. 2003;361(9361):909-17.
2. Pershad D, Verma SK. Hand Book of PGI Battery of Brain Dysfunction (PGIBBD). Agra: National Psychological Corporation; 1990.
3. Tripathi R, Kumar JK, Bharath S, Marimuthu P, Varghese M. Clinical validity of NIMHANS neuropsychological battery for elderly: A preliminary report. Indian J Psychiatry. 2013;55(3):279-82.
4. Das SK, Banerjee TK, Mukherjee CS, Bose P, Biswas A, Hazra A, et al. An urban community-based study of cognitive function among non-demented elderly population in India. Neurol Asia. 2006;11:37-48.
5. Sosa AL, Albanese E, Prince M, Acosta D, Ferri CP, Guerra M, et al. Population normative data for the 10/66 Dementia Research Group cognitive test battery from Latin America, India and China: A cross-sectional survey. BMC Neurol. 2009;9:48.
6. Iyer G, Paplikar A, Alladi S, Dutt A, Sharma M, Mekala S, et al. Standardising dementia diagnosis across linguistic and educational diversity: study design of the Indian Council of Medical Research-Neurocognitive Tool Box (ICMR-NCTB). J Int Neuropsychol Soc. 2020;26(2),172-86.
7. Basu J. Present status and challenges of intellectual assessment in India. Int J School Educ Psychol. 2016;4:231-40.
8. Porselvi AP, Shankar V. Status of cognitive testing of adults in India. Ann Indian Acad Neurol. 2017;20(4):334-40.
9. Shah U. Neuropsychological assessment in the Indian elderly. Indian J Private Psychiatry. 2009;3:59-66.
10. Chandra V, Ganguli M, Ratcliff G, Pandav R, Sharma S, Belle S, et al. Practical issues in cognitive screening of elderly illiterate populations in developing countries. The Indo-US Cross National Dementia Epidemiology Study. Aging Clin Exp Res. 1998;10:349-57.
11. Chan D, Gallaher LM, Moodley K, Minati L, Burgess N, Hartley T. The 4 Mountains Test: A Short Test of Spatial Memory with High Sensitivity for the Diagnosis of Pre-dementia Alzheimer's Disease. J Vis Exp. 2016;(116):54454.
12. Litvan I, Goldman JG, Troster AI, Schmand BA, Weintraub D, Petersen RC, et al. Diagnostic criteria for mild cognitive impairment in Parkinson's disease: Movement Disorder Society Task Force guidelines. Mov Disord. 2012;27(3):349-56.
13. Chakraborty M, Klooster N, Biswas A, Chatterjee A. The scope of using pragmatic language tests for early detection of dementia: A systematic review of investigations using figurative language. Alzheimers Dement. 2023;19(10):4705-28.

CHAPTER 7

Cornerstones in the Diagnosis of Epileptic Seizures in Children and Adolescents: Their Pitfalls and Mimics

Ambar Chakravarty

INTRODUCTION

The most important factor contributing to making a wrong diagnosis of epilepsy is obtaining an inadequate and inaccurate history. Observers of spells should be queried directly. All too often, a story within the confines of the clinic proves to be very inaccurate. "Dizzy spells" without loss of consciousness (LOC) may be revealed by witnesses as full tonic-clonic seizures. A careful history is an unbiased history, told in the patient's and observer's own words. Trainees, relatives, and patients must learn to avoid use of too technical terms while presenting the history to the treating physician. Young children are often not expected to mention every details of a spell experienced by them and hence parental account of the incidents observed, assumes paramount importance. By the time multiple physicians have asked a patient the very same question, especially a child (e.g., getting a bad odor before an attack), they often get confused and tend to give a positive answer, even if that was not the case. Witness observations of the sequence of events preceding during and after the event/events contribute a lot in making a proper diagnosis.

This has been assessed very scientifically recently in UK by Reuber and his colleagues[1] using the paroxysmal event observer (PEO) questionnaire. The study concluded that witness reported factors alone differentiated better between syncope and epilepsy than patient-reported factors (accuracy: 96% vs. 85%, $p = 0.0004$). This data improved accuracy of differentiation very significantly not only between epilepsy and syncope but also between syncope and psychogenic nonepileptic seizures (PNES).

The combination of a shaky history and an over interpreted electroencephalogram (EEG) is especially pernicious. As a consequence of this combination of errors, patients may be treated inappropriately for years with anticonvulsants and subjected to a variety of unnecessary social restrictions.

Box 1 lists some very useful queries which may be asked to older children or parents of younger children for making a clinical diagnosis of the event experienced by the child. Box 2 lists some hallmark clinical character of the events experienced and Box 3 lays out a road map to arrive at the most likely clinical diagnosis of the event in a logical manner (called a deductive approach by DiMario[2]).

Confusion may arise as to the cause of the seizure. There may be instances where whether a neurological deficit had resulted from a seizure or had been the cause of the seizure, become difficult to decide.

BOX 1: Basic queries for elucidation of clinical history.

- Age at onset?
- Is there more than one type of event?
- What happens just prior to the event?
- Does the child get a warning or any change in behavior noted?
- What is the exact sequence of the event?
- Is the pattern stereotyped or the pattern variable?
- What are the child's posture, tone, respiratory pattern, color, and behavior before, during and after the event?
- Is there any relationship of the event to activity, attention, play, temperament, sleep, and diet?
- Any precipitant of event?
- Any relieving factor?
- Can the events be suppressed by the child?
- Can the child be distracted during the event?
- Any concurrent motor activity, sensory phenomenon, or autonomic feature evident during the event?
- What does the child do immediately afterwards?
- Can the child recall the event in detail?
- The duration, frequency, and periodicity of the event?
- Any family history of similar illness?
- Can the child or observer mimic the event?
- Any video recording done?

> **BOX 2: Hallmark clinical character of event.**
> - Paralysis
> - Collapse/drop attack
> - Generalized posturing/jerking/twitching
> - Focal posturing/jerking/twitching
> - Ocular movement/deviation
> - Autonomic phenomenon
> - Sensory phenomenon

> **BOX 3: Road map to logical thinking.**
> - Accurate statement of the problem
> - Aggregation of facts (based on **Boxes 1 and 2**)
> - Identification of the nodal point (clinically the most important issue determining the possible causes of the event, e.g., generalized/focal jerking)
> - Generate list of possibilities
> - Trim list to most probable ones
> - Identify the most probable one
> - Validate the diagnosis by appropriate investigations

Focal seizures can cause a postictal transient hemiparesis (Todd's paresis), but cerebrovascular disease can also directly cause hemiparesis and may present as a seizure in about 15% of cases. Bilateral carotid occlusive disease can also cause brief LOC. Differentiating idiopathic epilepsy from epilepsy secondary to cerebrovascular disease can be difficult. The latter diagnosis as the primary diagnosis as the primary causative one may be helped by such features like presence of stroke risk factors while the diagnosis of a primary epileptic condition may be suggested by finding a past history of seizure or a positive family history of epilepsy. Similarly, seizures can induce cardiac arrhythmias, as well as result from them.

The inexperienced clinician tends to overemphasize the rare and obscure. This is particularly easy to do in the differential diagnosis of epilepsy. Most staring spells are simple daydreaming. Most explosive outbursts in children are temper tantrums. Most episodes of abrupt falls or drop attacks in the elderly are either tripping or syncopal—vasovagal or cardiogenic. The paradigm of approach gets altered when it is known that the individual concerned suffers from epilepsy. The first condition to be considered if such a person presents with only a brief LOC would always be epilepsy; however, if he had not had prior history of epilepsy, such conditions like vasovagal or cardiac syncopes should be considered and excluded much before a diagnosis of epileptic seizure be considered.

Great difficulties are often encountered in patients who exhibit features suggestive of mixed seizures. This is not very uncommon. A certain percentage of individuals with documented psychogenic seizures, varying from 10 to 37% or more,[1,3,4] may at other times exhibit epileptic seizures and vice versa. Presumably, the epileptic seizures and their aftermath somehow became a "template" for subsequent nonepileptic spells. By absence of EEG changes during a generalized seizure-like episode, video EEG monitoring can show that the episode under observation is nonepileptic in origin, but it can never show that prior episodes were not epileptic seizures. Inference by analogy is imprecise. Even after establishing a diagnosis of nonepileptic attacks, the experienced clinician should continue to look for the possibility of a mixed disorder. He may, if circumstances so demand, withdraw anticonvulsants (only in hospitalized patients) with the understanding that epileptic seizures may emerge and properly characterized.

Improvement of spells with anticonvulsants need not necessarily mean that the patient has epilepsy and nothing other than that. Placebo response may occur, especially in those with psychogenic components. The efficacy of antiepileptic drugs is not limited to seizures alone. Carbamazepine and sodium valproate are useful mood stabilizers. Phenobarbitone and benzodiazepines are effective both as antiepileptics and as well as anxiolytics. Phenytoin can suppress ventricular arrhythmias. When a positive response to an antiepileptic agent is encountered, the clinician should consider what else besides epilepsy might have been treated. Conversely, some patients with presumed epilepsy may worsen with increasing doses of antiepileptic drugs. This generally should call for looking for presence of associated psychogenic seizures in some cases but not in all. It is well known that absence seizures and juvenile myoclonic epilepsy may worsen following treatment with carbamazepine or phenytoin.

Perhaps the greatest source of mistakes in epilepsy diagnosis is the performance of EEGs.[5,6] Very often these are ordered by general practitioners, who for no uncertain reason lack adequate knowledge what they would really be looking for in the report and performed by technicians not really adequately trained (common problems include for the technician to understand the difference between a sleep EEG and a sleep deprived EEG; problems of interpretation relating to routinely using monopolar montages with reference electrode on ear lobules, inability to recognize common artifacts like electrode pops, pulse artefacts, 60 Hz AC artefacts, etc., and how to minimize them during recording) and lastly and most importantly, the final interpretation by a trained (at least by qualification) neurologist, who often had no clue as to the clinical condition for which EEG had been ordered and who, perhaps trying to play safe, interprets anything which "strikes out" as "dysrhythmic" and subsequently puts the

TABLE 1: Age-wise distribution of common seizure mimics in children.

Neonate	Infancy/Toddler	Children/Adolescents
• Neonatal sleep myoclonus • Jitteriness • Hyperekplexia	• Benign myoclonus/shuddering • Self-gratification • Breath holding spell • Benign paroxysmal vertigo • Gastroesophageal reflux/Sandifer syndrome • Benign tonic upgaze • Benign paroxysmal torticollis • Stereotypies • Parasomnias • Infantile colic	• Syncope • Psychogenic nonepileptic seizures • Tics • Migraine equivalents • Parasomnias

final impression as "seizure disorder". Such a term does not exist in the International League Against Epilepsy (ILAE) nomenclature!

Result

Parents and relatives get panicky; move from doctor to doctor and the poor patient (often a child), gets loaded up with unnecessary antiepileptic drugs almost all of which have potential side effects, especially in relation to cognition and behavior. It is very strongly felt that the reporting neurologist must exhibit some degree of restraint in "wording" the conclusive sentence. One must remember that *it is always better to underinterpret an EEG than overinterpreting them.* If a patient really has got epilepsy, it would reveal its true nature in due course of time.

Table 1 depicts the age-wise distribution of common conditions which are often mistaken as epileptic seizures in children.

PHYSICAL AND NEUROLOGICAL STATUS

Head injuries, shoulder dislocation, and tongue bite involving the lateral aspect of the tongue are strongly suggestive of epileptic seizures.[7] Bilateral extensor plantar responses are common in the postictal stuporous state.

ELECTROENCEPHALOGRAM

The pitfalls in EEG diagnosis of epileptic seizures had already been touched upon. It is an important diagnostic tool as paroxysmal changes are seen in 34% cases after a first seizure and as much as 50–70% if performed within 24 hours.[8,9] A sleep-deprived EEG can reveal additional spike discharges in additional 13–31% cases. EEG has got a low sensitivity and should be used as a test to exclude epilepsy but it is very useful in the classification of different types of seizures and epilepsy syndromes (**Appendix 1**). Minor EEG findings should not be over interpreted as 2.8% children and 0.4% adults may display minor paroxysmal changes in absence of epilepsy.[10] The request for EEG should come from a specialist as a survey in a district hospital has revealed that as many as 56% of EEG done were unnecessary.[11]

BRAIN IMAGING

The CT scan of the brain is widely available but in absence of focal neurological signs its yield is relatively low (4–6%).[12,13] MRI scan of the brain with appropriate sequences is the investigation of choice, but it should be ordered only by specialists in the field. In a case series of 166 patients with first unprovoked seizures, MRI was positive in 47% cases.[14]

LABORATORY TESTS

Routine blood tests like blood glucose, electrolytes, calcium, and blood counts are of clinical significance in only a small proportion of cases.[15,16] In patients with generalized tonic-clonic seizure (GTCS), serum lactate levels were higher than in patients with syncope and PNES. Serum lactate levels in male patients with GTCS were higher than females. It has been suggested that a cutoff value of 2.43 mol/L may be considered appropriate to distinguish GTCS from nonepileptic events. This cutoff value was less sensitive for female patients. If the serum lactate value is determined within 2 hours from ictus then this cutoff value can be useful in differentiating GTCS from other nonepileptic events such as syncope and psychogenic nonepileptic events in male patients.[10] In addition to astute clinical observation, imaging, and EEG, serum lactate can also be a helpful diagnostic tool in assessing patients with impaired consciousness. However, this needs to be tested in larger population of patients before its routine clinical use.

SERUM PROLACTIN IN SEIZURE DIAGNOSIS

Ever since the original report by Trimble in 1978 about the role of prolactin in seizure diagnosis is still remains unsettled. In a series of 200 patients undergoing video EEG monitoring in an epilepsy clinic, serum prolactin was measured within 20 minutes of the seizure or seizure-like event. Abubakr and Wambacq found serum prolactin to be elevated in all 22 patients with GTCS, in 27 out of 32 patients with complex partial seizures but in only 42 out of 146 patients with psychogenic seizures.[11] Sensitivity was 100% for tonic-clonic seizures and 84.6% for complex partial seizures. Serum prolactin was elevated in 84.4% of cases with epileptic events but only in 28.8% of patients with nonepileptic events. The American Academy of Neurology Technology and Assessment Subcommittee reviewed 10 studies and found a sensitivity of 52.6% and specificity of 92.8% for all types of epileptic seizures. The criteria for establishing an elevated prolactin level was unclear as some studies took doubling of base line serum prolactin values whereas others considered an absolute value of 16–45 ng/mL. The absolute value is important as doubling of value from 1 to 2 ng/mL is unlikely to be of any significance. So, ideally the serum prolactin level must double and also reach a minimum value of 15 ng/mL to be of clinical significance. Clinical conditions that interfere with prolactin levels such as pregnancy and lactation and intake of neuroleptic and dopaminergic drugs should be carefully taken into account. Serum prolactin levels really do not actually provide any significant additional information and it is often the case of the glass being half full or half empty. They do not really help in distinguishing psychogenic nonepileptic events from organic ones. The serum prolactin estimation does not help in coming to a diagnosis in an epilepsy monitoring unit as the issue is usually solved with the integration of the clinical and electrophysiologic data. In some settings, the serum prolactin estimation can be of value where epilepsy is strongly considered. A negative prolactin level can be useful in an outpatient setting with suspected tonic-clonic seizures. Therefore, serum prolactin estimation plays only a minor role in the diagnosis of epileptic seizures where an astute clinical observation and history plays a far more important role. All laboratory tests with the exception of video EEG play only a minor supplementary role with false positives and false negatives and do not substitute a clinical observation which is still considered a gold standard in the diagnosis of epilepsy.

EXCLUSION OF OTHER PAROXYSMAL EVENTS MIMICKING EPILEPTIC SEIZURE

Anoxic/Hypoxic Paroxysmal Event (Syncope)

Syncope is almost ten times more common than epilepsy.[12] This is particularly relevant in the elderly, and in patients above 70 years they have a 23% chance of having a syncope in the next 10 years.[13] A standard 12-lead ECG is the initial investigation for the evaluation of syncope. Echocardiography is positive only in patients with a suggestive cardiac history and with abnormalities in their ECG.[14] The tilt table test can only be recommended in patients with an atypical history of LOC according to the guidelines of the European Society of Cardiology.[15] When syncope is accompanied by jerking movements, it may be confused with epilepsy. This was frequently seen in a group of 56 medical students with self-induced syncope.[16] Syncope generally has a prodromal phase of lightheadedness, gradual fading of the visual and auditory surroundings, blurred vision, and generalized weakness. The patient is usually pale with epigastric discomfort with a lot of sweating. There is no cyanosis or a rising feeling in the epigastric region as seen in seizures. There is loss of postural tone with a fall usually without injuries and a brief LOC. There may be a tonic phase and a few clonic jerks but only after a few seconds and never accompanying the fall. There may be some vocalizations and automatisms, but they are usually very brief. If there is prolonged cerebral hypoxia there may be decorticate posturing and opisthotonos. Urinary incontinence may also occur. According to the Lempert's study on intentionally provoked syncope, clonic jerks are multifocal, arrhythmic, and are probably less frequent than those observed in "spontaneous" syncope. Jerking movements range from 12 to 46%[17,18] among blood donors who faint. Recovery is usually rapid and eye contact is very quickly established. But occasionally recovery may be delayed and some degree of postictal confusion may occur which may mimic a seizure. Eyes are usually open during the episode as also occurs during a seizure. However, eyes usually roll upward during a syncope whereas eyes usually turn laterally to either side during a seizure depending on the side of location of the epileptic focus. The patient may still feel very weak after recovery, look pale, and have a lot of diaphoresis. A large number of patients have a precipitating factor like emotional stress, prolonged standing in a hot crowded place, carotid sinus stimulation, low salt intake or dehydration or raised intrathoracic pressure like during coughing. The common causes of syncope are listed in **Box 4** and may include benign causes like vasovagal attacks or malignant life-threatening causes like dangerous cardiac arrhythmias. If the syncope occurs a few moments after exercise, it may indicate reflex syncope but an attack during exercise indicates a more sinister cause like cardiomyopathy or a conduction defect. Neurally mediated vasovagal syncope generally occurs in the upright position but venepuncture-induced syncope can occur in supine position as well. Abdominal pain, that may be confused with epigastric aura of temporal lobe seizures, may occur at onset. Auras comprising epigastric, vertiginous, visual, or somatosensory experiences may occur in both vasovagal and cardiogenic syncope.

> **BOX 4: Classification of syncope.**
>
> - *Insufficient pumping action of the heart:*
>   - Arrhythmia (atrioventricular block, paroxysmal supraventricular and ventricular tachycardia, and long QT syndrome)
>   - Structural cardiac disease (valvular disease, congenital heart disease, obstructive cardiomyopathy, cardiac tamponade, pulmonary embolism, and global myocardial ischemia)
> - *Insufficient vascular tone, leading to orthostatic hypotension:*
>   - Autonomic failure
>   - Primary (multiple system atrophy and pure autonomic failure)
>   - Secondary (diabetic and other neuropathies)
>   - Drugs (antidepressants and beta-blockers)
> - *Insufficient circulatory volume:*
>   - Hypovolemia (Addison's disease, diuretics, and hemorrhage)
> - *Inappropriate neural control over the circulation:*
>   - Reflex syncope (vasovagal syncope, carotid sinus syndrome, visceral syncopes, micturition, deglutition, glossopharyngeal, cough, Valsalva, and sneeze)

Transient Ischemic Attack

A transient ischemic attack (TIA) involving the vertebrobasilar territory can involve the ascending reticular activating system and cause transient LOC. Such events are accompanied by other brainstem features such as dysarthria, diplopia, vertigo, ataxia, or hemiparesis and be easy to distinguish. More than 75% of TIAs last longer than 5 minutes and this is longer than either a seizure or a syncope.[19]

Carotid Sinus Syncope

Carotid sinus hypersensitivity is a common cause of unexplained falls in elderly people generally above the age of 60 years. Testing for such hypersensitivity should be part of routine workup of elderly subjects with falls and transient LOC of very brief duration. Such testing should always be done with ECG and blood pressure monitoring in a hospital setting. Some subjects with carotid sinus hypersensitivity may have falls without definite LOC where sinus pressure may occur from head turning or tight collars. Sinus hypersensitivity causes peripheral vasodilatation causing hypotension as well as slowing of heart rate. Both these features need to be looked for during a carotid massage test **(Fig. 1)**. However, such tests carry the risks prolonged asystole, transient or permanent neurological deficits, stroke, and sudden death; hence, the justification of the aforementioned warning.

Long QT Syndrome

This form of cardiogenic syncope needs special mentioning as it may be associated with convulsive syncopes that cause unexplained sudden death in a young person and may closely mimic a GTCS. The condition is often familial with autosomal dominant inheritance resulting from a mutation affecting sodium or potassium channels. Syncope results from ventricular tachyarrhythmia, generally torsades de pointes triggered by fear, fright, emotionally charged exercises, and sleep. ECG is diagnostic.

Brugada syndrome is characterized by three types of ST segment anomalies and is another type of genetic ion channel disorder caused usually by SCN5A mutation. This

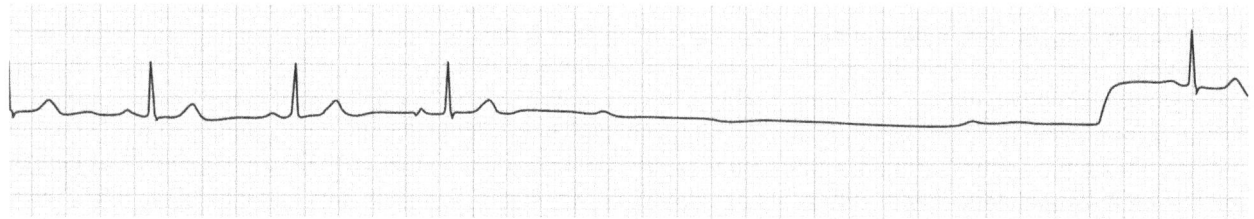

FIG. 1: Sinus arrest induced by carotid massage.

may imitate an epileptic attack and may cause sudden death.[20]

Such conditions highlight the need for a proper ECG recording in every subject presenting with a history suggestive of a convulsion for the first time. A recent report highlights the need for searching for occult cardiac arrhythmias (asystole/complete heart block) in some subjects presenting with intractable "epileptic seizures" with implantable loop recorder (ILR) on a long-term basis.[21]

Anoxic Epileptic Seizures

At times, not very commonly though, true epileptic seizures can be triggered by nonepileptic syncope, and hence the name. This is not synonymous with reflex anoxic seizure, which is a syncope. Neurally mediated syncope may trigger a prolonged clonic seizure with myoclonic jerks and Valsalva maneuver-induced syncope can trigger a vibratory tonic epileptic seizure in children. On the other hand, epileptic seizures may manifest with syncope like attacks in Panayiotopoulos syndrome (*epileptic seizure imitating syncope*).

PSYCHOGENIC PAROXYSMAL EVENT

Psychogenic pseudosyncope and dissociative seizures remain diagnostic challenges to general practitioners and specialists. They constitute about 30% of cases in syncope clinics and about 25% cases who are referred for refractory epilepsy in tertiary epilepsy centers.[22-24] These events start by external or internal triggers like unpleasant people or surroundings and flashback of traumatic internal events. The prodromal phase is characterized by symptoms such as tachycardia, epigastric discomfort, and difficulty in breathing with tachypnea. Such patients may have neurological symptoms such as tremor, weakness, headache, or sensory changes. They may also present with pure psychogenic features such as visual and auditory hallucinations, intense fright, depersonalization, dreamlike states, or feeling of impending death. The patient may stare blankly, have bizarre movements, and may fall down very slowly without any injury. Unresponsiveness may be very prolonged and last for >10 minutes. Some patients may have pseudostatus epileptics. Movements are asynchronous and demonstrative and usually out of phase with intermittent vocalizations. Pelvic thrusting, side-to-side head movements, and forcible eye closure are commonly seen. *La grande courbure* of Charcot or intense opisthotonus like body arching is not commonly seen nowadays. There may be quick return of consciousness after the ictus and patient may only be partially amnestic about it. Total amnesia is rare.[25] The "eye sign" is important. Convulsive movements with closed eyes are highly suggestive of PNES. Eyes are generally open during GTCS and syncope and if closed before, would open during the event The resistance offered to passive opening of eyes is also an important feature to note in psychogenic cases.

These events have been named differently but the accepted terminology is PNES as decided by epilepsy experts. The American Psychiatry Association names them as conversion disorders [the Diagnostic and Statistical Manual of Mental Disorders, fourth edition (DSM-4)—somatoform section].[25] The most suitable term could be dissociative convulsion. The International Classification of Diseases, Tenth Revision (ICD-10) states that the common theme shared by dissociative disorders is a partial or complete loss of the normal integration between memories of the past, awareness of identity, and immediate sensation and control of body movements (World Healing Organization 1992).[26] Dissociative convulsions may begin in early life and usually begin in a specific situation caused by external (place, time, and witness) or internal triggers (flash backs and emotions). Bowman and Markand's[27] study of 45 cases revealed that dissociative convulsions begin in the young adulthood (20-30 years of age) and are mostly seen in women (78%). Past history of a traumatic event is mentioned by 84% of patients (sexual abuse 67%, physical abuse 67%, and other trauma 73%). Psychiatric comorbidity is common. These include somatoform disorders (89%), dissociative disorders (91%), affective disorders (64%), personality disorders (62%), posttraumatic stress disorders (49%), and other anxiety disorders (47%).[27]

Suggestive features of PNES are given in **Box 5**.

PAROXYSMAL EVENTS OCCURRING DURING SLEEP

Electric shock-like movements, called hypnic/hypnagogic jerks/myoclonus, can occur at the onset of sleep. Body rocking, head banging, or rolling can occur at the sleep-wake transition.[28,29] In adults above 50 years, rapid eye movement (REM) sleep behavior disorders are seen. These conditions often resemble frontal lobe seizures and are difficult to differentiate. In the pediatric age group, sleep walking, sleep talking, nocturnal terrors, and different types of non-rapid eye movement (NREM) parasomnias can be seen. Some motor phenomenon of different types of nocturnal seizures can mimic these various parasomnias. This could be due to cortical release of subcortical motor

> **BOX 5: Psychogenic nonepileptic seizures (PNES)—suggestive features.**
>
> - Atypical auras
> - Preictal behavior changes
> - Gradual onset
> - "Pseudo sleep" at onset
> - Eye closure during unresponsiveness
> - Eye fluttering
> - Discontinuous seizure activity
> - Gradual cessation
> - Absence of postictal state
> - High seizure frequency
> - Excessive variation in seizure manifestations
> - Funny vocalization
> - Resistance to eye opening
> - Prolonged duration
> - Occurrence during clinic visits
> - Suggestibility
> - Precipitation of typical attack by suggestion
> - Attacks only in the presence of others
> - Vocalizations consisting of gagging, retching, gasping, screaming, crying, or moaning
> - Emotional display during events
> - Emotional triggers
> - Retained consciousness and recollection of events with bilateral jerking activity

learned patterns during such episodes.[30] Night terrors happen in the first 3 hours of sleep, when the child suddenly wakes up from sleep, screams, and is terrified. This may last up to 10 minutes. Sleepwalking is found in children of 5-10 years of age and in the first half of sleep. The child walks about in a trance like state with eyes often open and may wander out of the room but usually returns to bed. Several other clinical conditions may resemble epileptic events and will be discussed later on in the appropriate context. Distinctive features of sleep parasomnias and nocturnal frontal lobe epilepsy are depicted in **Table 2**.

CONCLUDING REMARKS

The present chapter would hopefully serve to reinforce three principles: (1) The primacy of the clinical history in the determination of epilepsy diagnosis; (2) the utility of the EEG is at its maximum when the prior probability can be shifted from the extremes (by a good history); and (3) many of the pitfalls can only be avoided by secure knowledge of normal maturational patterns and variation in childhood EEGs. Some of the common errors in pediatric EEG reporting include misinterpreting movement artifacts, high amplitude delta slowing during hyperventilation, and normal sleep markers including vertex waves, spindles, K-complexes, and hypnagogic

TABLE 2: Sleep parasomnias and nocturnal frontal lobe epilepsy.

Feature	Non-REM parasomnias (somnambulism; night terrors)	Nocturnal frontal lobe epilepsy
Onset age	<10 years	*Variable*: Generally childhood or adolescence
Positive family history	60–90%	<40%
Number of attacks/day	1–2	>3
Attacks/month	<1–4	20–40
Clinical course	Disappear by adolescence	Frequency generally stable
Duration of disorder	Around 7 years	Around 20 years
Duration of episodes	Seconds to 30 minutes	Seconds to 2–3 minutes
Semiology	Variable complexity	Very stereotyped on VEEG
Triggering factors	Sleep deprivation; fever; stress	Usually none
Associated conditions	Obstructive sleep apnea	Usually none
Ictal EEG	Slow waves; no epileptiform features	Usually normal; often obscured by muscle artifacts; epileptiform features in <10%
Timing of sleep	First half of night—generally after first 30 minutes	Any time
PSG stage	Stage III–IV	Generally stage II; may be later

(EEG: electroencephalogram; PSG: polysomnography; REM: rapid eye movement; VEEG: video electroencephalogram)

hypersynchronous discharges as epileptiform discharges. In children, benign variants such as wicket waves, benign epileptiform transients of sleep (BETS), and rhythmic midtemporal theta bursts of drowsiness (RMTD) can all mimic epileptiform discharges to an inexperienced reader. The diagnosis of epilepsy is still based on careful elicitation of history from patient (if not too young) and relatives and often repeated analyses of seizure semiology, either physically or videographically (home videos/mobile phones). This still would constitute the closest to a gold standard for diagnosis, although currently often combined with video EEG monitoring. Video EEG, of course, has its own limitations such as its inability to record seizures arising from inaccessible areas like supplementary motor seizures, recording only one form of seizure discharge in children with polymorphic seizure semiologies, and occasional precipitation of generalized seizures (even status) during recording (with a drug withdrawal protocol). Detailed history elicitation by an experienced clinician is more sensitive than EEG or almost any other investigation in the evaluation of epilepsy. Finally, the use of EEG should be framed within a consideration of the costs and consequences of a falsely positive or falsely negative result.

LEARNING POINTS

- The art of listening has to be mastered in differentiating seizures from close mimics. This is time consuming and can be acquired with practice.
- If a dissociative disorder is suspected then suggestive questions like depersonalization and derealization can be helpful. Sense of panic and dissociation are common in the prodromal phase but not often volunteered by patients.[31]
- Patients with a first seizure should ideally be seen by an epileptologist with experience in that field. This gives a diagnostic yield of about 96%.[33] Patient should not be treated in case of diagnostic uncertainty; it is better to adopt a policy of "wait and see".
- Video EEG is very useful in diagnosis particularly in dissociative seizures and a 48-hour recording may clinch the diagnosis in the majority of cases.[32] There indeed are pitfalls with this technique as well. In difficulty to diagnose cases, a combined tilt table test and carotid massaging done under EEG control may be helpful.[33,34] Provocation of a seizure by an experienced clinician under protected environment with proper counseling is accepted ethically.

REFERENCES

1. King MA, Newton MR, Jackson GD, Fitt GJ, Mitchell LA, Silvapulle MJ, et al. Epileptology of the first-seizure presentation: clinical, electroencephalographic, and magnetic resonance imaging study of 300 consecutive patients. Lancet. 1998;352:1007-11.
2. Schreiner A, Pohlmann-Eden B. Value of the early electroencephalogram after a first unprovoked seizure. Clin Electroencephalogr. 2003;34:140-6.
3. Walczak TS, Jayakar P. Interictal EEG. In: Engel J Jr, Pedley TA (Eds). Epilepsy: A Comprehensive Textbook. Philadelphia: Lippincott-Raven; 1997. pp. 831-48.
4. Smith D, Bartolo R, Pickles RM, Tedman BM. Requests for electroencephalography in a district general hospital: retrospective and prospective audit. BMJ. 2001;322:954-7.
5. Ramirez-Lassepas M, Cipolle RJ, Morillo LR, Gumnit RJ. Value of computed tomographic scan in the evaluation of adult patients after their first seizure. Ann Neurol. 1984;15:536-43.
6. Breen DP, Dunn MJG, Davenport RJ, Gray AJ. Epidemiology, clinical characteristics, and management of adults referred to a teaching hospital first seizure clinic. Postgrad Med. 2005;81:715-8.
7. Pohlmann-Eden B, Schreiner A. Epileptology of the first seizure presentation. Lancet. 1998;352:1855-6.
8. Turnbull TL, Vanden Hoek TL, Howes DS, Eisner RF. Utility of laboratory studies in the emergency department patient with a new-onset seizure. Ann Emerg Med. 1990;19:373-7.
9. Dunn MJ, Breen DP, Davenport RJ, Gray AL. Early management of adults with an uncomplicated first generalised seizure. Emerg Med J. 2005;22:237-42.
10. Doğan EA, Ünal A, Ünal A, Erdoğan Ç. Clinical utility of serum lactate levels for differential diagnosis of generalized tonic–clonic seizures from psychogenic non-epileptic seizure and syncope. Epilepsy Behav. 2017;75:13-7.
11. Abubakr A, Wambacq I. Diagnostic value of serum prolactin levels in PNES in the epilepsy monitoring unit. Neurol Clin Pract. 2016;6(2):116-9.
12. Soteriades ES, Evans JC, Larson MG, Chen MH, Chen L, Benjamin J, et al. Incidence and prognosis of syncope. N Engl J Med. 2002;347:878-85.
13. Sararin FP, Louis-Simonet M, Carballo D, Slama S, Rajeswaran A, Metzger JT, et al. Prospective evaluation of patients with syncope: a population based study. Am J Med. 2001;111:177-84.
14. Sarasin FP, Junod AF, Carballo D, Slama S, Unger PF, Louis-Simonet M. Role of echocardiography in the evaluation of syncope: a prospective study. Heart. 2002;88:363-7.
15. Brignole M, Alboni P, Benditt DG, Bergfeldt L, Blanc JJ, Thomsen PE, et al. Task Force on Syncope, European Society of Cardiology. Guidelines on management (diagnosis and treatment) of syncope–update 2004. Executive Summary. Eur Heart J. 2004;25:2054-72.
16. Lempert T, Bauer M, Schmidt D. Syncope: a videometric analysis of 56 episodes of transient cerebral hypoxia. Ann Neurol. 1994;36:233-7.
17. Lin JT, Ziegler DK, Lai CW, Bayer W. Convulsive syncope in blood donors. Ann Neurol. 1982;11:525-8.
18. Newman BH, Graves S. A study of 178 consecutive vasovagal syncopal reactions from perspective of safety. Transfusion. 1982;41:1475-9.

19. Warlow CP, Dennis M, van Gijn J, Hankey G, Bamford J, Sandercock P, et al. Stroke: A Practical Guide to Management, 2nd edition. Malden: Wiley–Blackwell; 2000. pp. 28-105.
20. Kanjwal K, Karabin B, Kanjwal Y, Grubb BP. Differentiation of convulsive syncope from epilepsy with an implantable loop recorder. Int J Med Sci. 2009;6(6):296-300.
21. Mattson RH. Value of intensive monitoring. In: Wada HA, Penry JK (Eds). Advances in epileptology. New York: Raven Press; 1980. pp. 43-51.
22. Gates JR, Ramani V, Whalen S, Loewenson R. Ictal characteristics of psychogenic seizures. Arch Neurol. 1985;42:1183-7.
23. Benbadis SR, O'Neill E, Tatum WO, Heriaud L. Outcome of prolonged video-EEG monitoring at a typical referral epilepsy center. Epilepsia. 2004;45:1150-3.
24. Bowman ES. Why conversion seizures should be classified as a dissociative disorder. Psychiatr Clin N Am. 2006;29:185-211.
25. American Psychiatric Association. Diagnostic and statistical manual of mental disorders, 4th edition. Washington, DC: American Psychiatric Association; 1994. p. 477.
26. World Health Organization. The ICD-10 classification of mental and behavioural disorders. Clinical description and diagnostic guidelines. Geneva, Switzerland: World Health Organization; 1992;151:737-9.
27. Bowman ES, Markand ON. Psychodynamics and psychiatric diagnoses of pseudoseizure subjects. Am J Psychiatry. 1996;153:57-63.
28. American Academy of Sleep Medicine. The International Classification of Sleep Disorders (revised). Chicago, IL: American Sleep Disorders Association; 2001.
29. Tassinari CA, Rubboli G, Gardella E, Cantalupo G, Calandra-Buonaura G, Vedovello M, et al. Central pattern generators for a common semiology in fronto-limbic seizures and parasomnias. A neuroethologic approach. Neurol Sci. 2005;26:225-32.
30. Stone J, Carson A, Sharpe M. Functional symptoms and signs in neurology: assessment and diagnosis. J Neurol Neurosurg Psychiatry. 2005;76:2-12.
31. Deacon C, Wiebe S, Blume WT, McLachlan RS, Young GB, Matijevic S. Seizure identification by clinical description in temporal lobe epilepsy: how accurate are we? Neurology. 2003;61:1686-9.
32. Lobello K, Morgenlander JC, Radtke RA, Bushnell CD. Video-EEG monitoring in the evaluation of paroxysmal behaviour events: duration, effectiveness and limitations. Epilepsy Behav. 2006;8:261-6.
33. Zaidi A, Clough P, Cooper P, Scheepers B, Fitzpatrick AP. Misdiagnosis of epilepsy: many seizure-like attacks have a cardiovascular cause. J Am Coll Cardiol. 2000;36:181-4.
34. Grubb BP, Gerard G, Roush K, Temesy-Armos P, Elliott L, Hahn H, et al. Differentiation of convulsive syncope and epilepsy with head-up tilt testing. Ann Intern Med. 1991;15:871-6.

APPENDIX 1

Epilepsy Imitators

There are a range of conditions associated with recurrent paroxysmal events that may imitate and be misdiagnosed as epilepsies. It is important that these disorders are considered in the evaluation of paroxysmal events as misdiagnosis rates in epilepsy are high throughout the world. History remains the key to a correct diagnosis with video recordings very helpful. There are some conditions in which epileptic and nonepileptic events can coexist. The following is a list of conditions whose clinical manifestations may closely mimic those of epileptic seizures and these conditions may be designated as epilepsy imitators by the ILAE in 2017.

- *Syncope and anoxic seizures*:
  - Vasovagal syncope
  - Reflex anoxic seizures
  - Breath-holding attacks
  - Hyperventilation syncope
  - Compulsive Valsalva
  - Neurological syncope
  - Imposed upper airways obstruction
  - Orthostatic intolerance
  - Long QT and cardiac syncope
  - Hypercyanotic spells
- *Behavioral, psychological, and psychiatric disorders*:
  - Daydreaming/inattention
  - Self-gratification
  - Eidetic imagery
  - Tantrums and rage reactions
  - Out of body experiences
  - Panic attacks
  - Dissociative states
  - Nonepileptic seizures
  - Hallucinations in psychiatric disorders
  - Fabricated/factitious illness
- *Sleep-related conditions*:
  - Sleep-related rhythmic movement disorders
  - Hypnagogic jerks
  - Parasomnias
  - REM sleep disorders
  - Benign neonatal sleep myoclonus
  - Periodic leg movements
  - Narcolepsy–cataplexy
- *Paroxysmal movement disorders*:
  - Tics
  - Stereotypies
  - Paroxysmal kinesigenic dyskinesia
  - Paroxysmal nonkinesigenic dyskinesia
  - Paroxysmal exercise-induced dyskinesia
  - Benign paroxysmal tonic upgaze
  - Episodic ataxias
  - Alternating hemiplegia
  - Hyperekplexia
  - Opsoclonus-myoclonus syndrome
- *Migraine-associated disorders*:
  - Migraine with visual aura
  - Familial hemiplegic migraine
  - Benign paroxysmal torticollis
  - Benign paroxysmal vertigo
  - Cyclical vomiting
- *Miscellaneous events*:
  - Benign myoclonus of infancy and shuddering attacks
  - Jitteriness
  - Sandifer syndrome
  - Nonepileptic head drops
  - Spasmus nutans
  - Raised intracranial pressure
  - Paroxysmal extreme pain disorder
  - Spinal myoclonus

Utility of Sleep in Seizure Diagnosis

Ambar Chakravarty

INTRODUCTION

It had been emphasized on numerous occasions that diagnosis of an epileptic seizure is essentially a clinical one. A number of adjunctive tests are available, of which electroencephalogram (EEG) is the one most commonly used. Its role is primarily in confirming the clinical suspicion of epilepsy. However, it need to be remembered that interictal EEG, which is the one most commonly done, may be entirely normal in around 40% of cases of proved epilepsy patients. Increasing the recording time can certainly increase the yield and this has prompted the development of continuous ambulatory EEG recording as well as the development of long-term video EEG (VEEG). The latter has the unique advantage of correlating the clinical semiology with its EEG counterpart. Various activation procedures have been introduced to increase the yield of routine EEG recording. Two such measures include sleep (natural or induced) EEG and sleep-deprived awake EEG recording. This commentary would briefly address these two issues.

The Greek philosopher Aristotle believed that during sleep there occurs a dissociation between body and soul and that helps in prophecy. Gowers[1] in late 1800 noted that about 20% of subjects with epilepsy have seizures solely during sleep. He also noted that the crucial times were the onset of sleep and end of sleep. Similar observations were made by Janz[2] and others several years later. In relation to EEG, Gibbs and Gibbs[3] noted increase in epileptiform activity during sleep, especially in those with generalized tonic-clonic seizures.

The author would briefly examine the effect of sleep on epilepsy and vice versa first before discussing the effects of sleep deprivation on epilepsy and EEG in particular.

EFFECT OF SLEEP ON EPILEPSY

Janz[2] noted that 10% of daytime epilepsies later become exclusively sleep epilepsies whereas only 6% became diffuse epilepsies in long follow-up. According to Janz,[2] sleep and diffuse epilepsies lasting for >2 years, rarely become daytime awake epilepsy. Later on, an analysis of a number of studies revealed that idiopathic epilepsy is generally wake onset, epilepsies with structural lesions are of the diffuse type and exclusive sleep onset ones are of the intermediate types.

Classically epileptiform discharges are more likely to be recorded in the non-rapid eye movement (NREM) stage of sleep along with such features as sleep spindles and high amplitude delta waves. In rapid eye movement (REM) stage when EEG becomes more asynchronous, epileptic discharges are less evident. Generalized epileptic discharges in particular become more explicit during NREM stage, but focal discharges also become more frequent and prominent. It is interesting to note that while EEG epileptic discharges are more prominent in deeper stages of sleep, clinical seizures are more common in the early NREM stages.

It would not be out of place to mention here a few epilepsy syndromes which almost exclusively or more commonly occur during sleep. Such epilepsies are often of pediatric or juvenile age onset. These include benign epilepsy of childhood with centrotemporal spikes (BECTS), juvenile myoclonic epilepsy (JME), Landau–Kleffner syndrome of speech retardation with continuous spikes and waves during sleep (CSWS), and adult onset focal epilepsies, especially nocturnal frontal lobe epilepsy as also temporal lobe seizures.

Why this Predilection for Sleep Onset of such Seizures?

Possible explanations include hypersynchronization of brain electrical activity during NREM sleep promoting seizures; such hypersynchronization may also cause seizure onset on arousal (as in JME) and lastly circadian mechanisms playing a part in activating interictal seizures discharges.[4]

What Effect does Epilepsy have on Sleep Architecture?

These may be summarized as follows: A reduction in REM sleep; an increase in wake after sleep onset (WASO); increased instability of sleep states, like unclassifiable sleep epochs; an increase in NREM stages I and II; a decrease in NREM stages III and IV; a reduction in density of sleep spindles; and an increase of sleep onset latency.[5,6]

The problem in assessing such changes in sleep architecture is that most patients in whom such studies have been performed had been on various types of antiepileptic drugs (AEDs) and hence the possibility of some of these changes being related to the drugs remain.[7]

Can Epilepsy Lead to a Sleep Disorder?

This is a complex question. General impression is that sleep disorders in persons with epilepsy is the direct effect of severity of epilepsy, combined with the effect of having seizures during sleep. Experimental evidence suggests a role of the amygdala. Clinical evidence suggests that proper treatment of epilepsy with effective AEDs and/or surgery normalizes sleep patterns in most subjects with epilepsy.[8,9]

EFFECTS OF SLEEP DEPRIVATION

This is the most important facet in relation to sleep and epilepsy. Activation of EEG revealing unmasking of epileptiform features by sleep deprivation was first demonstrated by Janz[2] in persons with JME. Subsequent studies have revealed that:[10,11]

- Sleep deprivation can facilitate epileptiform discharges in patients with idiopathic generalized epilepsy.
- Comparison drug-induced sleep versus sleep deprivation-induced sleep revealed that epileptic discharges are more commonly recorded in activated patients with sleep deprivation than during drug-induced sleep recording.
- Awake EEGs after sleep deprivation tend to show more epileptiform features than sleep EEGs after sleep deprivation. This possibly suggests that sleep deprivation is an independent activator of epileptic discharges.

The aforementioned observations would suggest using sleep-deprived EEG as an useful activating tool to unmask latent epileptiform discharges in subjects with history of probable epileptic seizures, but with normal interictal EEG recording. Furthermore, sleep deprivation may at times be used to assess effect of drug treatment in seizure-free individuals again by unmasking latent epileptic discharges. Lastly, the present author feels (and uses) that sleep deprivation may be used to identify individuals where drug withdrawal may be considered, of course, along with other established criteria.

What should be the Duration of Sleep Deprivation?

As of now there are no uniform criteria. For adult patients, the present author suggests whole night sleep deprivation and both awake and sleep EEGs performed the following morning. In children, waking them up about 4 hours before their normal waking time and keeping them awake till the EEG is done seems readily acceptable to the parents.

PITFALLS OF SLEEP EEG AND SLEEP-DEPRIVED EEG IN SEIZURE DIAGNOSIS

- Sleep EEGs (natural or induced), especially in children, are very often overinterpreted. In countries like India, where medical reports are often directly handed over to parents/relatives, the psychological effects of seeing use of such terms such as "seizure disorder" and "epileptiform discharges" on the report are often deleterious. Such practice need to be stopped and great care need to be taken to identify which feature is pathological and which one is a normal feature in a sleep EEG.
- The following normal features recorded in sleep EEGs, especially in children, are often reported as "epileptiform discharges": Hypnagogic hypersynchronous discharges (reported as generalized epileptic discharges); vertex sharp waves and K-complexes; benign epileptiform transients of sleep (BETS); positive occipital sharp transients of sleep (POSTS); various artifacts, e.g., arising from electrode, muscle, movements, and pulse/ECG; and 60 Hz electromagnetic radiation, etc. Lastly, it needs to be remembered that classical hypsarrhythmic pattern of EEG seen in children with infantile spasms (West syndrome) with a chaotic background and multifocal spikes and sharp waves disappears in sleep and is

replaced by a pattern characterized by a semi-periodic generalized symmetrical bursts of spikes and sharp waves with flattening of the intervening background (mimicking a burst suppression pattern). Such features are very often reported as suggestive of generalized epileptic discharges and the diagnosis of infantile spasm missed and institution of appropriate therapy delayed **(Figs. 1A to C)**.

An epileptiform discharge should meet several criteria: (1) Must be paroxysmal meaning that it must stand out clearly from the background; (2) must be spiky meaning that the transition from ascending and descending phase must be abrupt with a short duration (<200 ms); (3) must have a clear field meaning that it should not be confined to one electrode, generally should have a negative polarity; and lastly (4) generally followed by a slow wave. It is, however, true that epileptiform discharges may have different morphologies depending upon the syndrome with which they are associated.

BRIEF NOTES ON OSAS AND SUDEP

Excessive daytime sleepiness is a common complaint among patients with epilepsy. This is independent of the number of AEDs prescribed, their dosage, severity and frequency of seizures, type of epilepsy, and lastly occurrence of nocturnal seizures. Sleep disordered breathing problem, especially obstructive sleep apnea syndrome (OSAS), is common and its incidence could be as high as 30% among patients admitted in epilepsy monitoring units with refractory seizures. Early detection of this treatable condition is essential from history of snoring spells elicited from bed partners and further confirmation by polysomnography. Control of OSAS with nocturnal continuous positive airway pressure (CPAP) or bilevel positive airway pressure (BiPAP) can reduce the frequency of seizures in many such subjects.[12]

Sudden unexpected death in epilepsy (SUDEP)[13] is defined as a *"sudden, unexpected, witnessed or unwitnessed, nontraumatic, and nondrowning death in patients with epilepsy with or without evidence for a seizure and excluding documented status epilepticus in which postmortem examination does not reveal a toxicologic or anatomic cause for death."* This is a serious problem whose exact incidence is not known but could be as high as about 9% among patients with epilepsy. This is much common in patients with uncontrolled seizures and in those having nocturnal seizure. Getting smothered by a pillow while having a seizure during sleep in persons sleeping alone may be one factor related to death in a small subset of patients. But the real pathogenic mechanism in the vast majority is unknown. Current research hints toward

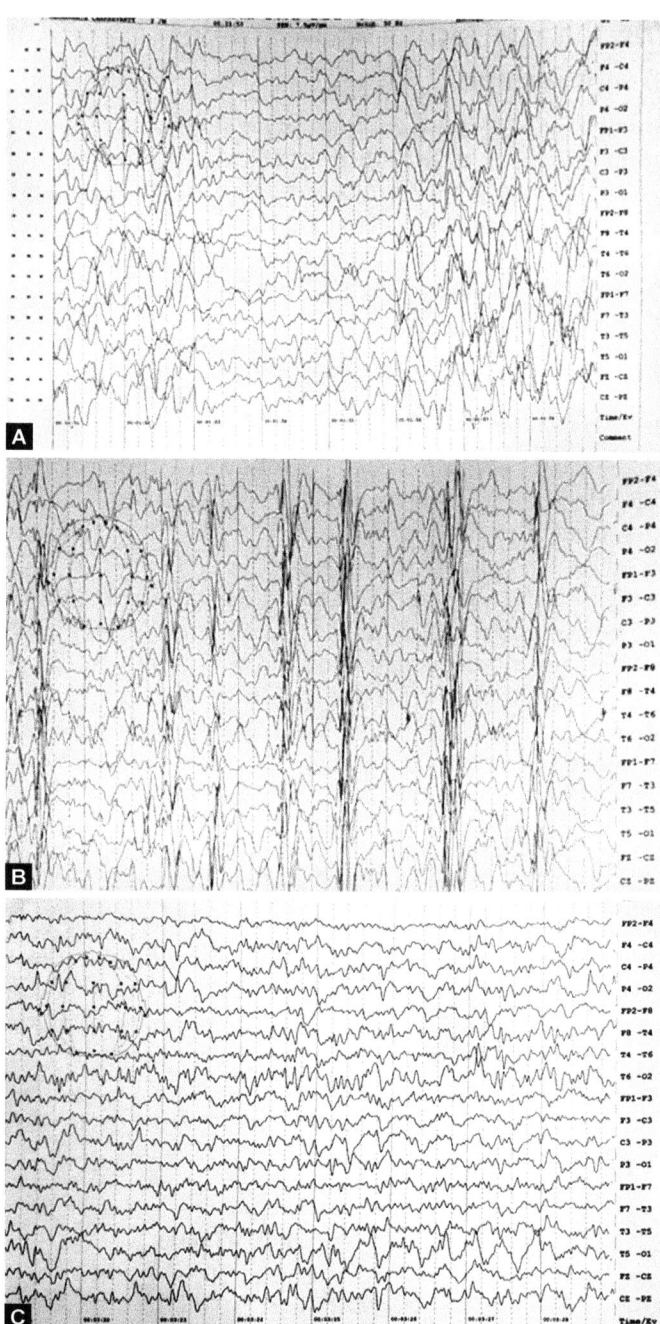

FIGS. 1A TO C: EEGs of a 2-year-old child with West syndrome, delayed milestones, and speech retardation. [(A) February 2016 and (B) March 2016] Sleep records illustrating the modified hypsarrhythmic pattern as mentioned in the text; (C) Sleep EEG (September 2017) illustrating significant improvement in the epileptic discharges after treatment with ACTH and vigabatrin.

various mechanisms such as seizure-related respiratory depression, cardiac arrhythmia, cerebral depression, and autonomic dysfunction. The last mentioned may be the most important—changes in autonomic function during sleep increasing vulnerability to cardiorespiratory decompensation during seizure accounting for increased occurrence of SUDEP during sleep. Simple measures such as not sleeping alone, keeping door unlocked, and avoidance of using pillow at night are generally advised to all patients with epilepsy as precautionary measures. Their real benefits have never been worked out yet.

REFERENCES

1. Gowers WR. Epilepsy and Other Chronic Convulsive Disorders: Their Causes, Symptoms, and Treatment, 1st edition. London: Churchill Livingstone; 1881.
2. Janz D. The grand mal epilepsies and the sleep waking cycle. Epilepsia. 1962;3:69-109.
3. Gibbs EL, Gibbs FA. Diagnostic and localising value of electroencephalographic studies in sleep. Res Publ Assoc Res Nerv Ment Dis. 1947;26:366-76.
4. Kellaway P. Sleep and epilepsy. Epilepsia. 1985;26(suppl 1):S15-30.
5. Touchon J, Baldy-Moulinier M, Billiard M, Besset A, Cadilhac J. Sleep organization and epilepsy. Epilepsy Res Suppl. 1991;2:73-81.
6. Chokroverty S. Sleep and epilepsy. In: Chokroverty S (Ed). Sleep Disorders Medicine. Boston: Butterworth–Heinemann; 1994.
7. Jain SV, Glauser TA. Effects of epilepsy treatments on sleep architecture and daytime sleepiness: An evidence-based review of objective sleep metrics. Epilepsia. 2014;55:26-37.
8. Hallböök T, Lundgren J, Köhler S, Blennow G, Strömblad LG, Rosén I. Beneficial effects on sleep of vagus nerve stimulation in children with therapy resistant epilepsy. Eur J Paediatr Neurol. 2005;9:399-407.
9. Serafini A, Kuate C, Gelisse P, Velizarova R, Gigli GL, Coubes P, et al. Sleep before and after temporal lobe epilepsy surgery. Seizure. 2012;21:260-5.
10. Dinner DS, Luders HO. Epilepsy and Sleep: Physiological and Clinical Relationships. San Diego: Academic Press; 2001.
11. Degen R, Rodin EA. Epilepsy, Sleep, and Sleep Deprivation. Amsterdam: Elsevier; 1991.
12. Vaughn BV, D'Cruz OF, T Beach R, Messenheimer JA. Improvement of epileptic seizure control with treatment of obstructive sleep apnoea. Seizure. 1996;5:73-8.
13. Shorvon S, Tomson T. Sudden unexpected death in epilepsy. Lancet. 2011;378:2028-38.

Geriatric Seizure Mimics: A Problem Oriented Approach

Ambar Chakravarty

INTRODUCTION

The following clinical situations are not very uncommonly encountered in general neurological practice. The present chapter aims at giving practical tips to young clinicians in their day-to-day work.

AN ELDERLY SUBJECT FOUND UNCONSCIOUS ON THE FLOOR

In general, in many such cases, historical details are seldom available as such people often live alone. If the clinician is fortunate enough, he might get some insight into the subject's past medical history, mental status, and drug intake history from neighbors and relatives visiting him from time to time. Information obtained from a local physician may also be useful. Seldom one may notice motor movements suggestive of a seizure or loss of movements in one side of body which would be of localizing value: A stroke on the opposite hemisphere or perhaps a subdural hematoma. The age-old question would always be there: Did he lose consciousness and fell or did he simply slip on a wet floor, fell, and sustained a head injury. The duration of unconsciousness is usually not known, but some idea may be made from onlookers as to when was he last seen, when did he answer the phone last, or when did he use to go out for a walk. It is possible that the subject may be recovering when found; he may or may not be confused, but mostly he would have loss of memory for the event as well as for any premonitory symptoms. In most such cases, therefore, the attending clinician has to totally depend on his own examination findings and clinical acumen.

The important features to look for include:
- *The vitals and assess the airway, breathing, and circulation (ABC)*: Any disturbance of these would merit immediate transfer to a hospital emergency room (ER). On arrival, check capillary blood glucose, oxygen saturation (SpO_2), arterial blood gas (ABG), electrocardiogram (ECG) and cardiac monitoring, drug screen in urine, full blood biochemistry, especially renal and liver functions and serum electrolytes, chest X-ray and X-ray of any other relevant body part based on examination findings, and a CT scan of brain for any evidence of recent stroke or head injury. Exclusion of hypoglycemia is of paramount importance in the elderly.
- A careful search for any evidence of bodily injury needs to be made which include cuts and bruises or hematomas, fractures which may masquerade as a paralyzed limb due to immobility of the affected limb.
- A thorough medical and neurological examination is mandatory whether the subject would remain at home or hospitalized.
- Does he need an electroencephalogram (EEG)? It is unlikely in most such cases to get a positive past history of having had seizures, but it is not uncommon for epilepsy to start later in life. Such seizures are generally symptomatic; commonly related to remote/chronic cerebrovascular disease (acute strokes may also present with a seizure, especially, if it is a hemorrhagic one), recent or past head injury, brain tumors, and metabolic encephalopathies. An EEG is often needed if aforementioned investigations fail to throw adequate light to make a definitive diagnosis of the cause of loss of consciousness and fall. In awake patients, the finding of localizing or lateralizing features like spike discharges would give a clue as also the finding of generalized epileptic discharges. The latter, of course, is uncommon in the present clinical scenario. In unconscious or confused cases, EEG may help to establish a diagnosis of nonconvulsive status epilepticus (NCSE)[1] which is a treatable condition.

A brief discussion on its recognition and management would not out of place here.

- NCSE may occur in two forms: (1) Absence type—seen mostly in children and hence would not be discussed here; and (2) complex partial type—which is more relevant in this case scenario. Apart from the present scenario, possibility of NCSE should be considered in the following situations:
  - Failure to recover full awareness after prolonged general anesthesia (GA)
  - Cerebral hypoxia from any cause, e.g., cardiac arrest, pulmonary embolism, and prolonged systemic hypotension
  - Multisystem diseases such as sepsis, hepatorenal failure, and metabolic encephalopathies
  - *Drug withdrawal*: Benzodiazepines and psychotropics
  - Prolonged postictal confusional state following a generalized tonic-clonic seizure (GTCS)

Diagnostic features in the EEG include:

- Generalized rhythmic bifrontally dominant high voltage sharp waves and spikes
- *Configuration may be mono-, bi-, or triphasic*: Needs differentiation from triphasic waves of hepatic encephalopathy
- *Variable rhythmicity*: Regular runs alternating with more irregular sequences
- Random focal or multifocal sharp or spike discharges
- Occasional cessation of discharges for brief periods and replaced by a relatively low voltage background with dominance of theta waves
- Bifrontal rhythmic delta waves with sharp contours without any obvious sharp wave/spike discharges—need differentiation from encephalopathic pattern by the presence of rhythmicity
- Decrease in rhythmicity and discharges with small dose of intravenous (IV) lorazepam or sodium valproate

AN ELDERLY MAN PRESENTING WITH BLACKOUTS[2]

The term "blackouts" is commonly used to mean one of three things: (1) A brief period of unawareness, (2) A brief period of memory loss, and (3) Thirdly, a brief period of getting disoriented. The differentials would include syncope, seizure, and other causes of intermittent memory disturbances. Apart from a thorough general medical and neurological examination, such subjects need two essential investigations namely:

1. A 48-hour Holter ECG monitoring, and
2. A prolonged EEG recording preferably 24–48 hours video EEG (VEEG).

The former would confirm or exclude the diagnosis of cardiac rhythm disturbance causing a syncope. Failing this, if the story is strongly suggestive of a syncopal attack, a carotid massage test and a head-up tilt test (HUTT) need to be undertaken with utmost care and in a hospital setup in an elderly subject. One, however, should never forget to elicit the drug history as several drugs may cause postural hypotension and orthostatic syncope. Routine checking of supine and standing blood pressure (BP) is essential in the elderly.

A positive EEG, especially VEEG, would clinch the diagnosis of a seizure disorder. However, the pitfalls of routine interictal EEG recording as well as those of VEEG are well-known; other possibilities such as transient global amnesia and a posterior circulation transient ischemic attack (TIA) need consideration. Both these phenomenon result from transient focal cerebral hypoperfusion due to cardiac or artery-to-artery embolism and appropriate investigations need to be carried out and therapeutic measures are instituted.

What to do when everything mentioned earlier fail to reveal the cause of the "blackout"? It is always best to adopt a wait and watch policy rather than prescribe an antiepileptic drug (AED) purely on empirical ground. These agents are more likely to produce serious side effects in the elderly than in younger subjects. Perhaps from the practical point of view, an exception may be made in case of elderly subjects who live alone. If the story is highly suggestive, such subjects, considering the risks involved from having a blackout and fall at home or outside, when nobody is around, may possibly be considered for putting them on an AED like sodium valproate which is less likely to produce very significant adverse effects like drowsiness or dizziness.

AN ELDERLY PERSON IN WHOM RELATIVES NOTICED TO HAVE BRIEF STARING LOOKS AT TIMES

There is no doubt that people do stare frequently. Such a brief staring spell, especially when not accompanied by any motor activity, is very difficult to characterize: Is it daydreaming? Is the person in deep thought? Is the person just absent minded? or Is the person having a true absence seizure like spell? The last possibility is the one which all doctors try to exclude in an absent minded child, when complaints of these come from school teachers and the child's educational performance declines.

However, what is not understood by many is that such staring spells, not very infrequently, may be the sole manifestation of epileptic seizure in the elderly. The difference from a child's staring due a true absence seizure is that in children, such seizures are of the idiopathic generalized seizure (IGS) whereas in the elderly, they are more likely to be of complex partial seizure (CPS), now called focal unaware seizures. The elderly person concerned, when asked during such a spell, would always deny being "unaware", although he would have missed out part of a conversation or might have failed to respond to a question. Close observation during such a spell might reveal very subtle automatism, much less marked than what one usually finds during a classic CPS in an adult or child. Furthermore, such staring spells are always stereotyped in the sense that their duration does not vary from one spell to another. An ictal EEG would reveal focal or lateralized epileptiform discharges confirming the diagnosis. What to do if the EEG does not reveal a classical epileptiform abnormality? If the physician concerned is fully satisfied about the stereotypic nature of such staring spells, he is justified to start the subject on an appropriate AED.

EPISODIC MEMORY LOSS AND FUGUES[3]

Intermittent lapses of memory are very common complaints in the elderly. It is very difficult to demarcate the dividing line between age-related memory problem and that due to organic brain disease. Memory loss is an early feature of dementia of Alzheimer type. Brief episodic lapses of memory may also be due to epileptic seizures of complex partial type. So, whom to send for a long-term EEG monitoring? Again, one needs to consider the stereotypic nature of these spells. That perhaps is the only clinical clue to consider the epileptic nature of such brief spells of memory impairment. Wandering, going out of the house and moving about aimlessly, is a feature of advanced dementia and causes very significant stress on caregivers. On the other hand, on occasions, elderly people with fairly intact cognition may behave in a similar fashion when such episodes are labeled as fugues. Such fugues generally are psychogenic in origin related mostly to depression, but rather rarely they may be a manifestation of epileptic seizure when these are called poriomania or wandertrieb. These subjects manifest compulsive aimless wandering with total loss of memory for a prolonged period and are often robbed of their possessions by miscreants and often they are ultimately picked up by the police. This may represent a form of hyperkinetic seizure. It is debatable whether the wandering phase represents the ictal phase or the postictal phase. Bitemporal discharges are generally recorded during the wandering phase. In contrast, in psychogenic wandering, the EEG during the fugue state is normal or might show nonspecific changes.

Lastly, it is important to remember that excess alcohol intake (not uncommon in elderly people living alone) may simulate (causing unconsciousness, drop attacks, blackouts, and episodic memory loss) as well as precipitate epileptic seizures.

REFERENCES

1. Kaplan PW. Nonconvulsive status epilepticus. Semin Neurol. 1996;16:33-40.
2. Olsky M, Murray J. Dizziness and fainting in the elderly. Emerg Med Clin North Am. 1990;8:295-30.
3. Spiegel D, Lewis-Fernandez R, Lanius R, Vermetten E, Simeon D, Friedman M. Dissociative disorders in DSM-5. Annu Rev Clin Psychol. 2013;9:299-326.

CHAPTER 8

Seizures and Epilepsy Syndromes: What a Psychiatrist should Know?

Neenu Alexander, Chaturbhuj Rathore

INTRODUCTION

Epilepsy is one of the most common neurological disorders across all age groups and presents a considerable diagnostic and therapeutic challenge. Epilepsy is a broad group of disorders encompassing various subtypes and syndromes with diverse etiologies and prognoses. Establishing a correct syndromic diagnosis of epilepsy is an essential step toward optimal management and prognostication. Epilepsy is essentially a clinical diagnosis supplemented by few tests including electroencephalogram (EEG) and magnetic resonance imaging (MRI). There is no test to confirm the diagnosis of epilepsy in all the patients and the available tests have important limitations including low sensitivity. Many other disorders, both organic and nonorganic, can present with episodic manifestations mimicking epilepsy. Hence, a careful and meticulous clinical history remains the most important tool for the diagnosis of epilepsy. Many psychiatric disorders, most notably psychogenic nonepileptic seizures (PNES), can mimic epileptic seizures. On the other hand, epilepsy is associated with various psychiatric comorbidities including depression and psychosis in many patients. Thus, epilepsy represents a disease that falls between the domains of neurology and psychiatry, making it essential for psychiatrists to be aware of the common epilepsy syndromes, their diagnosis, various differential diagnoses, and the broad aspects of epilepsy management.

EPIDEMIOLOGY OF EPILEPSY

Various epidemiological studies of epilepsy have shown a prevalence rate of 5 per 1,000 person-years and an incidence rate of 50 per 100,000 person-years.[1,2] There are estimated 5–8 million people with epilepsy in India. The prevalence of epilepsy is higher in children and elderly with a prevalence rate of 1% and incidence of 50–150 per 1,000 person-years in these age groups.[3]

Many studies have also evaluated the incidence of various seizure types in the population. These studies involving patients with newly diagnosed epilepsy have shown that 50–60% patients have focal seizures, 30–40% have generalized seizures, whereas epilepsy type remains undetermined in 5–10% of the patients **(Fig. 1)**.[1,2] Regarding the etiology, in a recent hospital-based study focusing on etiology in children, the etiology was considered as genetic in 22% of the cases, structural/metabolic in 28% of the cases, and undetermined in 50% of the cases **(Fig. 2)**.[4]

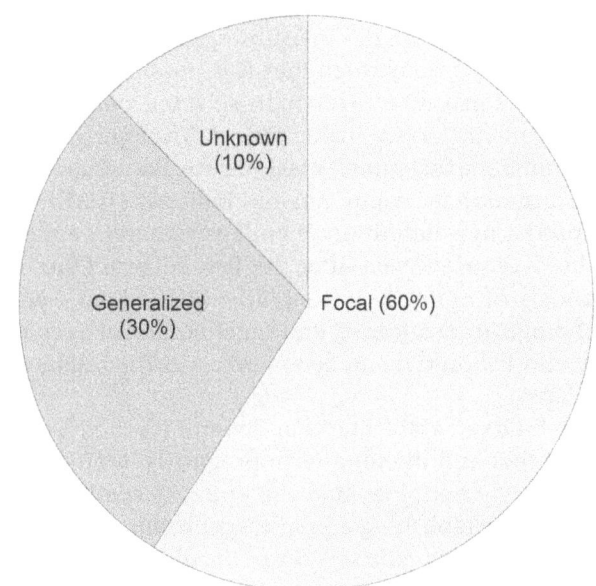

FIG. 1: Distribution of different epilepsy types in patients with new-onset epilepsy.

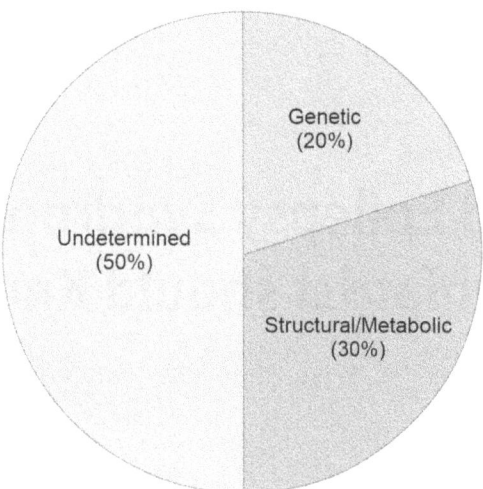

FIG. 2: Distribution of different epilepsy etiologies in patients with new-onset epilepsy in a hospital setting.

> **BOX 1: Practical and clinical definition of epilepsy.**
>
> Epilepsy is a disease of the brain defined by any of the following conditions:
> - At least two unprovoked (or reflex) seizures occurring >24 hours apart
> - One unprovoked (or reflex) seizure and a probability of further seizures similar to the general recurrence risk (at least 60%) after two unprovoked seizures, occurring over the next 10 years
> - Diagnosis of an epilepsy syndrome
>
> Epilepsy is considered to be resolved for individuals who had an age-dependent epilepsy syndrome but are now past the applicable age or those who have remained seizure-free for the last 10 years, with no seizure medicines for the last 5 years

EPILEPSY DEFINITION AND CLASSIFICATION

Conceptually, epilepsy is defined as "a disorder of the brain characterized by an enduring predisposition to generate epileptic seizures and by the neurobiological, cognitive, psychological, and social consequences of this condition."[5] For practical purposes, this translates into a patient experiencing recurrent (at least two) and unprovoked seizures. Based on this, the practical definition of epilepsy is proposed as "occurrence of two or more unprovoked seizures, 24 hours apart." The subsequent natural history studies have demonstrated that it is possible to predict the risk of seizure recurrence in selected patients and certain patients have a higher risk of developing second seizure after the first unprovoked seizure. Based upon this, the International League Against Epilepsy (ILAE) have proposed a new definition of epilepsy wherein epilepsy can be diagnosed even after the first seizure **(Box 1)**.[6] Diagnosis of epilepsy has significant medical, social, psychological, economic, and legal consequences and every effort should be made to make a correct diagnosis of epilepsy.

The fundamental factor that determines the response to treatment and the long-term prognosis in epilepsy is the underlying etiology and the epilepsy syndrome. In this regard, establishing a proper syndromic diagnosis is crucial for assessing the severity of the disease, predicting the prognosis, and making short- and long-term therapeutic decisions. The features aiding in diagnosing an epilepsy syndrome include the type of seizures, age at onset, mode of inheritance, associated comorbidities, as well as EEG and MRI findings.

The broad differentiation between focal and generalized seizures has been known for more than a century. Recent advances in neuroimaging, genetics, and molecular biology have improved our understanding of the pathogenesis of seizures and epilepsies. With these advances, many new epilepsy syndromes and etiologies have been defined. Still, the broad differentiation of seizures and epilepsies into focal and generalized types remains the basic fulcrum for epilepsy classification.

Based upon recent advances, the ILAE has proposed a revised classification of seizures and epilepsies in 2017.[7,8] The current system allows epilepsy classification at three levels and also includes the concept of comorbidities and etiology at each level.

Epilepsy Classification Level I: Seizure Type

The first step in epilepsy classification is to ascertain the seizure type based upon the clinical history and often added by the EEG. The present seizure classification system retains the two broad-spectrum categories of focal and generalized onset seizures while adding another category of unknown onset **(Flowchart 1)**. The term "unknown onset" is used when a patient presents with a generalized tonic-clonic seizure (GTCS) or a seizure with only behavior arrest, and it is not possible to classify as focal or generalized onset seizure. The focal seizures are further classified as focal-aware seizures when consciousness is preserved (previously simple partial seizures) and the patient is able to respond to external stimuli, and as "focal-seizures with impaired awareness" (previously complex partial seizures) when the patient is not able to respond appropriately. Both types of focal seizures can have motor manifestations such as tonic or clonic movements or automatisms and nonmotor manifestations such as sensory and emotional experiences. The secondarily

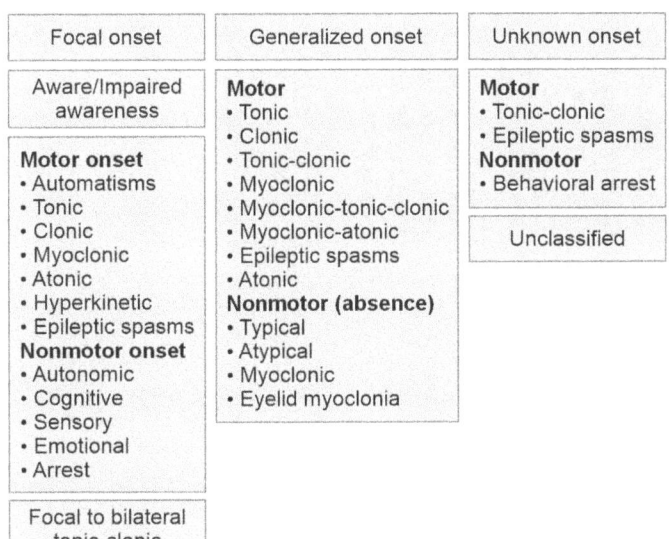

FLOWCHART 1: New seizure classification proposed by the International League Against Epilepsy.

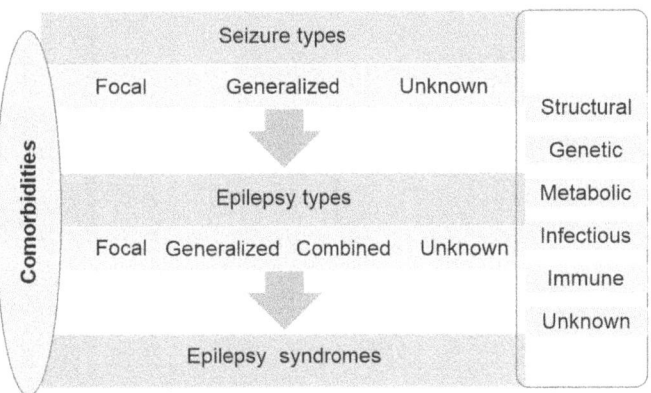

FLOWCHART 2: New epilepsy classification proposed by the International League Against Epilepsy.

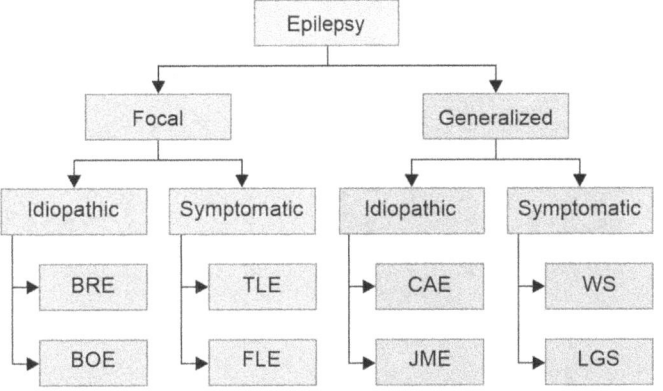

FLOWCHART 3: A simplistic classification of epilepsy syndromes.
(BOE: benign occipital epilepsy; BRE: benign rolandic epilepsy; CAE: childhood absence epilepsy; FLE: frontal lobe epilepsy; JME: juvenile myoclonic epilepsy; LGS: Lennox–Gastaut syndrome; TLE: temporal lobe epilepsy; WS: West syndrome)

generalized seizures have been renamed as focal to bilateral tonic-clonic seizures. Similarly, generalized seizures can have motor and nonmotor (absence seizures) manifestations. As determining the seizure type is the most important step in diagnosis of epilepsy, every effort should be made to differentiate between focal and generalized seizures.

Epilepsy Classification Level II: Epilepsy Type

Similar to seizure types, epilepsies are also classified into two broad types: (i) Focal and (ii) generalized epilepsies **(Flowchart 2)**. Focal epilepsies are associated with seizures that originate from the networks confined to one hemisphere. On the other hand, generalized epilepsies are characterized by seizures that originate at some point within, or rapidly engage bilaterally distributed networks. The 2017 classification recognizes that some epilepsies cannot be clearly dichotomized into either focal or generalized epilepsies.[8] Thus, certain epilepsies, especially early-onset severe epilepsies in children such as Lennox–Gastaut syndrome and Dravet syndrome, have both focal and generalized seizures. On the other hand, certain epilepsies cannot be clearly classified into focal or generalized epilepsies due to the lack of information. Such epilepsies are classified as unknown epilepsies.

Epilepsy Classification Level III: Epilepsy Syndrome

An epilepsy syndrome represents a complex of clinical features, signs, and symptoms that together define a distinctive, recognizable clinical seizure disorder. Apart from the seizure type (focal or generalized), the underlying etiology largely determines the epilepsy syndrome. While some of the epilepsy syndromes have a single specific etiology (SCN1A mutation in Dravet syndrome), others have multiple etiologies leading to similar clinical phenotype such as West syndrome. The important clinical features that are helpful for ascertaining syndromic diagnosis include the history of any antecedent event, age at onset, seizure type/s, seizure frequency, family history, and response to the treatment. This has to be supplemented by the information obtained from EEG, MRI, and in some cases from genetic studies. The simple two-tier classification system of epilepsy syndromes involves the initial categorization of epilepsy into either focal or generalized epilepsy. Subsequently, each type is further classified as idiopathic (either unknown or presumed genetic etiology) or symptomatic (known or presumed symptomatic etiology) epilepsy **(Flowchart 3)**. The common epilepsy syndromes according to the age of onset are summarized in **Table 1** and the major categories are discussed here.

TABLE 1: Epilepsy syndromes defined into broad categories.

Broad category	Specific syndrome	Age at onset	Seizure types	Development	EEG and MRI features	Medical management	Surgery	Prognosis
Benign neonatal and infantile epilepsies	Benign familial neonatal convulsions	Newborn	Focal, tonic or clonic ± apnea and cyanosis	Normal	Normal: AD Inheritance: KCNQ2 mutations; rarely KCNQ3 or SCN2A mutations	PB, LVT	No	Good; remission by 6 months; 10–30% develop late epilepsy
	Benign familial infantile convulsions	Infant	Brief focal seizures; often in clusters	Normal	Normal: PRRT2, SCN2A, KCNQ2 or 3 mutations in few cases	PB, CBZ, and LVT	No	Remission within 1 year of onset
	Benign infantile seizures (nonfamilial)	Infant	Brief focal seizures; often in clusters	Normal	Normal	PB, CBZ, and LVT	No	Remission within 1 year of onset
	Benign myoclonic epilepsy in infancy	3 months to 3 years	Myoclonic seizures; often reflex in response to tactile or auditory stimuli	Often normal: 10% may develop delay later on	EEG often shows generalized discharges; MRI is normal	VPA and CLB	No	Remission by 3–5 years; 10% develop late epilepsy
Idiopathic focal epilepsies of childhood	Benign rolandic epilepsy	3–13 years	Infrequent nocturnal hemiclonic seizures with facial jerks and salivation	Normal: 10% may have attention deficits	EEG: Typical centrotemporal spikes with frontal dipole; MRI: Normal	LVT, OXCBZ, and VPA	No	Good; remission by 2 years in most; 10% may have difficult to control seizures
	Benign early onset occipital epilepsy (Panayiotopoulos syndrome)	2–8 years	Nocturnal focal seizures with eye deviation, vomiting, and autonomic features	Often normal	EEG: Typical occipital, centroparietal or multifocal spikes in sleep	LVT, OXCBZ, and VPA	No	Good; remission by 2 years in most
	Benign early onset occipital epilepsy (Gastaut syndrome)	6–17 years	Typical focal occipital seizures with visual aura	Often normal	EEG: High amplitude bi-occipital spikes during sleep with scotosensitivity	LVT, OXCBZ, and VPA	No	Good; remission by 18 years in most; 10% have difficult to control seizures

Continued

Continued

Broad category	Specific syndrome	Age at onset	Seizure types	Development	EEG and MRI features	Medical management	Surgery	Prognosis
Genetic generalized epilepsies	Epilepsy with myoclonic astatic seizures (Doose syndrome)	3–5 years	Myoclonic-atonic seizures with falls are defining features; patients may have atypical absences and GTCS	Normal at onset; slows down during the disease course	Normal at onset and then evolves into high amplitude slowing and 2–5 Hz generalized spike-wave discharges	VPA, CLB, LTG, and TPM	No	Variable; two-thirds remit by 10 years; one-third have protracted course
	Childhood absence epilepsy	5–6 years	Typical absence seizures	Normal; few have ADHD and learning problems	Typical 3 Hz spike-wave discharges precipitated by hyperventilation	ETX, VPA, LTG, and LVT	No	Good; most remit by late childhood; 10–20% evolve into juvenile myoclonic epilepsy
	Epilepsy with myoclonic absences (Tassinari syndrome)	1–12 years	3 Hz unilateral or bilateral shoulder myoclonic jerks superimposed on tonic arm abduction; May have GTCS	50% may have mild intellectual disability	Generalized spike-wave discharges; Ictal EEG shows 3 Hz generalized spike-wave discharges	VPA, LTG, LVT, and CLB	No	Variable; 40% may have remission
	Juvenile absence epilepsy	10–12 years	Typical absence seizures; GTCS later on	Normal; few have ADHD and learning problems	Typical 3 Hz and atypical, 4–6 Hz, generalized spike-wave discharges	VPA, LVT, LTG, and TPM	No	Drug responsive; usually do not remit
	Juvenile myoclonic epilepsy	12–18 years	Early morning myoclonic jerks (100%); GTCS (80%); absences (20%)	Normal	Atypical, 4–6 Hz, generalized spike-wave discharges; 30% have photosensitivity	VPA, LVT, LTG, and TPM	No	Drug responsive; usually do not remit
	Epilepsy with generalized tonic-clonic seizures only	12–18 years	GTCS often precipitated by sleep deprivation	Normal	Generalized spike and polyspike wave discharges	VPA, LVT, LTG, and TPM	No	Drug responsive; usually do not remit
	Eyelid myoclonia with absences (Jeavons syndrome)	3–12 years	Frequent eyelid myoclonia with absences; GTCS	Half of the patients may have mild intellectual disability	Generalized spike and polyspike-wave discharges; photosensitivity and eye-closure sensitivity	VPA, LVT, LTG, and TPM	No	Often drug resistant and do not remit

Continued

Continued

Broad category	Specific syndrome	Age at onset	Seizure types	Development	EEG and MRI features	Medical management	Surgery	Prognosis
Symptomatic focal epilepsies	Migrating partial seizures of early infancy	Infancy	Focal, often subtle, tonic or clonic seizures with autonomic features	Severe delay	EEG: Slow background with multifocal spikes; often genetic (KCNT1, SCN2A) etiology	PB, PHT, CBZ, TPM, VPA, and BDZ	No	Drug resistant; early mortality
	Mesial temporal lobe epilepsy with hippocampal sclerosis	8–14 years;	Febrile seizures in 30–50% cases; typical automotor focal seizures; rare secondarily generalized seizures	Memory decline with increasing duration	Anterior temporal spike-wave discharges; MRI shows mesial temporal sclerosis	CBZ, LCM, LVT, and CLB	ATL	Drug resistant; very good outcome with surgery
	Mesial temporal lobe epilepsy associated with other lesions	Variable	Automotor seizures with motor features; frequent secondary generalization and seizure clustering	Memory decline with increasing duration	Anterior and mid-temporal spikes; MRI shows dysplasia; low grade tumors; vascular lesions	CBZ, LCM, LVT, and CLB	ATL	Drug resistant; very good outcome with surgery
	Neocortical epilepsies associated with focal cortical dysplasia	Variable; 1–10 years	Extratemporal seizures depending upon the location	Frequent learning disability, ADHD, and cognitive problems	EEG: Rhythmic spikes over the location; MRI: Type I or II FCD	CBZ, LCM, LVT, and CLB	Lesionectomy	Drug resistant; often good outcome with surgery
	Neocortical epilepsies associated with other lesions	Variable	Extratemporal seizures depending upon the location	Frequent learning disability, ADHD, and cognitive problems	EEG: Spikes over the location; MRI shows gliosis, low-grade tumors or vascular lesions	CBZ, LCM, LVT, and CLB	Lesionectomy	Drug resistant; often good outcome with surgery
	Cryptogenic focal epilepsies	Variable	Seizure semiology according to site of origin; temporal or extratemporal	Cognitive and memory problems if seizures are uncontrolled	MRI is normal while EEG shows focal spikes	CBZ, LCM, LVT, and CLB	Selected drug-resistant cases	60% remit; 40% have drug resistance
	Rasmussen's encephalitis	6–12 years	Focal motor seizures progressing to epilepsia partialis continua	Normal at onset; subsequent progressive hemiparesis, hemianopia, and dominant hemispheric language deficits	MRI: Progressive hemispheric atrophy; EEG shows focal spikes with increasing slowing	CBZ, LCM, LVT, and CLB	Hemispherotomy	Drug resistant; very good outcome with surgery

Continued

Continued

Broad category	Specific syndrome	Age at onset	Seizure types	Development	EEG and MRI features	Medical management	Surgery	Prognosis
Symptomatic focal epilepsies	Gelastic epilepsy with hypothalamic hamartoma	1–4 years	Gelastic seizures in early stage; later on focal and generalized seizures	Normal development at onset; regression with onset of epileptic encephalopathy	Normal at onset; later on multifocal and generalized spikes; MRI shows hypothalamic hamartoma	CBZ, LCM, LVT, and CLB	Hamatoma resection	Drug resistant; good outcome with surgery
	Hemiconvulsion-hemiplegia-epilepsy syndrome	1–5 years	Initially prolonged episode of focal clonic seizures leading to hemiplegia; drug-resistant focal seizures later on	Hemiparesis; cognitive problems in all	Uni-hemispheric atrophy and gliosis	CBZ, LCM, LVT, and CLB	Hemispherotomy	Drug resistant; very good outcome with surgery
Epileptic encephalopathies	Early myoclonic encephalopathy	Newborn-infant	Multifocal myoclonus; focal seizures	Severe impairment	EEG: Burst-suppression pattern; MRI usually normal; mainly metabolic or genetic etiology	Steroids, VPA, and CLB	No	Drug resistant; early mortality
	Ohtahara syndrome	Newborn-Infant	Tonic spasms; focal seizures	Severe delay	EEG: Burst-suppression pattern; mainly structural etiology in form of malformation of cortical development	Steroids, VPA, and CLB	Possible if focal pathology	Drug resistant; early mortality; better outcomes if amenable to surgery
	West syndrome	Infant	Epileptic spasms; may be asymmetrical	Severe delay	EEG: hypsarrhythmia; MRI may show structural lesion	Steroids, VGB, VPA, LTG, and CLB	Possible if focal pathology	One-third have favorable outcome; others progress to LGS and have severe impairment
	Lennox–Gastaut syndrome	2–9 years	Multiple seizures; tonic; atonic; complex absences; focal and focal to bilateral tonic clinic seizures	Severe delay and regression	EEG: Slow background; multifocal and generalized slow spike-wave discharges; MRI may show structural lesion	Broad-spectrum drugs	Possible if focal pathology/callosotomy for drop attacks	Drug resistant; one-third have favorable outcome; others have severe impairment

Continued

Continued

Broad category	Specific syndrome	Age at onset	Seizure types	Development	EEG and MRI features	Medical management	Surgery	Prognosis
Epileptic encephalopathies	Dravet syndrome	Infant	Febrile hemiclonic seizures; myoclonia	Severe delay and regression	EEG: Multifocal and generalized spikes; MRI: Normal	VPA, CLB, TPM, and CNB	No	Drug resistant; unfavorable prognosis
	Landau–Kleffner syndrome	3–6 years	Focal and generalized seizures; atonic	Auditory agnosia and language regression	EEG: Continuous dominant hemispheric or generalized spike–wave discharges during sleep	Broad-spectrum drugs; immunotherapy	Multiple subpial transections in selected cases	May remit by 6–12 years; guarded language outcome
	Epilepsy with continuous spike waves in slow sleep	4–7 years	Seizure often infrequent; may be focal, generalized, and atonic seizures	Regression and behavioral problems	Rare focal or multifocal spikes in wakefulness; almost continuous generalized spike–wave discharges during sleep	Broad spectrum drugs; Immunotherapy	None	Remit by 8–12 years; guarded cognitive outcome
Familial (autosomal dominant) epilepsies	Autosomal dominant nocturnal frontal lobe epilepsy	Childhood	Nocturnal hypermotor frontal seizures; often frequent	Normal	Often normal	CBZ, LCM, CLB, and TPM	None	Variable
	Familial lateral temporal lobe epilepsy	Childhood-adolescent	Temporal seizures with auditory and experiential auras	Normal	EEG shows temporal spikes	CBZ, LCM, CLB, and TPM	None	Variable
	Generalized epilepsies with febrile seizures plus (except Dravet syndrome)	Childhood-adolescent	Variable phenotype; generalized febrile and afebrile seizures	Often normal	Often normal; EEG may show generalized spike–wave discharges; SCN mutations	VPA and CLB	None	Variable; often remit by adulthood
Progressive myoclonus epilepsies	Unverricht–Lundborg, Lafora, neuroceroid lipofuscinoses (NCL)	Late infant–adolescent	Multifocal myoclonus, focal and generalized seizures	Regression	EEG: Multifocal and generalized spikes, slow background; generalized atrophy on MRI	Broad-spectrum drugs	None	Drug resistant; progressive course; early mortality

(BDZ: benzodiazepines; CBZ: carbamazepine; CLB: clobazam; ETX: ethosuximide; GTCS: generalized tonic-clonic seizures; LCM: lacosamide; LTG: lamotrigine; LVT: levetiracetam; OXCBZ: oxcarbazepine; PB: phenobarbitone; PHT: phenytoin; TPM: topiramate; VPA: valproate; VGB: vigabatrin; ZNS: zonisamide)

Symptomatic Generalized Epilepsies

This group of epilepsies basically include epileptic and developmental encephalopathies. Epileptic and developmental encephalopathies are a broad group of disorders where seizures, epileptiform abnormalities on EEG, or both contribute to progressive cerebral dysfunction leading to severe cognitive and behavioral impairments.[9] These conditions are classically seen in young children and share certain common features: (1) Drug-resistant polymorphic seizures where a patient has multiple seizure types in various combinations including epileptic spasms, tonic and atonic seizures, focal seizures, GTCS, and complex absence seizures; (2) developmental delay or psychomotor regression; (3) EEG showing multifocal and generalized spike-wave discharges superimposed on slow background activity and poorly formed sleep architecture **(Fig. 3)**.

The various syndromes under this category are summarized in **Table 1**. The two most common and prototype syndromes in this category include West syndrome and Lennox–Gastaut syndrome. Rather than a single etiology, these syndromes represent age-specific response of the brain to various insults. The etiologies of epileptic encephalopathies are variable and include genetic, structural, and metabolic causes. These are most severe form of epilepsies where seizures are very frequent and resistant to pharmacological treatment. The resective surgery is an option in a selected group of patients where a focal substrate can be identified either through MRI or functional imaging. Prognosis is universally poor and only a small proportion of patients can achieve independent living.

Psychiatric Comorbidities in Epileptic Encephalopathies

Children with developmental and epileptic encephalopathies have poorly controlled seizures and multiple psychiatric comorbidities. By definition, these patients have psychomotor delay or regression and almost all the patients have moderate-to-severe cognitive or intellectual disability.[9] These patients have developmental delay involving cognitive, motor, social-emotional, communicative, and adaptive domains. In addition, majority of the patients have behavioral problems including attention-deficit/hyperactivity disorder (ADHD), autism spectrum disorder (ASD), and aggressive behavior including self-harm behavior. Various surveys among the caregivers of patients with Dravet syndrome and Lennox–Gastaut syndrome have shown that approximately two-thirds of the children have autistic features, about half of them have ADHD, and approximately one-fourth children have diagnosed ASD.[10] In addition, majority of these children have motor impairment and sleep disturbances while older children often have features of anxiety.

The pathogenesis of psychiatric comorbidity in patients with epileptic encephalopathies is multifactorial and is contributed by the underlying etiology of epilepsy, frequent drug resistant seizures, and continuous epileptiform discharges on EEG. The behavioral problems can be aggravated or precipitated by certain antiseizure medicines (ASMs) such as phenobarbitone, clobazam, levetiracetam, brivaracetam, and perampanel and these drugs should be used with caution in patients with epileptic encephalopathies.[11]

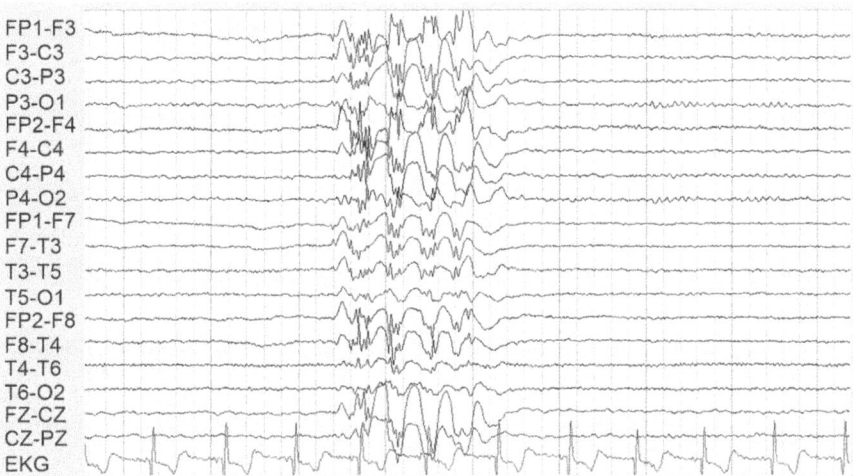

FIG. 3: Typical electroencephalogram in a patient with Lennox–Gastaut syndrome showing disorganized background activity and multifocal and generalized, slow (2–2.5 Hz), spike-wave discharges (common average montage; low frequency filter: 1.0 Hz, high frequency filter: 70 Hz, sensitivity: 10 μv/mm).

Benign Focal Epilepsies of Childhood

These have been termed as self-limited focal epilepsies of childhood in the new 2017 epilepsy classification.[8] These epilepsies as a group are characterized by: (1) An age-specific onset; (2) infrequent seizures; (3) normal cognition; (4) typical EEG features with activation of EEG spikes during sleep **(Fig. 4)**; (5) pharmacoresponsiveness; and (6) favorable prognosis with age dependent remission.[12]

The two broad syndromes under this category are benign epilepsy with centrotemporal spikes (BECTS, benign rolandic epilepsy) and benign occipital epilepsies. Benign epilepsy with centrotemporal spikes typically starts at 3–13 years of age. The seizures are typically nocturnal and are characterized by unilateral facial and upper limb jerks with salivation. Approximately 10% of patients can present with focal status epilepticus. The seizures are usually infrequent, respond to low doses of ASMs, and remit within 2–3 years of onset in the majority of the cases. However, approximately 10% of patients can have atypical features in the form of early age of onset, frequent drug resistant atonic seizures, and cognitive difficulties. However, these patients also remit by the age of adolescence. The early onset occipital lobe epilepsy typically starts between 3–7 years of age. The seizures in these patients have atypical features in the form of autonomic manifestations such as episodic pallor and syncope such as episodes and repeated vomiting lasting for 15–30 minutes. Seizures are infrequent and respond well to medicines with majority of the patients undergoing remission within 2–3 years. Late-onset occipital epilepsies present with typical occipital seizures in the form of visual auras and versive motor seizures. Prognosis is variable in these patients with one-third of the patients having drug-resistant epilepsy.

Psychiatric Comorbidities in Benign Focal Epilepsies

Although considered benign, recent evidence suggest that a small proportion of children with benign focal epilepsies of childhood can have development and language delay, behavioral problems, and anxiety. Various studies have shown that approximately 10% of the children with benign focal epilepsies of childhood have cognitive disabilities, language delay, features of autism, attention deficit, and anxiety.[13,14]

Genetic Generalized Epilepsies

Genetic generalized epilepsies (GGE) are a group of epilepsies with presumed genetic basis and no underlying structural or anatomical substrate. GGE make up one-fourth of all epilepsies and usually have onset at a young age. These epilepsies have three types of seizures in various combinations: GTCS, absence seizures, and myoclonic seizures. These epilepsies are classified by the predominant seizure type, age at the onset, and to a certain extent by EEG features **(Box 2 and Fig. 5)**.[15] The ILAE recognizes four well-established syndromes of GGE, namely childhood absence epilepsy (CAE), juvenile absence epilepsy (JAE), juvenile myoclonic epilepsy (JME), and GTCS alone (GTCA). These four syndromes are grouped together as idiopathic generalized epilepsies (IGE). In addition, there are many other rare epilepsy syndromes that share the features of GGE but are not recognized by the ILAE such as eyelid myoclonia with absences. Seizures in patients with GGE typically begin at early age and are easy to control. While absences and myoclonic seizures can be quite frequent in untreated patients, GTCS are typically infrequent. Diagnosis of GGE is based on the typical seizure semiology, classical EEG features, and positive family history in selected patients. It is important to inquire about the minor seizures such

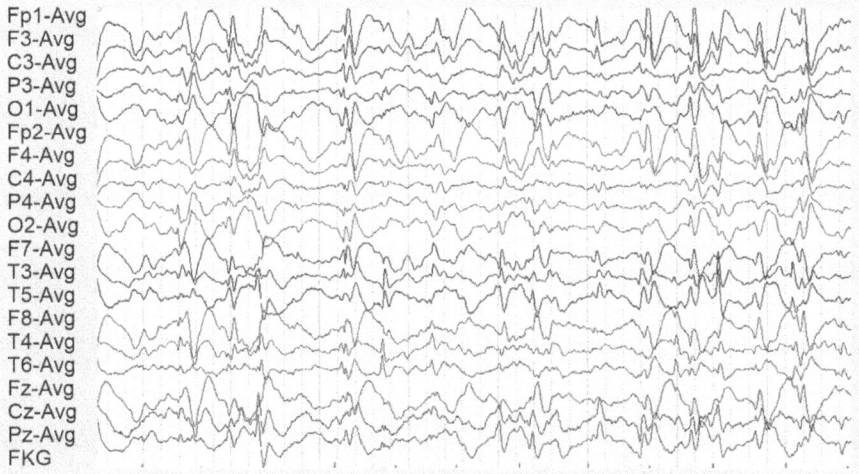

FIG. 4: Typical sleep electroencephalogram in a patient with benign rolandic epilepsy showing frequent bilateral centrotemporal spikes (longitudinal bipolar montage; low frequency filter: 1.0 Hz, high frequency filter: 70 Hz, sensitivity: 10 μv/mm).

BOX 2: General features of genetic generalized epilepsies.

- Have underlying genetic predisposition
- Onset in early age, usually during childhood or adolescent age
- Infrequent generalized seizures
- Have absence, myoclonic, and generalized tonic-clonic seizures in various combination
- Early morning seizure occurrence and evidence of photosensitivity
- Normal IQ and neurological examination
- Electroencephalogram (EEG) shows bilateral, symmetrical, and synchronous generalized spike-wave and polyspike-wave discharges
- EEG discharges are often precipitated by hyperventilation, photic stimulation, and eye closure
- Good response to antiseizure medicines in 80–90% of the patients

as absences and myoclonic jerks in all the patients with apparent GTCS as wrong diagnosis is often the cause for the uncontrolled seizures in patients with GGE.

Psychiatric Comorbidities in Genetic Generalized Epilepsies

Prevalence and nature of various psychiatric and cognitive comorbidities have been well studied in patients with CAE and JME. Although considered a benign epilepsy syndrome, patients with CAE have significant associated comorbidities. In a study of 69 children with CAE and 103 controls who were evaluated with a semistructured psychiatric interview and language and cognitive assessment, 25% of patients had subtle cognitive deficits, 43% had linguistic difficulties, and 61% had a psychiatric diagnosis.[16] The psychiatric diagnoses consisted of ADHD in 26% patients and anxiety in 20% patients. In addition, 30% of the children had significant behavioral problems as evaluated through child behavioral checklist. The longer duration of disease, higher seizure frequency, and the use of ASMs were associated with higher cognitive and psychiatric comorbidities. Similarly, in a study of 49 patients with JME, 35% patients had psychiatric comorbidity mainly in the form of personality disorders in 23% and axis I disorder in 19% patients.[17] In a review of 20 studies, Filho and Yacubian reported that approximately one-third of the patients with JME have psychiatric disorders mainly in the form of anxiety, mood disorders, and psychosis.[18] Additionally, these patients also have personality disorders predominantly in the form of impulsive behavior and borderline personality. There is substantial data to suggest that patients with longer duration of disease and those with drug-resistant JME have a higher risk of developing psychiatric comorbidity.[19]

Symptomatic Focal Epilepsies

This is the largest group and approximately 50% of patients with epilepsy belong to this group. The epilepsies in this group occur at all ages and have diverse etiologies and variable prognoses. Still, a definite etiology can be determined in only approximately 20% of the patients either with MRI and/or genetic studies. These patients experience focal and/or focal with bilateral tonic-clonic seizures and the seizure symptoms are largely determined by the site of seizure origin, e.g., temporal, frontal, and occipital **(Table 2)**. Approximately 50–60% of patients have temporal lobe epilepsy (TLE) while others have

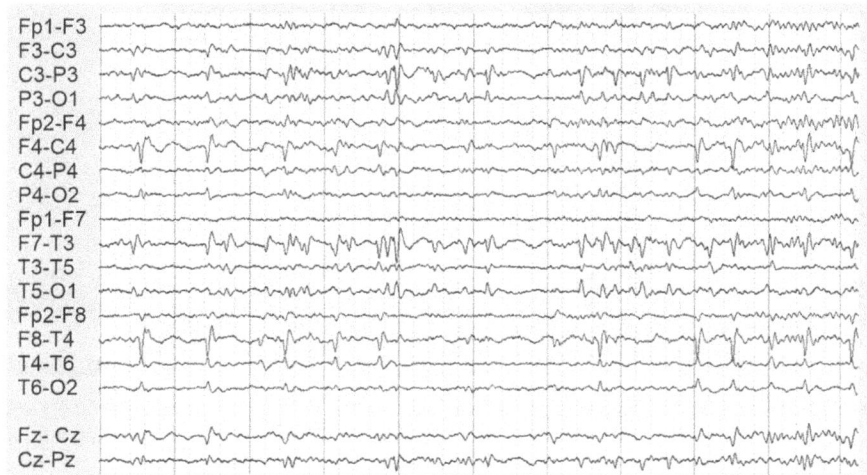

FIG. 5: Typical electroencephalogram of a patient with juvenile myoclonic epilepsy showing frontally, dominant, generalized, spike, and polyspike wave discharges (Longitudinal bipolar montage; low frequency filter: 1.0 Hz, high frequency filter: 70 Hz, sensitivity: 10 μv/mm).

TABLE 2: Differentiation between temporal and extratemporal seizures.

Characteristics	Temporal seizures	Extratemporal seizures
Auras	Limbic (epigastric, fear, and Déjà vu)	Visual, sensory, none, nonspecific
Ictal behavior	Hypomotor (arrest, stare)	Hypermotor; vocalization
Motor movements	Complex (automatisms)	Primary (tonic, clonic, and myoclonic)
Posturing	Dystonic	Tonic
Evolution	Slow	Rapid
Duration	Longer (>1 minute)	Brief
Frequency	Low (1–4/month)	High
Clustering/ Generalization	Rare	Frequent

epilepsies originating from extratemporal areas. The etiologies differ according to the age of the onset. The main etiologies include hippocampal sclerosis, malformations of cortical development including focal cortical dysplasia (FCD), gliosis related to birth injury, head trauma or stroke, tumors, and vascular malformations such as cavernoma and arteriovenous malformations **(Figs. 6A to F)**. Approximately 30–40% of the patients in this group have drug-resistant epilepsies and are potential candidates for epilepsy surgery. The mesial temporal lobe epilepsy associated with hippocampal sclerosis (MTLE-HS) is the most well characterized syndrome in this group and is briefly discussed here.

Approximately 80–90% of the patients with MTLE-HS have drug-resistant epilepsy and the hippocampal sclerosis is the most common etiology in patients with drug-resistant epilepsy **(Fig. 6A)**. In large series of patients with drug-resistant epilepsy undergoing surgery, 50–70%

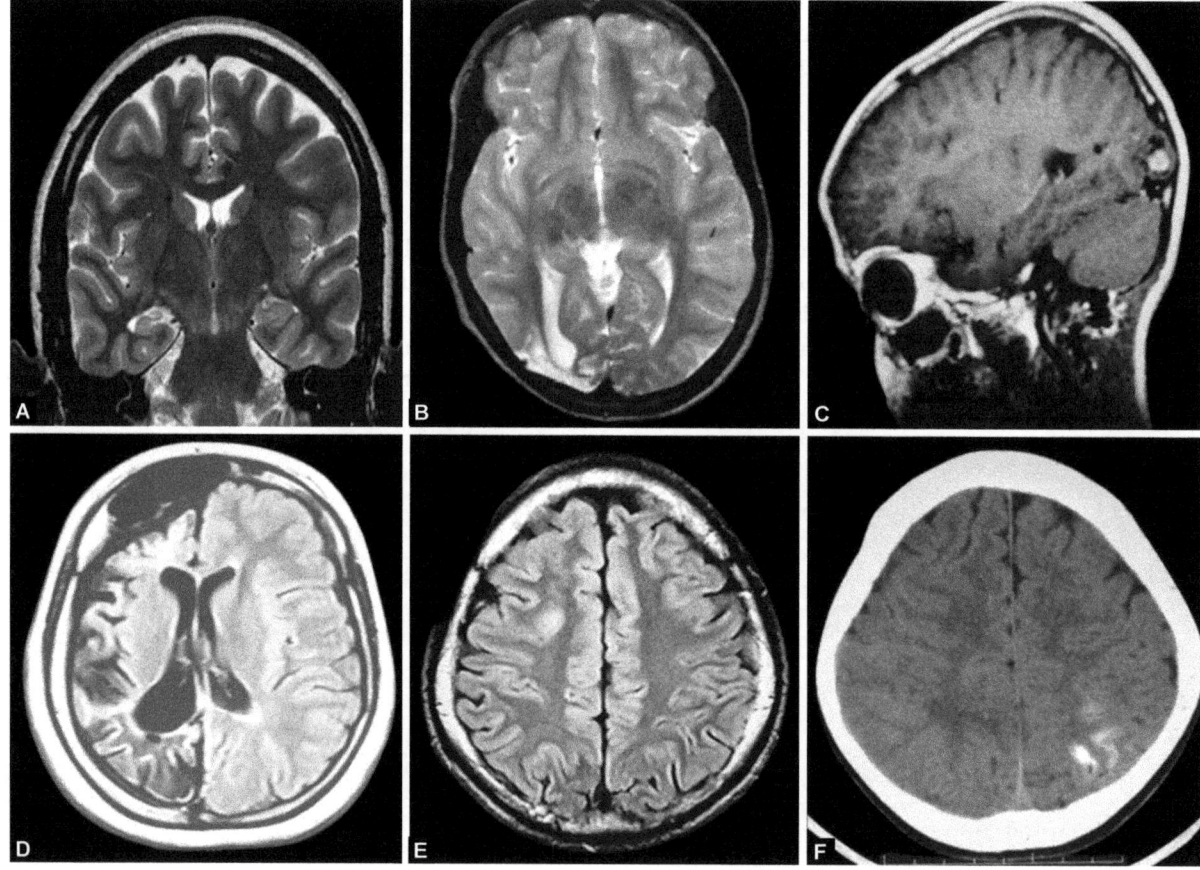

FIGS. 6A TO F: Common substrates for epilepsy; (A) right mesial temporal sclerosis; (B) right occipital gliosis; (C) left occipital ganglioglioma; (D) right hemispheric gliosis; (E) right frontal focal cortical dysplasia; and (F) Sturge–Weber syndrome involving left parieto-occipital region.

> **BOX 3: Syndrome of mesial temporal lobe epilepsy associated with hippocampal sclerosis.**
>
> - History of febrile seizures in 50–60% of the patients aged between 1 and 3 years
> - Latent period of 5–10 years before the onset of habitual seizures
> - Seizures onset between 10–15 years of age
> - Typical temporal complex partial seizures: Aura, Arrest, Automatisms, Amnesia (4A's)
> - Seizure frequency of 2–4 per month
> - Rare bilateral tonic clonic seizures
> - Rare seizure clustering
> - Magnetic resonance imaging shows unilateral mesial temporal sclerosis
> - Interictal and ictal electroencephalogram shows typical temporal patterns **(Fig. 7)**
> - 90% of patients do not respond to antiseizure medicines
> - Progressive memory decline and behavioral problems
> - Excellent response to surgical treatment

cases are due to MTLE-HS.[20] The syndrome of MTLE-HS have well-defined clinical course and prognosis[21] **(Box 3)**. Febrile seizures in childhood occur in 50–60% of the patients with MTLE-HS. Seizures are typically characterized by initial limbic aura (fear, epigastric rising sensation, and Déjà vu) followed by behavioral arrest, oral and manual automatisms, loss of awareness with surroundings, and amnesia. The seizures are typically resistant to medical therapy and epilepsy course in often progressive with gradual decline in memory and appearance of psychiatric and behavioral symptoms. The response to surgical treatment is excellent with 70–80% of the patients becoming seizure free.[22,23] Due to this fact, epilepsy surgery should be considered early in these patients once they fail to respond to optimal medical therapy.

Focal cortical dysplasias **(Fig. 6E)** and gliosis **(Figs. 6B and D)** are another common etiologies of drug-resistant focal epilepsy especially in children.[24,25] FCDs are focal malformations of cortical development resulting from abnormal neuronal organization and proliferation. These are common causes of drug-resistant epilepsy and represent 25% of the cases in various surgical series and 50% of cases in pediatric epilepsy surgery series.[24] The majority of patients with FCD have epilepsy onset before 2 years of age and have frontal lobe epilepsy. These children do not have any initial precipitating injury and have focal motor seizures, which occur multiple times a day. The majority of the patients with FCD have drug-resistant epilepsy, which is amenable to surgical treatment.

Psychiatric Comorbidities in Temporal Lobe Epilepsy

Being the most common and chronic epilepsy, the psychiatric comorbidities have been extensively studied and well characterized in patients with TLE. Overall, psychiatric comorbidities are more common in patients with TLE compared to other epilepsies. Psychiatric comorbidities are present in approximately 50% of the patients with chronic TLE mainly in the form of mood disorders (25%), anxiety (15%), and psychosis (10%).[18,26] The psychosis in patients with TLE has features different from schizophrenia and has been referred as schizophreniform psychosis or psychosis of epilepsy.[27,28] The main differences are lack of negative symptoms of schizophrenia particularly flattening of affect and personality deterioration, better premorbid personality, presence of paranoid delusions and delusions of reference, uncommon command hallucinations, and a more benign course. The only factor which has been consistently shown to be associated with the development of psychosis is the longer duration of epilepsy.[28,29] Mood disorders, especially depression, are present in 25% of the patients with TLE.[30,31] The symptoms of depression in patients with TLE are different from primary depression and are characterized by fewer neurotic traits, more psychotic traits, higher anxiety scores, more abnormal affect and chronic dysthymic disorder, high hostility scores especially for self-criticism and guilt, waxing and waning course, and sudden onset and brief duration of symptoms. Due to these differences, it has been termed as "dysthymic-like disorder of epilepsy".[30,31] Children with TLE and depression can present with unusual symptoms such as aggression, irritability, anger, and oppositionality.[32] Both depression and psychosis are under recognized in patients with TLE as both the patients and physicians are often reluctant to discuss psychiatric comorbidity and the main focus remains on seizure control. However, depression is associated with poor quality of life in these patients and proper treatment of depression can improve the quality of life.[33]

DIFFERENTIAL DIAGNOSIS OF EPILEPSY

Diagnosis of epilepsy is usually ascertained on clinical grounds and is based on the accurate history and precise description of the event by an eye witness. There are no confirmatory tests to positively diagnose epilepsy in all the patients. Epilepsy can have variable manifestations which can cause diagnostic confusion **(Box 4)**. On the other hand, many other conditions can have episodic manifestations, which can closely mimic epilepsy. The first step in the proper management of epilepsy is to confirm that patient

> **BOX 4: Uncommon manifestations in epilepsy.**
>
> - Atypical auras with minimal or no impairment of consciousness, e.g., abdominal pain, déjà vu, jamais vu, fear
> - Status emeticus in temporal lobe epilepsy (TLE)
> - Fugue like state in TLE
> - Apnea and cyanosis in neonates
> - Bimanual automatisms with preserved responsiveness in nondominant TLE
> - Hypermotor frontal lobe seizures with preserved responsiveness
> - Visual auras followed by headache in occipital lobe epilepsy mimicking migraine
> - Autonomic manifestations in Panayiotopoulos syndrome
> - Pure sensory seizures in patients with parietal lobe epilepsy
> - Gelastic and dacrystic seizures in hypothalamic hamartoma
> - Absence seizures with oral and hand automatisms
> - Eyelid myoclonia with preserved responsiveness
> - Absence and complex partial status epilepticus
> - Self-induced seizures in photo and pattern sensitive epilepsy
> - Clustering of brief seizures with preserved responsiveness
> - Drug-induced episodic cerebellar dysfunction related to peak drug levels

> **BOX 5: Clinical features of syncope that may result in misdiagnosis as epileptic seizures.**
>
> - Convulsive movements (myoclonic jerks, tonic posturing of limbs, and automatisms) can occur in 70–90% of patients with syncope
> - Eyes are commonly open and rolled upward during syncope
> - Visual and auditory hallucinations can occur in 60% patients with syncope
> - Serious injuries are common in patients with syncope
> - Rarely generalized seizure can occur following prolonged hypoxia
> - Urinary and fecal incontinence is common in syncope

has definite epilepsy and not an epilepsy mimicker. A careful evaluation is important to suspect and confirm various conditions, which can mimic seizures. Some of the common nonepileptic events are summarized here.

Syncope

Syncope is one of the most common conditions misdiagnosed as epilepsy. The misdiagnosis often results from failure to take a detailed history. Children often have syncopal episodes while standing in the school assembly for prolonged periods. A typical episode of syncope is preceded by prodromal symptoms of lightheadedness, visual blurring, uneasiness, nausea, and sweating. Following these symptoms, the patient usually slumps to the ground associated with cold and pale skin, sweating, and flaccid limbs. Although the majority of syncopal episodes last less than a minute and the patient immediately regains full consciousness, variations in these symptoms can occur **(Box 5)**.[34] Hence, a detailed analysis of all symptoms together, along with the analysis of the setting and situation in which an episode has occurred, is important for the correct diagnosis of syncope.

Psychogenic Nonepileptic Seizures

Psychogenic nonepileptic seizures are commonly misdiagnosed as epilepsy. Approximately 30% of the patients undergoing video EEG (VEEG) monitoring have PNES while 10% of the patients with apparent drug-resistant epilepsy have a combination of true seizures and pseudoseizures. Based on clinical manifestations, PNES can be divided into four major categories: (1) Events with generalized motor movements, (2) akinetic events or pseudosyncope, (3) axial dystonic events, and (4) trembling events.[35,36] The clinical features that are helpful in the diagnosis of PNES are listed in **Table 3**. Overall, a high degree of suspicion coupled with careful analysis of symptoms and settings is greatly helpful in the diagnosis of PNES.

Migraine

Migraine is the most common neurological disorder with episodic manifestations. While the diagnosis of classical migraine with and without aura is easy, the diagnosis of complicated migraine and "acephalgic" migraine often presents diagnostic challenges.[37] Patients with migraine may have atypical auras such as unilateral limb paresthesias, limb pain, unilateral weakness, and blindness.[38] Patients with basilar migraine can have episodic symptoms of brain stem dysfunction, which may even progress to loss of consciousness. Isolated recurrent vertigo may be the only manifestation of migraine. All these manifestations can lead to a diagnosis of the seizures. On the other hand, patients with occipital lobe epilepsy can have visual auras and postictal headache, which can be confused with migraine. It is useful to remember that symptoms of migraine develop gradually and last over hours compared to seizures where symptoms develop rapidly and are brief.

Sleep Disorders (Parasomnia)

The common disorders causing diagnostic confusion are nonrapid eye movement (NREM) sleep parasomnias such as sleep terror, confusional arousals, and sleep walking.

These are commonly confused with frontal lobe seizures. Various features can help in differentiating parasomnias from frontal lobe seizures **(Table 4)**. A composite scale, FLEP (Frontal Lobe Epilepsy and Parasomnia) scale, is highly sensitive and specific for differentiating frontal lobe seizures from parasomnia.[39]

TABLE 3: Differences between epileptic and psychogenic nonepileptic events.

	True seizures	**Psychogenic seizures**
Setting	Unpredictable	Often in stressful situation; in the presence of witnesses
Time duration	Rarely more than 2 minutes	Often more than 2 minutes
Stereotypy	Always	May occur
Episodes during sleep	Common	Cannot occur in true sleep
Course of episodes:		
• Onset	• Abrupt	• Gradual
• Fluctuating course	• Rare	• Common
• Eyes closed	• Very rare	• Common
• Violent thrashing movements	• Rare	• Common
• Side to side head movements	• Rare	• Common
• Pelvic thrusting	• Rare	• Can occur
• Opisthotonus posturing	• Very rare	• Can occur
• Asynchronous movements	• Very rare	• Common
• Automatisms	• Common	• Rare
• Recovery	• Gradual	• Abrupt
• Postictal confusion	• Common	• Not present
• Recall	• Rare	• Common
Tongue bite	Common; sides of tongue	Rare; mild; tip of tongue
Examination during episode:		
• Resistance to eye opening	• No	• Present
• Visual tracking (placing a mirror in front of patient)	• Absent	• Present
• Dropping of hand over face	• Hand falls on face	• Avoids face
• Corneal and plantar reflex	• May be impaired	• Intact

TABLE 4: Differentiating between frontal lobe seizures and parasomnia.

	Parasomnias	**Frontal lobe seizures**
Age at onset	Early childhood	Adolescence or later
Timing in night	Usually during first third of night	Unpredictable
Numbers per night	Usually single	Multiple
Aura	Absent	May be present
Motor movements	Complex and nonstereotyped	Stereotyped
Tonic or dystonic posturing	Absent	May be present
Wandering outside the room	May be present	Absent
Complex directed behavior	May be present	Absent
Duration	2–30 minutes	<2 minutes
Recall	Absent	Present
Sleep stage	Stage III or IV of NREM sleep; REM sleep	Stage II NREM sleep
Full arousal after the event	Common	Rare
Positive family history	Common	Rare

(NREM: nonrapid eye movement sleep; REM: rapid eye movement; RBD: sleep behavior disorder)

CLINICAL APPROACH TO EPILEPSY DIAGNOSIS

After confirming that the patient has seizures, the next step is to establish the epilepsy type and epilepsy syndrome. A stepwise approach for patients presenting with seizure/s is provided in **Figure 7**. It is equally important to ascertain associated comorbidities in a patient with epilepsy so as to provide holistic management of epilepsy. A good clinical history is the most important tool in differentiating epilepsy from nonepileptic events while investigations help in confirming the syndromic diagnosis and ascertaining the etiology of epilepsy.

Clinical History

A detailed history should be obtained from the patient and from those who have witnessed the event regarding the onset, duration, progression, and termination. Patients and caregivers should be encouraged to record the events on mobile video phones, which can make diagnosis easy. However, recording may not be possible in brief or infrequent events. It is important to emphasize that attention should be paid to the combination and sequence of different features to reach a diagnosis rather than relying on one feature.

Role of Electroencephalogram and Video Electroencephalogram

Electroencephalogram plays an important role in confirming the diagnosis of epilepsy and epilepsy syndrome. It also provides useful prognostic information regarding the risk of seizure recurrence after the first seizure and after ASM withdrawal in patients with epilepsy in remission. To obtain the maximum yield from an EEG, it should be properly done and correctly interpreted. An EEG should be done for a minimum period of 30–40 minutes and every attempt should be made to obtain a sleep record. True epileptiform abnormalities are very rare in normal people and their presence is a strong indicator of the diagnosis of epilepsy.[40] In patients with epilepsy, a single awake plus sleep record will reveal epileptiform abnormalities in about 80% of individuals; however, about 10–20% of patients with epilepsy never show epileptiform abnormalities on repeated EEGs.[41] Therefore, a normal EEG does not exclude the diagnosis of epilepsy. However, epileptiform abnormalities are present in 10–20% of patients with cerebral palsy, mental retardation, and autisms even when these patients do not have seizures and EEG alone cannot be used for the diagnosis of epilepsy in such patients.[42]

Long-term VEEG monitoring is the gold standard test for the characterization of the nature of paroxysmal events, confirming the epilepsy syndrome in selected cases, and for presurgical evaluation in patients with drug-resistant epilepsy. However, the utility of VEEG is limited in patients with infrequent episodes. Long-term VEEG is a cost and labor-intensive investigation, is not freely available, and is technically demanding. A high degree of experience and expertise is required for the correct interpretation of VEEG data. Hence, it should be judiciously used in indicated cases.

Neuroimaging

Neuroimaging provides an important clue for the diagnosis of the etiology of epilepsy. For all practical purposes, an MRI is a preferred investigation compared to a CT scan

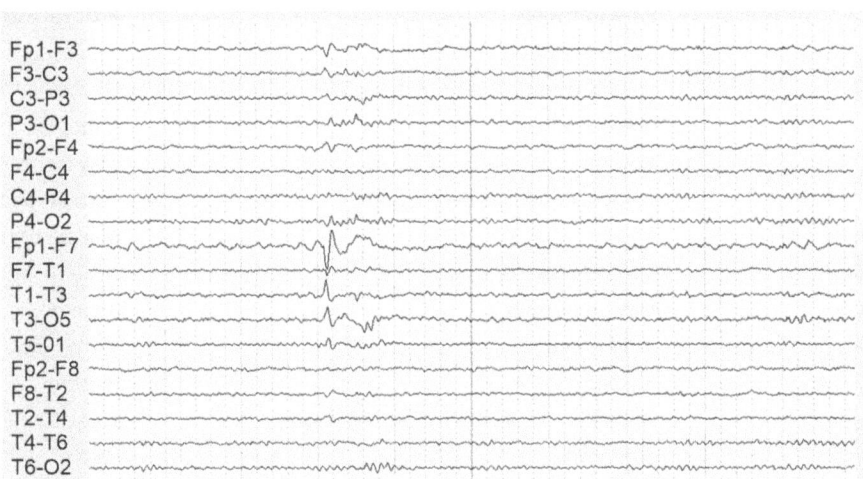

FIG. 7: An electroencephalogram in a patient with left medial temporal epilepsy with hippocampal sclerosis showing typical left anterior temporal spike (Longitudinal bipolar montage; low frequency filter: 1.0 Hz, high frequency filter: 70 Hz, sensitivity: 10 μv/mm).

for the evaluation of epilepsy. However, in a resource-poor setting, a CT scan can be done to rule out potential lesions such as tumors, which may require additional intervention. Emergent imaging is indicated only in cases with acute symptomatic seizures or when acute brain pathology such as a stroke or neuroinfection is suspected. In all other cases, an elective MRI should be done whenever indicated. Patients with simple febrile seizures, well-defined generalized epilepsy syndromes, and those with benign focal epilepsies do not require neuroimaging, and an MRI can be avoided in such patients. An MRI should be done with a proper epilepsy protocol, which is optimized for the evaluation of hippocampi and the detection of small malformations of cortical development. A 3T MRI should be obtained in patients with drug-resistant epilepsy for proper evaluation and detection of subtle lesions. Common substrates for epilepsy on MRI are presented in **Figures 6A to F**.

TREATMENT OF EPILEPSIES

Planning appropriate treatment in patients with epilepsy is crucial for ensuring an optimal outcome. Pharmacotherapy with ASMs remains the cornerstone of epilepsy treatment. Choosing an appropriate ASM for a given patient requires consideration of multiple factors including the underlying epilepsy syndrome, age and gender of the patient, effectiveness and tolerability of the ASMs, socioeconomic status, and associated comorbidities. Doses of ASMs should be slowly titrated and kept at a minimum with avoidance of over-treatment and polytherapy. Patients tend to become overtly anxious after epilepsy diagnosis and hence proper counseling regarding the nature of the disease, need of long-term treatment, and expected outcomes is a must to alleviate anxiety.

The majority of the evidence for the use of ASMs in the treatment of epilepsy is derived from uncontrolled case series and unblinded randomized controlled trials. There are very few class I or class II studies evaluating the efficacy of ASMs in patients with epilepsy.

Treatment of Focal Epilepsies

The introduction of many new ASMs in the last decade has made the choice of ASM for the initial therapy of patients with focal epilepsy wider as well as difficult. As stated earlier, there is a lack of double-blind, randomized class I trials comparing the efficacy of various ASMs as initial monotherapy for focal epilepsy. The only class I trial has reported better tolerability and equal efficacy of oxcarbazepine compared to phenytoin in children.[43] Recently Standard Versus New Antiepileptic drugs (SANAD I and II) trials have evaluated the efficacy of various ASMs as initial monotherapy for focal epilepsy in patients aged ≥5 years.[44,45] Both SANAD I and SANAD II are unblinded, randomized, pragmatic trials where treating physicians managed the patients and made decisions as per the clinical requirements after randomization. In SANAD I, 1,721 patients with focal epilepsy were randomly assigned to receive carbamazepine, gabapentin, lamotrigine, oxcarbazepine, or topiramate.[44] In this study, lamotrigine was found to have the same efficacy as carbamazepine while it was better tolerated than carbamazepine. Based on these results, the authors suggested that lamotrigine is clinically better and is a cost-effective alternative for patients with focal seizures. Subsequently, a recently published SANAD II trial has evaluated the efficacy of lamotrigine, levetiracetam, and zonisamide in 990 patients with newly diagnosed focal epilepsy. In this study, lamotrigine was found to be superior to both the other drugs and it remains the first drug of choice for the initial monotherapy of patients with focal epilepsy.[45]

For practical purposes, lamotrigine is a difficult drug to use, requires a long period of titration, and is associated with a higher risk of allergic reaction. Due to these reasons, we usually do not use lamotrigine as initial monotherapy for patients with focal epilepsy. Hence, in practice, we use either levetiracetam or carbamazepine as a first-line drug in patients with newly diagnosed focal epilepsy due to their ease of use **(Table 5)**. Lacosamide is a drug with emerging evidence of its efficacy for focal epilepsy and likely to become an alternative to other drugs as initial monotherapy of focal epilepsy.[46] Drugs such as topiramate, zonisamide, and phenobarbitone are associated with cognitive side effects and are not preferred as initial monotherapy or first add-on in patients with epilepsy. Once a drug is chosen as initial monotherapy, it should be started at a low dose and should be titrated slowly to a moderate maintenance dose **(Table 6)**. In case of seizure recurrence, the dose should be slowly titrated to the maximally tolerated dose.

If a patient does not respond to the maximally tolerated dose of initial monotherapy, the choice is between an alternative monotherapy and the addition of a new ASM. Few small studies have not reported any difference in seizure outcomes between the two approaches.[47] Practically, if the first ASM has not produced any benefit then it needs to be replaced by an alternative ASM. We believe that carbamazepine is the most effective drug for focal epilepsy and we usually switch over to carbamazepine if it has not been tried as the initial monotherapy. However, in cases of carbamazepine failure, we usually prefer to add another ASM. There are no comparative trials of different ASMs as adjuvant therapy. In patients with focal

TABLE 5: Choice of ASMs according to the epilepsy syndrome.

Syndrome	First-line ASMs	Second-line ASMs	ASMs to avoid
Absence epilepsy	ETX, VPA	LTG, LVT	CBZ, PHT, OXCBZ
Other GGE	VPA, LTG, LVT	TPM, PRM, ZNS	VGB, CBZ, PHT, OXCBZ
Focal epilepsies	CBZ, LTG, LCM	LVT, TPM, CLB, PHT	
West syndrome	ACTH, VGB	VPA, TPM, LTG, CLB	CBZ, OXCBZ
Lennox–Gastaut syndrome	VPA, LTG, TPM	CLB, CLP, LVT, ZNS	CBZ, OXCBZ
Dravet syndrome	VPA, TPM, CLB	LVT, ZNS	LTG, CBZ
Landau–Kleffner syndrome CSWS	VPA, CLB, Steroids	LVT, LTG, TPM, IVIG	CBZ, OXCBZ

(ASM: antiseizure medications; CBZ: carbamazepine; CLB: clobazam; CSWS: continuous spike-wave discharges in slow sleep; ETX: ethosuximide; GGE: genetic generalized epilepsies; LCM: lacosamide; LTG: lamotrigine; LVT: levetiracetam; OXCBZ: oxcarbazepine; PB: phenobarbitone; PHT: phenytoin; TPM: topiramate; VGB: vigabatrin; VPA: valproate; ZNS: zonisamide)

TABLE 6: Commonly used antiseizure medicines, their average daily doses, and daily cost of therapy.

Antiseizure medicine	Usual maintenance dose (mg/kg/day)	Maximum dose (mg/kg/day)	Dosing	Daily cost in INR
Phenobarbitone	2–3	8	OD	5–6
Phenytoin	4–5	8	OD	5–6
Carbamazepine	15	20	BID	6–8
Sodium valproate	20	40	BID	10–12
Lamotrigine	4–5	15	BID	15–20
Topiramate	4–5	8	BID	20
Levetiracetam	20	40–50	BID	20–30
Zonisamide	4–5	8	OD/BID	15
Oxcarbazepine	20	35	BID	20–30
Lacosamide	4–5	12	BID	15–20
Perampanel	0.6–0.9 (4–6 mg)	0.18 (10–12 mg)	OD	20–30
Brivaracetam	1.6–2.0	3.0–3.2	BID	20–30
Clobazam	0.5	1	OD/BID	10

(BID: twice daily; OD: once daily)

epilepsy, we usually prefer to add clobazam as an add-on therapy to carbamazepine because of its ease of use, lower risk of side effects, and possible synergistic effect with carbamazepine.[48]

Treatment of Genetic Generalized Epilepsies

While the overall principles of management in patients with GGE are similar to other epilepsies, certain treatment protocols are specific to GGE.[15] As the majority of the patients with GGE have multiple seizures types **(Flowchart 4)**, the chosen ASM should be effective for all types of seizures. Importantly, certain drugs especially those acting through sodium channel blockade can aggravate seizures in patients with GGE.[49] These narrow-spectrum drugs, notably carbamazepine and phenytoin, can lead to worsening of seizure control in GGE and are not recommended in these patients. Based on these observations, patients with GGE or those with unclassified epilepsy are usually treated with broad-spectrum ASMs. Seizures in the majority of the patients with GGE can be controlled with small doses of appropriate ASMs, and hence these patients should be initiated at low doses of ASMs. Lastly, the majority of the patients with GGE, except CAE, require long-term treatment. Hence, proper choice of ASM and patient counseling are essential to avoid long-term side effects and to ensure compliance.

Many early observational studies in patients with GGE established the efficacy of valproate in the management of patients with GGE.[50] Subsequently, two major randomized trials (SANAD I and II) have specifically examined the efficacy of various broad-spectrum ASMs in patients with

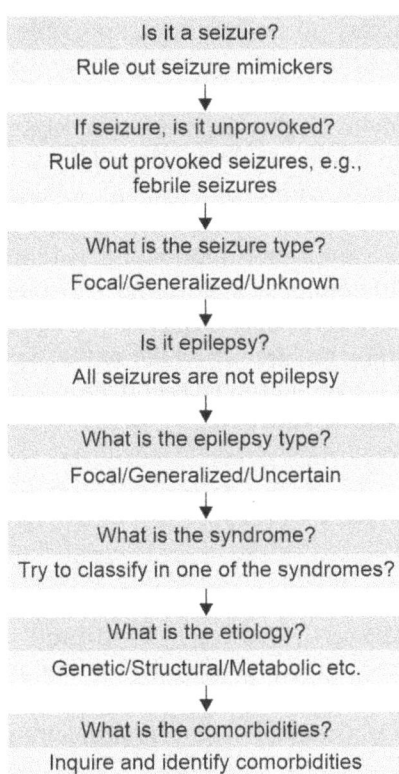

FLOWCHART 4: Stepwise approach to a patient with new-onset seizures.

BOX 6: Surgically remediable epilepsy syndromes.

- Mesial temporal lobe epilepsy associated with hippocampal sclerosis
- *Circumscribed potentially* epileptogenic lesions:
  - Benign neoplasms:
    - *Ganglioglioma*
    - *Dysembryoplastic neuroepithelial tumor*
    - *Low-grade astrocytoma*
    - *Oligodendroglioma*
  - Focal cortical dysplasias
  - Vascular malformations
  - Atrophic scars
- *Large unihemispheric epileptogenic lesions (for hemispherectomy)*:
  - Hemiconvulsion-hemiplegia-epilepsy (HHE) syndrome
  - Sturge–Weber syndrome
  - Rasmussen encephalitis
  - Hemimegalencephaly
- *Epileptic encephalopathies and multifocal disease (for corpus callosotomy)*:
  - Lennox–Gastaut syndrome

GGE.[51,52] Both these trials in a large group of patients have shown that valproate is the most effective ASM as initial monotherapy in patients with GGE. However, because of the significant risk of teratogenicity with valproate, it is not recommended in young and adolescent girls,[53,54] where levetiracetam or lamotrigine should remain the drugs of first choice **(Table 5)**. The results of a class I randomized trial comparing valproate, lamotrigine, and ethosuximide in patients with CAE showed that ethosuximide should be considered as first-choice for CAE.[55] Valproate is the most effective drug in patients with GGE and those patients not responding to valproate do not respond to any other medicine. There is good evidence for using the combination of valproate and lamotrigine in resistant cases of GGE.[56]

DRUG-RESISTANT EPILEPSY

Approximately one-third of the patients with newly diagnosed epilepsy do not achieve seizure control with an adequate trial of two ASMs and develop drug-resistant epilepsy.[57] Various long-term follow-up studies have shown that the chances of sustained seizure freedom are remote (<5%) after the failure of an adequate trial of two ASMs.[57] In a selected group of patients where a definite focal epileptogenic zone can be localized, epilepsy surgery can produce seizure freedom in a large majority of the patients with drug-resistant epilepsy. As continuing seizures can have significant deleterious effects on the developing brain, children with drug-resistant epilepsy should be identified early and referred for early presurgical evaluation and epilepsy surgery. Undertaking epilepsy surgery is a complex process that requires inputs from multiple modalities and multiple specialties.[58] Certain epilepsy syndromes that have a natural history of drug resistance from beginning, progressive course, and excellent outcomes following surgery have been termed as surgically remediable syndromes.[20] Early epilepsy surgery is indicated in patients with well-defined surgically remediable syndromes **(Box 6 and Fig. 6C)**.

The efficacy and safety of epilepsy surgery have been well established through three randomized controlled trials, several systematic reviews and meta-analyses, and multiple open label studies. Epilepsy surgery is associated with long-term seizure freedom in 80–90% of the patients undergoing hemispheric resections, 70–80% of the patients undergoing temporal resections, and 60–70% of children undergoing extratemporal resections.[22,23,59-61] Antiseizure medicine can be completely withdrawn in 40–50% of the patients following successful surgery.[23,60]

ANTISEIZURE MEDICINE WITHDRAWAL IN REMITTED EPILEPSY

Approximately two-thirds of the patients with newly diagnosed epilepsy will easily enter into long-term remission with one or two ASMs. The decision to withdraw the ASMs in such patients needs to be individualized and largely depends upon the estimated risk of seizure recurrence after ASM withdrawal. The single most important factor determining successful drug withdrawal is the underlying epilepsy syndrome. While ASM can be successfully withdrawn in >90% of the patients with benign focal epilepsies and CAE, they can never be withdrawn in the majority of the patients with epileptic encephalopathies.[62] Similarly, patients with JAE and JME require long-term therapy usually up to the age of 40 years or even longer. However, the majority of the patients fall in between two extremes and individualized decision-making is often indicated in such patients.

Various studies and meta-analyses have shown that the relapse rate following ASM withdrawal at 2 years varies from 20 to 40%.[63,64] The relapse rate is higher when ASMs are withdrawn before 2 years of completed remission. Hence, ASM withdrawal is advised in children after 2 years of seizure freedom. In adults, we usually withdraw ASM after 4 years of seizure freedom. Patients with neurological deficits, abnormal EEG, structural abnormality on MRI, and those with difficult initial control have a higher risk of seizure relapse.[62-64] ASM withdrawal should be cautiously attempted in such patients and only after a longer period of remission. We usually attempt withdrawal after 5 years of seizure freedom in such patients.

CONCLUDING REMARKS

Epilepsy is a group of disorders with variable etiologies and prognoses. Establishing a syndromic diagnosis in epilepsy is essential for choosing the appropriate therapy and for assessing the long-term prognosis. Every effort should be made to positively establish the epilepsy diagnosis while ruling out any mimickers. History remains the most important tool for epilepsy diagnosis supplemented by EEG and MRI. A holistic approach is needed during the management of epilepsy to optimize the outcomes. Patients with epilepsy have significant comorbidities including psychiatric comorbidities. The treatment approach should not be centered on seizure control alone but should also focus on optimizing developmental and cognitive outcomes as well as recognition and management of comorbidities. A proper counseling should form an integral part of epilepsy management in all the patients. ASMs should be used only if necessary and in the lowest possible doses while avoiding overtreatment. Carbamazepine, levetiracetam, lamotrigine, and lacosamide are drugs of choice for initial therapy of focal epilepsies while valproate remains the preferred drug in patients with GGE except in young women. Patients with drug-resistant epilepsy should be identified early and referred for epilepsy surgery. Overall, patients free on long-term follow-up. An understanding of the specific epilepsy syndromes expected outcomes and associated comorbidities goes in a long way to ensure optimal therapy and quality of life in these patients with epilepsy have a good prognosis and approximately three-fourths become seizure free.

LEARNING POINTS

- Epilepsy is a group of disorders with variable etiologies and prognoses.
- Determining the epilepsy syndrome is the most important step in planning the optimal management and prognostication.
- Epilepsy is a clinical diagnosis supplemented by EEG and MRI.
- Careful analysis of history is the most important tool for epilepsy diagnosis.
- Both EEG and MRI have important limitations including low sensitivity.
- False diagnosis of epilepsy is common; approximately 20–30% patients diagnosed with epilepsy have nonepileptic events.
- Psychogenic nonepileptic events and syncope are two most common conditions misdiagnosed as epilepsy in adults.
- A broad differentiation between focal and generalized seizures should always be attempted and is starting point for epilepsy management.
- Lamotrigine, carbamazepine, levetiracetam, and lacosamide are preferred first-line drugs for focal epilepsy.
- Valproate is the most effective drug for generalized epilepsy but should be avoided in women of reproductive age group.
- Carbamazepine and clobazam is an effective combination for focal epilepsy while valproate and lamotrigine combination is effective for generalized epilepsy.
- 70% of patients with epilepsy achieve long-term remission and have good prognosis.
- One-third patients with epilepsy have drug-resistant epilepsy.
- Epilepsy surgery should be considered in all the patients with drug-resistant epilepsy.

REFERENCES

1. Sander JWAS, Shorvon SD. Epidemiology of the epilepsies. J Neurol Neurosurg Psychiatry. 1996;61(5):433-43.
2. Sridharan R, Murthy BN. Prevalence and pattern of epilepsy in India. Epilepsia. 1999;40(5):631-6.
3. Radhakrishnan K, Pandian JD, Santhoshkumar T, Thomas SV, Deetha TD, Sarma PS, et al. Prevalence, knowledge, attitude, and practice of epilepsy in Kerala, South India. Epilepsia. 2000;41(8):1027-35.
4. Wirrell EC, Grossardt BR, Wong-Kisiel LCL, Nickels KC. Incidence and classification of new-onset epilepsy and epilepsy syndromes in children in Olmsted County, Minnesota from 1980 to 2004: a population-based study. Epilepsy Res. 2011;95(1-2):110-8.
5. Fisher RS, van Emde Boas W, Blume W, Elger C, Genton P, Lee P, et al. Epileptic seizures and epilepsy: definitions proposed by the International League Against Epilepsy (ILAE) and the International Bureau for Epilepsy (IBE). Epilepsia. 2005;46(4):470-2.
6. Fisher RS, Acevedo C, Arzimanoglou A, Bogacz A, Cross JH, Elger CE, et al. ILAE official report: a practical clinical definition of epilepsy. Epilepsia. 2014;55(4):475-82.
7. Fisher RS, Cross JH, French JA, Higurashi N, Hirsch E, Jansen FE, et al. Operational classification of seizure types by the International League Against Epilepsy: Position Paper of the ILAE Commission for Classification and Terminology. Epilepsia. 2017;58(4):522-30.
8. Scheffer IE, Berkovic S, Capovilla G, Connolly MB, French J, Guilhoto L, et al. ILAE classification of the epilepsies: Position paper of the ILAE Commission for Classification and Terminology. Epilepsia. 2017;58(4):512-21.
9. Hussain SA. Epileptic encephalopathies. Continuum (MinneapMinn) 2018;24(1,Child Neurology):171-85.
10. Villas N, Meskis MA, Goodliffe S. Dravet syndrome: characteristics, comorbidities, and caregiver concerns. Epilepsy Behav. 2017;74:81-6.
11. Strzelczyk A, Schubert-Bast S. Psychobehavioural and cognitive adverse events of anti-seizure medications for the treatment of developmental and epileptic encephalopathies. CNS Drugs. 2022;36(10):1079-111.
12. Panayiotopoulos CP, Michael M, Sanders S, Valeta T, Koutroumanidis M. Benign childhood focal epilepsies: assessment of established and newly recognized syndromes. Brain. 2008;131(Pt 9):2264-86.
13. Liu X, Han Q. Depression and anxiety in children with benign childhood epilepsy with centrotemporal spikes (BCECTS). BMC Pediatr. 2016;16:128.
14. Kwon S, Seo HE, Hwang SK. Cognitive and other neuropsychological profiles in children with newly diagnosed benign rolandic epilepsy. Korean J Pediatr. 2012;55(10):383-7.
15. Rathore C, Patel KY, Satishchandra P. Current concepts in the management of idiopathic generalized epilepsies. Ann Indian Neurol. 2022;25(1):35-42.
16. Caplan R, Siddarth P, Stahl L, Lanphier E, Vona P, Gurbani S, et al. Childhood absence epilepsy: behavioral, cognitive, and linguistic comorbidities. Epilepsia. 2008;49(11):1838-46.
17. Trinka E, Kienpointner G, Unterberger I, Luef G, Bauer G, Doering LB, et al. Psychiatric comorbidity in juvenile myoclonic epilepsy. Epilepsia. 2006;47(12):2086-91.
18. de Araujo Filho GM, Yacubian EM. Juvenile myoclonic epilepsy: psychiatric comorbidity and impact on outcome. Epilepsy Behav. 2013;28 (Suppl 1):S74-S80.
19. Stevelink R, Koeleman BPC, Sander JW, Jansen FE, Braun KPJ. Refractory juvenile myoclonic epilepsy: a meta-analysis of prevalence and risk factors. Eur J Neurol. 2019;26(6):856-64.
20. Engel J Jr. Surgery for seizures. N Engl J Med. 1996;334(10):647-52.
21. Sadler RM. The syndrome of mesial temporal lobe epilepsy with hippocampal sclerosis: clinical features and differential diagnosis. Adv Neurol. 2006;97:27-37.
22. Wiebe S, Blume WT, Girvin JP, Eliasziw M. A randomized, controlled trial of surgery for temporal lobe epilepsy. N Engl J Med. 2001;345(5):311-8.
23. Rathore C, Panda S, Sarma PS, Radhakrishnan K. How safe is it to withdraw antiepileptic drugs following successful surgery for mesial temporal lobe epilepsy? Epilepsia. 2011;52(3):627-35.
24. Fauser S, Huppertz HJ, Bast T, Strobl K, Pantazis G, Altenmueller DM, et al. Clinical characteristics in focal cortical dysplasia: a retrospective evaluation in a series of 120 patients. Brain. 2006;129(Pt 7):1907-16.
25. Dash GK, Rathore C, Jeyaraj MK, Wattamwar P, Sarma SP, Radhakrishnan K. Predictors of seizure outcome following resective surgery for drug-resistant epilepsy associated with focal gliosis. J Neurosurg. 2018;130(6):2071-9.
26. Filho GM, Rosa VP, Lin K, Caboclo LO, Sakamoto AC, Yacubian EM. Psychiatric comorbidity in epilepsy: a study comparing patients with mesial temporal sclerosis and juvenile myoclonic epilepsy. Epilepsy Behav. 2008;13(1):196-201.
27. Stagno SJ. Psychiatric aspects of epilepsy. In: Wyllie E (Ed). The Treatment of Epilepsy. Baltimore MD: Williams & Wilkins; 1997. pp. 1131-44.
28. Kanner AM. Psychosis of Epilepsy: A Neurologist's Perspective. Epilepsy Behav. 2000;1(4):219-27.
29. Adachi N, Matsuura M, Okubo Y, Oana Y, Takei N, Kato M, et al. Predictive variables of interictal psychosis in epilepsy. Neurology. 2000;55(9):1310-4.
30. Hermann BP, Jones JE. Depression in Epilepsy: What is the Extent of the Current Problem? Mood Disorders in Epilepsy: Bridging the Gap Between Psychiatry and Neurology. American Epilepsy Society and IntraMed Scientific Solutions; 2005. pp. 3-11.
31. Kanner AM. How to recognize depression in epilepsy. Mood Disorders in Epilepsy: Bridging the Gap Between Psychiatry and Neurology. American Epilepsy Society and IntraMed Scientific Solutions; 2005. pp. 13-21.
32. Jones JE, Hermann BP, Barry JJ, Gilliam FG, Kanner AM, Meador KJ. Rates and risk factors for suicide, suicidal ideation, and suicide attempts in chronic epilepsy. Epilepsy Behav, 2003;4 (Suppl 3):S31-8.
33. Tombini M, Assenza G, Quintiliani L, Ricci L, Lanzone J, Di Lazzaro V. Epilepsy and quality of life: what does really matter? Neurol Sci. 2021;42(9):3757-65.
34. Lempert T, Bauer M, Schmidt D. Syncope: a videometric analysis of 56 episodes of transient cerebral hypoxia. Ann Neurol. 1994;36(2):233-7.
35. Gröppel G, Kapitany T, Baumgartner C. Cluster analysis of clinical seizure semiology of psychogenic nonepileptic seizures. Epilepsia. 2000;41(5):610-4.

36. Hubsch C, Baumann C, Hingray C, Gospodaru N, Vignal JP, Vespignani H, et al. Clinical classification of psychogenic non-epileptic seizures based on video-EEG analysis and automatic clustering. J Neurol Neurosurg Psychiatry. 2011;82(9):955-60.
37. Parker C. Complicated migraine syndromes and migraine variants. Pediatr Ann. 1997;26(7):417-21.
38. Prakash S, Rathore C, Makwana P, Rathod M. Recurrent spontaneous paresthesia in the upper limb could be due to migraine: a case series. Headache. 2015;55(8):1143-7.
39. Derry CP, Davey M, Johns M, Kron K, Glencross D, Marini C, et al. Distinguishing sleep disorders from seizures: diagnosing bumps in the night. Arch Neurol. 2006;63(5):705-9.
40. Gregory RP, Oates T, Merry RTG. Electroencephalogram epileptiform abnormalities in candidates for aircrew training. Electroenceph Clin Neurophysiol. 1993;86(1):75-7.
41. Salinsky M, Kanter R, Dashieff RM. Effectiveness of multiple EEGs in supporting the diagnosis of epilepsy and operational curve. Epilepsia. 1987;28(4):331-4.
42. Mulligan CK, Trauner DA. Incidence and behavioral correlates of epileptiform abnormalities in autism spectrum disorders. J Autism Dev Disord. 2014;44(2):452-8.
43. Guerreiro MM, Vigonius U, Pohlmann H, de Manreza ML, Fejerman N, Antoniuk Sa et al. A double-blind controlled clinical trial of oxcarbazepine versus phenytoin in children and adolescents with epilepsy. Epilepsy Res. 1997;27(3):205-13.
44. Marson AG, Al-Kharusi AM, Alwaidh M, Appleton R, Baker GA, Chadwick DW, et al; SANAD Study group. The SANAD study of effectiveness of carbamazepine, gabapentin, lamotrigine, oxcarbazepine, or topiramate for treatment of partial epilepsy: an unblinded randomised controlled trial. Lancet. 2007;369(9566):1000-15.
45. Marson A, Burnside G, Appleton R, Smith D, Leach JP, Sills G, et al; SANAD II collaborators. The SANAD II study of the effectiveness and cost-effectiveness of levetiracetam, zonisamide, or lamotrigine for newly diagnosed focal epilepsy: an open-label, non-inferiority, multicentre, phase 4, randomised controlled trial. Lancet. 2021;397(10282):1363-74.
46. Sanmartí-Vilaplana F, Díaz-Gómez A. The effectiveness and safety of lacosamide in children with epilepsy in a clinical practice setting. Epilepsy Behav. 2018;79:130-7.
47. Millul A, Iudice A, Adami M, Porzio R, Mattana F, Beghi E; THEOREM Study Group. Alternative monotherapy or add-on therapy in patients with epilepsy whose seizures do not respond to the first monotherapy: an Italian multicenter prospective observational study. Epilepsy Behav. 2013;28(3):494-500.
48. Bresnahan R, Martin-McGill KJ, Williamson J, Michael BD, Marson AG, et al. Clobazam add-on therapy for drug-resistant epilepsy. Cochrane Database Syst Rev. 2019;10(10):CD004154.
49. Genton P, Gelisse P, Thomas P, Dravet C. Do carbamazepine and phenytoin aggravate juvenile myoclonic epilepsy? Neurology. 2000;55(8):1106-9.
50. Nicolson A, Appleton RE, Chadwick DW, Smith DF. The relationship between treatment with valproate, lamotrigine, and topiramate and the prognosis of the idiopathic generalized epilepsies. JNNP. 2004;75(1):75-9.
51. Marson AG, Al-Kharusi AM, Alwaidh M, Appleton R, Baker GA, Chadwick DW, et al; SANAD Study group. The SANAD study of effectiveness of valproate, lamotrigine, or topiramate for generalised and unclassifiable epilepsy: an unblinded randomised controlled trial. Lancet. 2007;369(9566):1016-26.
52. Marson A, Burnside G, Appleton R, Smith D, Leach JP, Sills G, et al; SANAD II collaborators. The SANAD II study of the effectiveness and cost-effectiveness of valproate versus levetiracetam for newly diagnosed generalised and unclassifiable epilepsy: an open-label, non-inferiority, multicentre, phase 4, randomised controlled trial. Lancet. 2021;397(10282):1375-86.
53. Meador K, Reynolds MW, Crean S, Fahrbach K, Probst C. Pregnancy outcomes in women with epilepsy: a systematic review and meta-analysis of published pregnancy registries and cohorts. Epilepsy Res. 2008;81(1):1-13.
54. Tomson T, Battino D, Bonizzoni E, Craig J, Lindhout D, Perucca E, et al; EURAP Study Group. Comparative risk of major congenital malformations with eight different antiepileptic drugs: a prospective cohort study of the EURAP registry. Lancet Neurol. 2018;17(6):530-8.
55. Glauser TA, Cnaan A, Shinnar S, Hirtz DG, Dlugos D, Masur D, et al; Childhood Absence Epilepsy Study Group. Ethosuximide, valproic acid, and lamotrigine in childhood absence epilepsy. N Engl J Med. 2010;362(9):790-9.
56. Baheti N, Rathore C, Bansal AR, Shah S, Veedu HK, Prakash S, et al. Treatment outcomes in drug resistant juvenile myoclonic epilepsy: Valproate resistance may not be the end of the road. Seizure. 2021;92:112-7.
57. Kwan P, Brodie MJ. Early identification of refractory epilepsy. N Engl J Med. 2000;342(5):314-9.
58. Rathore C, Radhakrishnan K. Concept of epilepsy surgery and presurgical evaluation. Epileptic Disord. 2015;17(1):19-31.
59. Dwivedi R, Ramanujam B, Chandra PS, Sapra S, Gulati S, Kalaivani M, et al. Surgery for drug-resistant epilepsy in children. N Engl J Med. 2017;377(17):1639-47.
60. Menon R, Rathore C, Sarma SP, Radhakrishnan K. Feasibility of antiepileptic drug withdrawal following extratemporal resective epilepsy surgery. Neurology 2012;79(8):770-6.
61. Tellez-Zenteno JF, Dhar R, Wiebe S. Long-term seizure outcomes following epilepsy surgery: a systematic review and meta-analysis. Brain. 2005;128(Pt 5):1188-98.
62. Rathore C, Paterson R. Stopping antiepileptic drugs in patients with epilepsy in remission: why, when and how? Neurol India. 2014;62(1):3-8.
63. Randomised study of antiepileptic drug withdrawal in patients in remission. Medical Research Council Antiepileptic Drug Withdrawal Study Group. Lancet. 1991;337(8751):1175-80.
64. Berg AT, Shinnar S. Relapse following discontinuation of antiepileptic drugs: a meta-analysis. Neurology. 1994;44(4):601-8.

CHAPTER 9

Neuropsychiatric Aspects of Epilepsy

Ambar Chakravarty

INTRODUCTION

Over the past two decades, the recognition of psychiatric comorbidities in people with epilepsy (PWE) has become increasingly important among neurologists and epileptologists. These comorbidities have been shown to have a negative impact on both the seizure disorder itself and the overall quality of life for the patients.[1] The proposed definition of epilepsy by the International League Against Epilepsy (ILAE) emphasizes the need to consider the existence of comorbid psychiatric conditions in the comprehensive management of PWE, as these conditions have a relatively high lifetime prevalence, with mood and anxiety disorders being the most common.[2] The presence of psychiatric disorders can contribute to the stigma associated with epilepsy, leading to discrimination, social withdrawal, and poor self-esteem. Additionally, limitations such as the loss of driving privileges and the unpredictable nature of seizures can further exacerbate depression and other psychiatric symptoms.[3]

Neuroimaging studies have revealed overlapping abnormalities in brain networks between primary psychiatric conditions, such as depression or schizophrenia, and temporal lobe epilepsy (TLE), specifically involving the amygdala and the hippocampi.[4] Furthermore, psychiatric symptoms can manifest peri-ictally, before, during, or after a seizure, or as a consequence of epilepsy treatment.[5] The origin of psychiatric problems in PWE can be attributed to shared neurobiological mechanisms, the presence of epilepsy itself, or the unfortunate coincidence of two conditions in the same individual. Nevertheless, the management of these individuals poses challenges regardless of the underlying causes, emphasizing the importance of identifying comorbid psychiatric disorders and adopting a multidisciplinary approach involving various healthcare professionals, such as psychiatrists, clinical psychologists, neuropsychologists, psychiatric nurses, and social workers, to ensure comprehensive care.[6]

EPIDEMIOLOGY

Cross-sectional studies have consistently shown that psychiatric disorders occur at a higher rate in both adults and children with epilepsy compared to those without epilepsy. Individuals with epilepsy and psychiatric disorders tend to have higher healthcare resource utilization, including increased emergency department admissions and outpatient visits.[7] Prospective observational studies have established a bidirectional relationship between epilepsy and psychiatric disorders. A large observational cohort study conducted in the UK, involving over 10 million subjects, found a 2.5-fold increased risk of developing epilepsy in individuals with depression and a 2.9-fold increased risk of suicide even before the diagnosis of epilepsy.[8] These findings suggest the presence of shared pathogenic mechanisms between epilepsy and major psychiatric disorders.

In the case of depression, potential mechanisms include hyperactivity of the hypothalamic pituitary-adrenal axis, which can modulate the expression and composition of gamma-aminobutyric acid (GABA) A receptors, leading to increased brain excitability and epileptogenesis.[9] It is also plausible to consider that psychiatric disorders may represent the premorbid phase of certain epileptic syndromes, which could have significant implications for future treatments and the development of disease-modifying agents.

PRACTICAL CONSIDERATIONS

The accurate definition of the epilepsy syndrome is crucial for the treatment and prognosis of epilepsy. Similarly, the same approach should be applied to psychiatric comorbidities, considering that certain psychiatric disorders are more commonly associated with specific epilepsy syndromes, such as temporal lobe epilepsy compared to generalized syndromes. However, it is important to note that psychiatric comorbidities do not necessarily adhere to such boundaries, and their presence must be considered when informing individuals about the long-term prognosis of epilepsy itself. Historically, psychiatric comorbidities in PWE have been associated with poor quality of life. However, recent data suggest that they also serve as prognostic indicators. For instance, a UK study demonstrated that depression is associated with high comorbidity rates, as measured by the Charlson Comorbidity Index, and the severity of depression correlates with lower odds of achieving seizure remission in a Canadian cohort.[10] Psychiatric comorbidities are linked to a higher risk of side effects, particularly cognitive complaints and psychiatric side effects, with depression being a significant cause of cognitive complaints.[11] Additionally, psychiatric comorbidities are associated with a four-fold increased risk of drug resistance in both focal and generalized epilepsies.[12] The impact of psychiatric comorbidities on seizure and psychiatric outcomes following epilepsy surgery is complex and yet to be fully established. Some studies have indicated a lower probability of achieving seizure freedom after temporal lobectomy, whereas others have refuted these findings.[13,14] Similarly, the effect on psychiatric outcomes varies, with some studies reporting an increased risk of recurrence of depression or anxiety during the first year after surgery, whereas others show long-term improvement. Psychiatric comorbidities are also associated with premature mortality in epilepsy, potentially due to factors such as increased substance or alcohol abuse, higher risk of injury, poor adherence to medications, and elevated suicide rates. A population-based study in Sweden involving over 57,000 individuals revealed that females with epilepsy and psychiatric comorbidities had a five-fold increased risk of sudden unexpected death in epilepsy compared to those without such comorbidities.[15]

DEPRESSION

The presence of psychiatric comorbidities in epilepsy has been recognized for centuries, and depression is one of the most common and impactful conditions in this population. Depression has been found to have a significant negative impact on the quality of life and prognosis of individuals with epilepsy. Studies have shown that depression is a stronger predictor of quality of life than the actual frequency of seizures. Additionally, PWE and depression are more likely to experience side effects of antiepileptic drugs (AEDs), have drug-refractory epilepsy, and have poorer outcomes after epilepsy surgery compared to those without depression.

Screening for psychiatric comorbidities in epilepsy is important for accurate diagnosis and appropriate management. Validated clinical instruments for depression and anxiety, such as the Hamilton Depression Rating Scale, the Hospital Anxiety and Depression Scale HADS (Hospital Anxiety and Depression Scale), and the Generalized Anxiety Disorder 7 (GAD-7), have been developed and shown to be effective in the epilepsy population. These screening tools are valuable in identifying individuals who may benefit from further evaluation and intervention.

It is worth noting that psychiatric symptoms in epilepsy can be influenced by various factors, including peri-ictal symptoms (occurring around the time of a seizure), side effects of antiseizure medications, and comorbid psychiatric disorders. The boundaries between these scenarios can be blurred, making the confirmation of diagnoses challenging. However, screening instruments, when used appropriately, can help differentiate between these scenarios and guide appropriate treatment.

The observation that the relationship between epilepsy and depression is not necessarily unidirectional, namely that some patients may present a mood disorder before the emergence of the seizures.[16,17] Major depressive episode occurred closer to the date of the first seizure. It may suggest that the depressive episode may have facilitated the onset of the seizure. Several factors may explain the bidirectional relationship between epilepsy and depression, including the development of epilepsy following suicidal attempts, alcohol or drug abuse, or head trauma. It is possible that common pathogenetic mechanisms are operant in both conditions, with the presence of one disorder may facilitate the development of the other. Such factors may include the following:

- Several neurotransmitters particularly serotonin, noradrenalin, dopamine, GABA, and glutamate may show abnormal activity.
- Structural changes in temporal and frontal lobe structures, amygdala, hippocampus, and entorhinal cortex demonstrable by neuroimaging.
- Functional abnormalities in temporal and frontal lobes, consisting of decreased 5-HT1A binding in the mesial structures, raphe nuclei, thalamus, and cingulate gyrus demonstrable by nuclear and molecular imaging.
- Abnormal function of the hypothalamic pituitary adrenal axis by hormone assays
- Hippocampal volume loss, which may induce seizures and at the same time can cause mood disorders by causing disturbance in the temporo-limbic circuit.[18]

Overall, the close association between epilepsy and depression suggests shared underlying mechanisms between the two conditions. Further research is needed to better understand the complex neurobiology of depression in epilepsy and to develop more targeted and effective treatments for individuals with epilepsy and comorbid psychiatric conditions.

Antiepileptic drugs have psychotropic effects beyond their primary antiseizure action, and their impact on mood and behavior needs to be thoroughly investigated in patients with epilepsy. While some AEDs, such as carbamazepine and valproic acid, have potential positive effects on mood, others have been associated with detrimental effects, particularly in relation to depressive symptoms.[19,20]

The AEDs most commonly associated with the occurrence of depressive symptoms in patients with epilepsy are those that act on the benzodiazepine-GABA receptor complex, including barbiturates, topiramate, and vigabatrin.[21] Zonisamide has limited available data, whereas AEDs such as tiagabine, levetiracetam, and felbamate appear to be associated with an intermediate risk of depression, with reported incidence rates of about 3% or lower. The majority of other AEDs have a low incidence of depression <1%.

Identifying clinical factors that may predispose individuals to developing mood symptoms during AED therapy is crucial for informing patients and their families and ensuring close monitoring. Using AEDs as monotherapy, adopting slow titration schedules, and employing low doses whenever possible can significantly reduce the incidence of depressive symptoms. Previous history of mood disorders or familial predisposition are important risk factors that should be considered when selecting the appropriate AED. **Table 1** highlights the psychotropic and mood effects of major AEDs.

It is important to mention the recent concern about the risk of suicide associated with AEDs. The US Food and Drug Administration (FDA) conducted a meta-analysis of 199 placebo controlled studies involving 11 AEDs used for seizure control or psychiatric indications. The analysis revealed that the odds ratio for suicidal behavior or ideation was 1.8 in individuals taking AEDs compared to those on placebo. The increased risk was significant for people taking AEDs for epilepsy but not for other indications.[22,23]

While the risk of suicidal ideation and behavior as side effects of AED treatment is very low, clinicians should inform patients and their families about the FDA's alert. However, it is important to put the reported increased risk into proper perspective. Some individuals with epilepsy may be more prone to developing psychiatric side effects with any AED, and these individuals should be closely monitored when starting a new AED. Nonetheless, the risk of suicidality associated with AEDs needs to be balanced against the risk of not treating the seizures, as discontinuing AEDs or refusing to start them for seizure control can have serious consequences, including harm and death to the patient.

PSYCHOSIS

Psychosis in epilepsy refers to a condition where individuals with epilepsy experience symptoms such as impaired thought content and coherence, reduced connection to reality, hallucinations, delusions, disorganized speech and behavior, and extreme changes in affect and motivation.

There are two main types of psychosis associated with epilepsy: Ictal psychosis and postictal psychosis (PIP).

1. *Ictal psychosis:*[24]
   - Occurs during a seizure and is rare.
   - Symptoms include cognitive, affective, and hallucinatory manifestations that combine to produce a psychotic state.

TABLE 1: Psychotropic effects of various antiepileptic drugs.

Antiepileptic drug	Psychotropic effects	Mood effects
Barbiturates	Depression and hyperactivity	Anxiolytic and hypnotic
Carbamazepine/ Oxcarbazepine	Irritability	Mood stabilizing and antimanic
Ethosuximide	Behavioral abnormalities and psychosis	–
Felbamate	Depression, anxiety, and irritability	–
Gabapentin	Behavioral problems in children	–
Lamotrigine	Insomnia and agitation	Mood stabilizing and antidepressant
Levetiracetam	Irritability and emotional lability	Antimanic?
Phenytoin	Encephalopathy	Antimanic?
Pregabalin	–	Anxiolytic
Tiagabine	Depression (nonconvulsive status epilepticus)	Antianxiety?
Topiramate	Depression, psychomotor slowing, and psychosis	Mood stabilizing
Valproate	Encephalopathy	Mood stabilizing and antimanic (anxiolytic)
Vigabatrin	Depression, aggression, and psychosis	–
Zonisamide	Agitation, depression, and psychosis	Antimanic

- Visual or auditory illusions and hallucinations are common, along with affective changes like agitation, fear, or paranoia.
- Other phenomena may include depersonalization, derealization, autoscopy, out of body experiences, or a sense of "someone behind."
- Temporal lobe involvement is often observed, with activation of limbic and neocortical areas
- Prolonged ictal psychotic states are rare and may occur as nonconvulsive status epilepticus.

2. *PIP*:[25]
- Occurs within 1 week after a seizure and affects 2-7.8% of epilepsy patients. Features hallucinations, delusions, and/or gross abnormalities of behavior or affect. Abnormal mood predominates, including depressed affect, manic symptoms, irritability, and aggression.
- First rank symptoms of schizophrenia (e.g., voices commenting or thought insertion) are rare.
- Negative symptoms are not prominent.
- Typically arises after >10 years of seizures and is more common in right and left temporal lobe epilepsy.
- Risk factors include age >30 years, localization-related epilepsy, bilateral seizure or interictal foci, seizure clustering, secondary generalization, and possibly a family history of mood disorders.

It is important to differentiate psychosis associated with epilepsy from other psychiatric conditions, as the management and treatment approaches may differ. Consulting with a healthcare professional is essential for accurate diagnosis and appropriate management of psychosis in individuals with epilepsy.

Chronic, Interictal Psychosis[26]

- Chronic, interictal psychosis (CIP) can develop in >5% of patients with a long history of uncontrolled seizures.
- It typically has an insidious onset and is characterized by paranoid delusions and hallucinations.
- CIP shares similarities with schizophrenia, with a less intense affective component and common persecutory auditory hallucinations.
- First rank symptoms (involving disintegration of mental boundaries) are usually absent in CIP.
- Thought disorder is uncommon in CIP.
- Some individuals with temporal lobe epilepsy and CIP may experience negative symptoms, such as increasing isolation and decreasing socialization, cognitive decline, and affective blunting.

Forced Normalization or Alternative Psychosis[27,28]

Forced normalization refers to the phenomenon where individuals experience personality and mood changes, and in some cases, psychosis, when their electroencephalograms (EEGs) become normalized.

The concept of forced normalization is controversial, and its occurrence varies among different types of epilepsy.

It is observed more frequently in absence epilepsy successfully treated with ethosuximide.

In some cases, forced normalization occurs when seizures are controlled or reduced with medication, and the psychosis could be a side effect of the medication rather than a direct result of EEG improvement.

De Novo Psychosis after Epilepsy Surgery[29]

After temporal lobectomy, depression is the most common psychiatric complication. Rates of de novo psychosis after epilepsy surgery range from <1 to 28.5%, with an average of 7% among reported cases.

Transient postoperative psychosis is typical, and it is important to assess and monitor patients during the high-risk period of the first 6 months after surgery. Risk factors for de novo psychosis after epilepsy surgery include a family history of psychosis, surgery after the age of 30 years, and preoperative psychosis.

Management of Epileptic Psychosis[30-38]

Timely pharmacotherapy and psychotherapy are crucial in managing epileptic psychosis.

Antipsychotic drugs (neuroleptics and major tranquilizers) are commonly used to treat psychotic symptoms associated with epilepsy.

Positive symptoms such as disordered thinking, anxiety, delusions, hallucinations, aggression, and insomnia respond well to antipsychotic drugs.

Negative symptoms such as apathy, aspontaneity, social withdrawal, and catatonia are more difficult to treat and may respond better to atypical antipsychotics. Achieving stringent seizure control is important, along with appropriate psychotherapeutic measures.

Creating a supportive environment with psychosocial supports for the patient and their family can help maintain functioning and prevent setbacks.

The treatment of psychiatric comorbidity in epilepsy should aim for full remission. Here are some key points regarding treatment.

PSYCHOLOGICAL INTERVENTIONS

Psychological interventions, particularly cognitive behavioral therapy, are recommended for PWE and mild-to-moderate depressive symptoms. Psychoeducation and psychological interventions are important for the management of psychogenic nonepileptic seizures (PNES) in PWE.

While the evidence is limited, psychological interventions can be considered as first-line treatments for anxiety disorders and mild-to-moderate depression in PWE.

PHARMACOLOGIC TREATMENTS

Antidepressants, such as selective serotonin reuptake inhibitors (SSRIs) and newer antidepressants, have shown safety and efficacy in treating depression in epilepsy. Limited studies exist on the effectiveness of drug treatments for anxiety disorders in epilepsy, but SSRIs are often considered as first-line treatment when medication is necessary.

Drug interactions can occur between antiseizure medications and psychotropic drugs. Enzyme-inducing antiseizure medications can affect the levels of antidepressants and antipsychotics, whereas some antidepressants can interact with epilepsy medications. Pharmacodynamic interactions, both positive and negative, can influence treatment response and side effects. Neurologists should be familiar with the side effects of psychotropic medications.

Seizure Risk

Psychotropic medications, when used appropriately, do not increase the risk of seizures significantly. High-dose clomipramine and clozapine have shown higher seizure risk. The incorrect overestimation of seizure risk with psychotropic medications has led to limited access to proper treatment for PWE and psychiatric comorbidities.[39,40]

Attention Deficit/Hyperactivity Disorder and Epilepsy

Attention deficit/hyperactivity disorder (ADHD) is frequently associated with epilepsy as a comorbid condition. ADHD is associated with significant psychosocial and academic consequences. ADHD is found in 12–39% of patients with newly diagnosed epilepsy to as high as 70% of patients with drug-resistant epilepsy. The diagnosis of ADHD requires parent-validated and teacher-validated rating scales, based on the Diagnostic and Statistical Manual of Mental Disorders (DSM)-IV and DSM-V, to confirm the information in the rating scales by interviewing parents and to exclude other causes of symptoms. At present, there is no specific treatment of ADHD associated with epilepsy and its treatment is based on the usual treatments of ADHD. Such treatments have been found to be safe in patients with epilepsy. Treatment with methylphenidate results in clinically significant improvement of ADHD symptoms in 60–75% of patients. Current data suggest that ADHD medications do not increase risk of seizures, even in patients with epilepsy. In addition, it is recommended to include multidisciplinary involvement in transition clinics for patients with both comorbid ADHD and epilepsy.[41]

CONCLUDING REMARKS

The treatment of epileptic seizure disorders is not restricted to the achievement of seizure freedom, but must also include the management of comorbid medical, neurological, psychiatric, and cognitive comorbidities. Psychiatric and neurological comorbidities are relatively common and often coexist in PWE. For example, depression and anxiety disorders are the most common psychiatric comorbidities in PWE, and they are particularly common in PWE who also have a neurological comorbidity, such as migraine, stroke, traumatic brain injury, or dementia. Moreover, psychiatric and neurological comorbidities often have a more severe impact on the quality of life in patients with treatment-resistant focal epilepsy than do the actual seizures. Epilepsy and psychiatric and neurological comorbidities have a complex relationship, which has a direct bearing on the management of both seizures and the comorbidities: the comorbidities have to be factored into the selection of AEDs, and the susceptibility to seizures has to be considered when choosing the drugs to treat comorbidities.

LEARNING POINTS

- Psychiatric and neurological comorbidities are relatively common and often coexist in PWE. The relationship between these two happens to be bidirectional.
- The treatment of psychiatric comorbidity in epilepsy should consider psychological interventions, appropriate use of pharmacologic treatments, potential drug interactions, and the accurate assessment of seizure risk associated with psychotropic medications.

REFERENCES

1. Fiest KM, Dykeman J, Patten SB, Wiebe S, Kaplan GG, Maxwell CJ, et al. Depression in epilepsy: a systematic review and meta-analysis. Neurology. 2013;80(6):590-9.
2. Scott AJ, Sharpe L, Hunt C, Gandy M. Anxiety and depressive disorders in people with epilepsy: A meta-analysis. Epilepsia. 2017;58(6):973-82.
3. Clancy MJ, Clarke MC, Connor DJ, Cannon M, Cotter DR. The prevalence of psychosis in epilepsy; a systematic review and meta-analysis. BMC Psychiatry. 2014;14:75.
4. Kutlubaev MA, Xu Y, Hackett ML, Stone J. Dual diagnosis of epilepsy and psychogenic nonepileptic seizures: systematic review and meta-analysis of frequency, correlates, and outcomes. Epilepsy Behav. 2018;89:70-8.
5. Reilly C, Atkinson P, Das KB, Chin RF, Aylett SE, Burch V, et al. Neurobehavioral comorbidities in children with active epilepsy: a population-based study. Pediatrics. 2014;133(6):e1586-93.
6. Aaberg KM, Bakken IJ, Lossius MI, Lund Søraas C, Håberg SE, Stoltenberg C, et al. Comorbidity and childhood epilepsy: A nationwide registry study. Pediatrics. 2016;138(3):e20160921.
7. Josephson CB, Lowerison M, Vallerand I, Sajobi TT, Patten S, Jette N, et al. Association of depression and treated depression with epilepsy and seizure outcomes: A multicohort analysis. JAMA Neurol. 2017;74(5):533-9.
8. Hesdorffer DC, Ishihara L, Webb DJ, Mynepalli L, Galwey NW, Hauser WA. Occurrence and recurrence of attempted suicide among people with epilepsy. JAMA Psychiatry. 2016;73(1):80-6.
9. MacKenzie G, Maguire J. Chronic stress shifts the GABA reversal potential in the hippocampus and increases seizure susceptibility. Epilepsy Res. 2015;109:13-27.
10. Stephen LJ, Wishart A, Brodie MJ. Psychiatric side effects and antiepileptic drugs: observations from prospective audits. Epilepsy Behav. 2017;71(Pt A):73-8.
11. Nogueira MH, Yasuda CL, Coan AC, Kanner AM, Cendes F. Concurrent mood and anxiety disorders are associated with pharmacoresistant seizures in patients with MTLE. Epilepsia. 2017;58(7):1268-76.
12. Stevelink R, Koeleman BPC, Sander JW, Jansen FE, Braun KPJ. Refractory juvenile myoclonic epilepsy: a meta-analysis of prevalence and risk factors. Eur J Neurol. 2019;26(6):856-64.
13. Bell GS, de Tisi J, Gonzalez-Fraile JC, Peacock JL, McEvoy AW, Harkness WFJ, et al. Factors affecting seizure outcome after epilepsy surgery: an observational series. J Neurol Neurosurg Psychiatry. 2017;88(11):933-40.
14. Altalib HH, Berg AT, Cong X, Vickrey BG, Sperling MR, Shinnar S, et al. Presurgical depression and anxiety are not associated with worse epilepsy surgery outcome five years postoperatively. Epilepsy Behav. 2018;83:7-12.
15. Fazel S, Wolf A, Långström N, Newton CR, Lichtenstein P. Premature mortality in epilepsy and the role of psychiatric comorbidity: a total population study. Lancet. 201; 382(9905):1646-54.
16. Hesdorffer DC, Hauser WA, Annegers JF, Cascino G. Major depression is a risk factor for seizures in older adults. Ann Neurol. 2000;47(2):246-9.
17. Forsgren L, Nyström L. An incident case-referent study of epileptic seizures in adults. Epilepsy Res. 1990;6(1):66-81.
18. Kanner AM. Depression and epilepsy: a new perspective on two closely related disorders. Epilepsy Curr. 2006;6(5):141-6.
19. Kanner AM. Epilepsy and mood disorders. Epilepsia. 2007;48 (Suppl 9):20-2.
20. Cramer JA, Blum D, Reed M, Fanning K; Epilepsy Impact Project Group. The influence of comorbid depression on quality of life for people with epilepsy. Epilepsy Behav. 2003;4(5):515-21.
21. Mula M, Sander JW. Negative effects of antiepileptic drugs on mood in patients with epilepsy. Drug Saf. 2007;30(7):555-67.
22. Mula M, Kanner AM, Schmitz B, Schachter S. Antiepileptic drugs and suicidality: an expert consensus statement from the Task Force on Therapeutic Strategies of the ILAE Commission on Neuropsychobiology. Epilepsia. 2013;54(1):199-203.
23. Katz R. FDA update. Epilepsy Res. 2006;68(1):85-94.
24. Wells CE. Transient ictal psychosis. Arch Gen Psychiatry. 1975;32(9):1201-3.
25. Logsdail SJ, Toone BK. Post-ictal psychoses. A clinical and phenomenological description. Br J Psychiatry. 1988;152: 246-52.
26. Trimble MR, Schmitz B. Forced Normalisation and Alternative Psychoses of Epilepsy. Petersfield: Wrightson Biomedical Publishing Ltd; 1998.
27. Landolt H. Serial electroencephalographic investigations during psychotic episodes in epileptic patients and during schizophrenic attacks. In: Lorentz de Haas AM (Ed). Lectures on Epilepsy. Amsterdam: Elsevier; 1958. pp. 91-133.
28. Schmitz B. Forced normalization: History of a concept. In: Trimble MR, Schmitz B (Eds). Forced Normalization and Alternative Psychoses of Epilepsy. Petersfield, UK: Wrightson Biomedical Publishing Ltd; 1998. pp. 7-24.
29. Glosser G, Zwil AS, Glosser DS, O'Connor MJ, Sperling MR. Psychiatric aspects of temporal lobe epilepsy before and after anterior temporal lobectomy. J Neurol Neurosurg Psychiatry. 2000;68(1):53-8.
30. Michaelis R, Tang V, Goldstein LH, Reuber M, LaFrance WC Jr, Lundgren T, et al. Psychological treatments for adults and children with epilepsy: Evidence-based recommendations by the International League Against Epilepsy Psychology Task Force. Epilepsia. 2018;59(7):1282-302.
31. Gasparini S, Beghi E, Ferlazzo E, Beghi M, Belcastro V, Biermann KP, et al. Management of psychogenic non-epileptic seizures: a multidisciplinary approach. Eur J Neurol. 2019;26(2):205-e15.
32. Maguire MJ, Weston J, Singh J, Marson AG. Antidepressants for people with epilepsy and depression. Cochrane Database Syst Rev. 2014;2014 (12):CD010682.
33. Mula M, Sander JW. Current and emerging drug therapies for the treatment of depression in adults with epilepsy. Expert Opin Pharmacother. 2019;20(1):41-5.
34. Agrawal N, Mula M. Treatment of psychoses in patients with epilepsy: an update. Ther Adv Psychopharmacol. 2019;9:2045125319862968.
35. Kerr M, Linehan C, Brandt C, Kanemoto K, Kawasaki J, Sugai K, et al. Behavioral disorder in people with an intellectual disability and epilepsy: A report of the Intellectual Disability Task Force of the Neuropsychiatric Commission of ILAE. Epilepsia Open. 2016;1(3-4):102-11.
36. Italiano D, Spina E, de Leon J. Pharmacokinetic and pharmacodynamic interactions between antiepileptics and antidepressants. Expert Opin Drug Metab Toxicol. 2014;10(11): 1457-89.

37. Mula M. The pharmacological management of psychiatric comorbidities in patients with epilepsy. Pharmacol Res. 2016;107:147-53.
38. Baldwin DS, Anderson IM, Nutt DJ, Allgulander C, Bandelow B, den Boer JA, et al. Evidence-based pharmacological treatment of anxiety disorders, post-traumatic stress disorder and obsessive-compulsive disorder: a revision of the 2005 guidelines from the British Association for Psychopharmacology. J Psychopharmacol. 2014;28(5):403-39.
39. Alper K, Schwartz KA, Kolts RL, Khan A. Seizure incidence in psychopharmacological clinical trials: an analysis of Food and Drug Administration (FDA) summary basis of approval reports. Biol Psychiatry. 2007;62(4):345-54.
40. Brikell I, Chen Q, Kuja-Halkola R, D'Onofrio BM, Wiggs KK, Lichtenstein P, et al. Medication treatment for attention-deficit/hyperactivity disorder and the risk of acute seizures in individuals with epilepsy. Epilepsia. 2019;60(2):284-93.
41. Auvin S, Wirrell E, Donald KA, Berl M, Hartmann H, Valente KD, et al. Systematic review of the screening, diagnosis, and management of ADHD in children with epilepsy. Consensus paper of the Task Force on Comorbidities of the ILAE Pediatric Commission. Epilepsia. 2018;59(10):1867-80.

Psychogenic Nonepileptic Seizures: Psychobiology, Clinical Aspects, and Management

LG Viswanathan, Sanjib Sinha

■ INTRODUCTION

Psychogenic nonepileptic seizures (PNES), also known as psychogenic seizures or nonepileptic attack disorder, represent a complex and challenging phenomenon at the intersection of psychiatry and neurology. These seizures bear a resemblance to epileptic seizures in their clinical presentation but not due to abnormal electrical discharges in the brain. Instead, they stem from psychological reasons, often reflecting underlying emotional distress or unresolved psychological trauma.

Understanding the psychobiology, clinical aspects, and management of PNES is of paramount importance in providing appropriate care and support for affected individuals. This chapter aims to explore the multifaceted nature of PNES, encompassing its psychological, biological, and social dimensions. Understanding the intricacies of this condition will enhance the approach to diagnosis, treatment, and long-term management.

■ EPIDEMIOLOGY

Epidemiological information on PNES is scarce and constrained. The mean incidence of PNES was predicted by another study to be around 3/100,000 in Ohio, USA,[1] and the prevalence of PNES is 1.4/100,000 people in Iceland, with symptoms typically appearing in young adulthood (between 20 and 40 years).[2] In rural India, a community-based survey found the prevalence to be much higher (2.9/1,000 population).[3] Large-scale multi-center studies that may reliably estimate the prevalence and incidence are lacking. Approximately 75% of PNES cases are females, which is presumably owing to variations in neurobiology and social factors.[4]

■ CLINICAL FEATURES AND DIAGNOSIS OF PSYCHOGENIC NONEPILEPTIC SEIZURES

There are a number of paroxysmal neurologic conditions that can affect consciousness, but the majority of patients are diagnosed with either syncope, epilepsy, or PNES. In one study, a correct diagnosis could be made in 158 consecutive patients 87% of the time.[5] More than half of the patients who presented to healthcare providers after experiencing a blackout were diagnosed with epilepsy, 22.3% with syncope, and 18% with PNES, according to the authors of another study.[6,7]

Psychogenic nonepileptic seizures are not clearly understood, and therefore poorly treated.[6] Delay in diagnosis, misinterpretation of PNES as epileptic attacks (or less frequently, epilepsy as PNES), and inadequate doctor-patient communication are still common. Neurologists are essential in assisting patients in understanding their illness.

Clinically, PNES are characterized by periods of abnormal behavior, bodily sensations, or experiences that look like epileptic seizures but are not associated with ictal electrical activity. The most typical semiology comprises uncontrollable limb, trunk, and head movements that resemble tonic-clonic seizures. PNES can also include rigidity, tremor, atonia, and unresponsiveness. Pertinent features of PNES semiology have been enlisted in **Box 1**. It is also important to keep in mind that bizarre seizure semiology may be seen in some forms of frontal lobe epilepsy and the features listed here are only indicative and not specific. Scales and prediction scores for the diagnosis of PNES have been devised with varying degrees of sensitivity and specificity.[8-10]

> **BOX 1: Features of psychogenic nonepileptic seizures (PNES) semiology.**
>
> - Variable semiology
> - Asynchronous limb movements
> - Opisthotonos
> - Hyperventilation
> - Crying/shutting eyes tight
> - Side-to-side movements of the head
> - Protruding tip of tongue (tongue bite if present usually on the tip)
> - Pelvic thrusting
> - Prolonged duration of ictus/loss of consciousness
> - Inducible at bedside with suggestions

TABLE 2: Classification of psychogenic nonepileptic seizures (PNES).

Hubsch et al.[15]	Dhiman et al.[16]

- Dystonic attack with primitive gestural activity or pauci-kinetic attack
- Pseudosyncope
- Hyperkinetic
- Axial dystonic
	- *Abnormal motor*:
	  ○ Hypermotor
	  ○ Partial
	- Affective
	- Dialeptic
	- Aura
	- Mixed

TABLE 1: Diagnostic certainty of PNES.

Diagnostic level	History	Witnessed event	EEG
Possible	±	By witness or self-report/description	No epileptiform activity in routine or sleep-deprived interictal EEG
Probable	±	By clinician who reviewed video/in person, showing semiology typical or PNES	No epileptiform activity in routine or sleep-deprived interictal EEG
Clinically established	±	By clinician experienced in diagnosis of epilepsy (video/in-person), showing semiology typical of PNES, while not on EEG	No epileptiform activity in routine EEG or ambulatory ictal EEG, capturing a typical ictus
Documented	±	By clinician experienced in diagnosis of epilepsy, showing semiology typical of PNES, on video-EEG	No epileptiform activity immediately before, during or after ictus captured on ictal video EEG with typical PNES semiology

(EEG: electroencephalogram; PNES: psychogenic nonepileptic seizures)

The definitive test for the diagnosis of PNES is by video electroencephalogram (EEG). Semiology can be documented clearly and normal EEG/absence of abnormal ictal EEG activity will affirm the diagnosis. The duration of video EEG should be at least 24 hours or up till events are captured. Approximately 77% of patients would have had their first PNES within 24 hours of recording and 96% by the end of 48 hours.[11] PNES may be induced during telemetry after informed consent from patient's relatives to reduce the total duration of video EEG recording. Common noninvasive methods of inducing seizures are hyperventilation, photic stimulation, using a tuning fork or torchlight or verbal suggestions.[12] Nonhabitual events that occur while induction must be interpreted with caution. Invasive methods are discouraged. Interictal EEG abnormalities may be seen up to 9% of patients with PNES.[13] Their presence should not obviate the diagnosis of PNES, rather one must reappraise the history to ascertain if the patient also has epileptic seizures. The diagnostic level of certainty in the diagnosis of PNES[14] has been elucidated in **Table 1** and PNES classification has been enumerated in **Table 2**.

PSYCHOBIOLOGY OF PSYCHOGENIC NONEPILEPTIC SEIZURES

Psychogenic nonepileptic seizures are influenced by a complex interplay of psychobiological factors, including stress, trauma, and the conversion of emotional stress into physical phenomena. PNES manifest in diverse ways. No unifying mechanism or supporting factor has been recognized that is sufficient and necessary to explain PNES in all patients. The biopsychosocial, multifactorial etiologic model best explains PNES **(Fig. 1)**.[6]

Genetic Predisposition

The obvious and apparent "genetic" risk factor for the developing PNES is the female gender. Lesser[17] analyzed the gender distribution in 21 studies and discovered 734 females and 250 males with PNES. In contrast to other somatoform disorders, women are three times more likely than men to develop PNES. This difference between sexes cannot be completely explained by apparent observed

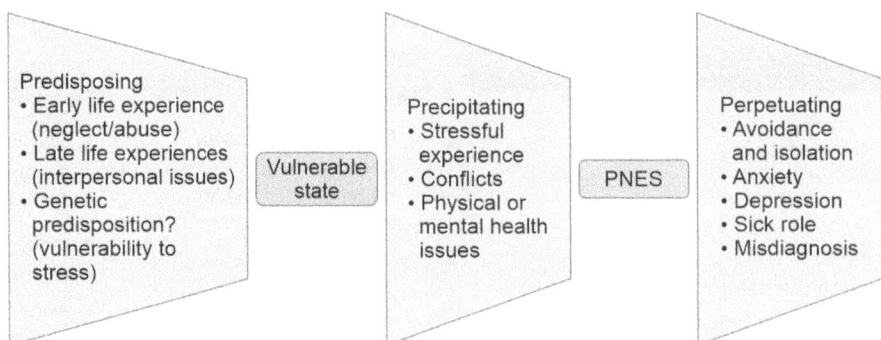

FIG. 1: Multifactorial model of psychogenic nonepileptic seizures (PNES) etiology.
Source: Adapted from Reuber et al (2009).[6]

demographic variations between men and women, such as higher rates of sexual abuse in women and girl children. However, there may be more direct biological factors why women are more probable to suffer from PNES than men, which are yet to be ascertained.

Childhood Sexual Abuse

The possible link between sexual abuse in childhood (CSA) and PNES has garnered considerable interest and been emphasized. CSA illustrates the unique association between a remote antecedent and appearance of psychopathology in adult life. A large study comparing CSA rates between patients with PNES ($n = 71$) and those with epilepsy ($n = 140$) found substantially high occurrence of sexual (24.0% vs. 7.1%) and physical (15.5% vs. 2.9%) abuse in childhood in patients with PNES.[18] Although the etiologic significance of CSA for PNES is debatable, these results have been reproduced by other studies on this topic.[19,20]

Similar to other psychiatric disorders associated with CSA, the unpleasant experience in childhood must likely interact with other extrinsic or intrinsic factors to cause PNES in adulthood. Holman et al.[21] demonstrated that, unlike epilepsy-affected controls, patients with PNES have a fearful style of attachment, making it more difficult for them to develop and sustain secure interpersonal relationships as adults. An apprehensive style of attachment was correlated with an adverse childhood experience. Patients with PNES and a history of CSA were also more probable to experience adult sexual abuse, indicating that a history of CSA may be indicative of a more ubiquitous adverse event. It has also been observed that >90% of patients with PNES probably had alexithymia on standardized tests, indicating that they had difficulty experiencing or perceiving emotions.[22]

Epilepsy with Psychogenic Nonepileptic Seizures

Epileptic seizures may coexist in up to 36% of PNES cases.[23] However, the mechanisms by which epilepsy increases the risk of PNES remain unknown. In a study comparing patients with epilepsy ($n = 590$) and those with epilepsy and PNES ($n = 90$), no clinical characteristics that increased the likelihood of comorbid PNES could be identified. Epilepsy may increase the risk of PNES through certain biological mechanisms and the experience or observation of epileptic seizures may enable model learning. Studies demonstrating that patients with PNES report a familial history more than those with epilepsy and are more likely to have witnessed someone else having a seizure prior to developing their own seizure disorder lend support to this theory.[23]

Psychogenic nonepileptic seizures have also been reported to occur after epilepsy surgery. "Forced normalization" after surgery and abandonment of the sick role may lead to the development of psychogenic seizures. In a study that looked into 697 patients who had seizures post epilepsy surgery, 4% of patients had PNES. It was noted that low full scale IQ and preoperative psychiatric comorbidities were associated with the same.[24]

Patients frequently report that their seizures began for no apparent reason, but significant risk factors for the onset of PNES can frequently be identified. In a small study evaluating individuals suffering from recent-onset PNES to those with epilepsy, the PNES group described more (typically negative or traumatic) life events in the 12 months preceding the onset of seizures than the epilepsy group.[25]

Stress has been identified as a significant contributor to the development and exacerbation of PNES. Studies have demonstrated that individuals with PNES often experience high levels of chronic stress, including life events, interpersonal conflicts, and financial difficulties. Increased stress levels have been associated with alterations in the hypothalamic-pituitary-adrenal (HPA) axis, leading to dysregulation of cortisol release and subsequent vulnerability to PNES.[6]

Furthermore, approximately 75-90% of patients with PNES report a significant history of trauma,[26] and there is evidence to suggest that a history of such trauma is more closely linked with the occurrence of PNES than other functional neurologic symptoms. It is evident that these potential precipitants are not specific for the development of PNES.

> **BOX 2: Differential diagnosis of psychogenic nonepileptic seizures (PNES).**
>
> - Epileptic seizures
> - Paroxysmal movement disorders, e.g., paroxysmal
> - Kinesigenic/nonkinesigenic dyskinesia
> - Syncope
> - Panic attack
> - Episodic vertigo

Dissociation and Somatization

Dissociation refers to a disruption in normal integration of consciousness, memory, and identity, often observed in individuals with PNES. Dissociative symptoms, such as depersonalization and derealization, have been implicated in the pathogenesis of PNES.[6] Moreover, somatization, the conversion of emotional distress into physical symptoms, plays a crucial role in the presentation of PNES. These psychobiological mechanisms highlight the complex interplay between psychological and physiological factors in PNES.

Neuroimaging studies have provided insights into the neural correlates of PNES, further supporting the psychobiological nature of the condition. Functional magnetic resonance imaging (fMRI) studies have demonstrated alterations in brain regions involved in emotion regulation, including the prefrontal cortex, amygdala, and hippocampus, in individuals with PNES. In a metanalysis and systematic review that looked into neuroimaging findings in PNES, none of the findings of the included studies were convergent. It is likely that brain alterations in PNES are heterogeneous and to identify biomarkers using small sample sizes may be difficult.[26]

By understanding the psychobiological factors involved in PNES, healthcare professionals can adopt a comprehensive and individualized approach to diagnosis and treatment. Integrating therapeutic interventions that address stress management, trauma processing, and the reduction of dissociative symptoms can significantly contribute to the overall management of PNES.

MANAGEMENT OF PSYCHOGENIC NONEPILEPTIC SEIZURES

It is essential to firmly establish the diagnosis of PNES before planning management. Common differential diagnoses to be considered are listed in **Box 2**. The management of PNES requires a comprehensive and multidisciplinary approach aimed at addressing the underlying psychological factors, improving coping mechanisms, and enhancing overall well-being. This section explores various strategies and interventions employed in the acute intervention and long-term management of PNES. A summary of studies that dealt with the treatment of PNES has been summarized in **Table 3**.

The management of PNES necessitates collaboration between mental health professionals, neurologists, and other healthcare providers. Establishing an interdisciplinary team facilitates comprehensive assessment, accurate diagnosis, and individualized treatment planning. The team may include psychiatrists, psychologists, neurologists, social workers, and nurses, all working together to address the complex needs of individuals with PNES.

Providing psychoeducation about PNES is a crucial aspect of management. Educating individuals, their families, and caregivers about the nature of PNES, its distinction from epilepsy, and psychogenic etiology helps reduce stigma, improve understanding, and foster self-management. Psychoeducation can include information about the neurobiological basis of PNES, triggers and stressors, coping strategies, and the importance of adherence to treatment plans.[27-29]

Cognitive behavioral therapy (CBT) has shown promising results in the management of PNES by targeting the underlying psychological factors and maladaptive coping mechanisms. CBT focuses on identifying and challenging cognitive distortions, addressing emotional regulation difficulties, and developing adaptive coping strategies. Through cognitive restructuring, relaxation techniques, and exposure therapy, CBT aims to reduce seizure frequency and improve overall functioning.[30,31]

While there is no specific medication for treating PNES, psychopharmacological interventions may be considered for comorbid psychiatric conditions. Antidepressants, anxiolytics, and mood stabilizers may be prescribed to alleviate symptoms of depression, anxiety, or other associated disorders. However, it is crucial to carefully evaluate the benefits and risks of medication use and ensure ongoing monitoring of their effects.[12]

TABLE 3: Management of PNES: Summary of pertinent studies.

Study	Type of study	Study participants	Intervention and duration	Intervention outcome (seizure frequency)
CBT				
Goldstein et al. (2004), UK	Before-after, noncontrolled study	n = 16	Individual CBT (12 × 1/week or fortnightly)	25% reported seizure freedom; 81% reported seizure reduction
Goldstein et al. (2020), UK	Pragmatic, parallel-group multicenter randomized controlled trial	n = 313	CBT plus standardized medical care (12 × 1/week or fortnightly) (n = 186) vs. standardized medical care alone (n = 182)	At 12 months, no significant difference in monthly dissociative seizure frequency was identified between the groups
LaFrance et al. (2009), USA	Before-after, noncontrolled study	n = 21	Individual CBT (12 × 1/week)	65% reported seizure freedom. 94% reported seizure reduction
LaFrance et al. (2014), USA	Multicenter pilot randomized controlled trial	n = 34	CBT-only: Individual CBT (60 min/week × 12) TAU; CBT w/sertraline; sertraline-only	33% reported seizure freedom. 55% reported seizure reduction
Myers et al. (2017), USA	Before-after, noncontrolled study	n = 16	Prolonged exposure psychotherapy. 12–15, 90-minute weekly sessions	81% reported seizure freedom
Mindfulness				
Baslet et al. (2020), USA	Prospective uncontrolled trial	n = 26	Individual mindfulness-based psychotherapy (12 × 1/week or fortnightly)	50% reported seizure freedom. 23% reported sustained cessation of PNES
Interpersonal therapy				
Mayor et al. (2010), UK	Before-after, noncontrolled study	n = 108	Psychodynamic IPT (19 × 50 min/week or fortnight)	25% reported seizure freedom
Psychoeducation				
Mayor et al. (2013), UK	Multicenter before-after, noncontrolled study	n = 13	Manualized psychoeducation (4 × 60 min/week)	31% reported seizure freedom. 54% reported seizure reduction
Chen et al. (2013), USA	Randomized controlled trial	n = 64	Three successive monthly, 1.5-hour long group sessions	No significant group difference in seizure frequency/intensity
Zaroff et al. (2004), USA	Before-after, noncontrolled study	n = 10	Group psychoeducational program 3 groups (10 × 1 hour/week)	75% reported seizure freedom
Cope et al. (2017), UK	Before-after, noncontrolled study	n = 19	3-session CBT-informed psychoeducation group	40% reported seizure freedom at the end of treatment. 63% reported seizure reduction during the intervention period
Sharpe et al. (2011), UK	Randomized controlled efficacy trial	n = 125	CBT-based self-help workbook and face-to-face guidance sessions	No data available about seizure frequency
Sarudiansky et al. (2020), Argentina	Before-after noncontrolled study	n = 12	3-group session cognitive behavioral based psychoeducation	42% reported a reduction in seizure frequency after the intervention
Group therapy				
Barry et al. (2008), USA	Before-after, noncontrolled study	n = 7	Group psychodynamic therapy (1 × week for 32 weeks)	57% reported seizure freedom

Continued

Continued

Study	Type of study	Study participants	Intervention and duration	Intervention outcome (seizure frequency)
Other interventions				
de Oliveira Santos et al. (2014), Brazil	Before-after, noncontrolled study	n = 37	Individual psychoanalysis (1 × 50 min/week for 12 months)	30% reported seizure freedom
Kuyk et al. (2008), Netherlands	Before-after, noncontrolled study	n = 22	Elective psychotherapy (individual, group, and family)	27% reported seizure freedom; 68% reported seizure reduction
Metin et al. (2013), Turkey	Before-after, noncontrolled study	n = 9	Group psychoanalytic and behavioral therapy (12 sessions)	67% reported seizure freedom
Paradoxical interventions				
Ataoglu et al. (2003)	Randomized controlled trial	n = 30	Individual IPT (2 times/day for 3 weeks)	93% reported seizure freedom

(CBT: cognitive behavioral therapy; PNES: psychogenic nonepileptic seizures; IPT: interpersonal psychotherapy)

Psychodynamic therapy, including individual or group therapy, can help individuals explore the underlying emotional and psychological issues contributing to PNES. By addressing unresolved trauma, conflicts, and maladaptive coping mechanisms, psychodynamic therapy aims to promote insight, enhance emotional regulation, and facilitate symptom reduction.[32]

Recently, retraining and control therapy has been proven to be useful in pediatric PNES.[33] Supportive interventions play a vital role in the management of PNES by providing emotional support, fostering self-esteem, and improving social functioning. Support groups, peer support networks, and individual counseling can offer a safe space for individuals with PNES to share experiences, gain validation, and develop coping strategies (LaFrance & Baker, 2010).[34]

The management of PNES necessitates a holistic and integrated approach that addresses the underlying psychogenic factors, provides psychoeducation, employs evidence-based psychotherapeutic interventions, and promotes self-management strategies. By adopting a collaborative treatment approach, healthcare professionals can optimize outcomes and improve the quality of life for individuals living with PNES.

CONCLUDING REMARKS

Psychogenic nonepileptic seizures represent a significant clinical challenge that requires an integrated approach bridging the gap between psychiatry and neurology. Increased knowledge in the domains of psychobiological mechanisms, clinical aspects, and management strategies will empower healthcare professionals to provide appropriate care, reduce diagnostic delays, and offer effective interventions to individuals living with PNES.

LEARNING POINTS

- Differentiating PNES from epileptic seizures is essential for accurate diagnosis.
- Understanding the psychobiological factors (stress, trauma, dissociation, and somatization) helps comprehend PNES etiology.
- Collaboration among mental health professionals, neurologists, and healthcare providers optimizes PNES management.
- Evidence-based interventions, including CBT, psychopharmacology, and psychodynamic therapy, enhance treatment outcomes

REFERENCES

1. Szaflarski JP, Ficker DM, Cahill WT, Privitera MD. Four-year incidence of psychogenic nonepileptic seizures in adults in hamilton county, OH. Neurology. 2000;55(10):1561-3.
2. Sigurdardottir KR, Olafsson E. Incidence of psychogenic seizures in adults: A population-based study in Iceland. Epilepsia. 1998;39(7):749-52.
3. Kokkat AJ, Verma AK. Prevalence of seizures and paralysis in a rural community. J Indian Med Assoc. 1998;96(2):43-5.
4. Alsaadi TM, Marquez AV. Psychogenic nonepileptic seizures. Am Fam Physician. 2005;72(5):849-56.
5. Angus-Leppan H. Diagnosing epilepsy in neurology clinics: a prospective study. Seizure. 2008;17(5):431-6.

6. Reuber M. The etiology of psychogenic non-epileptic seizures: toward a biopsychosocial model. Neurol Clin. 2009;27(4):909-24.
7. Kotsopoulos IAW, de Krom MCTFM, Kessels FGH, Lodder J, Troost J, Twellaar M, et al. The diagnosis of epileptic and non-epileptic seizures. Epilepsy Res. 2003;57(1):59-67.
8. Kerr WT, Janio EA, Braesch CT, Le JM, Hori JM, Patel AB, et al. An objective score to identify psychogenic seizures based on age of onset and history. Epilepsy Behav EB. 2018;80:75-83.
9. Rao SR, Slater JD, Kalamangalam GP. A simple clinical score for prediction of nonepileptic seizures. Epilepsy Behav EB. 2017;77:50-2.
10. Baroni G, Martins WA, Rodrigues JC, Piccinini V, Marin C, de Lara Machado W, et al. A novel scale for suspicion of psychogenic nonepileptic seizures: development and accuracy. Seizure. 2021;89:65-72.
11. Bettini L, Croquelois A, Maeder-Ingvar M, Rossetti AO. Diagnostic yield of short-term video-EEG monitoring for epilepsy and PNESs: A European assessment. Epilepsy Behav. 2014;39:55-8.
12. Baslet G, Bajestan SN, Aybek S, Modirrousta M, D Clin Psy JP, Cavanna A, et al. Evidence-based practice for the clinical assessment of psychogenic nonepileptic seizures: A report from the American Neuropsychiatric Association Committee on Research. J Neuropsychiatry Clin Neurosci. 2021;33(1):27-42.
13. Reuber M, Fernández G, Bauer J, Singh DD, Elger CE. Interictal EEG abnormalities in patients with psychogenic nonepileptic seizures. Epilepsia. 2002;43(9):1013-20.
14. LaFrance Jr. WC, Baker GA, Duncan R, Goldstein LH, Reuber M. Minimum requirements for the diagnosis of psychogenic nonepileptic seizures: A staged approach. Epilepsia. 2013;54(11):2005-18.
15. Hubsch C, Baumann C, Hingray C, Gospodaru N, Vignal JP, Vespignani H, et al. Clinical classification of psychogenic non-epileptic seizures based on video-EEG analysis and automatic clustering. J Neurol Neurosurg Psychiatry. 2011;82(9):955-60.
16. Dhiman V, Sinha S, Rawat VS, Vijaysagar KJ, Thippeswamy H, Srinath S, et al. Children with psychogenic non-epileptic seizures (PNES): A detailed semiologic analysis and modified new classification. Brain Dev. 2014;36(4):287-93.
17. Lesser RP. Psychogenic seizures. Neurology. 1996;46(6):1499-507.
18. Alper K, Devinsky O, Perrine K, Vazquez B, Luciano D. Nonepileptic seizures and childhood sexual and physical abuse. Neurology. 1993;43(10):1950-3.
19. Duncan R, Oto M. Predictors of antecedent factors in psychogenic nonepileptic attacks: multivariate analysis. Neurology. 2008;71(13):1000-5.
20. Sharpe D, Faye C. Non-epileptic seizures and child sexual abuse: a critical review of the literature. Clin Psychol Rev. 2006;26(8):1020-40.
21. Holman N, Kirkby A, Duncan S, Brown RJ. Adult attachment style and childhood interpersonal trauma in non-epileptic attack disorder. Epilepsy Res. 2008;79(1):84-9.
22. Bewley J, Murphy PN, Mallows J, Baker GA. Does alexithymia differentiate between patients with nonepileptic seizures, patients with epilepsy, and nonpatient controls? Epilepsy Behav EB. 2005;7(3):430-7.
23. Reuber M, Qurishi A, Bauer J, Helmstaedter C, Fernández G, Widman G, et al. Are there physical risk factors for psychogenic non-epileptic seizures in patients with epilepsy? Seizure. 2003;12(8):561-7.
24. Asadi-Pooya AA, Asadollahi M, Tinker J, Nei M, Sperling MR. Post-epilepsy surgery psychogenic nonepileptic seizures. Epilepsia. 2016;57(10):1691-6.
25. Reuber M, Howlett S, Khan A, Grünewald RA. Non-epileptic seizures and other functional neurological symptoms: predisposing, precipitating, and perpetuating factors. Psychosomatics. 2007;48(3):230-8.
26. Mcsweeney M, Reuber M, Levita L. Neuroimaging studies in patients with psychogenic non-epileptic seizures: A systematic meta-review. NeuroImage Clin. 2017;16:210-21.
27. Zaroff CM, Myers L, Barr WB, Luciano D, Devinsky O. Group psychoeducation as treatment for psychological nonepileptic seizures. Epilepsy Behav EB. 2004;5(4):587-92.
28. Chen DK, Maheshwari A, Franks R, Trolley GC, Robinson JS, Hrachovy RA. Brief group psychoeducation for psychogenic nonepileptic seizures: a neurologist-initiated program in an epilepsy center. Epilepsia. 2014;55(1):156-66.
29. Sarudiansky M, Pablo Korman G, Lanzillotti AI, Areco Pico MM, Tenreyro C, Paolasini GV, et al. Report on a psychoeducational intervention for psychogenic non-epileptic seizures in Argentina. Seizure. 2020;80:270-7.
30. Goldstein LH, Chalder T, Chigwedere C, Khondoker MR, Moriarty J, Toone BK, et al. Cognitive-behavioral therapy for psychogenic nonepileptic seizures: a pilot RCT. Neurology. 2010;74(24):1986-94.
31. Goldstein LH, Robinson EJ, Chalder T, Reuber M, Medford N, Stone J, et al. Six-month outcomes of the CODES randomised controlled trial of cognitive behavioural therapy for dissociative seizures: A secondary analysis. Seizure. 2022;96:128-36.
32. Bajestan SN, LaFrance WC. Clinical approaches to psychogenic nonepileptic seizures. Focus J Life Long Learn Psychiatry. 2016;14(4):422-31.
33. Fobian AD, Long DM, Szaflarski JP. Retraining and control therapy for pediatric psychogenic non-epileptic seizures. Ann Clin Transl Neurol. 2020;7(8):1410-9.
34. LaFrance WC, Baker GA, Duncan R, Goldstein LH, Reuber M. Minimum requirements for the diagnosis of psychogenic nonepileptic seizures: a staged approach: a report from the International League Against Epilepsy Nonepileptic Seizures Task Force. Epilepsia. 2013;54(11):2005-18.

Psychogenic Nonepileptic Seizure and Psychogenic Movement Disorder: Are they Really Different?

Ambar Chakravarty

INTRODUCTION

Psychogenic nonepileptic seizures (PNES) are very common and constitute a major differential diagnosis of epileptic seizures, perhaps only second to syncopes. In contrast, psychogenic movement disorders (PMDs) are much rarer constituting about 2–3% of all cases seen in a movement disorder clinic. Diagnosis of both PNES and PMD are essentially clinical, generally easy but on occasions extremely difficult; while absence of ictal epileptic discharges in video electroencephalogram (EEG) almost always can exclude the diagnosis of epileptic seizure, there is no such easily available standardized test to diagnose PMD (except complex electrophysiological tests).[1-4]

Similar to PNES, PMD is much more commonly encountered in women in the third or fourth decades of life; but unlike PNES, these are not very common in younger girls. However, both conditions share similar comorbidities. 10–15% of cases with PMD have additional neurological disorders, and 80% have psychiatric comorbidities. But as a fair proportion of patients may harbor both epilepsy and PNES, co-occurrence of an organic movement disorder along with a PMD must be extremely rare. However, both PNES and PMD share similar risk factors including history of sexual abuse, surgery, trauma, and major emotional stress. Somatoform disorders are very common in PMD, including somatization disorder, conversion disorder, and hypochondriasis, followed by depression, anxiety, and personality disorders.[5-10]

Psychogenic tremor is the most common form of PMD encountered in practice and this generally involves the hands and arms and rather rarely the head and legs. Clues to diagnosis include distractibility, entrainment (a change in the original tremor frequency to match the frequency of a repetitive task performed in another limb), and the presence of coactivation (the co-contraction sign). Psychogenic tremor almost never affects the face, tongue, and fingers. Psychogenic dystonia is the second most common form and its distinction from organic dystonia may be very difficult. A painful fixed dystonia following trauma and localized to one body part (causalgia–dystonia) is almost always functional in nature. Other commonly cited functional dystonias include blepharospasm, limb focal dystonia, and abductor laryngeal dystonia or paradoxical vocal cord dysfunction. With advancement in molecular genetics and functional neuroimaging, many such conditions are now falling in the borderland zone between functional/psychogenic and organic disorder. Myoclonus constitutes an unique entity: It may be an organic movement disorder, a psychogenic movement disorder, and can even be epileptic in origin. Clinical differentiation may not always be possible and one has to rely on combined electromyography (EMG) and EEG with back averaging technique to ascertain its nature and origin.

Myoclonus also needs differentiation from startles which again may be organic (hyperekplexia in children and autoimmune encephalitis in adults) or psychogenic in origin. Startles almost always are stimulus induced and occasionally culture specific (Latah and Jumping Frenchman of Maine).

Table 1 compares the levels of diagnostic certainty between PNES[7] and PMD.

Coming back to the question of relationship between PNES and PMD, the current overall impression is that PNES and PMD, despite differences in their phenomenology and demographics, share the same psychiatric symptoms, suggesting that PNES and PMD represent different presentations of a single disorder. The only clinical difference between the two being preservation of consciousness in patients with PMD and its apparent loss in cases with PNES. Ganos et al.[10] in an editorial commented that these disorders occupy a gray

TABLE 1: Categories of diagnostic certainty.

	PNES	PMD
Documented	No epileptiform activity immediately before, during, or after an event with typical PNES semiology captured on video EEG	Complete resolution of PMD following psychotherapy, psychological suggestion, physiotherapy or administration of a placebo, or presence of data from electrophysiologic tests proving a PMD (primarily evidence of premovement potentials before jerks or data from tremor studies)
Clinically established	By neurologist experienced in epilepsy (on video or in person) showing typical semiology of PNES, while not on EEG	PMD is inconsistent over time or incongruent with the typical presentation of a classical movement disorder plus one of the following additional features: Other psychogenic neurologic signs, multiple somatizations, obvious psychiatric disturbance, disturbance of PMD with distraction
Probable	By clinician who reviewed video recording or in person, showing typical semiology of PNES	PMD is incongruous and inconsistent in the absence of any of the other features listed above (clinically established) or symptoms that are consistent and congruent with a classical movement disorder but in the presence of other features, such as disappearance of the movement with distraction or other psychogenic neurologic disorders and multiple somatizations
Possible	By witness of self-report/description	Clinical features suggesting PMD and occurring in the presence of an emotional disturbance

(PNES: psychogenic nonepileptic seizures; PMD: psychogenic movement disorder)

Source: Reproduced with modification from Erro R, Brigo F, Trinka E, Turri G, Edwards MJ, Tinazzi M. Psychogenic nonepileptic seizures and movement disorders. A comparative review. Neurol Clin Pract. 2016;6:138-49.

area between neurology and psychiatry and commented on the poor level of integration between neurologists and psychiatrists. Somewhere else, Professor Stanley Fahn commented "What's in a name?" and quite rightly so.[11] Interestingly a group of subjects with PNES at times exhibits other disorders of movement, that is to suggest coexistence of PNES and PMD—adding more fuel to the debate between Lumpers and Splitters. Advancement in functional neuroimaging techniques and our knowledge of brain neurotransmitter localization and functions would soon mar the differences between neurology and psychiatry.

From the therapeutic point, cognitive behavioral therapy remains the treatment of choice for both conditions, though the evidence is stronger for PNES than PMD.

REFERENCES

1. Factor SA, Podskalny GD, Molho ES. Psychogenic movement disorders: frequency, clinical profile, and characteristics. J Neurol Neurosurg Psychiatry. 1995;59(4):406-12.
2. Munhoz RP, Zavala JA, Becker N, Teive HA. Cross-cultural influences on psychogenic movement disorders: a comparative review with a Brazilian series of 83 cases. Clin Neurol Neurosurg. 2011;113(2):115-18.
3. Kranick S, Ekanayake V, Martinez V, Ameli R, Hallett M, Voon V. Psychopathology and psychogenic movement disorders. Mov Disord. 2011;26(10):1844-50.
4. Shill H, Gerber P. Evaluation of clinical diagnostic criteria for psychogenic movement disorders. Mov Disord. 2006;21(8):1163-8.
5. Driver-Dunckley E, Stonnington CM, Locke DE, Noe K. Comparison of psychogenic movement disorders and psychogenic nonepileptic seizures: is phenotype clinically important? Psychosomatics. 2011;52(4):337-45.
6. Erro R, Tinazzi M. Functional (psychogenic) paroxysms: the diagnosis is in the eye of the beholder. Parkinsonism Relat Disord. 2014;20(3):343-4.
7. Kanemoto K, LaFrance WC Jr, Duncan R, Gigineishvili D, Park SP, Tadokoro Y, et al. PNES around the world: Where we are now and how we can close the diagnosis and treatment gaps-an ILAE PNES Task Force report. Epilepsia Open. 2017;2(3):307-16.
8. Gupta A, Lang AE. Psychogenic movement disorders. Curr Opin Neurol. 2009;22(4):430-6.
9. Hallett M, Weiner WJ, Kompoliti K. Psychogenic movement disorders. Parkinsonism Relat Disord. 2012;18(suppl 1):155-7.
10. Ganos C, Aguirregomozcorta M, Batla A, Stamelou M, Schwingenschuh P, Münchau A, et al. Psychogenic paroxysmal movement disorders: clinical features and diagnostic clues. Parkinsonism Relat Disord. 2014;20(1):41-6.
11. Fahn S, Olanow C. Reply to: psychogenic movement disorders: what's in a name? Mov Disord. 2014;29(13):1699-701.

COMMENTARY 7

Psychogenic Nonepileptic Seizures: Is it All in the Mind?

Ambar Chakravarty

INTRODUCTION

In the preceding chapter, Viswanathan and Sinha discussed in detail the psychobiological factors involved in the precipitation of psychogenic nonepileptic seizures (PNES) and only mentioned in passing the role of structural changes in the brain (determined by gender and genetic factors), which might be responsible for the genesis of PNES in susceptible subjects. This commentary aims to provide a brief overview of the brain mechanisms underlying PNES, with a special focus on analyzing brain networks.

The various cognitive and behavioral functions that humans are blessed with are performed by the complex network of interconnected regions in the human brain.[1,2] White matter tracts, which are bundles of myelinated axons and dendrites, in the brain maintain the connectivity between the different functional areas of the brain. These tracts transfer information from one brain area to another. Hence, knowledge about the structure and organization of the brain's white matter network is essential for gaining insights into the brain's functional architecture. Current research suggests that abnormal brain activity may play a role in the development and maintenance of PNES. The limbic system, consisting of structures such as the amygdala and the hippocampus, is involved in emotional processing and memory formation, and has been shown to be affected in patients with PNES. Morphological magnetic resonance imaging (MRI) studies have not reported large abnormalities in these regions,[3] but functional and white matter fiber abnormalities have been reported by several workers. For example, abnormalities in uncinate fasciculus (UF) fibers have suggested increased connectivity in subjects with PNES. The prefrontal cortex, controlling executive functioning and decision-making, has also been implicated in the pathophysiology of PNES. Reductions in the gray matter volume and cortical thickness in prefrontal areas such as the cingulate gyrus, middle frontal gyrus, and superior frontal gyrus have been recorded,[4,5] suggesting dysregularity functioning in this patient population. ^{18}F-fluorodeoxyglucose (FDG) positron emission tomography (PET) or cerebral blood flow based on single-photon emission computerized tomography (SPECT) have also reported reduced uptakes in prefrontal cortex.[6,7] In addition, several functional MRI (fMRI) studies have reported abnormal neural activities in this area.[8,9] These studies would suggest disturbances in cognitive, emotional, and behavioral control difficulties in PNES patients. Additionally, abnormalities have been noted in the insular cortex and supplementary motor area (SMA) by both structural and fMRI,[10-13] which would support the involvement of emotional and cognitive dysfunctions in PNES. All in all, these studies suggest that abnormal brain activity in regions involved in emotional processing, cognitive control, and motor and autonomic regulation may contribute to the development and maintenance of PNES, although the exact mechanisms are not yet very clear.

Network analysis has been used as a powerful tool for characterizing the complex organization of brain connectivity. In the human brain, which has about 86 billion neurons and 100 trillion synapses, pathological changes are rarely confined to an isolated area and often spread to other adjacent areas via axons.[14,15] Dysfunctions in the brain networks that control emotional and cognitive processing can lead to the manifestation of PNES symptoms.

Hence, network analysis may help localize the specific brain regions and pathways that are involved in PNES and how they are connected to each other.[16] In fMRI, connectivity can be assessed by correlating signal changes over time in each region, and in diffusion MRI, connectivity can be gauged from the strength of white matter fibers connecting different regions. In structural MRI and perfusion/metabolic imaging, connectivity can be measured from the correlation of gray matter volume and blood flow at each site. Diffusion tensor imaging (DTI) is a noninvasive neuroimaging technique that has markedly enhanced our ability to investigate the white matter integrity of the brain.[17]

This information can be used to construct a structural network model of the brain's white matter connectivity and abnormalities in which may be correlated with the symptoms of PNES.

There are already several neuroimaging studies on PNES using network analysis, mostly based on fMRI studies. Despite the relatively small sample size in each study, these studies have provided important initial evidence into the neural mechanisms of PNES. Basically, these studies identified abnormal connectivity in the insula and other areas controlling emotions and movement such as the amygdala and the prefrontal cortex and also visual areas.[18]

Abnormal structural network area in PNES involving the right precuneus and parahippocampal gyrus noted in DTI studies suggest some specific involvement of this region such as default mode network dysfunction.[19]

These studies are still in their infancy and studies with larger number of subjects are the need of the day. Making a diagnosis of PNES with long term video electroencephalogram (EEG) is a practical problem. In addition, there are issues with improper attention to and under recognition of the condition.

It seems likely that emotion regulation problems are involved in the development of symptoms in PNES. But this may be a matter of speculation. The same would be true for other functional neurological disorders (FNDs).

REFERENCES

1. Rubinov M, Sporns O. Complex network measures of brain connectivity: uses and interpretations. NeuroImage. 2010;52(3):1059-69.
2. Sporns O. Structure and function of complex brain networks. Dialogues Clin Neurosci. 2013;15(3):247262.
3. McSweeney M, Reuber M, Levita L. Neuroimaging studies in patients with psychogenic non-epileptic seizures: a systematic meta-review. Neuroimage Clin. 2017;16:210-21.
4. Labate A, Cerasa A, Mula M, Mumoli L, Gioia MC, Aguglia U, et al. Neuroanatomic correlates of psychogenic nonepileptic seizures: a cortical thickness and VBM study. Epilepsia. 2012;53(2):377-85.
5. Perez DL, Matin N, Williams B, Tanev K, Makris N, LaFrance WC Jr, et al. Cortical thickness alterations linked to somatoform and psychological dissociation in functional neurological disorders. Hum Brain Mapp. 2018;39(1):428-39.
6. Varma AR, Moriarty J, Costa DC, Gaćinovic S, Schmitz EB, Ell PJ, et al. HMPAO SPECT in non-epileptic seizures: preliminary results. Acta Neurol Scand. 1996;94(2):88-92.
7. Arthuis M, Micoulaud-Franchi JA, Bartolomei F, McGonigal A, Guedj E. Resting cortical PET metabolic changes in psychogenic non-epileptic seizures (PNES). J Neurol Neurosurg Psychiatry. 2015;86(10):1106-12.
8. Ding J, An D, Liao W, Wu G, Xu Q, Zhou D, et al. Abnormal functional connectivity density in psychogenic non-epileptic seizures. Epilepsy Res. 2014;108(7):1184-94.
9. van der Kruijs SJ, Jagannathan SR, Bodde NM, Besseling RM, Lazeron RH, Vonck KE, et al. Resting-state networks and dissociation in psychogenic non-epileptic seizures. J Psychiatr Res. 2014;54:126-33.
10. Neiman ES, Noe KH, Drazkowski JF, Sirven JI, Roarke MC. Utility of subtraction ictal SPECT when video-EEG fails to distinguish atypical psychogenic and epileptic seizures. Epilepsy Behav. 2009;15(2):208-12.
11. van der Kruijs SJ, Bodde NM, Vaessen MJ, Lazeron RH, Vonck K, Boon P, et al. Functional connectivity of dissociation in patients with psychogenic non-epileptic seizures. J Neurol Neurosurg Psychiatry. 2012;83(3):239-47.
12. Li R, Liu K, Ma X, Li Z, Duan X, An D, et al. Altered functional connectivity patterns of the insular subregions in psychogenic nonepileptic seizures. Brain Topogr. 2015;28(4):636-45.
13. Diez I, Ortiz-Teran L, Williams B, Jalilianhasanpour R, Ospina JP, Dickerson BC, et al. Corticolimbic fast-tracking: enhanced multimodal integration in functional neurological disorder. J Neurol Neurosurg Psychiatry. 2019;90(8):929-38.
14. Pakkenberg B, Pelvig D, Marner L, Bundgaard MJ, Gundersen HJ, Nyengaard JR, et al. Aging and the human neocortex. Exp Gerontol. 2003;38(1-2):95-9.
15. Herculano-Houzel S. The human brain in numbers: a linearly scaled-up primate brain. Front Hum Neurosci. 2009;3:31.
16. Liao X, Vasilakos AV, He Y. Small-world human brain networks: perspectives and challenges. Neurosci Biobehav Rev. 2017;77:286-300.
17. Smith SM, Jenkinson M, Johansen-Berg H, Rueckert D, Nichols TE, Mackay CE, et al. Tract-based spatial statistics: voxelwise analysis of multi-subject diffusion data. NeuroImage. 2006;31(4):1487-505.
18. Foroughi AA, Nazeri M, Asadi-Pooya AA. Brain connectivity abnormalities in patients with functional (psychogenic nonepileptic) seizures: a systematic review. Seizure. 2020;81:269-75.
19. Ding JR, An D, Liao W, Li J, Wu GR, Xu Q, et al. Altered functional and structural connectivity networks in psychogenic non-epileptic seizures. PLoS One. 2013;8(5):e63850.

CHAPTER 11

Psychiatric Mimics of Epileptic Seizures: Part 1—Episodic Dyscontrol Syndrome: The Concept

Ambar Chakravarty

INTRODUCTION

The term episodic dyscontrol syndrome (EDS) had been in use in psychiatric literature for several years. It was Elliot who probably tried to make neurologists familiar to this condition in 1984 in his superb review of the subject in Neurology Clinics.[1] He defined the condition as *"recurrent attacks of uncontrollable rage, usually with minimal provocation and often out of character; and it can be a symptom of both psychogenic and physical disorders"*. The recurrent attacks of uncontrollable rage usually occur with minimal provocation and often completely out of context. It is not regarded as a specific disorder but rather a symptom of many other disorders, including antisocial personality disorder, psychoses, neurosis, and organic brain syndromes.

Episodic dyscontrol is important on account of its social and legal implications. It has been shown to be one of the causes of unplanned suicide, meaningless attacks on strangers, social and echo-vandalism, battering of spouses, child abuse, criminally aggressive driving, meaningless destruction of property, and savage attacks on animals. It is different from planned aggression, or habitual aggressive maneuvering, seen in some communities living in slums, where these behavioral outbursts are used as a means of survival or social protest. It is also different from the use of physical aggression as a means of settling problems or issues by some people, living in states of continued deprivation. This is also different from unexplained rage and rage encountered in overt or borderline psychotics, true psychopaths, mentally retarded persons, or from isolated acts of extreme violence sometime seen in an individual who has been otherwise normal. It is also different from aggressive and explosive behavior triggered by intake of drugs or alcohol or noticed in persons who deliberately use aggressive behavior to manipulate situations to suit them.

CLINICAL CHARACTERISTICS

Since, these patients do not exhibit their violence and anger in a doctor's clinic, the diagnosis is based on the history provided by them or their relatives and eyewitnesses. But it is more or less similar story in each of the attacks, in a given patient with only minor variations. The episodes of dyscontrol usually come on abruptly, without any warning, but sometimes they may be preceded by dysphoric symptoms, which is evident to the onlooker within a short while. Without any provocation, the explosions occur. There is a Dr Jekyll and Mr Hyde like transformation of patient's behavior which reaches its peak within minutes and continues over a period of several minutes or in some cases hours. Once in an attack, the subject is uncontrollable and does not listen to any arguments, explanations, advices, or instructions. The type of physical violence has a savage quality. He often kicks, scratches, and bites his spouses or children. If the patient is a male, as is often the case, he may pick up his wife's bodily and throw her against the wall or to the floor. Next moment, he may smash windows or kick the doors and smash them. If the patient is a female, she might bite her husband's arms and tear his clothes. If he is driving a car he may use it as weapon against pedestrians or other cars or animals on the road. Pets such as small cats and dogs may be one of the worst victims. They are often swung by their tails and their heads smashed against a wall or a hard furniture. They may assault another person with a knife and might try to kill him with a single stab to his heart and may then give several more stabs to the dead body.

Women might use verbal violence as well, they use obscene, abusive, and absurd language, which is totally out of context. This they might do, even in social gatherings, without any apparent reason and without any regard to the presence of other people. Their speech is often garbled while they are verbally violent and their lips may be flecked with foam. They may snarl with their lips retracted baring their teeth and they growl like a dog.

During these attacks, patients often display remarkable strength and speed in their violent acts and do not give their victims a chance of self-defense. They look absolutely mad, although only for a short while. In some cases, however, there is enough self-control left, so that instead of attacking the main object in their mind, such as the wife or the child they attack the furniture or a family pet.

Once the attack is over, patients often feel exhausted and they have partial amnesia for the event. Remorse then usually appears, hours later in majority of patients and they are apologetic about their behavior and often begin to cry, and it might be sometime so profound that it has led to suicide or attempts at suicide.[2] But not all patients have remorse; particularly, the adolescents are less likely than adults, to feel guilty. Some of the males who assault their wives do not have a remorse because they believe that it is their privilege to beat or assault their wives. There are others who might try put the blame on others for their violence, using some excuse. Episodic dyscontrol can be triggered by consumption of even very small quantities of alcohol or they might occur on the morning following an evening spent in excessive drinking.[3] This has been attributed to a possible hypoglycemia resulting from the hangover.

In some women, attacks may occur usually in the week before the start of their menstruation.[4] Between attacks, the patient may appear psychiatrically unremarkable.

Not all people who act violently have the syndrome.[5] The differentiation of the EDS from temper tantrums may be a matter of semantics, although the less provocation there is, for attack provocation, more likely, it is EDS.

Disturbances of consciousness have been reported,[3] but in these patients the possibility of epilepsy must be considered. It is more understandable that the subject has no memory of the event, as can occur when violent emotions are involved. As outbursts stem from minimal provocation, it is unlikely that they are premeditated attacks.

It is difficult to estimate the frequency of episodic dyscontrol in the general population for several reasons. Firstly, an uncontrollable burst of temper is often taken as a part of an individual's personality and is hardly ever regarded as a medical or psychiatric disorder, particularly, in the society, in which domestic violence is common where it does not generate much public comment. Second, few people would be willing to admit that they have bursts of uncontrollable temper and several of them are pleasant enough between their attacks of rage so their family often tends to cover up these episodes of abnormal temper and often tries to offer excuses to account for them. Thirdly, study of violent behavior often does not find a place in the usual courses of studies for doctors, neurologists, and psychiatrists. Fourth, even physicians are not quite comfortable when they come across a patient who has been known to have a violent behavior and they tend to camouflage the bursts using much milder terms such as "irritable" and "hyperexcitable". Lastly, there is a lack of reliable information, as to how often organic disorders of the brain may contribute to family or street violence which is important. It is only after a detailed neurological search that a very significant number of individuals with *unprovoked* episodic dyscontrol, are found to have evidence of organic cerebral diseases.

ORGANIC CORRELATES OF EPISODIC DYSCONTROL

The syndrome is seen in different age groups in different forms, from tantrums of early childhood to the explosive behavior noticed in some senile individuals, but it is socially most disruptive in adolescence and early adult life. It is more common among males than in females. A correlation between male aggressiveness and high testosterone level has been suggested in some studies and it has also been reported that in violent and aggressive females the testosterone level is often higher than in nonviolent females.[6,7]

Genetic factors have also been reported to play a role, as in some cases there is clear family history of explosive rage involving three or more generations and affecting nearly half the siblings.[8] On the other hand, it has also been suggested that the aggressive behavior is learned from the parents and peers and is not genetically related.

Minimal brain dysfunction, temporal lobe epilepsy, and head injuries have been shown to account for the majority of cases. In the study of Elliot[9] in 102 individuals with episodic dyscontrol, the attacks of rage began and following a brain injury in a previously emotionally stable individual and it appeared reasonable to assure that the rage was a direct sequelae to the brain damage caused by head injury.[9]

Minimal brain dysfunction is a condition that embraces a wide variety of developmental and acquired disorders that do not amount to cerebral palsy or mental retardation. It has been accepted as a common precursor of social deviation in some adolescents and adults. Many children get over the problem but in some, it may continue in later life. One does not, however, know the number of people with adult minimal brain dysfunction, who are free of emotional and behavioral problems.

Relationship between Episodic Dyscontrol and Complex Partial Seizures

Clinical symptomatology of complex partial seizures of temporal lobe origin, is very variable. And it is no wonder that some features of episodic dyscontrol look very similar to those seen in complex partial seizures. These similarities account for episodic dyscontrol to come close in differential diagnosis of complex partial seizures. Even a past history of generalized tonic-clonic seizures, quite different from the febrile convulsions of childhood, has been found in some.[10-12] It has also been suggested by some as an epilepsy equivalent, although this term is rather ill defined and not always acceptable.[11,12] The prevalence of epilepsy amongst the delinquent and the criminal population is somewhat above normal, but there is no evidence to suggest that disruptive aggression is an epileptic phenomenon. Therefore, the developmental or acquired lesions that are responsible for epileptic seizures are not necessarily the ones that are responsible for the explosive rage. In majority of cases of episodic dyscontrol, the anatomic site of lesion responsible for the rage cannot be identified with precision. Tumors have sometimes been seen but not in a particular brain area. They seem to have been scattered all over and have been seen in limbic structures, hypothalamus, thalami, and cerebellum.[13] Apart from the limbic system, it has been suggested that emotional control can be modified by brainstem and midline cerebellar structures, and that in phylogenetic terms more primitive behavior may emerge.[1]

The role of alcohol in promoting and triggering aggression is obvious but is largely ignored. Alcohol is known to reduce inhibition and release the limbic system from cortical control, thus leading to primitive animal-like behavior.

CURRENT NOSOLOGICAL STATUS OF EPISODIC DYSCONTROL SYNDROME

The term EDS has not been mentioned in the DSM5.[14] An umbrella term "disruptive, impulse control, and conduct disorders" has been used to include "conditions involving problems in the self-control of emotions and behaviors". The condition "intermittent explosive disorder", having the same connotation as EDS, has been described under this category. The diagnostic criteria include:

- "Recurrent behavioral outbursts representing a failure to control aggressive impulses as manifested by either of the following:
  - Verbal aggression (e.g., temper tantrums, tirades, verbal arguments, or fights) or physical aggression toward property, animals, or other individuals, occurring twice weekly, on average, for a period of 3 months. The physical aggression does not result in damage or destruction of property and does not result in physical injury to animals or other individuals.
  - Three behavioral outbursts involving damage or destruction of property and/or physical assault involving physical injury against animals or other individuals occurring within a 12-month period.
- The magnitude of aggressiveness expressed during the recurrent outbursts is grossly out of proportion to the provocation or to any precipitating psychosocial stressors.
- The recurrent aggressive outbursts are not premeditated (i.e., they are impulsive and/or anger-based) and are not committed to achieve some tangible objective (e.g., money, power, and intimidation).
- The recurrent aggressive outbursts cause either marked distress in the individual or impairment in occupational or interpersonal functioning, or are associated with financial or legal consequences.
- Chronological age is at least 6 years (or equivalent developmental level).
- The recurrent aggressive outbursts are not better explained by another mental disorder (e.g., major depressive disorder, bipolar disorder, disruptive mood dysregulation disorder, a psychotic disorder, antisocial personality disorder, and borderline personality disorder) and are not attributable to another medical condition (e.g., head trauma and Alzheimer's disease) or to the physiological effects of a substance (e.g., a drug of abuse and a medication). For children ages 6–18 years, aggressive behavior that occurs as part of an adjustment disorder should not be considered for this diagnosis."

Important exclusions include:
- Disruptive mood dysregulation disorder
- Antisocial personality disorder or borderline personality disorder

- Delirium, major neurocognitive disorder, and personality change due to another medical condition, aggressive type
- Substance intoxication or substance withdrawal
- Attention-deficit/hyperactivity disorder, conduct disorder, oppositional defiant disorder, or autism spectrum disorder

CONCLUDING REMARKS

The fundamental presenting problem to a neurologist or psychiatrist would be similar—disproportionate uncontrollable rage. It is important to assess the severity of the triggering factor and the underlying psychiatric and neurological developmental status. Only on these would depend whether the episode could be labeled as organic or psychiatric. Whether the subject needs further evaluation or not.

LEARNING POINTS

- In EDS recurrent attacks of uncontrollable rage, usually occur with minimal provocation and often completely out of context.
- It is not regarded as a specific disorder but rather a symptom of many other disorders, including antisocial personality disorder, psychoses, neurosis, and organic brain syndromes.
- Episodic dyscontrol is important on account of its social and legal implications. It has been shown to be one of the causes of unplanned suicide, meaningless attacks on strangers, social and echo-vandalism, battering of spouses, child abuse, criminally aggressive driving, meaningless destruction of property and savage attacks on animals.
- Identifying a provocative element is the key to making a diagnosis of EDS in contrast to organic brain disorders like epilepsy.

REFERENCES

1. Elliot FA. The episodic dyscontrol syndrome and aggression. Neurol Clinics. 1984;2:113-25.
2. Mark VH, Ervine FR. Violence and Brain. New York: Harper and Row; 1970.
3. Maletzky BM. The diagnosis of pathological intoxication. J Stud Alcohol 1976;37:1210-28.
4. Dalton K. The premenstrual syndrome and progesterone therapy. London: Heinemann; 1977.
5. Maletzky BM. The episodic dyscontrol syndrome. Dis Nerv Syst. 1973;34:178-85.
6. Valzelli L Psychobiology of Aggression and Violence, New York: Raven Press; 1981.
7. Ehlers CL, Ricklar KC, Hovey JE. A possible relationship between plasma testosterone and aggressive behaviour in a female outpatient populations. In: Girais M and Kiloh L (eds). Limbic Epilepsy and the Dyscontrol Syndrome. New York: Elsevier/North Holland; 1979.
8. Davenport CB. The feebly inhibited. Violent temper and its inheritance. J Nerv Ment Dis. 1915;42:593-605.
9. Elliot FA. Neurological findings in adult minimal brain dysfunction and the dyscontrol syndrome. J Nerve Ment Dis. 1982;170:680-7.
10. Bach-Y-Rita G, Lion JR, Climent CF, Ervin FR. Episodic dyscontrol. A study of 130 violent patients. Am J Psychiat. 1971;217:1473-5.
11. Monroe RR. Brain Dysfunction in Aggressive Criminals. Lexington: MassLexington Books; 1978.
12. Monroe RR. The Episodic Behavioural Disorders. Cambridge. Mass, Harvard University Press; 1970.
13. Malamud M. Psychiatric disorders in intracranial tumours of the limbic system. Arch Neurol. 1967;17:113-23.
14. Diagnostic and Statistical Manual. Washing DC: American Psychiatric Association; 2013.

CHAPTER 12

Psychiatric Mimics of Epileptic Seizures: Part 2—Epilepsy, Rage, Tantrums, and Violence

Ambar Chakravarty

■ INTRODUCTION AND HISTORICAL ASPECTS

Society and medicine have long argued the purported association between epilepsy and violence. In ancient Greece, Hercules was believed to have murdered his family in a fit of uncontrollable "epileptic rage".[1] An early report in the modern era of violence associated with epileptic seizures was provided by Williams,[2] who identified 17 cases of ictal aggression among 100 cases of temporal lobe epilepsy. In modern times, the American public had been exposed to the case of Charles Whitman, a man with brain tumor and seizures, who climbed a tower at the University of Texas and opened fire on students. There have also been varied opinions about the relationships among epilepsy, brain injury, electroencephalogram (EEG) abnormalities, and violence in Jack Ruby, killer of Lee Harvey Oswald, the man who assassinated President Kennedy.[3] In Great Britain, a man with a known history of seizures was visiting a friend and proceeded to attack and kick him, with no recollection of the event. A British judge allowed a plea of not guilty by reason of insanity.[4]

Hindler[5] reported a case of a 19-year-old woman with epilepsy who killed a baby in a seizure allegedly triggered by the baby's crying. A causal association was difficult to establish, but the court accepted a plea of guilty to manslaughter with demisted responsibility. One well-publicized case had claimed to raise an association of epilepsy with arson.[6] A man suffered a subarachnoid hemorrhage and resulting personality change with violent outbursts. The EEG was paroxysmal and episodes of complex partial seizures were observed. After a night of drinking in a pub, he travelled home, shoveled burning coals from the fireplace around his living room, hastened his family out of the house, and returned to stand in the fire, although he subsequently escaped. The legal argument was made successfully that an organic cause was responsible, and no punishment or hospitalization was ordered by the Judge. Despite the article's title, "Epilepsy and Arson," evidence that this fire happened during and because of a seizure was very speculative.

Prevalence of aggression in population with epilepsy is poorly identified because case series discussing this association have severe referral and ascertainment bias. At a center such as the Maudsley Hospital in London (now closed), known to be interested in neuropsychiatric conditions and possible epilepsy surgery candidates, incidence of aggression in temporal lobe epilepsy may reach 27% of 100 cases[7] or 45% of 31 surgical referrals.[8] Patients with tumors and seizures have been reported to show a 27% incidence of violence in 90 cases of temporal lobe epilepsy,[9] but the contribution of the tumor may be important. Among a sample of 100 consecutive children with epilepsy referred to a program with interest in psychosocial complications of epilepsy, 36 exhibited rage attacks.[10]

Glaser[11] documented aggressive behavior in 56% of children with limbic epilepsy. In tertiary referral centers specializing in medical therapy, 7% of 666 patients[12] and 4.8% of 700 cases[13] were considered to show aggressive behavior. It may be presumed that these numbers substantially overestimate the incidence of aggression in community-based epilepsy studies. In general, psychopathology is more common in individuals with epilepsy.[14,15]

In reviews of epilepsy and violence, investigators have concluded that violence is no more common in epilepsy than in properly matched populations of people without epilepsy.[16-18] Ictal violence is rare and "resistive" in nature.

There is, however, little doubt that violence can occur during seizures, rarely even with fatalities.[19] Mark and Ervin[20] described a patient, Julia, who stabbed a bystander who had bumped into her at the start of a seizure. On another occasion, she stabbed a nurse with a pair of scissors.

The International League Against Epilepsy (2017) considers *"Tantrums and rage reactions" to be almost never part of an epileptic seizure. Tantrums are common in young children and are usually easy to distinguish from an epileptic seizure. Rage reactions, episodic dyscontrol or intermittent explosive disorder describe situations in which there are recurrent episodes of rage which seem to be out of proportion to relatively minor stimuli. Sustained outbursts of aggression may occur for many minutes, sometimes for up to half an hour or longer. There may be screaming, swearing, aggression, damage to property, and physical violence. Through the event it may seem that the individual is not normally responsive. Individuals often report no memory for an event afterward, and may express remorse for their actions. Rage reactions are usually much longer and are only very broadly stereotyped when compared to focal seizures. A rage reaction, when closely analyzed is likely to include a series of complex directed motor tasks, which would be exceptionally rare for an epileptic seizure. Aggressive or violent behaviors in an epileptic seizure are very rare, and if seen are typically confused and nondirected actions.*

The question remains: Is violence more common in people with Epilepsy? Methodological flaws in studies of aggression and temporal lobe epilepsy make it impossible to determine whether or not there is a higher incidence of violence in patients with epilepsy. Often epilepsy is diagnosed loosely (e.g., on the basis of déjà vu experiences), the seizure type poorly characterized, EEG abnormalities not critically examined, violence and aggression poorly defined, proper control/comparison groups not established, small numbers expanded to grand conclusions, referral and selection biases ignored, and other confounding factors not considered.

The claim of a relationship between violence and epilepsy has been used to provide an "excuse" for antisocial behavior. Psychomotor seizures are said to be more prevalent in violent populations.[21]

The "epilepsy defense" argues that a defendant is innocent because his or her alleged crime resulted from epilepsy and not from voluntary misbehavior.[22] Because neurologists are at times asked to make a judgment as to whether an alleged act may have been the result of an epileptic condition, it is worthwhile to review the evidence that such acts may occur, and to ask what criteria should be used to decide that a given act was, or could have been, the result of an epileptic seizure.

At first, answers to the following questions must be known:
- What are characteristics of an epileptic seizure? How can we decide a paroxysmal event is ictal?
- Is there any evidence that directed violence may be part of an epileptic seizure?
- Is there any evidence that violent behavior occurs more frequently in individuals with epilepsy or that epilepsy is more frequent in violent criminals?
- Is there evidence that interictal violence occurs in individuals with epilepsy, and that the violence is an intrinsic part of the epileptic syndrome?
- What criteria should be used by neurologists when assessing whether an episode of violence was a part of an epileptic seizure?

In the second step, detailed information regarding the accused's seizure semiology must be elicited and a detailed sequence of events leading to committing the alleged crime must be obtained specially in relation to the behavior of the accused individual during preictal, ictal, and postictal states. Answers to the following questions are essential for a neurologist called as an expert witness or a defense lawyer:
- What was the accused doing at the time of the event?
- What was the first thing noted by him or her and by observers?
- What happened next?
- Was there any apparent alteration of consciousness, any automatic behavior,
- If so, in what sequence did each component occur?
- Did the alleged crime occur before or after other components of the seizure?
- Was the seizure or the crime in any way provoked?
- Was there any evidence of premeditation and planning for the crime?

Three types of aggressive behavior may be associated with ictal activity. These include:[23]
1. *"Nonaggressive violent automatisms that were stereotyped and repetitive* from seizure to seizure; or,
2. *Reactive automatisms manifested by directed aggression after the onset of clearly identifiable stereotyped complex partial seizures; or*
3. *Resistive violence at the end of a complex partial or generalized tonic-clonic seizure when the individual was being restrained while still in a confused state."*

Forensic consultants to St. Elizabeth's Hospital in Washington DC, USA, have asserted that *"It is our belief that the presence of a documented neurological deficit in an individual suffering from episodic dyscontrol should be considered strong evidence, under certain circumstances, for inability of the individual to conform his conduct to the requirements of the law by virtue of a mental defect."*[24]

With few exceptions, the epilepsy defense has been notoriously unsuccessful. Use of the epilepsy defense is highly objectionable to most advocates of people with epilepsy, because it casts people with epilepsy as dangerous or deranged. Only very rarely, if at all, can an epilepsy defense be a justification for violence. Treiman wrote *"there have been no adequately documented cases of ictal aggression in which an organized, directed attack toward another individual or object occurred as the initial or sole manifestation of an epileptic seizure"*.

In a recently published review of Epilepsy and Law, Arjundas and Arjundas,[25] commented on epilepsy defense (termed by them "helpful law") and cited two instances in India where the accused were acquitted on ground of epilepsy (Satwant Singh vs. State of Punjab and Ahmadullah vs. Madhya Pradesh).

Treiman and Delgado-Escueta[26] suggested the following guidelines for neurologists when asked to give expert testimony in connection with *epilepsy defense*:

- *"The diagnosis of epilepsy should be established by at least one neurologist with special competence in epilepsy.*
- *The presence of epileptic automatisms should be documented by the history and closed circuit television (CCTV)-EEG.*
- *The presence of aggression during epileptic automatisms should be verified in a video-recorded seizure, in which ictal epileptiform patterns also are recorded on the EEG.*
- *The aggressive or violent act should be characteristic of the patient's habitual seizures as elicited in the history. The act should occur suddenly and not in response to any external stimulus except, perhaps, and restraint. It should be of short duration, fragmentary, and unsustained and it should be associated with other features typical of a complex partial seizure.*
- *A clinical judgment should be made by the neurologist attesting to the possibility that the act was part of a seizure. In making such a judgment the neurologist should consider whether the act followed the known sequence of behavioral changes in complex partial seizures or whether it was too complex to have been carried out by an individual suffering from an epileptic automatism."*

CONCLUDING REMARKS

It is almost a routine practice by psychiatrists in this country, to order an EEG in all patients with aggressive or violent behavior. Minor, usually nonspecific changes, are often overinterpreted as "dysrhythmic" and the patients treated with antiepileptic medication. This practice is certainly not ideal. Neurologists need to show some degree of restraint in not overinterpreting EEGs specialty in patients with aggressive behavior disorders. Unprovoked aggression or violence is very rarely truly epileptic in nature.

LEARNING POINTS

- The claim of a relationship between violence and epilepsy has been used to provide an "excuse" for antisocial behavior.
- Neurologists are at times asked to make a judgment as to whether an alleged act may have been the result of an epileptic condition, it is worthwhile to review the evidence that such acts may occur, and to ask what criteria should be used to decide that a given act was, or could have been, the result of an epileptic seizure.

REFERENCES

1. Penfield W, Jasper H. Epilepsy and the Functional anatomy of the Human Brain. Boston: Little, Brown; 1954.
2. Delgado JMR. Physical Control of the Mind. New York: Harper and Row; 1969.
3. State V. Jack ruby. Trauma. 1964;6:5-268.
4. Brahams D. Medicine and the law. Epilepsy and insanity at common law. Lancet. 1983;1:309.
5. Hindler CG. Epilepsy and violence. Br J Psychiat. 1989;155:246-9.
6. Carpenter PK, King AL. Epilepsy and arson (see comments). Br J Psychiat. 1989;154:554-6.
7. Falconer MA. Reversibility by temporal-lobe resection of the behavioral abnormalities of temporal-lobe epilepsy. N Engl J Med. 1973;289:451-5.
8. Herzberg JL, Penwick PB. The aetiology of aggression in temporal-lobe epilepsy. Br J Psychiat. 1988;153:50-5.
9. Bingley T. Mental symptoms in temporal lobe epilepsy and temporal gliomas with special reference to laterality of lesion and the relationship between handedness and braindness. Acta Neurol Scand. 1958;33(Supp 120):1-151.
10. Ounsted C. Aggression and epilepsy rage in children with temporal lobe epilepsy. J Psychosom res 1969;13:237-42.
11. Glaser GH. Limbic epilepsy in childhood. J Nervment Dis. 1967;144:391-7.
12. Currie S, Heathfield W, Henson R, Scott D. Clinical course and prognosis of temporal lobe epilepsy: A survey of 666 patients. Brain. 1971;94:173-90.
13. Rodin EA. Psychomotor epilepsy and aggressive behavior. Arch Gen psychiat. 1973;28:210-3.
14. Perrine KR. Psychopathology in epilepsy. Sem Neurol. 1991;11:175-81.
15. Walker AE, Blumer D. Behavioral effects of temporal lobectomy for temporal lobe epilepsy. In: Bensor DF, Blumer D (eds.) Psychiatric Effects of Epilepsy. Washington DC: American Psychiatric Press; 1984. pp. 295-321.
16. Blurner D. Epilepsy and Violence. In: Madden DJ. Lion JR (eds.). Rage, Assault, and other Forms of Violence. Jamaica, NY: Spectrum Publications; 1976.
17. Daly DD. Ictal clinical manifestations of complex partial seizures. Adv Neurol. 1975;11:57-84.

18. Treiman DM. Epilepsy and violence: Medical and legal issues. Epilepsia. 1986;27(Suppl 2):S77-104.
19. Oliver JE. Successive generations of child maltreatment. The children. Br Psychiat. 1988;153:543-53.
20. Mark VH, Ervin FR. Violence and the Brain. New York: Harper & Row; 1970.
21. Lewis DO. Neuropsychiatric vulnerabilities and violent juvenile delinquency. Psychiatric Clin N Am. 1983;6:707-14.
22. Beresford HR, Legal implications of epilepsy. Epilepsia. 1988;29 (Supp 2):S114-21.
23. Treiman DM. Aggressive behavior and violence in epilepsy: Guidelines for expert testimony. Rosner R (ed): Principles and Practice of Forensic Psychiatry: A Comprehensive Textbook. New York: Chapman and Hall; 1994. pp. 451-60.
24. Ratner RA, Shapiro D. The episodic dyscontrol syndrome and criminal responsibility. Bull Am Acad Psychiat Law. 1979;7: 422-31.
25. Arjundas G, Arjundas D. Epilepsy and Indian Law. In: Singhal BS, Nag D (Eds). Epilepsy in India. India: Indian Epilepsy Association. 2001. pp. 388-97.
26. Treiman DM, Delgado-Escueta AV. Violence and epilepsy: A critical review. In: Pedley TA, Meldrum BS (eds): Recent Advances in Epilepsy. London: Churchill Livingstone; 1983. pp. 179-209.

CHAPTER 13

An Overview of Stroke Medicine for the Psychiatrist

Neetu Ramrakhiani

INTRODUCTION

A stroke is a medical emergency which occurs due to damage to the brain due to interruptions in blood supply. It often results in a sudden loss of focal brain functions. The World Health Organization (WHO) defines stroke as "rapidly developing clinical signs of focal (at times global) disturbances in cerebral function, lasting for more than 24 hours or leading to death with no apparent cause other than a vascular origin."[1]

A stroke that occurs due to a block of blood supply to the brain is called ischemic stroke and the one which occurs due to sudden bleeding in the brain is called hemorrhagic stroke. Ischemic stroke is more common than hemorrhagic stroke **(Flowchart 1)**.

PATHOPHYSIOLOGY

Normal cerebral blood flow (CBF) in the adult brain is usually 50–55 mL/100 g/min. When blood flow reaches 18 mL/100 g/min a threshold for *electrical failure* is reached consisting of salvageable nonfunctional neurons which are an important part of the penumbra. The second level is reached when blood flow reaches 8 mL/100 g/min which is the threshold for *membrane failure* when cell death occurs rapidly. Ischemic stroke occurs due to a reduction or complete blockage of blood flow. Severe stenosis or occlusion of a blood vessel and/or decreased systemic perfusion can be the cause of stroke. Cerebral autoregulation is impaired during the process of ischemic stroke. As cerebral perfusion falls, blood vessels dilate which increases the blood flow. Decreasing perfusion pressure beyond the ability of the brain to compensate results in a significant reduction in CBF. The infarcted brain appears pale. The brain develops neuronal swelling followed by pyknosis, endothelial swelling, and neutrophilic infiltration. This is followed by a phase of neovascularization.

Intracranial bleeds most commonly occur due to hypertension. Vascular lesions produced by lipo-

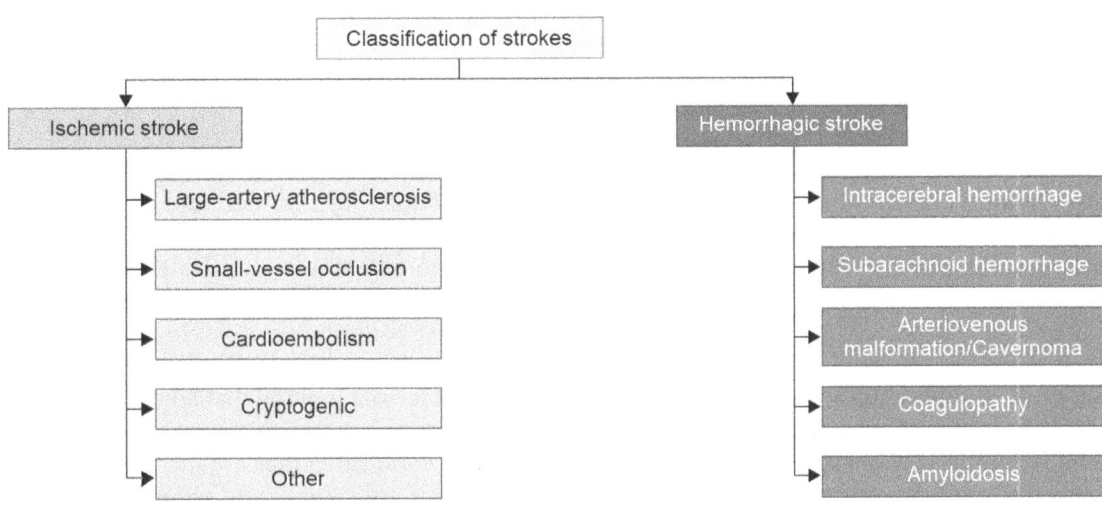

FLOWCHART 1: Classification of strokes.

hyalinosis of small arteries followed by arterial rupture are the presumptive mechanism of such bleeding in the brain. Small vascular malformations such as small arteriovenous malformation (AVM) and cavernomas can cause nontraumatic hemorrhage typically in young nonhypertensive females presenting with lobar hemorrhage. In bleeding diathesis, the use of anticoagulants causes a higher incidence of bleeding. The presence of cerebral microbleeds predisposes to the development of intracranial bleeding post-thrombolysis. Cerebral amyloid angiopathy (CAA) causes selective deposition of beta-amyloid in walls of cerebral vessels and is the cause of lobar bleeds in the elderly population. Subarachnoid hemorrhage (SAH) occurs due to a weakness in the wall of an artery resulting in ballooning which can rupture over time. Pathophysiologically they can be divided into saccular, fusiform, and dissecting subtypes.

TYPES OF ISCHEMIC STROKE

Determination of the type of ischemic stroke can influence the treatment offered to the patient. They are often subclassified using the system developed by investigators of the TOAST trials.[2] Ischemic stroke represents approximately 80% of all strokes. In India, a significant percentage of stroke occurs in young and is believed to be due to the presence of traditional risk factors such as hypertension, diabetes, and presence of intracranial atherosclerosis (ICAD).

Atherothrombosis

Atherosclerosis occurs due to blockage of a blood vessel which may happen acutely or gradually. Atherosclerosis may cause the narrowing of the diseased vessel which can affect intracranial and extracranial vessels at times the same process occurs due to a hypercoagulable state. Atheroma can produce stasis and vessel wall abnormalities leading to the development and propagation of a thrombus. Lacunar infarcts occur as a result of small vessel disease. Small penetrating vessels, due to chronic high blood pressure, lead to the deposition of fibrinoid material with luminal narrowing and occlusion. These strokes typically occur in the subcortical area of the brain.

Embolism

Embolism refers to a blood clot or any other material that travels away from the site of origin and blocks distal vessels causing ischemia. The heart is a common source of these vessels but artery-to-artery embolism can also occur. Air, fat globule, tumors, and venous clots can also result in such strokes.

Nonatherosclerotic Abnormalities

They can be inherited or acquired and are an important cause of stroke particularly in younger adults and children. These include arterial dissection, vasculitis, sickle cell disease, fibromuscular dysplasia, and moyamoya disease.

BRAIN HEMORRHAGE

There are two main subtypes. Intracranial hemorrhage (ICH) occurs due to bleeding in the brain parenchyma. SAH happens due to bleeding in cerebrospinal fluid (CSF) within the subarachnoid space that surrounds the brain.

Intracranial Hemorrhage

It usually occurs due to bleeding from small arteries which leads to the formation of localized hematoma which continues to grow until the pressure surrounding it limits its spread or it decreases itself emptying into the ventricular system. Common causes of ICH include hypertension, trauma, amphetamines and cocaine, angiopathy, and vascular malformations. Headache, vomiting, and decreased level of consciousness can develop if intracranial pressure increases.

Subarachnoid Hemorrhage

They occur commonly due to rupture of arterial aneurysms which release blood into CSF under high arterial pressure. This blood causes significant increases in intracranial pressure. It is often abrupt in onset compared to the more gradual onset of ICH and may or may not be accompanied by focal signs **(Fig. 1)**.

RISK FACTORS

Risk factors can be broadly classified into modifiable and nonmodifiable. Age, gender, and genetics are among the most important nonmodifiable risk factors for stroke. Modifiable risk factors can be subdivided further into behavioral and nonbehavioral subtypes. Hypertension is the most common modifiable risk factor for ischemic stroke and intracranial bleeding **(Fig. 2)**. Other modifiable risk factors include diabetes, atrial fibrillation (AF), cardiac disease, obstructive sleep apnea, and dyslipidemia. The behavioral categories are inactivity, smoking, alcohol abuse, illicit drug abuse, and sedentary lifestyle.

DIAGNOSIS

Stroke is suspected clinically based on the sudden onset of focal neurological deficits. A lot of prehospital stroke scales can help in detection and diagnosis including Los Angeles Prehospital Stroke Screen (LAPSS), CPSS (Cincinnati Prehospital Stroke Scale), and face, arm, speech, time (FAST). The important components in these scales include sudden onset of facial drooping, arm/leg weakness, and speech abnormalities. For differentiating stroke subtypes the pace of onset and offset of consolation of symptoms and signs of stroke is helpful. An embolic stroke occurs suddenly. Thrombotic strokes often fluctuate. Penetrating artery stroke cause symptoms that develop during a short period. ICH causes symptoms that progress from minutes to a few hours. SAH develops in an instant and is very severe. On clinical evaluation, presence of AF favors embolism from the heart. Urgent neuroimaging helps confirm the diagnosis in most cases and also helps in excluding some stroke mimics. The choice of imaging noncontrast computed tomography/computed tomographic angiography (NCCT/CTA) and MRI depends on availability and patient eligibility for reperfusion therapies.

STROKE LOCALIZATION

In the case of ischemic stroke, knowledge of basic brain anatomy and blood supply helps in stroke localization. Broadly blood supply is divided into anterior (paired) and posterior circulation. They are subdivided into their intracranial and extracranial parts. The main supply of anterior circulation arises from the carotid artery which travels from the neck into the brain and gives off the ophthalmic artery to the eye, middle cerebral artery (MCA) and anterior cerebral artery (ACA) to the anterolateral cerebral cortex, anterior choroidal, and posterior communicating arteries **(Fig. 3)**.

Transient ischemic attacks (TIAs) are defined as transient episodes of neurologic dysfunction caused by focal brain, spinal cord, or retinal ischemia without acute infarction. In this newer definition, an arbitrary 24-hour line has been replaced tissue-based definition. High-risk TIA is defined as per *ABCD2* score which consists of *A*ge, *B*lood pressure, *C*linical features, *D*uration of symptoms, and *D*iabetes. Although not perfect same provides a practical scale for routine practice.

Middle cerebral artery infarcts **(Fig. 4)** are the most common in clinical practice. The MCA is the most common artery involved in ischemic stroke. It supplies a large area of the brain and areas of the internal capsule

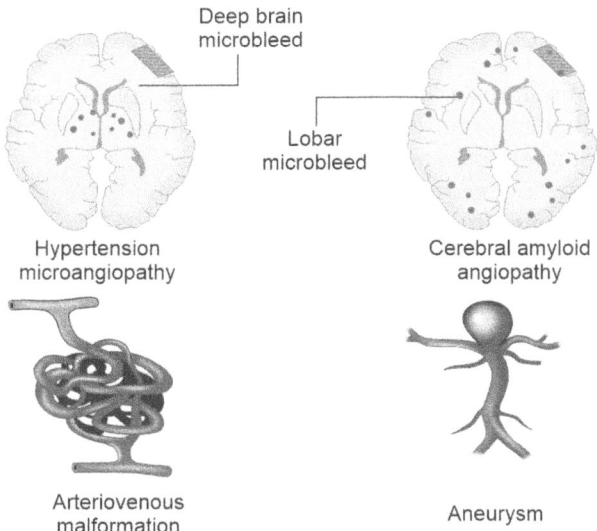

FIG. 1: Microbleed in brain.

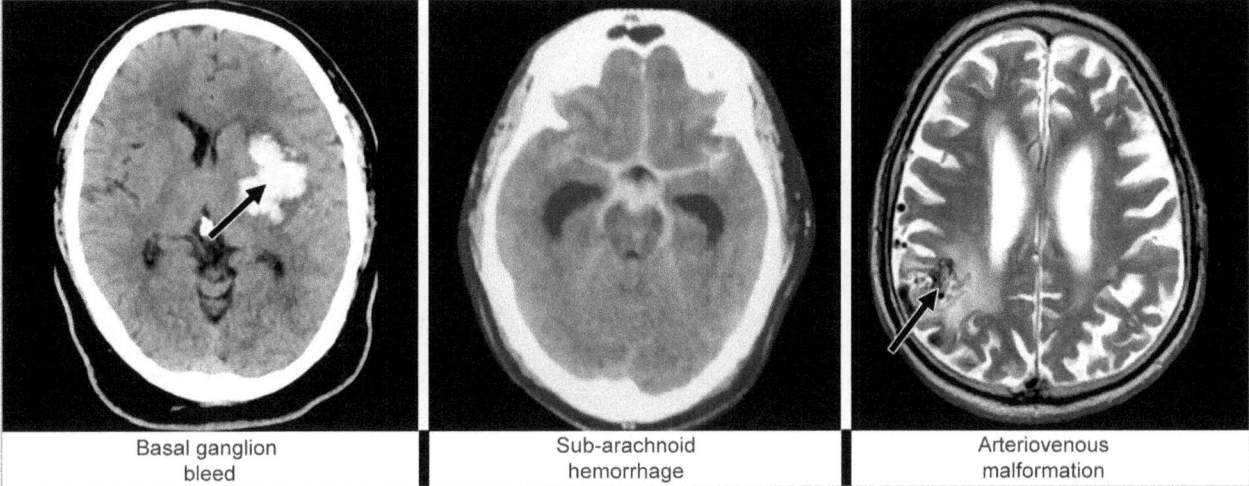

FIG. 2: Different pattern and etiology of bleeding in brain.

and basal ganglia. It is divided into four segments: i.e., M1 (horizontal segment), M2 (Sylvian segment), M3, and M4. Cortical signs such as aphasia, hemineglect, hemianopia, and gaze preference are often seen when the site of the infarct is cortical with large vessel occlusion (LVO) **(Fig. 4)**. Superior division MCA ischemia causes hemiplegia which is more severe in upper than lower limb with conjugate eye deviation to ipsilateral side and Broca's type aphasia with dominant lobe involvement. Inferior division MCA supplies inferior parietal and temporal lobe. Usually, these strokes do not have any elementary motor and sensory signs and are often presenting with Wernicke's aphasia, agitation, and field defect and can often end up in psychiatry units.

Occlusion of main stem MCA causes infarction of the basal ganglion and internal capsule before origin of lenticulostriate branch. Striatocapsular damage causes hemiparesis of face, dysarthria, and upper and lower limb weakness **(Fig. 5)**.

SYMPTOMS IN INFARCTS IN THE POSTERIOR CIRCULATION OF THE BRAIN

- *Lateral medullary (Wallenberg syndrome)* occurs due to occlusion intracranial vertebral artery. Common symptoms occur in form of vertigo, ataxia, sensory changes on ipsilateral face, and contralateral limbs for temperature and pain **(Fig. 6)**.
- *Medial medullary:* Contralateral hemiparesis and posterior tongue deviation.
- *Posterior cortical atrophy (PCA) syndrome*: Left side—ataxia without agraphia and Gerstmann syndrome and right side—prosopagnosia. Bilateral PCA stroke leads to Anton's syndrome.
- *Cerebellar syndrome*: Refer to **Figure 6**.

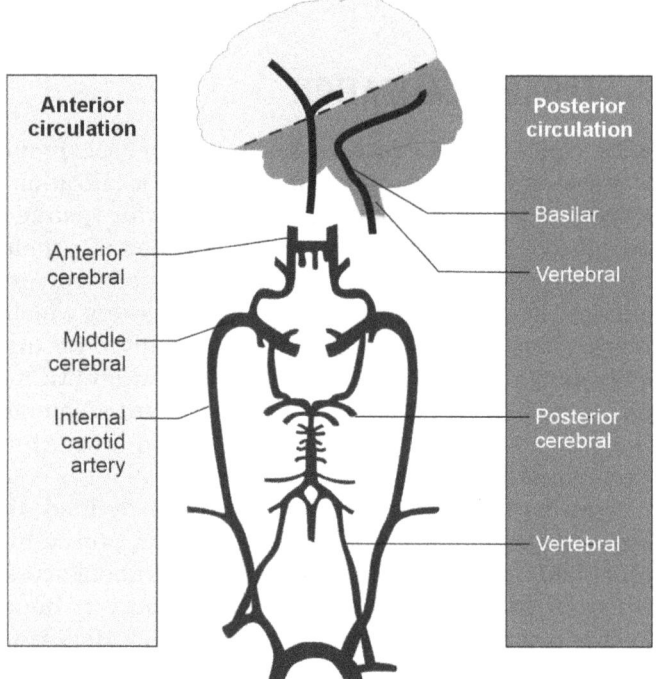

FIG. 3: Stroke localization.

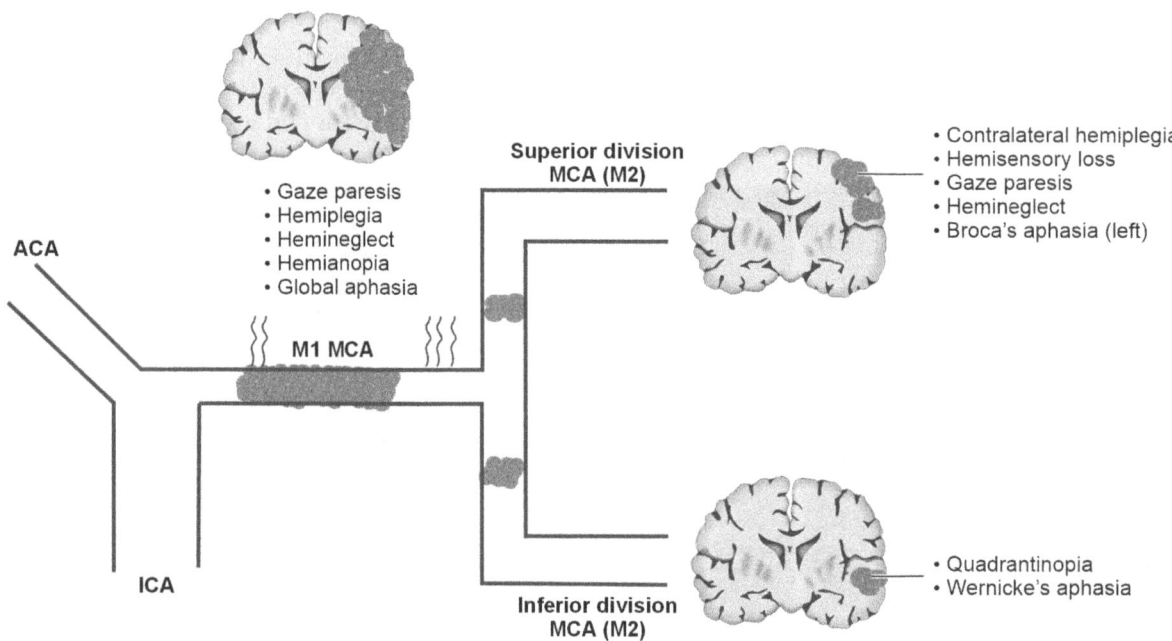

FIG. 4: Depicting localization and clinical features in middle cerebral artery infarcts.
(ACA: anterior cerebral artery; ICA: internal carotid artery; MCA: middle cerebral artery)

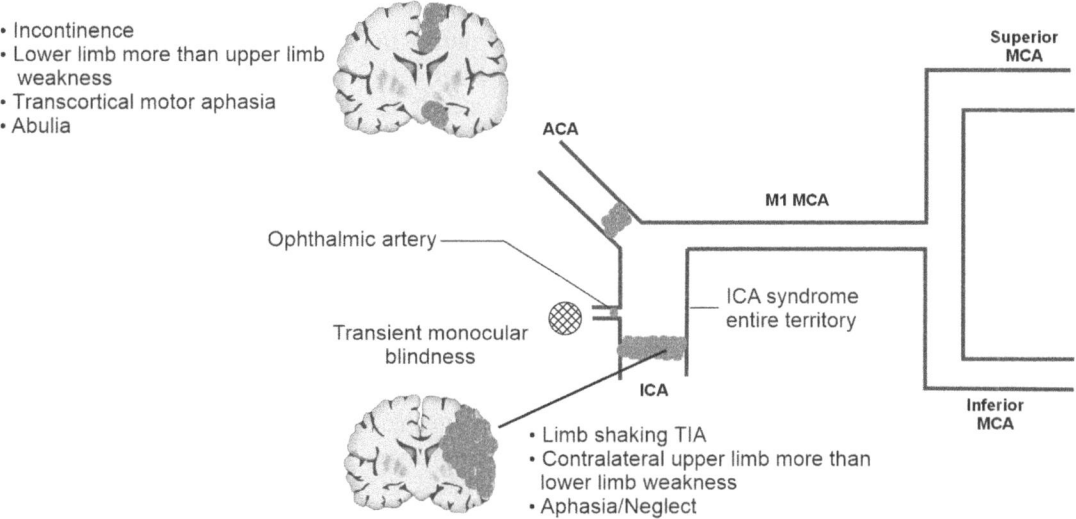

FIG. 5: Clinical symptoms and localization in case of ICA and ACA infarcts.
(ACA: anterior cerebral artery; ICA: internal carotid artery; MCA: middle cerebral artery; TIA: transient ischemic attack)

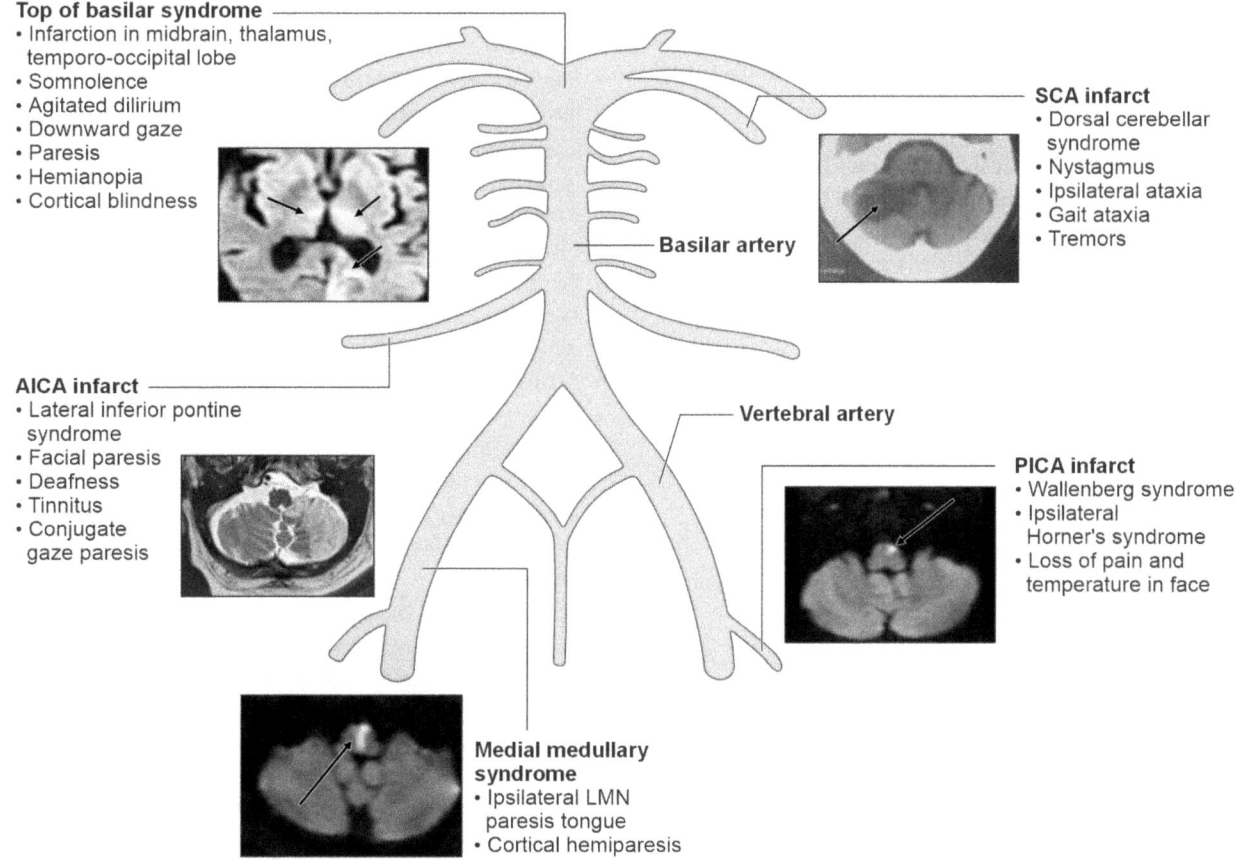

FIG. 6: Cerebellar syndrome.
(AICA: anterior inferior cerebellar artery; LMN: lower motor neuron; PICA: posterior inferior cerebellar artery; SCA: superior cerebellar artery)

Neuropsychiatric presentation of acute stroke (chameleons) is known to occur and should be recognized by all Wernicke's aphasia occurring commonly due to infarction in the posterior division of the MCA has a sudden onset of speech abnormality without motor manifestations and can be confused with psychiatric disorders. Similarly, ACA infarcts typically bilateral ACA infarcts can include prominent neuropsychiatric symptoms including abulia and mutism. Anton's syndrome with normally reactive pupils is another such syndrome of cortical blindness without awareness of same **(Fig. 7)**.

PRINCIPLES OF MANAGEMENT

A brief history, physical examination, blood sugar, and NCCT are enough in most cases as a guide for acute therapy. Diagnosis of an ICH can be aided by history on presentation and confirmed by an NCCT. A history of anticoagulant intake can help change the management in case of anticoagulant-induced ICH. CTA helps to assess for LVO and eligibility for thrombectomy.

- Attention to airway, breathing, and circulation (ABC) is of vital importance as in any other medical emergency. Patients with poor Glasgow Coma Scale (GCS) < 8, with bulbar dysfunction of hypoxia, need to be suitably inhibited and ventilated. Routine oxygen is not recommended in patients with ischemic stroke unless saturation is <94%.
- Assessing eligibility for revascularization in patients with ischemic stroke. Most revascularization therapies in acute stroke are time-dependent hence, the establishment of the exact time of onset is of critical importance. Thrombolysis is done within 4½ hours of onset of stroke and thrombectomy can be done without any advanced imaging within 6 hours of onset of stroke. Listed are the important criteria for thrombolysis and thrombectomy **(Box 1 and Table 1)**.

Other aspects of acute stroke management include blood pressure management. Blood pressure is usually elevated during stroke which can be due to sympathetic response or chronic hypertension. This however is protective in case of ischemic stroke to maintain brain perfusion in areas of borderline perfusion.[5] In case a patient is eligible for reperfusion therapy, blood pressure needs to be lowered to <185 mm Hg systolic

> **BOX 1: Eligibility criteria for the treatment of acute ischemic stroke with tissue plasminogen activator of tPA.[3]**
>
> *Inclusion criteria*
> - Clinical diagnosis of ischemic stroke causing measurable neurologic deficit
> - Onset of symptoms < 4.5 hours before beginning treatment: If the exact time of the patient was known to be normal or at neurologic baseline
> - Age ≥ 18 years
>
> *Exclusion criteria*
> Patient history:
> - Ischemic stroke or severe head trauma in the previous 3 months
> - Previous intracranial hemorrhage
> - Intra-axial intracranial neoplasm
> - Gastrointestinal hemorrhage in the previous 21 days
> - Intracranial or intraspinal surgery within the previous 3 months
>
> Clinical:
> - Symptoms suggestive of subarachnoid hemorrhage
> - Persistent blood pressure elevation (systolic ≥ 185 mm Hg or diastolic ≥ 110 mm Hg
> - Active internal bleeding
> - Presentation consistent with infective endocarditis
> - Stroke is known or suspected to be associated with aortic arch dissection
> - Acute bleeding diathesis, including but not limited to conditions defined under
>
> Hematologic:
> - Platelet count < 100,000/mm³
> - Current anticoagulant use with an INR > 1.7 or PT > 15 seconds or aPTT > 40 seconds
> - Therapeutic doses of molecular weight heparin received within 24 hours of prophylactic doses
> - Current use i.e., last dose within 48 hours in a patient with normal renal function inhibitor with evidence of anticoagulant effect by laboratory tests such as aPTT
>
> Head CT:
> - Evidence of hemorrhage
> - Extensive regions of obvious hypodensity consistent with irreversible injury
>
> (aPTT: activated partial thromboplastin time; INR: international normalized ratio; PT: prothrombin time; tPA: tissue plasminogen activator)

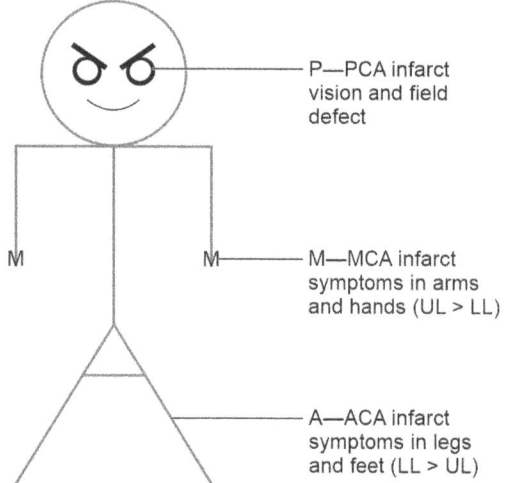

FIG. 7: A small cartoon depicting the important clinical finding which helps in stroke localization. P resembles spectacles (visual abnormalities), M for MCA (hand and arm), and A for legs.
(ACA: anterior cerebral artery; MCA: middle cerebral artery; PCA: posterior cortical atrophy)

TABLE 1: Criteria for intra-arterial thrombectomy based on the 2018 AHA/ASA guidelines categorized by evidence class and recommendation grade.[4]

1	Class Ia	Pre-stroke mRS 0–1
		For eligible patients, receiving IV alteplase within 4.5 hours of symptom onset
		Occlusion of the ICA or proximal M1-MCA segment
		Age 18 or older
		NIHSS score ≥ 6
		ASPECTS score ≥ 6
		Time to groin puncture within 6 hours of symptoms onset
		For selected patients within 6–16 hours of symptom onset with anterior circulation LVO who meet other eligibility criteria of the DAWN and DEFUSE-3 studies
2	Class IIa	For selected patients who were last seen normal 16–24 hours from symptom onset with anterior LVO occlusion who meet the other criteria of the DAWN study
3	Class IIb	Stent retrievers may be reasonable for M2 and M3 segments in patients for whom groin puncture is initiated within 6 hours
		Similarly, there may be benefit for select patients with occlusion of the ACA, PCA, or vertebral and basilar arteries
		There may be benefit of selected patients with mRS > 1, ASPECTS or NIHSS > 6 and ICA or M1 occlusions
		At the present time, stent retrievers are preferred to other endovascular devices

(ACA: anterior cerebral artery; AHA: American Heart Association; ASA: American Stroke Association; ASPECTS: Alberta Stroke Program Early CT Score; ICA: internal carotid artery; IV: intravenous; LVO: large vessel occlusion; MCA: middle cerebral artery; mRS: modified Rankin Score; NIHSS: National Institutes of Health Stroke Scale; PCA: posterior cortical atrophy)

and 110 mm Hg diastolic pressure. It also needs to be maintained below 180/105 mm Hg for 24 hours post-thrombolysis. For patients who are not a candidate for same permissive hypertension up to 220/120 mm Hg is permitted[6] unless there are specific contraindications such as cardiac failure, dissection of aorta, eclampsia, or preeclampsia. It is reasonable to restart antihypertensive medication if blood pressure is >140/90 mm Hg after 48 hours if patient is stable. Fluids need to be started in setting of intravascular volume depletion in acute stroke in older adults and usually isotonic saline is the first choice.[7] Blood sugar control is of particular importance as hypoglycemia can be a stroke mimic and hyperglycemia are associated with a poor outcome. Treatment is recommended or hyperglycemia to maintain a target of 140–180 mg/dL. Swallowing assessment is important to prevent aspiration pneumonia. Fever should be treated with antipyretics and cause of fever should be investigated. The Paracetamol in Stroke (PAIS) trial investigated the same. Stroke units have been started for the purpose of integrated care in patients with acute stroke.

Stroke Mimic

- Stroke mimics are commonly seen masquerading as strokes (8–43%). Common mimics include seizures, migraine, vertigo, metabolic, disorders, subdural hematoma, infections, and function disorders.
- Careful attention to history including hypertension and exact time of onset, bring well in the previous week's examination findings including the presence of gaze deviation, facial weakness, raised systolic blood pressure, older age, AF, and higher National Institutes of Health Stroke Scale (NIHSS) are factors which are in favor of a true stroke.
- Younger age, isolated sensory deficit, history of seizure, systolic blood pressure < 150 mm Hg, absence of facial droop, absence of focal neurological signs, and acute confusional state increase the probability of stroke mimic.
- Thrombolysis in stroke mimic should be avoided, although it may not carry a high risk of adverse effects.
- Negative CT does not exclude stroke. The use of MRI can help in differentiation with the use of multimodality CT like CTA/CT perfusion (CTP).
- Diagnosis of functional stroke mimics can be aided by clinical clues such as Hoover's sign, absence of pronator drift, and advanced imaging.

Secondary Prevention of Stroke

Most patients with ischemic stroke and TIA require control of risk factors such as hypertension, dyslipidemia, diabetes, and smoking and require antithrombotic therapy. Early short-term dual antiplatelets may be given for high risk TIAs and minor ischemic strokes. For long-term therapy either aspirin or clopidogrel can be given or a combination of aspirin extended-release dipyridamole can be used. Long-term anticoagulation can be used for chronic nonvalvular AF. Low-density lipoprotein (LDL) lowering therapy can be started with a target lowering below 70 mg/dL with high-dose statin. Glycemic control can be achieved with target glycosylated hemoglobin (HbA1c) of <7%. Lifestyle modification includes smoking and oral tobacco, alcohol intake, weight reduction, regular exercise, and decreased salt intake with a healthy diet.

CONCLUDING REMARKS AND LEARNING POINTS

- Acute stroke is a medical emergency and needs to be recognized with help of simple mnemonic like FAST (F–face, A–arm and leg, S–speech, and T–time.
- Most therapies of acute ischemic stroke are time-dependent and include thrombolysis and thrombectomy.
- Brain hemorrhage can either be intracranial due to hypertension, amyloid, AVM, cavernomas, or coagulopathy. Aneurysm can cause SAH which carries highest mortality among all stroke subtypes.
- Modifiable risk factors for stroke include hypertension, diabetes, smoking, dyslipidemia, AF, sedentary lifestyle, and obstructive sleep apnea (OSA). Hypertension is the most important risk factor for all types of stroke.
- Localization of ischemic stroke can be done through pattern of involvement. MCA strokes have greater facial and upper limb more than lower limb involvement. ACA stroke have lower limb more than upper limb involvement. PCA strokes often present with field defect in addition to other cortical deficits.
- Secondary prevention of stroke includes risk factor modification in case of ischemic stroke with use of antiplatelet medications and statins. In case of AF, anticoagulation may be done after assessment of risk benefit ratio for secondary prevention.

REFERENCES

1. Coupland AP, Thapar A, Qureshi MI, Jenkins H, Davies AH. The definition of stroke. J R Soc Med. 2017;110(1):9-12.
2. Adams HP Jr, Bendixen BH, Kappelle LJ, Biller J, Love BB, Gordon DL, et al. Classification of subtype of acute ischemic stroke. Definitions for use in a multicenter clinical trial. TOAST. Trial of Org 10172 in Acute Stroke Treatment. Stroke. 1993;24(1):35-41.
3. Powers WJ, Rabinstein AA, Ackerson T, Adeoye OM, Bambakidis NC, Becker K, et al.; American Heart Association Stroke Council. 2018 Guidelines for the Early Management of Patients With Acute Ischemic Stroke: A Guideline for Healthcare Professionals From the American Heart Association/American Stroke Association. Stroke. 2018;49(3):e46-110.
4. Demaerschalk BM, Kleindorfer DO, Adeoye OM, Demchuk AM, Fugate JE, Grotta JC, et al.; American Heart Association Stroke Council and Council on Epidemiology and Prevention. Scientific Rationale for the Inclusion and Exclusion Criteria for Intravenous Alteplase in Acute Ischemic Stroke: A Statement for Healthcare Professionals From the American Heart Association/American Stroke Association. Stroke. 2016;47(2):581-641.
5. Aiyagari V, Gorelick PB. Management of blood pressure for acute and recurrent stroke. Stroke. 2009:40(6):2251-6.
6. Powers WJ, Rabinstein AA, Ackerson T, Adeoye OM, Bambakidis NC, Becker K, et al. Guidelines for the Early Management of Patients with Acute Ischemic Stroke: 2019 update to 2018 Guidelines or the early management of acute ischemic stroke. A Guideline for Healthcare Professionals From the American Heart Association/American Stroke Association. Stroke. 2019;50(12):e344-418.
7. Den Hertog HM, van der Worp HB, van Gemert HM, Algra A, Kappelle LJ, van Gijn J, et al. The Paracetamol (Acetaminophen) in Stroke (PAIS) trial: a multicentric, randomized, placebo-controlled, phase III trial. Lancet Neurol. 2009;8(5);434-40.

Stroke Mimics and Chameleons

Ambar Chakravarty

STROKE MIMICS

The common notion on part of physicians to diagnose a stroke in any patient with acute onset of a focal neurological deficit with or without alteration in sensorium is utterly wrong. Stroke mimics are not uncommon (8–43%[1-4] in various studies). These are conditions which may look like a stroke apparently but these are not strokes. Common mimics include seizures, migraine (familial or sporadic hemiplegic migraine), vertigo, metabolic disorders (hypoglycemia), subdural hematoma/brain tumors, infections, and functional disorders. Attention to clinical history, demographic parameters, focused neurological examination, and neuroimaging including MRI and multimodal CT with CT angiography/CT perfusion (CTA/CTP) can help in differentiation. Various score including Frontal Assessment Battery (FAB) score and TeleStroke mimic (TM) can decrease the chances of thrombolysis in a stroke mimic. TM also evaluates six factors which include age, atrial fibrillation, hypertension, seizure, facial weakness, and the National Institutes of Health Stroke Scale (NIHSS) > 14. Careful attention to history including hypertension and exact time of onset, being well in previous week examination findings including presence of gaze deviation, facial weakness, raised systolic blood pressure, older age, atrial fibrillation, and higher NIHSS are factors which are in favor of a true stroke. In certain additional studies, presence of gaze deviation, facial paresis, raised blood pressure, and higher NIHSS increase the predictive value for a true stroke. Hyperacute MRI may help in detection of these mimics and also bring to light an alternative diagnosis. Development of certain biomarkers for commercial use may later help in diagnosis and evaluation the way troponin has done in the setting of acute myocardial infarction.

Younger age, isolated sensory deficit, history of seizure, systolic blood pressure < 150 mm Hg, absence of facial droop, absence of focal neurological signs, and acute confusional state increase the probability of stroke mimic.

Thrombolysis in stroke mimics should be avoided although it does not carry a high risk of adverse effect.

Negative CT does not exclude stroke. Use of MRI can help in differentiation with use of multimodality CT like CTA/CTP.

Diagnosis of functional stroke mimics can be aided by clinical clues like hoovers sign, absence of pronator drift, and advanced imaging.

Neurologic complications of coronavirus disease-2019 (COVID-19) vaccination are rare, but some cases of cerebral venous sinus thrombosis (CVST), Guillain-Barré syndrome, postural orthostatic tachycardia, and immunization stress-related response have been reported. Venous thrombosis is generally accompanied by a state of "thrombotic thrombocytopenia". Greinacher et al. (2021),[5] who coined this term, demonstrated their patients to test positive on a screening platelet factor 4 (PF4)-heparin immunoassay although none of them had received heparin in the past. Patients also tested positive on a platelet-activation assay in the presence of PF4 independent of heparin. Platelet activation was inhibited by high levels of heparin and immunoglobulin. These workers thus postulated that "the vaccine resulted in a rare thrombotic thrombocytopenia mediated by platelet-activating antibodies against PF4, which clinically mimics autoimmune heparin-induced thrombocytopenia (HIT)". However, no case of arterial thrombosis causally related to any of the available COVID 19 vaccines has yet been reported. A recent report from Thailand highlights on a large number of cases with a distinctive novel focal neurological syndrome to emerge nationwide among those receiving CoronaVac (an inactivated virus vaccine—Sinovac Biotech, China) but not among those who received the ChAdOx1 (AstraZeneca/Oxford, UK) adenovirus-associated vaccine.[6] The novel focal neurological syndrome developed within the first few days of the first dose of vaccination and consisted of transient (lasting few hours to few days) hemisensory (mostly) or hemimotor disturbances, at times associated with visual phenomenon developing in the corresponding hemifield of vision. No patient however developed any speech disturbance. Hemicranial or holocranial headaches were often associated. Diffusion-weighted MRI of brain and MR angiography excluded development of any brain infarction or cerebral vasculopathy. Single-photon emission computed tomography (SPECT) studies however demonstrated evidence of hypoperfusion on the contralateral hemisphere during the acute phase to be followed by hyperperfusion with clearing of symptoms. This has been likened to be suggestive of the phenomenon of cortical spreading depression (CSD) occurring in subjects with migraine with aura. In the patients, reported features consistent with CSD include initial positive followed by negative sensory symptoms, the frequent presence of a march of sensory symptoms over minutes, delayed headache in one-half of patients, and moderately large regions of hypoperfusion on SPECT. The exact trigger for this phenomenon had not been established but postulations include precipitation by stress related to vaccination and an immune response to the vaccine. Clinically speaking the syndrome certainly mimicked an ischemic stroke, but imaging failed to demonstrate an infarct in any patient.

STROKE CHAMELEONS: HOW DO THEY DIFFER FROM STROKE MIMICS?—IMPACT ON PRACTICAL EMERGENCY ROOM MANAGEMENT

The word chameleon is derived from the Saurian reptile of the genus *Chamaeleo*, a small sized lizard-like creature which can change the color of its skin to suit surroundings for camouflaging. A stroke chameleon is a clinical condition in which a stroke occurs with features which are unusual/uncommon in stroke leading to a missed diagnosis of stroke. A stroke mimic, on the other hand, is a situation in which a diagnosis of stroke at admission is suspected but on later evaluation, such a diagnosis could not be confirmed or some other pathology detected. What conditions may constitute stroke chameleons—that is they are indeed cases of stroke, mostly ischemic, but their presenting features at the emergency room (ER) or clinic may not be very typical or suggestive of a stroke (acute onset of a focal neurological deficit localizable to a particular vascular territory in the brain).[7] Some classic examples of stroke chameleons include a brainstem ischemic stroke presenting with an acute vestibular syndrome (AVS) when misdiagnosed as vestibular neuritis (MRI may be normal in many such cases); acute onset of a monoplegia, specially a crural monoplegia which may be mistaken as of spinal cord/plexus/peripheral nerve origin and the "wrong" body part is scanned; patients presenting with altered sensorium without any localizable signs, not very uncommon with brainstem ischemic strokes without any significant detectable abnormality in a CT scan or even on MRI at an early stage; headaches of acute or subacute onset without any clear localizable signs (about 15% of ischemic strokes may have only headache at the onset); presentation with one or more generalized seizures (again in 15% of ischemic strokes) without any localizable features (at times with a normal looking CT scan); and lastly presentation with a movement disorder like a unilateral ballistic movement where a tiny infarct in the basal ganglionic region (not necessarily in the subthalamic nucleus) may be missed in a CT scan and even in MRI which often reveal multiple small bright signals [in T2 or diffusion-weighted imaging (DWI) sequences] in patients with long-standing hypertension or diabetes or even migraine.

Crural monoplegia poses a tricky problem. Except for cases with a very flaccid monoplegia with lots of pain, the rule of the game is to exclude a cerebral cause first with appropriate neuroimaging. The same principle is applicable in cases of so called "spinal hemiplegias" where presentation is with a unilateral weakness/sensory alterations without any detectable cranial nerve involvement. While such a situation is theoretically possible with a high cervical cord lesion (akin to a partial Brown-Séquard syndrome, which in current times mostly result from a cervical cord demyelinating lesion), the vast majority of such cases ultimately prove to have an intracranial problem. So again the rule of the game is to exclude first a cerebral problem by appropriate neuroimaging modality.

What is the practical utility in differentiating between stroke mimics and stroke chameleons? The sheet anchor of therapy for ischemic stroke is thrombolysis within a specified time window. In our rush to reduce the door to needle time, it is possible to misdiagnose a stroke mimic as an ischemic stroke and perform thrombolysis. No great harm is done in the vast majority as the safety profile of intravenous thrombolysis (IVT) in patients who have stroke mimics is excellent, and intracranial hemorrhages are rare. Modern neuroimaging techniques help identifying most mimics. On the other hand, the situation is very different with stroke chameleons—the presenting features may not at all be suggestive of a stroke and appropriate neuroimaging studies are not performed in time. Such patients who actually harbor an ischemic infarct thus miss the opportunity to have the benefit of thrombolysis within the therapeutic window time.

Up to 25% of admissions for probable strokes are related to stroke mimics. The proportion of patients with stroke mimics decreases with use of MRI at baseline. Mimics cannot always be ruled out in emergency. The problem with mimics is that stroke facilities are inadequately used, and patients may receive IVT, when they do not need such treatment. However, thrombolysis is mostly well tolerated in mimics and we need not spend much time in all patients to improve diagnostic accuracy, knowing that the time lost is harmful in all patients. The problem with chameleons is more serious, because patients are not identified, and are not properly treated.

TRANSIENT GLOBAL AMNESIA: STROKE MIMIC OR STROKE CHAMELEON?

Case Vignette

A 65-year-old psychiatrist had been seeing patients in his clinic. After he had seen about six patients, the attending nurse noted that for subsequent patients he had been taking longer time for each patient than usual, had been repeating the same question more than once, and he seemed much less jovial than his usual self. After he had seen another half a dozen patients, he got up from his chair and started walking toward the door to leave his clinic although he still had three more patients to see. When the nurse reminded him about this, he simply ignored her and went upstairs to his living quarters. He had his lunch without talking much to his family members. Thereafter he watched the TV for about half an hour and then went to sleep. He woke up after about an hour and asked his son whether he had attended his clinic in the morning. His son was surprised and called the nurse to confirm. She confirmed his attending the clinic and also mentioned about a little change in his behavior in the clinic. The nurse, however, mentioned very categorically that there had not been any mistake made by the doctor in writing the prescriptions and the drugs and dosage written, were much the same as she had been used to see the doctor prescribing for a number of years. When the doctor was told about this, he was very surprised that he had seen so many patients and he could not recall any of them. The nurse mentioned to him about a few patients by their names, who had been seeing him for a number of years, but he could not remember at all if he had seen them on that morning. He also could not recollect what he had for lunch or the TV channel he had been watching before he went to bed. The total duration of memory loss had been approximately for 5-6 hours. He was seen by the Editor in the same evening when no focal neurological deficit could be detected. Barring the period of amnesia of around 6 hours, his memory, speech, behavior, orientation, writing, and problem solving capacity were all intact. An electroencephalogram (EEG) (wake record for 60 minutes) and a MRI scan (plain with diffusion-weighted sequence and contrast-enhanced study) along with a MR angiography and venography of brain were done, which were all essentially normal. He was mildly hypertensive but euglycemic.

This is a typical story of a patient who had an episode of transient global amnesia (TGA).[8-10] The point of interest here is the preservation of working memory and medical acumen in a doctor while treating his patients, in the backdrop of a transient global memory loss. In the present case, there had been some retrograde amnesia as well, as the doctor could not recall anything about his first six patients during which the nurse did not notice any alteration in his dealing with the patients or his behavior and mood.

Classically, TGA lasts for several hours during which the person may be able to carry out his work fairly normally and none would notice any deviation from his/her usual working manner, unless observed very critically. Such spells of long duration memory loss do not usually recur. The condition may be mistaken for complex partial seizure (CPS) (currently termed as focal unaware seizure) but CPS is usually of much shorter duration. The real differential would be from transient epileptic amnesia (TEA). These tend to be more numerous and of much briefer duration in general. Nearly 80% of TEA attacks last <1 hour compared to average duration of TGA attacks of 4-6 hours. TEA attacks characteristically occur on waking, but probably as frequently at other times. TEA may be associated with somewhat incomplete anterograde amnesia, in contrast to the dense amnesia of TGA. Thus some patients with TEA in one study were "able to remember not being able to remember". TEA may be due to epileptic discharges arising from the temporal lobes. Fisher and Adams[9] (1964) first reported a large series of patients with a stereotyped amnesic syndrome that they called "TGA". Currently, TGA is a well-recognized and defined clinical syndrome.

A single etiologic basis of the cause for TGA is not established. Although a vascular etiology is favored by many experts, it appears clear that an impressive variety of different disorders may be associated with TGA. Strokes or cerebral ischemia following cerebral angiography and thalamic hemorrhage or infarction have been reported to cause some cases of TGA, but most patients with TGA cannot be demonstrated to have experienced an acute vascular insult. Risk factors for TGA and transient ischemic attack (TIA) may overlap in some groups.

It has been postulated that TGA may be a migrainous type of vascular syndrome caused by dysfunction of the dominant or bilateral posterior cerebral arteries. Indeed both TGA and migraine share similar precipitants. The nature of the primary neuronal disorder in migraine is not established, but the phenomenon of a spreading depression of neuronal function (spreading depression of Leão) is considered as a possible mechanism. Spreading depression could also play a role in TGA. Specific precipitants could initiate this type of process by evoking intense volleys of sensory input into neuronal structures such as the hippocampus and initiating a spreading neuronal depression with associated impaired function.

The nature of the amnesic deficit in TGA suggests limbic system involvement.[10] The neuronal structures thought most likely to be affected in TGA are the medial temporal or diencephalic regions. A case report of a SPECT study during an episode of TGA described severe bitemporal hypoperfusion. Using diffusion tensor imaging (DTI), a reorganization of the brain network in patients with TGA, especially in such regions as the right superior and inferior orbitofrontal, the right inferior frontal operculum, the left superior parietal, and left postcentral gyrus have been demonstrated. These alterations of the brain network may have a contributory role in the genesis of TGA symptomatology and suggests that TGA is a network disease. Furthermore, by using diffusion-weighted MRI, 24–48 hours after a TGA episode, very small hyperintense lesions have been detected in the hippocampus, suggesting selective vulnerability of CA1 neurons of the hippocampus to metabolic stress causing clinical manifestations of TGA. In a relatively recent study, TGA patients have been shown to have higher prevalence of compression/stenosis of the bilateral internal jugular vein and the left brachiocephalic vein and transverse sinus hypoplasia. This is new evidence that supports the role of extracranial veins in TGA pathogenesis.

In observed subjects with TGA having classical features, rational approach may only include avoidance of overtesting, inappropriate medication, and uncalled for medical interventions; stress should be on observation, taking care of patient safety and reassurance of patients and their families. Data on long-term prognosis are limited, but available information suggests that the relapse rate is low, the risk of stroke and seizures is not considerably increased, and cognitive outcome is generally good. The patient described herein carried out his psychiatric for several years thereafter without experiencing any significant problem.

REFERENCES

1. Keselman B, Cooray C, Vanhooren G, Bassi P, Consoli D, Nichelli P, et al. Intravenous thrombolysis in stroke mimics: results from the SITS International Stroke Thrombolysis Register. Eur J Neurol. 2019;26(8):1091-7.
2. Liberman AL, Prabhakaran S. Stroke Chameleons and Stroke Mimics in the Emergency Department. Curr Neurol Neurosci Rep. 2017;17(2):15.
3. Natteru P, Mohebbi MR, George P, Wisco D, Gebel J, Newey CR. Variables That Best Differentiate In-Patient Acute Stroke from Stroke-Mimics with Acute Neurological Deficits. Stroke Res Treat. 2016;2016:4393127.
4. Chakravarty A. Between the devil and the deep blue sea. In: Chakravarty A (Ed). Neurology and Internal Medicine: A Case-based Study. New Delhi: Jaypee Brothers Medical Publishers (P) Ltd.; 2021. pp. 195-9.
5. Greinacher A, Thiele T, Warkentin TE, Weisser K, Kyrle PA, Eichinger S. Thrombotic Thrombocytopenia after ChAdOx1 nCov-19 Vaccination. N Engl J Med. 2021;384(22):2092-101.
6. Suwanwela1 NC, Kijpaisalratana N, Tepmongko S, Rattanawong W, Vorasayan P, Charnnarong C, et al. Prolonged migraine aura resembling ischemic stroke following CoronaVac vaccination: an extended case series. J Headache Pain. 2022;23:13.
7. Ray S, Chakravarty K, Kathuria H, Lal V. Errors in the Diagnosis of Stroke-Tales of Common Stroke Mimics and Strokes in Hiding. Ann Indian Acad Neurol. 2019;22(4):477-81.
8. Chakravarty A. The three musketeers: great mimickers of epileptic seizures. In: Chakravarty A (Ed). Mimics of Epileptic Seizures, 1st edition. New Delhi: Jaypee Brothers Medical Publishers (P) Ltd.; 2020.
9. Fisher CM, Adams RD. Transient global amnesia. Acta Neurol Scand. 1964;40:1-83.
10. Arena JE, Rabinstein AA. Transient global amnesia. Mayo Clin Proc. 2015;90(2):264-72.

CHAPTER 14

Neuropsychiatric Aspects of Cerebrovascular Disorders

Shashank Jaiswal, Subhash Kaul

INTRODUCTION

Cerebrovascular disease is the second most prominent contributor to both mortality and dependency on a global scale.[1,2] It constitutes nearly 5% of all disability-adjusted life years and is responsible for approximately 10% of all global fatalities.[3] The increased life expectancy beyond 60 years has made stroke as the fourth leading cause of death and fifth leading cause of disability in India.[4,5] Neuropsychiatric impairment after cerebrovascular disorders encompasses cognitive and psychiatric disorders. Stroke has been widely established to compromise the integrity of emotional and cognitive functioning, often disrupting an individual's premorbid self-directedness, quality of life, and meaningful existence. Yet, stroke outcomes research traditionally has focused on recovery of the basic activities of daily living, such as feeding oneself and walking. Although the understanding of poststroke cognitive and psychiatric symptoms may not be as tangible as that of physical disabilities, their existence has been firmly recognized as a hindrance to recovery. This is due to their potential to impede stroke survivors' adherence to the rehabilitation process and the necessary lifestyle adjustments.[6]

COGNITIVE EFFECTS OF CEREBROVASCULAR DISORDERS

Symptoms of cognitive impairment after stroke are heterogeneous from the clinical and pathogenic points of view. Infarcts may occur both in cortical and subcortical regions.[7] Hence, the clinical profile is characterized by a variable pattern of cognitive deficits, reflecting the size, location, and number of brain lesions. These patients can present with aphasia, hemineglect, visual field deficits, difficulty in calculation, ideomotor apraxia in the form of inability to carry out learned skills, frontal lobe syndromes comprising disinhibition, loss of initiative and executive dysfunction, or a combination thereof.

Evolution of the Concept of Vascular Cognitive Impairment

The link between age-related cognitive impairment and alterations in cerebral blood vessels was initially alluded to cerebrovascular insufficiency due to hardened arteries.[8] However, in the 1970s, the concept of multi-infarct dementia emerged, suggesting that cerebrovascular disease causes dementia through multiple brain infarcts. It was recognized that the term vascular dementia (VaD) was limited in encompassing the full range of cognitive changes arising from vascular factors. To address this, the term vascular cognitive impairment (VCI) was introduced[9] and later widely accepted.[10] VaD represents the most severe form of VCI.

Classification and Definitions

The VICCCS (Vascular Impairment of Cognition Classification Consensus Study) guideline definitions evolved from the American Heart Association/American Stroke Association[10] and the National Institute of Neurological Disorders and Stroke–Canadian Stroke Network[11] consensus statements, and aligned with revised terminology in The Diagnostic and Statistical Manual of Mental Disorders, Fifth Edition (DSM-5), which distinguishes between major and minor neurocognitive disorders. This scheme subclassifies VCI into mild and major types and also VCI existing alone or along with other comorbid pathologies such as Alzheimer's disease (AD) and dementia with Lewy bodies (DLB). The classification is depicted in **Flowchart 1**.

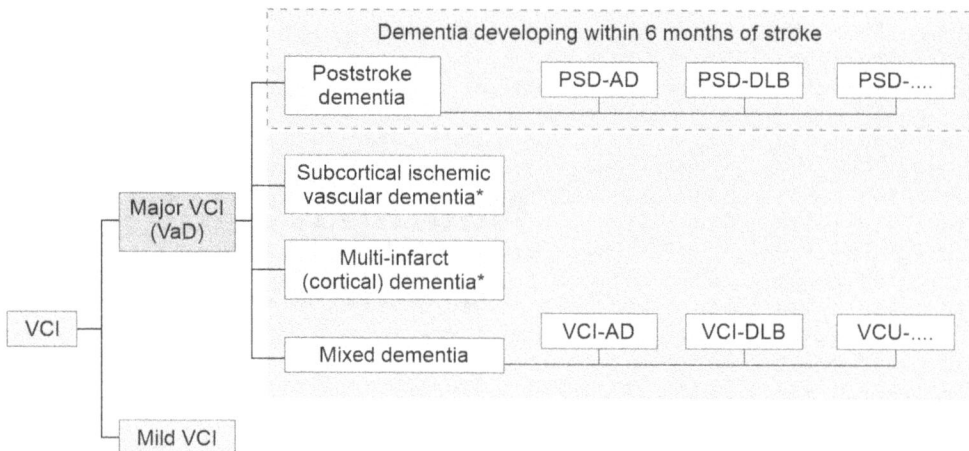

*Patients who also have evidence for comorbid pathology representing an established nonvascular cause of dementia such as Alzheimer's disease (AD) or dementia with Lewy bodies (DLB) are classified as mixed dementia. Mild VCI refers to impairment in at least one cognitive domain and mild to no impairment in instrumental activities of daily living or activities of daily living (independent of the motor/sensory sequelae of the vascular event).

FLOWCHART 1: Diagnostic classification for major vascular cognitive impairment (VCI) [major VCI = vascular dementia (VaD)]. The 6-month temporal basis for cognitive decline after stroke (dashed box) differentiates poststroke dementia from other forms of VaD.

Risk Factors

Shared risk factors between cognitive impairment and stroke support the idea of a common susceptibility. Advancing age is a significant risk factor for both conditions. While genetic factors, including Apolipoprotein E4, play a role in AD, their association with VaD and poststroke dementia requires further investigation, with only a few specific risk genes identified [particularly the rare *NOTCH3* gene mutation seen in cerebral autosomal dominant arteriopathy with subcortical infarcts and leukoencephalopathy (CADASIL)]. Modifiable risk factors for dementia can be categorized as protective factors and causative. Protective factors encompass cognitive reserve markers, such as higher education/intelligence quotient (IQ), occupation, social networks, and cognitive and physical activity, which enhance resilience against age- and disease-related changes.[12-14] This entails the concept of "cognitive reserve" which includes but is not limited to premorbid markers of brain susceptibility/reserve (educational level, premorbid dependency, and severity of leukoaraiosis). While the Mediterranean diet has been linked to reduced cognitive decline, its specific impact on VaD lacks sufficient data.[10] Factors that increase the risk include hypertension, diabetes, smoking, atrial fibrillation, and sedentary lifestyle.

Hemorrhagic stroke may carry slightly higher dementia risks than ischemic stroke for strokes of similar severity,[15] and risks are higher in superficial/lobar versus deep bleeding due to associations with cerebral amyloid angiopathy (CAA).[16]

Cognitive Domains Affected and Clinical Evaluation

There are currently no established guidelines specifying the optimal timing for conducting cognitive assessments after a stroke. Assessments are typically administered "a few weeks to 6 or more months following stroke."[17] VaD can occur in the setting of an "overt" stroke (stepwise following multiple sequential infarcts or following a single episode including infarcts in strategic regions) and "covert" gradual worsening [usually seen in the setting of small vessel disease (SVD)]. Considering the time elapsed since the injury and the commencement of testing, it is crucial to acknowledge that poststroke cognitive symptoms are not fixed entities. Many stroke survivors experience spontaneous recovery over time, while others may reach a plateau. The Hachinski ischemic score, validated against autopsy data predicts vascular contribution to dementia and distinguishes between VaD and AD.[18] Unlike AD, current diagnostic criteria of VCI do not mandate the presence of memory impairment.[12] Patients with vascular brain lesions often exhibit impairments in speed, praxis, executive function, and visual memory. Though deficits in delayed recall of word lists and visual content are also frequently observed[19] when compared to patients with similar cognitive dysfunction from AD, those with VaD perform better in verbal learning and recall but worse in frontal executive function. A study with autopsy confirmation showed that a combination of categorical fluency and word list recall differentiated VaD from AD with 85% sensitivity and 67% specificity, though the sample sizes were small.[20]

To conduct a comprehensive cognitive assessment, it is essential to evaluate five core domains: Executive function, attention, memory, language, and visuospatial function. While information on other domains such as learning, social cognition, and neuropsychiatry can be helpful in understanding the cognitive syndrome, they are not mandatory for diagnosing VaD. The evaluation of the five core domains aligns with the "60-minute" and "30-minute" protocols recommended by the National Institute of Neurological Disorders and Stroke-Canadian Stroke Network VCI harmonization standards. If deemed clinically appropriate, comprehensive testing can be postponed for about 3-6 months. An effective cognitive screening tool for individuals with vascular disease is the montreal cognitive assessment (MoCA), a concise 30-point test that can be conducted in approximately 10 minutes. The MoCA covers all the core domains mentioned earlier, is accessible in various languages, and has been validated in different contexts, including stroke patients.

Barriers to cognitive testing in the immediate post-stroke period include—(1) delirium, often fluctuating and present in up to 20% of hospitalized stroke patients, (2) aphasia-impaired comprehension and reliability of screening tests on language for assessment, and (3) premorbid cognitive status.

Strategic Infarcts and Cognitive Impairment

Single-strategic infarct dementia refers to the abrupt onset of cognitive impairment and behavioral changes caused by a single infarct in specific brain regions. Traditionally, infarcts in the left hemispherical white matter tracts, caudate nucleus, angular gyrus, and corpus callosum are implicated. The clinical picture is that of a frontal lobe syndrome with inattention, apathy, and psychomotor retardation and has been interpreted as a thalamocortical disconnection syndrome.[7] In a study using multivariate voxel-based support vector regression lesion-symptom mapping (SVR-LSM), the association between infarct volume and total MoCA was strongest for the anterior limb of the internal capsule.[21] Cognitive domain-specific strategic regions were also identified—(1) language was most strongly (but not exclusively) associated with left hemispheric cortical regions excluding the basal ganglia, (2) memory and executive functioning were associated with a widely distributed network of almost exclusively left hemispheric cortical and subcortical regions, (3) attention was exclusively associated with a left and right hemispheric white matter tract network and the left insula, and (4) visuospatial functioning involved a distributed left and right hemispheric subcortical network particularly right temporoparietal cortical regions. Anterior limb of the left internal capsule and the left fronto-occipital fasciculi were associated with all cognitive domains except language. MoCA global scores are possibly associated with left hemispheric lesions due to the test's reliance on verbal items and the language-dominant left hemisphere.

Neuroimaging

In routine clinical practice, a plain CT scan or MRI scan of brain is enough to support the diagnosis of stroke and VCI. However, at an advanced level quantification of infarcted tissue is promising, particularly in SVD-related cognitive impairment. The STRIVE (STandards for ReportIng Vascular changes on nEuroimaging) initiative has offered a comprehensive overview of the wide range of SVD-related lesions, along with agreed-upon terminology.[22]

Diagnosis

Consensus diagnostic criteria for VCI have been offered by several organizations, such as the American Heart Association, the DSM-5, and the International Society of Vascular Behavioral and Cognitive Disorders (VAS-COG) and include similar concepts.[10,23] For making a diagnosis, all the following three conditions need to be fulfilled:

1. Classification of VCI as either vascular mild cognitive impairment (MCI; referred to as "vascular minor neurocognitive disorder" in DSM-5) or VaD (vascular major neurocognitive disorder)
2. A requirement that cerebrovascular disease be identified either by history of stroke or by neuroimaging identification of silent cerebrovascular disease
3. A judgment that the cerebrovascular disease be considered sufficient to cause cognitive impairment

Management

Primordial prevention of VaD might include programs to improve education, promote healthy lifestyle awareness and physical exercise.

Vascular Risk Modification

Risk Factor Management

Despite lack of studies in risk factor management in VaD per se, there is sufficient data to suggest that recurrent stroke is associated with greater risk of cognitive decline, and PSD is associated with higher mortality. Treatment of blood pressure in older adults in general aligns with recommendations for secondary stroke prevention although intensively lowering systolic blood pressure to <120 mm Hg in patients with symptomatic VaD is *not* recommended. Similarly, glucose control is generally recommended for the prevention of complications associated with diabetes. For patients with VaD who have not had a clinical ischemic stroke or transient ischemic attack (TIA), statin therapy should be administered based on the patient's assessed cardiovascular risk.

Antithrombotic Therapy

Patients with VaD and a history of ischemic stroke or TIA, with or without the evidence on imaging, should be treated with antithrombotic therapy and/or anticoagulation based on the mechanism of stroke. In patients with no clinical history or imaging evidence of stroke or TIA, the Canadian Conference on Diagnosis and Treatment of Dementia and the European Stroke Organization recommend against using antiplatelet drugs for stroke or dementia prevention for patients with white matter lesions.[24,25]

Pharmacologic Therapy

Cholinesterase Inhibitors

Initiation of cholinesterase inhibitor therapy in patients with VaD is indicated in patients who have progressive cognitive decline that cannot be directly attributed to a clinical stroke, based on the possibility of concomitant AD. Though, a meta-analysis of six trials of cholinesterase inhibitors in patients with VaD concluded that the benefits were small and of uncertain clinical significance.[26] In patients who do receive cholinesterase inhibitor therapy, there is evidence to support the use of donepezil or galantamine over rivastigmine.

Memantine

An N-methyl-D-aspartate receptor antagonist similarly can be tried in patients with progressive cognitive decline. Doses up to 20 mg/day typically in combination with a cholinesterase inhibitor have been safely tolerated and shown benefits on cognitive scales.

Investigational Agents

These include nimodipine, ergot alkaloids (hydergine and nicergoline), cerebrolysin, ginkgo biloba, xanthine derivatives (propentofylline, pentoxifylline, and denbufylline), cytidinediphosphocholine, and piracetam; and lack conclusive results. Actovegin (a deproteinized hemoderivative of calf blood, 2,000 mg/day for ≤20 intravenous infusions followed by 1,200 mg/day orally) is licensed for poststroke cognitive impairment in some countries in Europe and Asia, based on a trial showing more improvement in the Alzheimer's Disease Assessment Scale-Cognitive Subscale (ADAS-Cog) at 6 months.[27]

Nonpharmacologic Therapy

Cognitive rehabilitation targets multiple cognitive domains, aiming to enhance various mental functions. Interventions for neglect focus on position sense and spatial representation deficits, utilizing prisms, eye-patching, hemispatial glasses, caloric and optokinetic stimulation, transcutaneous electrical nerve stimulation (TENS), and neck vibration. Certain language impairments such as phonological disorders, lexical semantic impairments, and syntactic impairments often exhibit significant recovery within the initial months after a stroke.

Predictors of Cognitive Outcomes

Age, the NIHSS (National Institutes of Health Stroke Scale), and stroke volume are important predictors for functional outcome but are less applicable to cognitive outcomes.[28-30] Addition of stroke location as an independent variable to the earlier-mentioned factors was found to significantly improve prediction in the latter.[31] Unilateral spatial neglect has been reported to have a negative impact on functional recovery, length of rehabilitation stays, and the need for assistance postdischarge. Individuals with higher education and bilingualism have been associated with slower cognitive aging and a later onset of dementia along with a better cognitive outcome after stroke, possibly by enhancing "cognitive reserve".[32]

PSYCHIATRIC EFFECTS OF CEREBROVASCULAR DISORDERS

This section highlights psychiatric effects of cerebrovascular disorders encompassing depressive disorders, anxiety disorders, post-traumatic stress disorder (PTSD), psychosis, and psychotic disorders.

Poststroke Depressive Disorders

Poststroke depression stands as the most prevalent treatable psychiatric complication of stroke occurring at any point after its onset. Clinical characteristics include depressed mood, anhedonia, loss of energy, decreased concentration, psychomotor retardation, decreased appetite, insomnia, suicidal thoughts, and guilt. The prospective prevalence rates of PSD up to 18 months are relatively consistent and meta-analysis incidence data ranges from 25–35%. No established diagnostic criteria exist for PSD and DSM-5 categorizes it as "depressive disorder due to another medical condition". According to the 2017 American Heart Association and American

Stroke Association, the Centre for Epidemiological Studies Depression Scale, Hamilton Depression Rating Scale, and particularly the Nine-item Patient Health Questionnaire (PHQ9) scores exhibit higher sensitivities in identifying PSD.[33] Neurological deficits such as expressive or receptive dysfunction, apathy, anosognosia, abulia, or lack of insight hinder the identification and diagnosis of PSD.

Poststroke depression showed a negative impact on survival rates, particularly short-term mortality. Early selective serotonin reuptake inhibitors (SSRIs) and serotonin and norepinephrine reuptake inhibitors (SNRIs) are recommended as a first-line antidepressant therapy once the definitive diagnosis of PSD has been made. The use of SSRIs such as escitalopram, paroxetine, fluoxetine, and sertraline are linked to various adverse effects including nausea, vomiting, anxiety, and weight changes, hence need to be monitored closely. Fluoxetine may be preferred when hypersexuality and weight gain is an issue. Tricyclic antidepressants (TCAs) such as mirtazapine and amitriptyline can cause dry mouth, blurred vision, and cardiac issues but may be preferred when sleep disturbances are present. SNRIs such as duloxetine and venlafaxine may result in nausea, headache, and ejaculation disorders but are reasonable when there is associated pain. Serotonin antagonist and reuptake inhibitors (SARIs) such as trazodone are associated with dry mouth and drowsiness. Dopaminergic drugs like bupropion may lead to side effects such as dry mouth, headache, and weight changes but have shown benefit with associated symptoms of apathy. CYP2C19-inhibiting SSRIs (fluoxetine and fluvoxamine) can decrease the therapeutic efficacy of clopidogrel and have been implicated in inhibiting warfarin metabolism by also competitively binding plasma proteins. In light of conflicting data on the heightened risk of both ischemic and abnormal bleeding events these drugs are best avoided in patients with PSD particularly those on anticoagulation.

Cognitive behavioral therapy (CBT) may be the most effective psychotherapeutic intervention. Mental and physical exercise could relieve most mood symptoms of PSD. Neuromodulation, such as transcranial magnetic stimulation and transcranial direct current stimulation, are promising adjunctive therapies. However, high quality randomized controlled trials using psychotherapy or neuromodulation are limited, and further research is needed.[34]

Poststroke Anxiety Disorders

Poststroke anxiety (PSA) disorders are the second most common psychiatric sequelae of stroke and manifest as generalized anxiety disorder, phobias, selective mutism, agoraphobia, social anxiety disorder, and panic disorders. Core psychological symptoms involve feelings of uneasiness, persistent and exaggerated worry, and fear frequently accompanied by noteworthy physical manifestations, some of which bear resemblance to neurological signs. The frequency of PSA studied until 6 months after stroke gradually rises over time and has been shown to be independent of incident depression.[35,36] The DSM-5 classifies PSA as an "anxiety disorder due to another medical condition". Patients suffer from persistent dependence with poorer quality of life and restricted social participation.[37] The Hamilton Anxiety Scale and the Hospital Anxiety and Depression Scale-Anxiety subscale are widely utilized to assess and quantify the severity of anxiety.

Several studies have shown PTSD as a common sequela among stroke survivors. Under the DSM-5, PTSD is categorized as a subtype of anxiety disorder characterized by: (1) Intrusive memories; (2) alterations in physical reactions and arousal; (3) avoidance; and (4) negative alterations in cognition and mood.[38] Incidence rates are reported as high as 37% with gradual decline over 1 year.[39,40] The most widely used scale in stroke patients is the PTSD checklist which specifically enquires about "stroke or TIA" as a stressor.[41-43]

There is no high-quality clinical evidence to guide PSA management[44] SSRIs, SNRIs, TCAs, mirtazapine, buspirone, benzodiazepines, and Z-drugs can be employed lacking large-scale randomized double-blind controlled trials. Self-help mindfulness and relaxation techniques have demonstrated efficacy as self-administered therapies in alleviating symptoms, particularly for patients facing communication challenges. Trauma-focused psychotherapies and exposure therapy hold promise for poststroke PTSD strategies, necessitating future efficacy studies.

Psychosis and Psychotic Disorders after Stroke

Poststroke psychotic disorders feature prominent hallucinations and delusions accompanied by disorganized speech and inappropriate motor behavior abnormalities.[45] These symptoms typically manifest within a week. Sparse studies have suggested that poststroke psychotic disorders are a rare complication of stroke. Lesions that were related to delusions are commonly in the right frontal, temporal, and parietal lobes. Poststroke psychosis appears to be the least studied neuropsychiatric sequelae probably due lack of a widely acknowledged diagnostic criteria and structured assessment that is suitable for a quantitative evaluation of psychosis.[46,47]

Second-generation antipsychotic drugs, such as risperidone, quetiapine, and olanzapine, are the most commonly used antipsychotic medications for poststroke psychoses. However, antipsychotic drugs, particularly olanzapine and clozapine, can negatively impact glucose and lipid metabolism. First-generation antipsychotics may increase the risk of stroke, especially in patients with VaD.[48,49] Postural hypotension and extrapyramidal side effects are well known with these group of drugs. CBT might help mitigate the distress caused by hallucinations or delusional beliefs.

Poststroke Delirium

Hallmark symptoms include reduced awareness of the surroundings, difficulties in maintaining attention, and disruptions in memory, orientation, language, and perception. Sleep-wake disturbances are frequent, leading to restless behavior at night and daytime sleepiness. Emotional disturbances, ranging from fear and anxiety to euphoria and apathy, are also common and can fluctuate rapidly. Delirium can manifest in three subtypes based on psychomotor activity, i.e., hyperactive, hypoactive, and mixed, with patients often transitioning between states.[50,51] Diagnosing delirium can be challenging due to its resemblance to dementia, psychotic disorders (e.g., schizophrenia), and psychiatric conditions (e.g., depression or mania). It is more prevalent in patients with cerebral hemorrhage rather than ischemic strokes.[52-54] Delirium can also occur after subarachnoid hemorrhage with a higher incidence associated with factors such as intraventricular bleeding, hydrocephalus, and basifrontal hemorrhage.[55,56] Incidence rates range from 10 to 48%.[52,57,58] Most cases of delirium occur within the first few days after a stroke.[59] Durations range from 3 days to a month with about one-third of medical inpatients still having delirium at the time of discharge.[60,61] Predictors of poststroke delirium include age, male gender, use of anticholinergic drugs, somatic or metabolic disorders, preexisting dementia, vision, and hearing impairment and location of stroke.[53,62,63] Management involves ruling out any potential metabolic causes followed by benzodiazepines, antipsychotics, and cholinesterase inhibitors based on severity and comorbidities.

Other Behavioral Manifestations not Included in DSM-5

Poststroke Mania

Prevalence of poststroke mania (PSM) is rather low (<2%) and is characterized by presence of elevated or irritable mood accompanied by pressured speech, grandiosity, hyperactivity, flight of ideas, distractibility, lack of judgment, and decreased sleep typically lasting for at least 1 week. Treatment of PSM is in line with treatment of an acute manic episode. Mood stabilizers (valproate, carbamazepine, and oxcarbazepine), antipsychotics (olanzapine, quetiapine, and risperidone), and benzodiazepines are the mainstay of treatment. Lithium is generally avoided due to potential drug-drug interactions. Choosing a mood stabilizer which allows antiepileptic coverage is beneficial.

Poststroke Emotional Lability/Pseudobulbar Affect

The pathology underlying this is not well understood but may be due to impairment of descending corticobulbar input and/or cerebellar modulation controlling emotional expression. Patients can present with sudden onset laughter or crying while speaking on a rather inconspicuous matter. Often transient, but if recurrent, it may result in distress, depression, social avoidance, and embarrassment. Patients and caregivers should be counseled that the symptoms of pseudobulbar affect do not reflect a psychological disorder. Often misdiagnosed as depression the prevalence of poststroke emotional lability varies between 8 and 32%.[64] Treatment options include dextromethorphan-quinidine (20/10 mg) up to twice daily. Dextromethorphan lozenges available in India are commonly used lacking the availability of the earlier-mentioned formulation. TCAs and SSRIs have also been used with modest benefit.[65]

Poststroke Fatigue

A prevalence of poststroke fatigue (PSF) between 25 and 85% has been reported. It is described as, subjective lack of mental and physical energy which interferes with individual's day to day activities.[66] Modafinil up to a dose of 400 mg/day has been found to be useful in PSF particularly in brainstem-diencephalic strokes because of its effect on reticular activating system.[67]

Poststroke Personality Disorders

Prominently, frontal lobe lesions can result in classified five types of personality changes (labile, disinhibited, aggressive, apathetic, and paranoid), and represent a change from the individual's previous personality pattern.

Poststroke apathy is characterized by diminished motivation with reduced goal-directed cognitive activity, goal-directed behavior, or emotions. It can be differentiated from PSD by lack of associated features such as anhedonia, low mood, lack of attention and concentration, negative cognition, and suicidal ideas although they can co-occur in about 40% of cases. If the patient is also depressed, antidepressants with dopaminergic activity (e.g., bupropion) or noradrenergic activity (e.g., reboxetine) could be used. A trial of donezepil, an acetyl cholinesterase inhibitor commonly used in dementia, is reasonable if there is VaD. Coping strategy training and problem-solving therapy both have shown promise for the prevention of apathy.

Poststroke aggression can be without feeling angry or, conversely, patients may experience only hostility without showing aggressive behavior. Individuals who have experienced infarcts in the dorsolateral prefrontal or basofrontal regions, such as those resulting from anterior communicating artery aneurysmal rupture, may exhibit changes in personality as a component of a dysexecutive syndrome. Likewise, individuals with severe Wernicke aphasia encounter a significant loss of language comprehension and may manifest heightened suspicion, anger, and aggressive conduct. In cases of severe aggressive behavior, neuroleptics (haloperidol or atypical) may be employed to prevent harm. Initiate with a low dose, adjusting based on aggression control and adverse effects intensity (sedation, confusion, cognitive impairment, rigidity, walking difficulties, and falls).

Denial of Illness

It occurs in several neurological conditions besides hemiplegia, e.g., in cortical blindness after bilateral occipital lesions, in some forms of amnesia after frontotemporal lesions, in aphasic syndromes (particularly of Wernicke type), or in other disturbances such as neglect or apraxia. Caloric vestibular stimulation and prism adaptation have shown a temporary benefit in anosognosia.

CONCLUDING REMARKS

Neuropsychiatric consequences, both cognitive and psychiatric, following stroke are common, but are often neglected due to entire focus on motor dysfunction. However, leaving these symptoms unaddressed can have serious consequences on recovery and rehabilitation of poststroke survivors. While pharmacological treatment, especially for depression, has shown promise, limitations in study methodologies persist, and integrating personality models and exploring biological factors are needed. Further investigation and innovative interventions are necessary for managing poststroke neuropsychiatric symptoms effectively.

LEARNING POINTS

- A variety of neuropsychiatric symptoms often occur in cerebrovascular disorders.
- The symptoms can be cognitive or psychiatric in nature or a combination of both.
- Cognitive symptoms range from mild mental slowing, impaired comprehension, difficulty in expression, inability to perform learnt tasks, and sometimes progressing to frank dementia.
- Psychiatric symptoms include depression, anxiety, PTSD, personality changes, anger, delirium, and sometimes psychotic behavior.
- Timely detection, counseling, cognitive rehabilitation, and pharmacotherapy are helpful.

REFERENCES

1. Feigin VL, Forouzanfar MH, Krishnamurthi R, Mensah GA, Connor M, Bennett DA, et al. Global and regional burden of stroke during 1990-2010: findings from the Global Burden of Disease Study 2010. Lancet. 2014;383(9913):245-54.
2. GBD 2017 Causes of Death Collaborators. Global, regional, and national age-sex-specific mortality for 282 causes of death in 195 countries and territories, 1980-2017: a systematic analysis for the Global Burden of Disease Study 2017. Lancet. 2018;392(10159):1736-88.
3. Horton R, Das P. Indian health: the path from crisis to progress. Lancet. 2011;377(9761):181-3.
4. Naik K. Challenges in delivering stroke care in India. Indian J Health Sci. 2016;9:245-6.
5. Ministry of Health and Family Welfare. (2019). National Programme for Prevention and Control of Cancer, Diabetes, Cardiovascular Diseases and Stroke. [online] Available from https://main.mohfw.gov.in/Major-Programmes/non-communicable-diseases-injury-trauma/Non-Communicable-Disease-II/National-Programme-for-Prevention-and-Control-of-Cancer-Diabetes-Cardiovascular-diseases-and-Stroke-NPCDCS. [Last accessed May, 2024].
6. Larsen PD. Rehabilitation 2030: A call for action. Philadelphia: Lippincott Williams & Wilkins; 2019. p. 129.
7. Tatemichi TK, Desmond DW, Prohovnik I, Cross DT, Gropen TI, Mohr JP, et al. Confusion and memory loss from capsular genu infarction: a thalamocortical disconnection syndrome? Neurology. 1992;42(10):1966-79.
8. Mast H, Tatemichi TK, Mohr J. Chronic brain ischemia: the contributions of Otto Binswanger and Alois Alzheimer to the mechanisms of vascular dementia. J Neurol Sci. 1995;132(1):4-10.
9. Hachinski V, Bowler J, Loeb C. Vascular dementia. Neurology. 1993;43(10):2159-60.
10. Gorelick PB, Scuteri A, Black SE, Decarli C, Greenberg SM, Iadecola C, et al. Vascular contributions to cognitive impairment and dementia: a statement for healthcare professionals from the American Heart Association/American Stroke Association. Stroke. 2011;42(9):2672-713.
11. Hachinski V, Iadecola C, Petersen RC, Breteler MM, Nyenhuis DL, Black SE, et al. National Institute of Neurological Disorders and Stroke–Canadian stroke network vascular cognitive impairment harmonization standards. Stroke. 2006;37(9):2220-41.

12. Skrobot OA, Black SE, Chen C, DeCarli C, Erkinjuntti T, Ford GA, et al. Progress toward standardized diagnosis of vascular cognitive impairment: Guidelines from the Vascular Impairment of Cognition Classification Consensus Study. Alzheimers Dement. 2018;14(3):280-92.
13. Dichgans M, Zietemann V. Prevention of vascular cognitive impairment. Stroke. 2012;43(11):3137-46.
14. Stern Y, Chételat G, Habeck C, Arenaza-Urquijo EM, Vemuri P, Estanga A, et al. Mechanisms underlying resilience in ageing. Nat Rev Neurosci. 2019;20(4):246.
15. Pendlebury ST, Rothwell PM. Incidence and prevalence of dementia associated with transient ischaemic attack and stroke: analysis of the population-based Oxford Vascular Study. Lancet Neurol. 2019;18(3):248-58.
16. Moulin S, Labreuche J, Bombois S, Rossi C, Boulouis G, Hénon H, et al. Dementia risk after spontaneous intracerebral haemorrhage: a prospective cohort study. Lancet Neurol. 2016;15(8):820-9.
17. Robinson RG, Jorge RE. Post-stroke depression: a review. Am J Psychiatry. 2016;173(3):221-31.
18. Moroney JT, Bagiella E, Desmond DW, Hachinski VC, Molsa PK, Gustafson L, et al. Meta-analysis of the Hachinski Ischemic Score in pathologically verified dementias. Neurology. 1997;49(4):1096-105.
19. Looi JC, Sachdev PS. Differentiation of vascular dementia from AD on neuropsychological tests. Neurology. 1999;53(4):670-8.
20. Ramirez-Gomez L, Zheng L, Reed B, Kramer J, Mungas D, Zarow C, et al. Neuropsychological Profiles Differentiate Alzheimer Disease from Subcortical Ischemic Vascular Dementia in an Autopsy-Defined Cohort. Dement Geriatr Cogn Disord. 2017;44(1-2):1-11.
21. Zhao L, Biesbroek JM, Shi L, Liu W, Kuijf HJ, Chu WW, et al. Strategic infarct location for post-stroke cognitive impairment: A multivariate lesion-symptom mapping study. J Cereb Blood Flow Metab. 2018;38(8):1299-311.
22. Wardlaw JM, Smith EE, Biessels GJ, Cordonnier C, Fazekas F, Frayne R, et al. Neuroimaging standards for research into small vessel disease and its contribution to ageing and neurodegeneration. Lancet Neurol. 2013;12(8):822-38.
23. Sachdev P, Kalaria R, O'Brien J, Skoog I, Alladi S, Black SE, et al. Diagnostic criteria for vascular cognitive disorders: a VASCOG statement. Alzheimer Dis Assoc Disord. 2014;28(3):206-18.
24. Smith EE, Barber P, Field TS, Ganesh A, Hachinski V, Hogan DB, et al. Canadian Consensus Conference on Diagnosis and Treatment of Dementia (CCCDTD)5: Guidelines for management of vascular cognitive impairment. Alzheimers Dement (N Y). 2020;6(1):e12056.
25. Wardlaw JM, Debette S, Jokinen H, De Leeuw FE, Pantoni L, Chabriat H, et al. ESO Guideline on covert cerebral small vessel disease. Eur Stroke J. 2021;6(2):CXI-CLXII.
26. Kavirajan H, Schneider LS. Efficacy and adverse effects of cholinesterase inhibitors and memantine in vascular dementia: a meta-analysis of randomised controlled trials. Lancet Neurol. 2007;6(9):782-92.
27. Guekht A, Skoog I, Edmundson S, Zakharov V, Korczyn AD. ARTEMIDA Trial (A Randomized Trial of Efficacy, 12 Months International Double-Blind Actovegin): A Randomized Controlled Trial to Assess the Efficacy of Actovegin in Poststroke Cognitive Impairment. Stroke. 2017;48(5):1262-70.
28. Konig IR, Ziegler A, Bluhmki E, Hacke W, Bath PM, Sacco RL, et al. Predicting long-term outcome after acute ischemic stroke: a simple index works in patients from controlled clinical trials. Stroke. 2008;39(6):1821-6.
29. Saposnik G, Guzik AK, Reeves M, Ovbiagele B, Johnston SC. Stroke Prognostication using Age and NIH Stroke Scale: SPAN-100. Neurology. 2013;80(1):21-8.
30. Vogt G, Laage R, Shuaib A, Schneider A, Collaboration V. Initial lesion volume is an independent predictor of clinical stroke outcome at day 90: an analysis of the Virtual International Stroke Trials Archive (VISTA) database. Stroke. 2012;43(5):1266-72.
31. Munsch F, Sagnier S, Asselineau J, Bigourdan A, Guttmann CR, Debruxelles S, et al. Stroke Location Is an Independent Predictor of Cognitive Outcome. Stroke. 2016;47(1):66-73.
32. Alladi S, Bak TH, Mekala S, Rajan A, Chaudhuri JR, Mioshi E, et al. Impact of Bilingualism on Cognitive Outcome After Stroke. Stroke. 2016;47(1):258-61.
33. Meader N, Moe-Byrne T, Llewellyn A, Mitchell AJ. Screening for poststroke major depression: a meta-analysis of diagnostic validity studies. J Neurol Neurosurg Psychiatry. 2014;85(2):198-206.
34. Starkstein SE, Hayhow BD. Treatment of Post-Stroke Depression. Curr Treat Options Neurol. 2019;21(7):31.
35. Cumming TB, Blomstrand C, Skoog I, Linden T. The High Prevalence of Anxiety Disorders After Stroke. Am J Geriatr Psychiatry. 2016;24(2):154-60.
36. Campbell Burton CA, Murray J, Holmes J, Astin F, Greenwood D, Knapp P. Frequency of anxiety after stroke: a systematic review and meta-analysis of observational studies. Int J Stroke. 2013;8(7):545-59.
37. Chun HY, Whiteley WN, Dennis MS, Mead GE, Carson AJ. Anxiety After Stroke: The Importance of Subtyping. Stroke. 2018;49(3):556-64.
38. Garton AL, Sisti JA, Gupta VP, Christophe BR, Connolly ES Jr. Poststroke Post-Traumatic Stress Disorder: A Review. Stroke. 2017;48(2):507-12.
39. Noble AJ, Baisch S, Mendelow AD, Allen L, Kane P, Schenk T. Posttraumatic stress disorder explains reduced quality of life in subarachnoid hemorrhage patients in both the short and long term. Neurosurgery. 2008;63(6):1095-104.
40. Utz KS, Kiphuth IC, Schenk T. Posttraumatic stress disorder in patients after transient ischemic attack: A one-year follow-up. J Psychosom Res. 2019;122:36-8.
41. Rutovic S, Kadojic D, Dikanovic M, Solic K, Malojcic B. Prevalence and correlates of post-traumatic stress disorder after ischaemic stroke. Acta Neurol Belg. 2021;121(2):437-42.
42. Goldfinger JZ, Edmondson D, Kronish IM, Fei K, Balakrishnan R, Tuhrim S, et al. Correlates of post-traumatic stress disorder in stroke survivors. J Stroke Cerebrovasc Dis. 2014;23(5):1099-105.
43. Kronish IM, Edmondson D, Goldfinger JZ, Fei K, Horowitz CR. Posttraumatic stress disorder and adherence to medications in survivors of strokes and transient ischemic attacks. Stroke. 2012;43(8):2192-7.
44. Knapp P, Campbell Burton CA, Holmes J, Murray J, Gillespie D, Lightbody CE, et al. Interventions for treating anxiety after stroke. Cochrane Database Syst Rev. 2017;5(5):CD008860.
45. Lieberman JA, First MB. Psychotic Disorders. N Engl J Med. 2018;379(3):270-80.

46. Stangeland H, Orgeta V, Bell V. Poststroke psychosis: a systematic review. J Neurol Neurosurg Psychiatry. 2018;89(8):879-85.
47. Joyce EM. Organic psychosis: The pathobiology and treatment of delusions. CNS Neurosci Ther. 2018;24(7):598-603.
48. Douglas IJ, Smeeth L. Exposure to antipsychotics and risk of stroke: self-controlled case series study. BMJ. 2008;337:a1227.
49. Wang S, Linkletter C, Dore D, Mor V, Buka S, Maclure M. Age, antipsychotics, and the risk of ischemic stroke in the Veterans Health Administration. Stroke. 2012;43(1):28-31.
50. Ferro JM, Caeiro L, Verdelho A. Delirium in acute stroke. Current opinion in neurology. 2002;15(1):51-5.
51. Oldenbeuving AW, de Kort P, Jansen B, Roks G, Kappelle L. Delirium in acute stroke: a review. Int J Stroke. 2007;2(4):270-5.
52. Gustafson Y, Olsson T, Eriksson S, Asplund K, Bucht G. Acute confusional states (delirium) in stroke patients. Cerebrovasc Dis. 1991;1(5):257-64.
53. Caeiro L, Ferro J, Claro M, Coelho J, Albuquerque R, Figueira M. Delirium in acute stroke: a preliminary study of the role of anticholinergic medications. Eur J Neurol. 2004;11(10):699-704.
54. Sheng AZ, Shen Q, Cordato D, Zhang YY, Yin Chan DK. Delirium within three days of stroke in a cohort of elderly patients. J Am Geriatr Soc. 2006;54(8):1192-8.
55. Caeiro L, Menger C, Ferro JM, Albuquerque R, Figueira ML. Delirium in acute subarachnoid haemorrhage. Cerebrovasc Dis. 2005;19(1):31-8.
56. Mobbs RJ, Chandran KN, Newcombe RL. Psychiatric presentation of aneurysmal subarachnoid haemorrhage. ANZ J Surg. 2001;71(1):69-70.
57. Melkas S, Laurila JV, Vataja R, Oksala N, Jokinen H, Pohjasvaara T, et al. Post-stroke delirium in relation to dementia and long-term mortality. Int J Geriatr Psychiatry. 2012;27(4):401-8.
58. Kostalova M, Bednarik J, Mitasova A, Dušek L, Michalcakova R, Kerkovsky M, et al. Towards a predictive model for post-stroke delirium. Brain Inj. 2012;26(7-8):962-71.
59. Mitasova A, Kostalova M, Bednarik J, Michalcakova R, Kasparek T, Balabanova P, et al. Poststroke delirium incidence and outcomes: validation of the Confusion Assessment Method for the Intensive Care Unit (CAM-ICU). Crit Care Med. 2012;40(2):484-90.
60. McManus J, Pathansali R, Hassan H, Ouldred E, Cooper D, Stewart R, et al. The course of delirium in acute stroke. Age Ageing. 2009;38(4):385-9.
61. Dostović Z, Smajlović D, Sinanović O, Vidović M. Duration of delirium in the acute stage of stroke. Acta Clin Croat. 2009;48(1):13-7.
62. Lipowski ZJ. Delirium in the elderly patient. N Engl J Med. 1989;320(9):578-82.
63. Edlund A, Lundström M, Karlsson S, Brännström B, Bucht G, Gustafson Y. Delirium in older patients admitted to general internal medicine. J Geriatr Psychiatry Neurol. 2006;19(2):83-90.
64. Kang SY, Paik JW, Sohn YH. Restlessness with Manic Episodes due to Right Parietal Infarction. J Mov Disord. 2010;3(1):22-4.
65. Ahmed A, Simmons Z. Pseudobulbar affect: prevalence and management. Ther Clin Risk Manag. 2013;9:483-9.
66. Allida S, Patel K, House A, Hackett ML. Pharmaceutical interventions for emotionalism after stroke. Cochrane Database Syst Rev. 2019;3(3):CD003690.
67. Hinkle JL, Becker KJ, Kim JS, Choi-Kwon S, Saban KL, McNair N, et al. Poststroke Fatigue: Emerging Evidence and Approaches to Management: A Scientific Statement for Healthcare Professionals from the American Heart Association. Stroke. 2017;48(7):e159-e70.

CHAPTER 15

An Overview of Movement Disorders for the Psychiatrist

Adreesh Mukherjee

INTRODUCTION

The realm of movement disorders includes several entities with characteristic presentations and underlying etiologies, which might appear daunting if approached impetuously. Instead, a systematic evaluation leads to the correct diagnosis which directs toward the appropriate treatment. Movement disorders, in essence, are syndromes characterized by either surplus (hyperkinesia) or scarcity (hypokinesia/bradykinesia) of movements, not explained by spasticity or weakness. Hyperkinetic movement disorders (HMDs) comprise a wide range of movements with respective defining characteristics, whereas, the various parkinsonian syndromes constitute the major portion of bradykinetic disorders. In this chapter, the author will present an overview and approach to movement disorders, including practical considerations from the aspect of a psychiatrist.

THE BASAL GANGLIA

The primary components of the basal ganglia include caudate, putamen, and globus pallidus (GP), along with subthalamic nucleus (STN), substantia nigra (SN) and pedunculopontine nucleus (PPN).[1] Caudate and putamen are collectively called the neostriatum or striatum, whereas putamen and GP together are called the lenticular/lentiform nucleus. The GP has two segments—(1) the external segment (GPe) and (2) the internal segment (GPi). The SN consists of pars compacta (SNc) and pars reticulata (SNr). The main input nuclei of the basal ganglia are the caudate nucleus and the putamen, whereas, the major output is through the GP. Although traditionally considered to be involved in motor tasks, the basal ganglia are also engaged in cognitive, behavioral, and emotional functions, via five parallel circuits, namely the (1) motor, (2) oculomotor, (3) orbitofrontal, (4) dorsolateral prefrontal, and (5) limbic loops.

The basal ganglia consist of three pathways—(1) direct (excitatory), (2) indirect (inhibitory), and (3) hyperdirect (inhibitory), which have different effects on the outflow neurons of the GPi and SNr. In general, the cerebral cortex connects to the striatum, which projects to the GP and SNr. The efferents from the basal ganglia project to the thalamus, which in turn projects to the cerebral cortex. In this construct, the basal ganglia are organized to work in a center-surround mechanism, which makes the movement more selective.[1]

Regarding the HMDs, in addition to the basal ganglia, a wider network of structures has been shown to be involved. In tremor genesis, the Guillain-Mollaret (dentato-rubro-olivary) triangle and the cerebello-thalamo-cortical network are considered to play an important role. Similarly, the network model of dystonia suggests that dystonia might arise from interference with any connection in the network between the basal ganglia, thalamus, cerebral cortex, and cerebellum.

THE PARKINSONIAN DISORDERS

Case 1

A 67-year-old man takes a laborious walk into the psychiatrist's office. He was on treatment for visual hallucinations and forgetfulness for last 8 months. Over the past few weeks, he started to walk slowly and talk softly. What happened to him?

Case 2

A 58-year-old woman developed tremulousness at resting position in her right hand followed by her left hand. There was slowness in her activities, and she started walking with short steps and a slightly stooped posture. Her symptoms responded well to levodopa, but gradually the dose had to be increased. After about 5 years, some new medications were added to control her symptoms. Few months later, she started experiencing visual hallucinations. How to address this issue?

These representative cases describe two patients with slowness of activities, but in different contexts. A rational approach to parkinsonian disorders will guide to the proper diagnosis in such cases.

Parkinsonism

Parkinsonism is a syndrome comprising six cardinal features—(1) tremor-at-rest, (2) rigidity, (3) bradykinesia, (4) loss of postural reflexes, (5) change in posture, and (6) freezing. The four chief characteristics of parkinsonism namely—(1) tremor, (2) rigidity, (3) akinesia, and (4) postural disturbances (TRAP) contribute to the majority of the disorders.

Bradykinesia refers to slowness of movement (akinesia refers to lack of movement) and may occur during both initiation and continuation of movement. The term hypokinesia is sometimes used to describe a reduction in amplitude of movement. Bradykinesia can be demonstrated on examination by slowness in rapid alternating movements where speed and amplitude are usually assessed. The performance of movements such as finger tapping, opening and closing the fist, pronation-supination of the forearm, and foot tapping is slow. Other manifestations of bradykinesia include monotonic and hypophonic dysarthria, loss of facial expression (masked facies/hypomimia), decreased blink rate, micrographia (handwriting becomes slower and smaller), and reduced arm swing when walking (loss of automatic movement). Rigidity is usually manifested by increased resistance throughout the range of movement (lead-pipe), however, cogwheeling (additional jerky quality) may be present, particularly if there is associated tremor. The rigidity may be enhanced during voluntary movement of a contralateral limb which is called activated rigidity (Froment sign). Rigidity may occur proximally (neck, shoulders, and hips) and distally (wrists and ankles), and it is important to note both axial and appendicular rigidity. The Movement Disorder Society-Unified Parkinson's Disease Rating Scale (MDS-UPDRS) is a standardized tool to assess the various functional domains in parkinson disease (PD).[2]

The most common form of parkinsonism is PD. The other less common entities comprise atypical parkinsonism [progressive supranuclear palsy (PSP), multiple system atrophy (MSA), corticobasal degeneration/syndrome (CBD/CBS), and dementia with Lewy bodies (DLB)], secondary parkinsonism, and genetic disorders which can present with parkinsonism **(Box 1)**. Evaluation of the symptoms and signs often leads to a basic clinical differentiation of PD from these other syndromes.

BOX 1: Parkinsonian disorders.[1]

- *Parkinson disease (PD)*:
  - Tremor-dominant PD
  - Postural instability gait disorder (PIGD)
  - Young onset PD (YOPD) (age of onset < 50 years)
- *Atypical parkinsonism (parkinsonism-plus)*:
  - Progressive supranuclear palsy (PSP):
    - PSP-Richardson syndrome (PSP-RS)
    - PSP-Parkinsonism (PSP-P)
    - Other subtypes of PSP
  - Multiple system atrophy (MSA):
    - MSA with predominant parkinsonism (MSA-P)
    - MSA with predominant cerebellar ataxia (MSA-C)
  - Corticobasal syndrome (CBS)
  - Dementia with Lewy bodies (DLB)
- *Genetic disorders with parkinsonism*:
  - Huntington disease (Juvenile HD and Westphal variant)
  - Wilson disease
  - Neurodegeneration with brain iron accumulation (NBIA)
  - Machado–Joseph disease (spinocerebellar ataxia 3)
- *Secondary (acquired) parkinsonism*:
  - Vascular parkinsonism
  - Normal pressure hydrocephalus
  - *Drugs*: Dopamine receptor blocking agents (antipsychotics and antiemetic), flunarizine, cinnarizine, and tetrabenazine
  - *Infectious cause*: Creutzfeldt–Jakob disease, postencephalitic parkinsonism
  - *Toxins*: Carbon monoxide and manganese
  - Trauma
  - *Metabolic/endocrine*: Parathyroid abnormalities
  - Neoplastic
  - Paraneoplastic/autoimmune

Parkinson Disease

The PD is the prototypic parkinsonian disorder, and usually presents with asymmetric onset bradykinesia, rigidity, and rest tremor. Bradykinesia is the most characteristic clinical hallmark of PD, and is initially manifested by slowness of daily activities. A painful shoulder is one of the most common early symptoms of PD, possibly related to decreased arm swing and rigidity, and is often misdiagnosed as bursitis, arthritis, or a rotator cuff disorder. Also, turning over in bed and adjusting the bedclothes become difficult. On examination, the movements are slow, with a gradual reduction in amplitude. In addition, there may be hesitation in initiating movement and arrests in ongoing movement (freezing). Initially, the rigidity is usually more prominent in the limbs than axial. The tremor of PD is typically a resting tremor, distal, asymmetric, usually starts in one upper limb (then spreading to the other side), and may be present in the lower limbs as well. The rest tremor has a supination-pronation, or pill-rolling character, and is exacerbated during walking or counting backward. About 50% of patients may also manifest a postural tremor that reoccurs with arms stretched outward after a pause of usually few seconds (re-emergent tremor). The PD patient shows a typical stooped posture with a forward tilt of the head, and flexion at the joints of upper and lower limbs. An extreme flexion at the waist is called camptocormia. There may also be postural deformities of the hands (striatal hand), and foot (striatal foot), and occasionally an extension of the great toe (striatal toe). Beyond the typical presentation of PD, two subtypes are recognized—(1) tremor-dominant PD and (2) postural instability gait disorder (PIGD).

The PD is now recognized to be a heterogeneous condition marked by both motor and nonmotor symptoms. The neuropsychiatric symptoms include depression, anxiety, apathy, impulse control disorders, psychosis, hallucinations, delusions, and abulia. Cognitive impairment in the form of slowness of thinking (bradyphrenia), trouble finding words ("tip of the tongue phenomenon"), executive dysfunction, and dementia may be present. Sleep disorders may manifest as insomnia, excessive daytime sleepiness, sleep attacks, restless legs syndrome (RLS), periodic limb movements of sleep, and rapid eye movement (REM) sleep behavior disorder (RBD). RBD is commonly seen in synucleinopathy (PD, MSA, and DLB) and it is an important prodromal marker of PD. Hyposmia and constipation are other associations seen in PD. Dysautonomia must be evaluated in PD and any parkinsonian syndrome, especially orthostatic hypotension, urinary urgency and incontinence, and sexual dysfunction.

Response to levodopa plays an important role in parkinsonism. PD is levodopa responsive, whereas, atypical parkinsonian syndromes are usually nonresponsive (although some forms may show improvement initially, it is usually partial and declines gradually). Additionally, after sustained treatment with levodopa, a patient of PD may develop dyskinesia related to the dose of levodopa.

Atypical Parkinsonian Syndromes

In general, the parkinsonian syndromes have been classified as synucleinopathy (PD, MSA, and DLB) and tauopathy (PSP and CBS). Atypical parkinsonism is considered when there are symptoms and signs which are unlikely in PD, termed as the "red flags" (**Box 2**).

> **BOX 2: Red flags suggesting an atypical parkinsonism.**
> - Rapid progression
> - Falls within the first year
> - Early instability (wheelchair within 5 years)
> - Early gait disorder
> - Symmetrical signs
> - Vertical supranuclear gaze palsy
> - Bulbar dysfunction-severe dysphonia, dysarthria, dysphagia
> - Prominent pyramidal tract or cerebellar signs
> - Abnormal posture—Pisa syndrome
> - Poor response to levodopa
> - Sleep apnea
> - Inspiratory stridor
> - Early prominent dementia
> - Apraxia
> - Cortical sensory loss
> - Early autonomic dysfunction

Progressive Supranuclear Palsy

The PSP is possibly the most common atypical parkinsonism. It is typically a symmetric levodopa-resistant akinetic-rigid parkinsonism, with prominent axial signs (and an extended posture). Vertical supranuclear gaze palsy (VSGP) is the clinical hallmark of PSP. Initially, the saccades are slow, and usually, downgaze is involved the earliest. Patients are unable to move their eyes voluntarily, but vertical eye movements can be elicited by the vestibulo-ocular reflex. There is early dysarthria, dysphagia, and postural instability with falls (tendency to fall backward). The patients have a wide-eyed, worried expression with furrowing of the brow (procerus sign). Tremor is less prominent, and postural rather than at-rest. Moreover, a frontal dysexecutive syndrome may accompany the clinical picture. However, recently several subtypes of PSP have been recognized which makes it a more heterogenous group. Thus, while the classical description of PSP [PSP-Richardson syndrome (PSP-RS)] still stands, the additional phenotypes add to the diagnostic dilemma. The PSP-P variant (PSP-parkinsonism) presents with asymmetric, limb-predominant parkinsonism, where the VSGP may be a late feature.[3] Interestingly, PSP pathology can have a cognitive-behavioral presentation similar to behavioral variant of frontotemporal dementia (bvFTD) or progressive nonfluent aphasia (PNFA), whereby the diagnosis may be delayed until the development of VSGP or the characteristic motor features.

Corticobasal Syndrome

Corticobasal syndrome is the preferred clinical term, whereas, CBD is a neuropathological diagnosis. This distinction is made because CBS presentation may have varied underlying pathology including CBD and PSP. The clinical picture of CBS usually includes features of both motor and cortical dysfunction. An asymmetric parkinsonism with rigidity and bradykinesia is the common presentation, and rarely, a postural tremor may be present. Limb dystonia, frequently unilateral, may be seen in CBS, and it may lead to contractures. The patient develops axial rigidity, postural instability, and falls. Myoclonus may also be observed. VSGP may be present, especially in a phenotypic overlap with PSP. Cognitive impairment (executive dysfunction, visuospatial deficits, agrammatism, and posterior cortical atrophy syndrome), neuropsychiatric symptoms, and limb apraxia are the common manifestations of cortical dysfunction in CBS.[4] Additionally, aphasia or cortical sensory loss may be present. The alien limb phenomenon is an interesting entity associated with CBS, in which the affected limb (usually an upper limb) appears to be out of the patient's voluntary control.

Multiple System Atrophy

Multiple system atrophy, as the name suggests, consists of a combination of parkinsonism, cerebellar dysfunction, autonomic dysfunction, and pyramidal signs (brisk reflexes and extensor plantar response). Two broad subtypes are recognized—(1) MSA with predominant parkinsonism (MSA-P) and (2) MSA with predominant cerebellar ataxia (MSA-C). Autonomic dysfunction is a distinctive feature in MSA, and predominantly occurs in the form of orthostatic hypotension (manifests as syncope), urinary incontinence, and erectile dysfunction. Although autonomic symptoms are also seen in PD, very early and prominent autonomic dysfunction is suggestive of MSA. A drop in blood pressure of ≥ 20 mm Hg systolic or ≥ 10 mm Hg diastolic after 3 minutes of standing from supine position is considered significant. Similar to the other atypical parkinsonian disorders, an akinetic-rigid syndrome with rare tremor (postural > rest) is characteristic for MSA. There is early gait impairment and falls. The parkinsonism is less responsive to levodopa and shows a rapid progression than PD. Examination of the eye movements may reveal impairment of smooth pursuit, and a gaze-evoked nystagmus. Other suggestive signs include anterocollis (forward flexion of the neck), early dysarthria and dysphagia. Although traditionally believed to be nonexistent, recent evidence suggests that cognitive impairment, especially executive dysfunction, can be seen in MSA.[5] Anxiety and depression may also be present.

Dementia with Lewy bodies

Dementia with Lewy bodies is a little different in this group as it has a predominant cognitive and behavioral presentation accompanied by parkinsonian symptoms. The cognitive impairment either precedes or occurs within 1 year of the onset of parkinsonism. While dementia is the essential criteria for the diagnosis of DLB, cognitive fluctuations are important core features. Prominent early neuropsychiatric features, especially hallucinations (visual) and delusions are characteristic for DLB. RBD, autonomic dysfunction (syncope), postural instability, and falls are the other key features. It is imperative to be careful about neuroleptic sensitivity in DLB, which occurs in the form of severe reaction to antipsychotics (such as haloperidol) with worsening of the motor and cognitive symptoms. From a clinicopathological point of view, PD, PD-mild cognitive impairment (PD-MCI), PD dementia (PDD), and DLB represent a spectrum of Lewy body disorders.[6]

Secondary Parkinsonism

Secondary causes of parkinsonism can be associated with both acute-subacute or chronic presentation **(Box 1)**. A chronic progressive course may be seen in vascular parkinsonism and normal pressure hydrocephalus. In any acute-subacute parkinsonism, a secondary cause should be intensively investigated. This is important as several of these etiologies are treatable.

Clinical Approach to Parkinsonism

Before establishing parkinsonism, careful examination is required to rule out the mimickers of bradykinesia (depression, hypothyroid, and painful conditions restricting movement), and to exclude other causes of hypertonia (spasticity, gegenhalten).[7] Along with the examination for the parkinsonian symptoms (TRAP), the following information is required—demography (age of onset, gender), temporal profile (onset, course and progression), neurological features, evaluation of other systems, nonmotor symptoms (including autonomic), family history, and treatment history (including levodopa responsiveness).[7] PD and the atypical parkinsonian syndromes usually have an older age of onset. However, a subset of PD patients has a considerably earlier onset (<50 years of age). This group, called young onset PD (YOPD), often has an underlying genetic etiology.

We look into the clinical features, and rule out the red flag signs suggesting a diagnosis other than PD. In general, a case of parkinsonism can be approached based

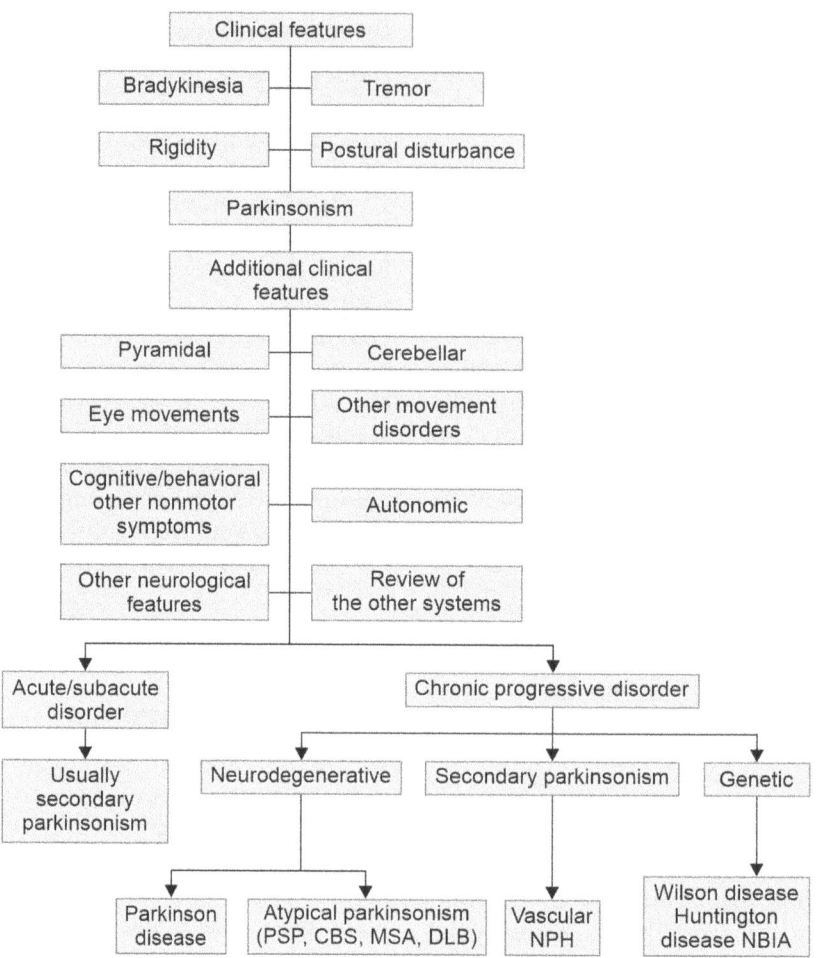

FLOWCHART 1: Approach to a patient with parkinsonism.

on the onset and course of the disease (acute/subacute/chronic) **(Flowchart 1)**. The investigation and treatment are accordingly guided by the clinical evaluation.

Investigations

The diagnosis of PD is mostly clinical. Neuroimaging such as magnetic resonance imaging (MRI) of the brain is useful to identify changes associated with atypical or secondary parkinsonism. Some of the typical findings include the hummingbird sign in PSP (midbrain atrophy with sparing of pons), and the hot cross bun sign (in the pons) in MSA. Signal intensity changes may be seen in the basal ganglia, thalamus, and other regions of the brain in the various secondary parkinsonian disorders. Other investigations including blood and cerebrospinal fluid (CSF) tests are guided by the clinical presentation. In young-onset cases, Wilson disease (WD) should be ruled out. Genetic study may be done in YOPD patients.

Treatment

Levodopa (with carbidopa) is the mainstay of treatment for PD and most other parkinsonian disorders. In PD, there is good levodopa responsiveness. In fact, a poor levodopa response indicates the possibility of an atypical parkinsonism. Other medications include dopamine agonists (ropinirole and pramipexole), monoamine oxidase B (MAO-B) inhibitor (rasagiline and safinamide), catechol-O-methyltransferase (COMT) inhibitor (entacapone), and amantadine. After prolonged treatment with levodopa, the PD patients may develop dyskinesia (levodopa-induced dyskinesia). In selected PD patients, deep brain stimulation surgery is useful. Other symptoms of parkinsonian syndromes should also be addressed, such as urinary symptoms, orthostatic hypotension, sleep disturbances, depression, and cognitive impairment. Antipsychotics should be used judiciously in parkinsonism patients, with close monitoring for any worsening or adverse effects. For the secondary causes, specific management will be guided by the individual diagnosis.

Case Discussion

Case 3

This patient presented with cognitive impairment and visual hallucinations followed by parkinsonism. The parkinsonian features may be part of the disease spectrum, or induced by any antipsychotic medication he may have received. While several other possibilities exist, these two appear to be the most plausible. We should consider the possibility of DLB at this point, and enquire about the core features such as cognitive fluctuations and RBD, and check for any autonomic dysfunction. The rest of the examination and corresponding investigations will thereby follow.

Case 4

This patient has the characteristic features of PD. The visual hallucinations appeared after several years of disease onset. Psychosis may be present in PD. However, some of the anti-parkinsonian medications such as Amantadine are known to precipitate such symptoms. Hence, in this patient, the first step would be to review the medications, especially those added recently. Additionally, any systemic or metabolic perturbation should be checked. Once these are excluded, she should be evaluated and managed in the line of PD psychosis.

■ HYPERKINETIC MOVEMENT DISORDERS

Case 1

A 15-year-old girl was brought by her parents to the psychiatrist for irritable and agitated behavior. About a month later, she developed progressive posturing and twisting movements in her limbs, and later, truncal posturing. What possibly caused this?

Case 2

A 12-year-old boy was reported by his school teacher for being disruptive in the class by making sounds and shaking his head and throwing his limbs. His parents assured the teacher that they would take care of the situation. But how should they do it?

The HMDs comprise a vast array of disorders, and identifying the phenomenology is the first step toward the correct diagnosis. Among the various HMDs **(Box 3)**, some are more commonly encountered, such as tremor, chorea, dystonia, myoclonus, and tics. It is important to have a basic knowledge of these disorders as the etiological workup and therapeutic approach vary according to the clinical diagnosis. While the clinical picture may appear

> **BOX 3: Hyperkinetic movement disorders.[1]**
> - Abdominal dyskinesia
> - Akathisia
> - Athetosis
> - Ballism
> - Chorea
> - Dystonia
> - Hemifacial spasm
> - Hyperekplexia
> - Myoclonus
> - Myokymia
> - Myorhythmia
> - Paroxysmal dyskinesia
> - Periodic movements in sleep
> - Restless legs
> - Stereotypy
> - Tics
> - Tremor

complicated in case of mixed movement disorders where more than one type of movement coexists, a systematic approach helps to identify the predominant movement disorder in such cases, which in turn guides further evaluation.

Tremor

Tremor may be defined as an involuntary, rhythmic, and oscillatory movement of a body part.[8] Tremors can be classified according to their phenomenology, distribution, frequency, or etiology. Phenomenologically, tremors are of two major types—(1) rest tremor and (2) action tremor. Action tremor is further classified into postural, kinetic, task-specific, position-specific, and isometric. Kinetic tremor is seen when moving a body part, and it may be present at the beginning, during the course, or at the terminal part (intention tremor when reaching near to the target) of the movement.[9] PD, essential tremor (ET), and cerebellar disorders are classically associated with rest tremor, postural tremor, and kinetic (intention) tremor, respectively.

Essential tremor is the prototypic syndrome associated with postural tremor. It shows a bimodal peak of age of onset (third and seventh decades of life). The tremor is predominantly in the bilateral distal upper limbs, and presents for at least 3 years' duration.[8] Tremor may also be evident in other parts of the body such as the head, voice, and lower limbs. Family history of tremor may be present.

Dystonia

Dystonia is characterized by sustained or intermittent muscle contractions causing abnormal, often repetitive, movements, postures, or both.[10] It is patterned or twisting, and may also be tremulous. Dystonia can be classified according to body distribution and temporal pattern. It can be focal, segmental, multifocal, generalized, or hemidystonia, and the temporal pattern may be persistent, diurnal, action-specific, or paroxysmal. While focal dystonia such as blepharospasm is common in adults, generalized dystonia is often seen in children (or adults) with genetic disorders.[9] A sensory trick or "geste antagoniste" is a useful feature seen in dystonia. It denotes the reduction of dystonia by voluntary touch, such as touching the chin may decrease the posturing in cervical dystonia.

Dopa-responsive dystonia (DRD) is commonly caused by mutation in the *GCH1* gene (DYT-*GCH1*) which is usually inherited in an autosomal dominant manner. It is typically a childhood-onset dystonia, starting from the lower limbs, and spreading upward, sometimes generalizing.[11] A characteristic diurnal variation may be seen, with worsening as the day progresses. Patients have an excellent response to levodopa, usually at a low dose.

Chorea

The term chorea represents involuntary, irregular, purposeless, nonrhythmic, rapid, unsustained movements that seem to flow from one body part to another.[1] The inability to maintain voluntary contraction is known as motor impersistence, and it is an important feature of chorea. It can manifest in actions such as manual grip (milkmaid grip) or tongue protrusion. The distribution of chorea provides clues, e.g., acute-onset hemichorea points toward nonketotic hyperglycemia or stroke. The list of etiologies is daunting in chorea, and the diagnostic process may become a little complicated. Several possibilities arise in sporadic forms of chorea such as Sydenham chorea, systemic lupus erythematosus (SLE), polycythemia, N-methyl-D-aspartate receptor (NMDAR) encephalitis, and paraneoplastic syndromes.[9]

Huntington disease (HD) is the most important genetic (autosomal dominant) cause of chorea. It is caused by a CAG repeat expansion in the huntingtin gene (*HTT*) on chromosome 4p16.3. Apart from the motor features (chorea, dystonia, etc.), cognitive and behavioral (anxiety, depression, impulsivity, and irritability) symptoms are also present in HD.[12] Juvenile HD (Westphal variant) occurs below 20 years of age, and may present with parkinsonism instead of chorea.

Myoclonus

Myoclonus denotes sudden, brief, and lightning-like involuntary movements, which may be evident at rest, on maintaining a posture or on movement.[13] Jerks may be triggered by external stimuli, which can be visual, auditory, or touch. Myoclonus may be confined to one particular region of the body (focal or segmental), or involve different parts of the body (multifocal), or it can be a generalized myoclonus. Importantly, myoclonus forms a meeting point of HMDs and epilepsy. Hence, its evaluation should be done carefully with relevant investigations.

Myoclonus may be present in several neurodegenerative disorders such as Alzheimer's disease, DLB, and CBS. A "slow" myoclonus is characteristic of subacute sclerosing panencephalitis (SSPE). Asterixis or negative myoclonus (brief inhibition of muscle activity) is classically present in hepatic and other metabolic encephalopathies, and forms the pathophysiological basis of the "liver flap".

Tics

Tics are brief, repetitive movements (motor tics) or vocalizations (phonic tics), which are usually suppressible for a short period of time, but at the expense of mounting inner tension (urge to move).[1,14] Tics may be simple or complex. Simple motor tics involve only one group of muscles, such as blinking and head jerking, whereas, complex motor tics may present in many forms such as trunk bending, arm straightening, touching, or jumping.[14] Simple phonic tics typically consist of sniffing, throat clearing, or other sounds, while complex phonic tics include verbalizations such as shouting of obscenities (coprolalia).

Tourette syndrome (according to DSM-5) is characterized by the presence of both motor and phonic tics, with onset before 18 years of age, and persisting for >1 year, without an apparent secondary cause.[15] It has a male preponderance, and may be associated with obsessive compulsive disorder or attention deficit hyperactivity disorder.

Wilson Disease

Any discussion on HMDs is incomplete without WD. It is a treatable autosomal recessive genetic disorder (*ATP7B* gene) not very uncommon in India. It is commonly seen in childhood and young adulthood, and the common modes of presentation include neurologic, psychiatric, and hepatic dysfunction. Psychiatric symptoms may remain unrecognized in the initial stages, and usually include personality change, depression, and anxiety.[16] Regarding movement disorders, WD can present in myriad ways, be it parkinsonism or HMDs such as dystonia and tremor. Indeed, WD should be considered in the differential diagnosis of most of the movement disorders presenting at an early age. Demonstration of corneal Kayser–Fleischer rings by slit-lamp examination is a useful clue to the diagnosis (present in nearly 99% of patients with neurological symptoms). MRI brain may show the "face of the giant panda" sign, with T2 hyperintensity in the midbrain. Additional MRI features include signal changes in the basal ganglia, thalamus, pons, and white matter.[16] Investigations include 24-hour urinary copper level (>100 μg/24 h), and a low serum ceruloplasmin (<20 mg/dL). Genetic study is also available. Treatment options in WD include zinc, d-penicillamine, and trientine.

Approach

In addition to a description of the motor symptoms, a thorough history should include information on the age at onset and course of the disease, nonmotor symptoms including cognitive or behavioral dysfunction, other neurological symptoms, any significant systemic symptoms, birth and developmental history, significant family history, any consanguinity, preceding drug (e.g., neuroleptics) history, and any response to treatment (as in the case of DRD).[9] The clinical examination should determine the HMDs, and in the case of a mixed phenomenology, the predominant movement present. It should also include a detailed neurological examination beyond the movements, and a review of the other systems **(Flowchart 2)**. This will guide the appropriate investigations required for the diagnosis.

Investigations

The investigations in HMDs are guided by the phenomenology and clinical diagnosis. It is not possible to generalize the tests required as each individual will be different. The investigations range from blood tests, to neuroimaging and genetic study. While MRI brain shows changes in several acquired causes of HMD, it may also provide clues to genetic disorders, such as the eye of the tiger sign in pantothenate kinase-associated neurodegeneration [a type of neurodegeneration with brain iron accumulation (NBIA)]. Additional tests may also be required such as a 24-hour urinary copper level for WD, or a CSF study in suspected autoimmune encephalitis. Special emphasis should be given to identify treatable causes.

Treatment

The treatment of HMDs depends on the phenomenology and the specific etiology. Stating briefly, for ET,

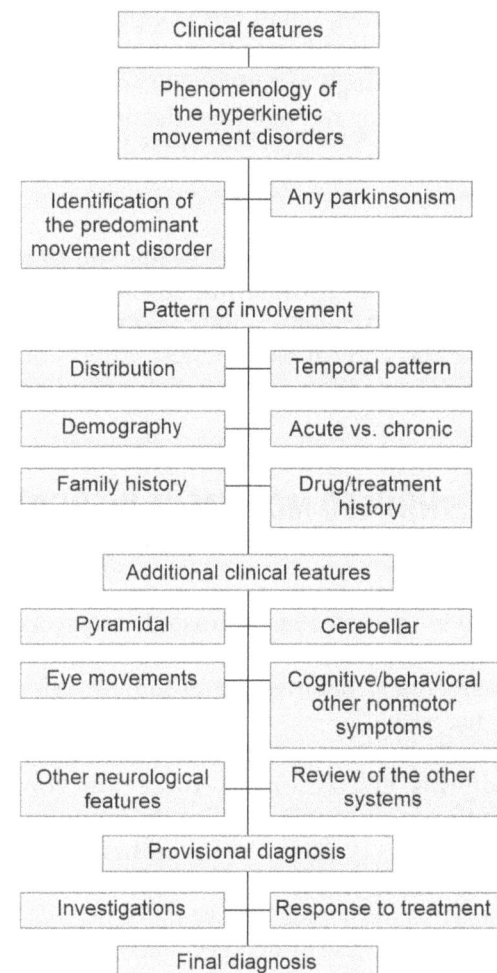

FLOWCHART 2: Approach to a patient with hyperkinetic movement disorders.

propranolol or primidone is used. For dystonia, several options are available, such as trihexyphenidyl, baclofen, tetrabenazine, and clonazepam. Botulinum toxin injection is useful in focal dystonia. Tetrabenazine is also used in chorea. Myoclonus may be treated with clonazepam, sodium valproate, and levetiracetam. Tic disorders require a multidisciplinary approach. The various acquired causes of HMDs should be treated according to the etiology. Importantly, there are genetic disorders with specific treatment, such as WD and DRD. Nonmotor symptoms, including the various psychiatric manifestations, should also be managed appropriately.

Case Discussion

Case 3

This patient presented with childhood-onset behavioral symptoms, followed by generalized dystonia. This may be due to a disorder which can manifest both psychiatric and movement disorders, such as WD. Another possibility is a drug-induced dystonia from any psychiatric medication she might have received for the behavioral symptoms. A thorough history and examination will be required followed by relevant investigations to reach the diagnosis.

Case 4

This patient will require careful evaluation to rule out a tic disorder. Often misinterpreted initially, a proper assessment should involve a neurologist together with psychiatrist and clinical psychologist. After a diagnosis of tic disorder is made, its treatment also requires a team approach.

DRUG-INDUCED MOVEMENT DISORDERS

Case 1

A 43-year-old man was being treated for psychosis for about a year. Recently, he developed excessive involuntary movements of his mouth and tongue. What is the possible diagnosis?

Drug-induced movement disorders form an important aspect of this discussion, as these are commonly associated with antipsychotic use. Dopamine receptor blocking agents (DRBA), both antipsychotics and antiemetics such as metoclopramide, can lead to a spectrum of manifestations. These may be acute-subacute or chronic **(Box 4)**. The acute presentations occur shortly after the introduction or a dose increase of a DRBA. Acute dystonia is the typical example, and in about a half of the patients it manifests within 48 hours of drug intake. Acute dystonia may take the form of orofacial dystonia, neck and back extension, oculogyric crisis (tonic conjugate ocular deviation), and rarely life-threatening laryngospasm.[17] While mostly the typical antipsychotics are associated with acute dystonia, it may also be seen with the use of atypical antipsychotics. Acute dystonic reactions respond rapidly to anticholinergic drugs. Parkinsonism may be caused or exacerbated by neuroleptics, and several other medications such as tetrabenazine and flunarizine. Although typically drug-induced parkinsonism is considered to be symmetric, in about one-third of patients it may be asymmetric. It usually develops between 2 and 4 weeks of neuroleptic use. Acute akathisia may start within hours or days (2 weeks) after the initiation of DRBA. It has two salient features, a subjective restlessness or inner tension, and the objective manifestations of restlessness in the form of movements of the limbs or body.

Tardive syndromes are antipsychotic-induced delayed-onset movement disorders. Orofacial (orobuccolingual) dyskinesia and stereotypies are the typical manifestations of tardive dyskinesia. These movements

> **BOX 4: Drug-induced movement disorders.[18]**
> - *Acute onset*:
>   - Acute dystonia/acute dystonic reactions
>   - Acute or subacute akathisia
>   - Neuroleptic malignant syndrome
> - Drug-induced parkinsonism
> - *Tardive syndromes (delayed onset)*:
>   - Tardive dyskinesia
>   - Tardive stereotypies
>   - Tardive chorea
>   - Tardive akathisia
>   - Tardive dystonia
>   - Tardive tics
>   - Tardive myoclonus
>   - Tardive tremor

are complex and appear as puckering, lip smacking, jaw movements, or abnormal protrusions of the tongue. Other forms of tardive syndrome consist of dystonia, akathisia, and tremor. Treatment of tardive syndromes include the VMAT2 inhibitors (tetrabenazine, valbenazine, and deutetrabenazine). Tapering or optimization of the dose of DRBA should be attempted. Switching to clozapine (or quetiapine) may be considered because of the low potential for such adverse effects.[18]

A drug-induced movement disorder emergency is the neuroleptic malignant syndrome (NMS), which develops acutely over hours to a few days. It is seen with both typical and atypical neuroleptics, although to a lesser extent with the latter.[19] It is characterized by hyperthermia (>100.4°F or >38.0°C), rigidity (with tremor, dystonia, and myoclonus), altered mental state, autonomic dysfunction, and increased serum creatine kinase. Treatment includes stopping the neuroleptic, and starting bromocriptine or other dopaminergic agents (pramipexole, ropinirole, and levodopa), and supportive care (in the intensive care unit for severe cases).[19]

Medications other than DRBA can also lead to movement disorders. For example, tremor may be seen with the use of valproic acid and lithium, while akathisia may be an adverse effect of SSRIs. Serotonin syndrome, resembling NMS, is caused by drugs increasing serotonin activity, such as SSRIs, SNRIs, and tricyclics. It has an acute presentation, and manifests as an altered mental state, autonomic dysfunction, hyperthermia, hyperreflexia, and movement disorders such as myoclonus and tremor (also rigidity). Treatment includes stopping the causative medication, supportive care (intensive care unit), using benzodiazepines or 5-HT2A receptor antagonists such as cyproheptadine.[19]

Case Discussion

Case 2

In this patient, the mouth and tongue movements may be due to dystonia, chorea, or an orobuccolingual dyskinesia. A phenomenological diagnosis is thus required as the first step. Considering the clinical setting of treatment with antipsychotics, a tardive syndrome is the likely possibility in this case.

FUNCTIONAL MOVEMENT DISORDERS

Case 1

A 31-year-old woman presented with acute-onset unsteadiness in walking. She was rushed to the hospital by her husband, who flew in from his new place of posting in another city. She had a wobbling gait with buckling of knees and tendency to fall, however, she never actually fell down. Interestingly, her husband noted from another room that she was walking without any difficulty while talking to her parents on cell phone. What is possibly happening?

Functional movement disorders (FMDs) form an intriguing group which can present with any movement disorder phenomenology, hypo- or hyperkinetic (**Box 5**). These often create a diagnostic dilemma, and both over- and underdiagnosis occur. The current understanding has shifted the approach to FMD from a diagnosis of exclusion to that based on positive clinical criteria. Although an important component, the DSM-5 no longer requires a psychological stressor for the diagnosis of a functional neurological disorder. Rather, the identification and demonstration of positive clinical signs are more helpful for the diagnosis. The neurological examination may identify inconsistency and incongruence of findings compared to "organic" disorders. Similarly, distractibility and suggestibility are other relevant features in FMD. In functional tremor, which is one of the most common FMD, the movement can show entrainment. In this, when the patient performs repetitive voluntary movement with the contralateral limb, the affected tremulous limb starts moving in the same frequency.[20] Functional gait disorders may be in the form of slowness, knee buckling, or astasia-abasia. The "huffing and puffing" sign denotes exceptionally slow movements, with tiredness, grimacing, and sighing. Interestingly, function gait disorder presenting with swaying and unsteadiness may actually demonstrate good balance on careful examination (**Box 6**).

Conversion reaction is the most common psychiatric disorder among patients with an FMD. Certain forms of personality disorders may also predispose to FMD. Other psychiatric disorders include factitious disorder, anxiety neurosis, and depression. According to recent studies, malingering is a relatively uncommon cause of FMD. An in-depth knowledge and awareness of these disorders are important for the clinician treating patients with suspected FMD.

Management of FMD entails an individualized multidisciplinary approach, including physical therapy, occupational therapy, psychotherapy (cognitive behavioral therapy), and pharmacotherapy (comorbid depression and anxiety). A positive approach with a positive diagnosis usually has a positive outcome.

BOX 5: Functional movement disorders.[20]

- Functional parkinsonism
- Functional hyperkinetic movement disorders
  - Functional tremor
  - Functional dystonia
  - Functional myoclonus
  - Functional tics
- Functional cranial movement disorders
- Functional gait disorder

BOX 6: A number of clinical characteristics are associated with FMDs.

- Abrupt onset
- Rapid progression to maximum symptom severity and disability
- History of a preceding event
- Movement abnormality not consistent with known organic disease (e.g., peculiar or difficult to classify)
- Involuntary movements vary over time with inconsistency in amplitude, frequency, or distribution
- Involuntary movements of the affected body part decrease with distraction
- Involuntary movements of the affected body part increase during observation
- Entrainment of involuntary movements to the frequency of repetitive movements (e.g., tremor)
- Coactivation sign of antagonist muscles
- Deliberate slowness of movement
- Disorders associated with false or "give-way" weakness or sensory loss and/or pain
- Disability due to FMD out of proportion to examination findings
- Unresponsiveness to drugs for organic movement disorders
- Responsiveness to placebo drugs and suggestion

Source: Hinson VK, Haren WB. Psychogenic movement disorders. Lancet Neurol 2006;5:695.

Case Discussion

Case 1

An acute gait disorder can have several etiologies across the central and peripheral nervous systems. In this patient, the typical knee buckling gait, with suggestions of inconsistency and distractibility, raises the possibility of a functional disorder. Her husband's transfer to another city might have acted as a precipitating event. However, the diagnosis should not be rushed. Rather, a thorough history and careful examination, followed by relevant investigations as required, will reveal the correct diagnosis.

CONCLUDING REMARKS AND LEARNING POINTS

- The presentation of movement disorders can be diverse, including the parkinsonian syndromes or the various HMDs.
- Identification of the phenomenology is essential for a proper clinical diagnosis. PD and the atypical parkinsonian disorders should be differentiated clinically, and in case of uncertainty, neuroimaging and other relevant investigations become useful.
- Etiological evaluation for the HMDs is guided by the predominant movement present and the associated clinical setting.
- While genetic study is useful to arrive at a diagnosis, thorough workup for any treatable cause should be performed. The nonmotor symptoms form an important component of PD and other movement disorders, and these should be managed appropriately.
- Drug-induced movement disorders are usually associated with the use of DRBA such as neuroleptics (and certain antiemetics). It can have either an acute-subacute, or a delayed (tardive) presentation.
- Patients with FMD can present with HMDs, parkinsonism, or gait disorder. A multidisciplinary approach is required for proper treatment of such patients.
- Thus, movement disorders can have different presentations from various etiologies, and a systematic clinical approach is required, followed by judicious investigations and rational treatment.

REFERENCES

1. Jankovic J, Hallett M, Okun MS, Comella C, Fahn S, Goldman JG. Principles and practice of movement disorders, 3rd ed. USA: Elsevier Inc.; 2022.
2. Goetz CG, Tilley BC, Shaftman SR, Stebbins GT, Fahn S, Martinez-Martin P, et al. Movement Disorder Society-sponsored revision of the Unified Parkinson's Disease Rating Scale (MDS-UPDRS): Scale presentation and clinimetric testing results. Mov Disord. 2008;23:2129-70.
3. Levin J, Kurz A, Arzberger T, Giese A, Höglinger GU. The Differential Diagnosis and Treatment of Atypical Parkinsonism. Dtsch Arztebl Int. 2016;113:61-9.
4. Saranza GM, Whitwell JL, Kovacs GG, Lang AE. Corticobasal degeneration. Int Rev Neurobiol. 2019;149:87-136.
5. Deutschländer AB, Ross OA, Dickson DW, Wszolek ZK. Atypical parkinsonian syndromes: A general neurologist's perspective. Eur J Neurol. 2018;25:41-58.
6. Weintraub D, Irwin D. Diagnosis and Treatment of Cognitive and Neuropsychiatric Symptoms in Parkinson Disease and Dementia With Lewy Bodies. Continuum (Minneap Minn). 2022;28:1314-32.
7. Mukherjee A. Approach to Parkinsonism. In: Ray BK (Ed). Bedside Neurology: Clinical Approach. 2nd edition. New Delhi: Jaypee Brothers Medical Publishers (P) Ltd; 2023. pp. 158-166.
8. Bhatia KP, Bain P, Bajaj N, Elble RJ, Hallett M, Louis ED, et al. Consensus Statement on the classification of tremors. from the task force on tremor of the International Parkinson and Movement Disorder Society. Mov Disord. 2018;33:75-87.
9. Mukherjee A. Approach to hyperkinetic movement disorders. In: Ray BK (Ed). Bedside Neurology: Clinical Approach, 2nd edition. New Delhi: Jaypee Brothers Medical Publishers (P) Ltd; 2023. pp. 167-72.
10. Albanese A, Bhatia K, Bressman SB, Delong MR, Fahn S, Fung VS, et al. Phenomenology and classification of dystonia: a consensus update. Mov Disord. 2013;28:863-73.
11. Segawa M. Dopa-responsive dystonia. Handb Clin Neurol 2011;100:539-57.
12. Stoker TB, Mason SL, Greenland JC, Holden ST, Santini H, Barker RA. Huntington's Disease: Diagnosis and Management. Pract Neurol. 2022;22:32-41.
13. Pena AB, Caviness JN. Physiology-based Treatment of Myoclonus. Neurotherapeutics. 2020;17:1665-80.
14. Efron D, Dale RC. Tics and Tourette syndrome. J Paediatr Child Health. 2018;54:1148-53.
15. American Psychiatric Association. Diagnostic and Statistical Manual Of Mental Disorders, 5th ed. Arlington: American Psychiatric Association; 2013.
16. Mulligan C, Bronstein JM. Wilson Disease: An Overview and Approach to Management. Neurol Clin. 2020;38:417-32.
17. Mehta SH, Morgan JC, Sethi KD. Drug-induced movement disorders. Neurol Clin. 2015;33:153-74.
18. Factor SA, Burkhard PR, Caroff S, Friedman JH, Marras C, Tinazzi M, et al. Recent developments in drug-induced movement disorders: A mixed picture. Lancet Neurol. 2019;18:880-90.
19. Burkhard PR. Acute and subacute drug-induced movement disorders. Parkinsonism Relat Disord. 2014;20(Suppl 1):S108-S112.
20. Galli S, Béreau M, Magnin E, Moulin T, Aybek S. Functional movement disorders. Rev Neurol (Paris). 2020;176:244-51.

Psychogenic Gait Disorders

Ambar Chakravarty

INTRODUCTION

Gait is the act and manner of walking. It is a complex motor skill that facilitates locomotion. It requires integration of mechanisms of locomotion with those of balance, motor control, cognition, and musculoskeletal function.[1]

Gait disorders have devastating consequences. Most notorious consequence is fall leading to physical injury. Other consequences are fear of falling, reduced mobility, and thus loss of independence and poor quality of life.[2] In this chapter, discussion will be made regarding potential pitfalls that can happen when analyzing different gait patterns.

Specific gait disorders cannot always be described accurately. Gait disorders can be classified in different ways but a sign-based approach may be more practical for the clinicians for managing patients in everyday practice. As gait disorders are complex and multifactorial caution must be exercised for their proper identification and evaluation so that organic gait disorders are not misinterpreted as functional gait problem and vice versa. During assessment, one must observe the pattern of movement of whole body when the patient walks and turns.[3-5]

The diagnostic features of specific gait syndromes are depicted in **Table 1**.

TABLE 1: Main features of specific gait syndromes.

Type	Main feature	Specific test	Associated symptoms and signs
Spastic gait	Circumduction/scissoring		Pyramidal signs
Cerebellar ataxic gait	Wide based	Not aggravated by eye closure	Cerebellar signs (nystagmus, dysarthria, and hypermetria)
Sensory ataxia gait	Wide based	Aggravated by eye closure	Proprioception loss
Vestibular gait	Deviation to one side	Aggravated by eye closure, Positive unterberger test	Vestibular features (nystagmus, abnormal tilt)
Hypokinetic rigid gait	Slow shuffling gait, hesitation, and freezing	Aggravation by secondary task	Resting tremor, rigidity, and bradykinesia
Dyskinetic gait	Extramovements that affect gait	Can be task specific (dystonic gait)	Features of dystonia, chorea, and myoclonus
Paretic/hypotonic gait	High steppage, waddling	Trendelenburg's sign	Lower motor neuron features
Antalgic gait	Reduced stance phase on affected limb, limping		• Pain • Limited range of movements
Cautious gait	Slow, wide base, and short steps	• Striking improvement with external support • Improvement in gait when performing dual task or when running or walking backward	• Excessive fear of falling • Seek support by objects that are actually quite far away

Continued

Continued

Type	Main feature	Specific test	Associated symptoms and signs
Higher level gait disorders	• Severe balance impairment (falling like a log) • Hesitation and freezing (ignition failure)	• No benefit from external aids or cues • Gait apraxia	• Frequent falls • Frontal release signs • Executive dysfunction

FEATURES SUGGESTIVE OF A PSYCHOGENIC GAIT DISORDER

These include:
- Variability in gait disorder severity over time
- Spontaneous remissions and exacerbations over time
- Lack of falls despite severe gait impairments
- Incongruous with known gait disorders
- Bizarre presentation
- Inconsistent pattern
- Abrupt onset and rapid progression
- Delayed onset of gait impairment after a trauma
- Sudden buckling of the knees
- Incongruous affect (belle indifference)

Care must be taken not to miss organic disorders that present with inconsistencies:
- Buckling gait (the knees giving way) is a common phenotype of a functional gait but can also occur in patients with negative myoclonus of the lower extremities.
- During pull test, patients with functional gait disorder can fall passively completely backward into the arms of the examiner. Patients with Parkinson disease usually take multiple steps to correct the balance but patients with advanced Parkinson disease and atypical parkinsonism can also show complete absence of balance correction during the pull test.[6-9]
- A marked discrepancy between a severely abnormal pull test and a much better or even normal forward push test point toward a functional gait disorder but patients with Parkinson disease can also show such discrepancies.[10]
- Improvement with walking backward can occur in patients with dystonic gait.[11]
- Marked improvement with running can occur in patients with freezing of gait.[12]
- Sometimes gestes antagonists (compensatory motor or sensory tricks to overcome or reduce dystonia) may also be incorrectly considered as an inconsistent gait feature.
- Chorea may also be misinterpreted as functional as also levodopa-induced dyskinesia, which can present with bizarre gait patterns. Stamping gait due to biphasic dyskinesias with dystonic elements can be seen in young men with Parkinson disease. This emphasize that a bizarre gait pattern should not be equated with functional gait disorders.[13]
- Walking pattern in patients with frontal lobe dysfunction can be mistaken for functional gait disorder because of highly variable gait pattern.[14]

A word or two about higher order gait disorders would not be out of place as psychiatrists who tend to see many patients with dementia who very often have gait disorders and history of falls related to unsteadiness. Higher level gait disorders should not be used as a dumping ground for all unclassifiable gait disorders. It is stressed that it indeed is a distinct clinical entity characterized by the presence of one or more core features which would include:[1]
- Gait disorders occurring in close temporal relation to cognitive dysfunction.
- Gait disorders with falls (not with impaired consciousness), not explained by any sensory modality dysfunction or hemodynamic disturbance.
- Severe balance impairment (no rescue reactions with the pull test; falling like a log).
- Inadequate synergies
- Inappropriate or bizarre foot placement
- Crossing of the legs
- leaning into wrong direction when turning
- Variable performance (influenced by environment and emotion)
- Hesitation and freezing (ignition failure)

Elderly people who had had experienced one or more falls due to unsteadiness and/or due to stumbling, poor vision, or simply due to frailty, tend to develop a sense of fear and often adopt extreme cautiousness while walking lest they fall. It is important to recognize this element of extreme caution in the gait pattern of elderly people as the only available would be encouragement and appropriate gait training and balancing exercises.

Human gait is a complex process and it can be involved in different disease process due to involvement of different areas of the neuraxis. Though gait disorders can be classified in different ways but a sign-based approach can be a good starting point for the clinicians in their daily practice. Subsequent examinations and investigations may elucidate the underlying gait disorder in a particular patient. There is considerable overlap of features between organic gait disorders and functional gait problems. Clinicians need to be aware of this major pitfall while assessing gait disorders. A detailed clinical history and a thorough physical examination are the keys to correct assessment and management.

REFERENCES

1. Nutt JG. Higher-level gait disorders: An open frontier. Mov Disord. 2013;28(11):1560-5.
2. Jorstad EC, Hauer K, Becker C, Lamb SE. Measuring the psychological outcomes of falling: a systematic review. J Am Geriatr Soc. 2005;53:501-10.
3. Morris J, Jankovic J. Neurological clinical examination. London: Hodder Arnold; 2012. pp. 1-128.
4. Snijders AH, van de Warrenburg BP, Giladi N, Bloem BR. Neurological gait disorders in elderly people: clinical approach and classification. Lancet Neurol. 2007;6(1):63-74.
5. Baizabal-Carvallo JF, Alonso-Juarez M, Jankovic J. Functional gait disorders, clinical phenomenology, and classification. Neurol Sci. 2019;41:911-5.
6. Giladi N, Shabtai H, Simon ES, Biran S, Tal J, Korcyn A. Construction of freezing of gait questionnaire for patients with Parkinson's disease. Parkinsonism Relat Disord. 2000;6:165-70.
7. Keus SH, Bloem BR, Hendriks EJ, Bredero-Cohen AB, Munneke M; Practice Recommendations Development Group. Evidence-based analysis of physical therapy in Parkinson's disease with recommendations for practice and research. Mov Disord. 2007;22(4):451-60.
8. Nonnekes J, Růžička E, Serranová T, Reich SG, Bloem BR, Hallett M. Functional gait disorders: A sign-based approach. Neurology. 2020;94(24):1093-9.
9. Nonnekes J, Goselink R, Weerdesteyn V, Bloem BR. The retropulsion test: a good evaluation of postural instability in Parkinson's disease? J Parkinsons Dis. 2015;5:43-7.
10. Boogaarts HD, Abdo WF, Bloem BR. "Recumbent gait: relationship to the phenotype of "astasia-abasia?" Mov Disord. 2007;22:2121-2.
11. Albanese A. The clinical expression of primary dystonia. J Neurol. 2003;250:1145-51.
12. Nonnekes J, Ruzicka E, Nieuwboer A, Hallet M, Fasano A, Bloem BR. Compensation strategies for gait impairments in Parkinson disease: a review. JAMA Neurol. 2019;76:718-25.
13. Ruzicka E, Zarubova K, Nutt JG, Bloem BR. "Silly walks" in Parkinson's disease: Unusual presentation of dopaminergic induced dyskinesias. Mov Disord. 2011;26:1782-4.
14. Nonnekes J, Goselink RJM, Ruzicka E, Fasano A, Nutt JG, Bloem BR. Neurological disorders of gait, balance and posture: a sign-based approach. Nat Rev Neurol. 2018;14:183-9.

Astasia–Abasia: Neurologic or Functional?

Ambar Chakravarty

INTRODUCTION

The phenomenon of astasia–abasia is commonly seen. There is inability to stand despite the apparently normal ability to control the legs. While sitting or standing, these patients progressively lean backward (not push as in pusher syndrome) and if standing, may fall like a tree or log of wood. Truncal tone is maintained throughout the fall and consciousness is never lost. Classically, this phenomenon is noted in progressive supranuclear palsy but is often encountered in advanced Parkinson's disease and in vascular lesion in the thalamus and lenticular nucleus and also at times in subjects with widespread subcortical ischemic lesions and occasionally in patients with communicating (normal pressure) hydrocephalus. It is possible that astasia is a form of neglect syndrome (body verticality in relation to space) rather than spatial disorientation as occurs in pusher syndrome.[1-5]

Astasia–abasia is a Greek term that refers to the inability to stand and to walk. First described in 1888 by Paul Blocq, who was an "interne des hôpitaux" at the Salpêtrière. Blocq's original description stressed on the inability to use the lower limbs during standing while their use was normal in the plane of the bed. Though initially considered a pure functional disorder (psychogenic), it has now been considered a higher level balance disorder seen in some extrapyramidal disorders as mentioned earlier and also in both focal and widespread vascular lesions of the brain. Thus cases with astasia–abasia can be divided into psychogenic and nonpsychogenic or organic causes. This differentiation is important for determining management principles and prognosis. The key clinical characteristics of psychogenic astasia-abasia described by Vercueil in 2010 include[5] "sudden onset; history of minor trauma; excessive slowness of movements; hesitations and pauses; uneconomic postures (narrow base of support, "at the edges" imbalance control); appropriate parachute reactions; genuflection without fall; psychogenic "Romberg's sign" (constant falls irrespective of position but avoided by clutching the physician, large amplitude body sway, and improvement of postural balance with distraction); tightrope walker posture (arms in abduction and extension); manifestations suggestive of great effort (grimaces, pain report); and associated psychogenic manifestations (psychogenic stuttering and psychogenic tremor)".

A word about apraxia of balance[1,2] would perhaps not be out of place. This is an occasionally observed phenomenon in patients with multi-infarct state or with widespread leukoaraiotic changes. Nutt, Marsden, and Thompson in 1993, used the term frontal and subcortical disequilibrium syndromes to refer to similar phenomena. However, it would probably be unwise to use anatomical terms in a phenomenological classification. Apraxia of balance is characterized by absence or distortion of normal postural responses. Rolling over and sitting up may be impaired. The patient tries to employ bizarre biomechanically impossible strategies. The patient cannot bring their legs under the chair when trying to get up from a chair and not able to place their weight over the feet making getting up physically impossible. Unusual responses such as crossing the legs when standing or an inability to sit down may be seen. The abnormalities are not stereotyped as occurs in freezing or march a petit pas. Disordered and inappropriate stepping which would fit the description of gait (locomotor) apraxia is present but generally masked by postural imbalance. Hence the term apraxia of balance is preferred over apraxia of gait. In essence, this is axial or truncal apraxia and much different from limb apraxia. The latter generally results from a unilateral brain lesion (commonly nondominant hemisphere) but in apraxia of balance bihemispheric pathologies seem mandatory (e.g., multifocal ischemic lesions). Norman Geschwind in 1985,[4] suggested that limb apraxia may be closely linked to the pyramidal system while axial apraxia may be associated with other systems.

Studies in experimental animals indeed suggested that lateral corticospinal (pyramidal) tracts controlled fine motor movements of the hands and anterior medial descending tracts controlled balance and ability to walk. Patients with apraxia of balance does not show any evidence of apraxia of leg movements. Unawareness about this condition, may lead to a wrong diagnosis of a functional disorder.[6,7]

REFERENCES

1. Nutt JG, Marsden CD, Thompson PD. Human walking and higher level gait disorders, particularly in the elderly. Neurology. 1993;43:268-79.
2. Nutt JG. Higher-order disorders of gait. In: Freund HJ, Jenneord M, Halett M, Leiguarda R (Eds). Higher order motor disorders. Oxford: Oxford University Press; 2005; 237-48.
3. Karnath HQ, Broetz D. Understanding and treating Pusher Syndrome. Phys Ther. 2003;88:1119-25.
4. Geschwind N, Damasio AR. Apraxia. In: AM Freedericks, (Ed.) Clinical Neuropsychology Vol.1 Amsterdam. Elsevier. 1985:423-32.
5. Vercueil L. Astasie-abasie: causes psychogène et nonpsychogènes. Revue Neurologique. 2010;166:221-8.
6. Okun MS, Koehler PJ. Paul Blocq and (psychogenic) astasia abasia. Mov Disord. 2007;22(10):1373-8.
7. Edwards MJ, Bhatia KP. Functional (psychogenic) movement disorders: merging mind and brain. Lancet Neurol. 2012;11(3): 250-60.

Diagnosis of Vascular Parkinsonism

Ambar Chakravarty

INTRODUCTION

Vascular parkinsonism (VP) can be defined as a clinical syndrome of a parkinsonian disorder associated with or temporally related to chronic ischemic cerebrovascular disease. "VP of insidious onset" is suggested by the presence of (1) parkinsonism; (2) relevant cerebrovascular disease by brain imaging; and (3) insidious onset with extensive subcortical/periventricular white matter lesions (leukoaraiosis), bilateral relatively symmetrical features at onset, generally absence of tremor and the presence of early short stepping gait (marche à petits pas) or early cognitive decline. The distinguishing features of this common form from the "acute or delayed progressive onset form" include clinical asymmetric signs, sites of lesion, and stroke onset.[1] Tremor is not a prominent feature in either of these two forms. In recent time, a third subgroup of VP has been identified as "mixed neurodegenerative parkinsonism and cerebrovascular disease". This term is used when a diagnostic overlap with neurodegenerative Parkinson's disease (PD) is suspected.[2] Such cases would have prominent asymmetric features including tremor. Such a diagnosis would be made when classical asymmetric PD phenotype would be associated with prominent features of ischemic cerebrovascular disease in their magnetic resonance imaging (MRI) scans.

The clinical heterogeneity in VP patients, as mentioned above, leads to a significant diagnostic overlap with idiopathic PD and other atypical or secondary parkinsonian disorders, including progressive supranuclear palsy (PSP) and idiopathic normal pressure hydrocephalus (iNPH).[3-5] Until now, there are, however, few instrumental biomarkers, imaging, or neurophysiological, supporting information which may help physicians in achieving diagnostic accuracy when VP is suspected.

VASCULAR PARKINSONISM VERSUS PARKINSON'S DISEASE

This is of utmost importance and the first step when evaluating patients with a possible diagnosis of VP. Barring clinical overlaps, the features favoring the latter diagnosis would be the presence of a pronounced lower-body involvement with postural instability and falls, a more frequent symmetric and akinetic-rigid presentation, additional features including corticospinal and pseudobulbar signs, urinary incontinence, and cognitive decline compared to PD patients.[6] About a third of patients with VP may report response to L-dopa treatment at times reporting long-term motor fluctuations possibly due to cerebral ischemic lesions in close proximity to nigrostriatal pathway. Hence, the diagnosis of idiopathic PD may get complicated, as the presence of a sustained L-dopa response as well as the detection of L-dopa-induced motor fluctuations and dyskinesia are considered to be hallmark features for the diagnosis of idiopathic PD.[7] The L-dopa short-term test looking for dyskinesias may give additional information for distinguishing VP from idiopathic PD,[8,9] since side effects have been recorded much more frequently among patients with atypical parkinsonian disorders compared with PD.[10] However, this happens to be a relative finding. By and large, information on pharmacological response in VP may be crucial for attaining diagnostic accuracy.[11] Lastly there may be subtle changes in the gait pattern between patients with VP and those with PD. The "shuffling gait" of the latter may not exactly be the same as the "short steppage' gait (marche à petits pas) of the former. "Heel grazing" may be an early feature in subjects prone to develop VP at a later date, while forefoot grazing may be an early indicator of a classical shuffling gait.

Dopamine transporter single-photon emission computed tomography (DAT-SPECT) study in VP may reveal abnormal striatal presynaptic dopamine transporter binding in almost 70% of patients.[12] A common symmetrical basal ganglia uptake reduction[13] may simulate the picture obtained in many idiopathic PD patients although asymmetrical uptake is typical of idiopathic PD. A quantitative approach using SPECT with [123I]FP-CIT based on ligand uptake in specific regions of interest has been used to compute a Striatal Asymmetry Index (SAI), which demonstrated to differentiate more specifically VP from PD.[14,15]

Hyposmia, rapid eye movement (REM) Sleep Behavior Disorder (RBD), slow colonic transit time as well as cardiac reduction in metaiodobenzylguanidine (MBT) cardiac uptake using SPECT imaging are classically associated with PD. These have not yet been adequately studied in patients with VP.[16]

VASCULAR PARKINSONISM VERSUS PROGRESSIVE SUPRANUCLEAR PALSY

Vascular parkinsonism patients may exhibit similar clinical cardinal features with PSP patients with dominant parkinsonian features (PSP-P), which may include marked postural instability (demonstrated by the pull test) and history of falls[6]—generally retropulsive. In VP patients, ischemic lesions in unilateral mesencephalic reticular formation or bilateral thalamic lesions have been proposed as the anatomical basis of vertical nuclear ophthalmoplegia much alike the classic vertical supranuclear ophthalmoplegia of PSP.[17] There are no definite clinical feature which can with certainty differentiate between PSP-P and VP.[18] In fact, within the first 2 years of disease, less than one-third of pathologically proven PSP patients could exhibit supranuclear gaze palsy and only approximately half of them would have falls—posing problems for early differentiation.[19,20] To complicate matters farther, in some PSP cases, supranuclear gaze palsy may be only observed in the later stages of the disease.[21] Some VP patients may present with freezing of gait as major clinical feature at the disease onset, and in this situation differentiation from the PSP-form which present with pure akinesia and gait freezing[22] would be needed. Morphometric analysis of selected brain structures (midbrain and superior cerebellar peduncle, pons, and middle cerebellar peduncle) using conventional MRI, specifically, when combined to compute a Magnetic Resonance Parkinsonism Index (MRPI), may be a reliable tool to differentiate PSP from PD and other atypical parkinsonian disorders including VP.[23-26]

VASCULAR PARKINSONISM VERSUS IDIOPATHIC NORMAL PRESSURE HYDROCEPHALUS

In VP patients, in addition to ischemic cerebrovascular lesions, neuroimaging may highlight ventricular enlargement[6] possibly attributable to a "central" cerebral atrophy. This radiological feature closely mimics that of iNPH. iNPH is clinically characterized by gait disturbance, cognitive impairment, and urinary incontinence, but parkinsonian features could also be common, making differentiating between VP and iNPH particularly challenging.[27] Diagnosis of iNPH is traditionally made on radiological evidence of enlarged cerebral ventricles with normal cerebrospinal fluid (CSF) pressure with no evidence of obstruction to the CSF flow from lateral to the fourth ventricle which may also be dilated **(Flowchart 1)**.

Improvement after ventricular shunting in iNPH remains still variable and thus not definitive in the differential diagnosis with VP. Successful outcome of shunting cannot always be accurately predicted but generally depend on age, response to external lumbar

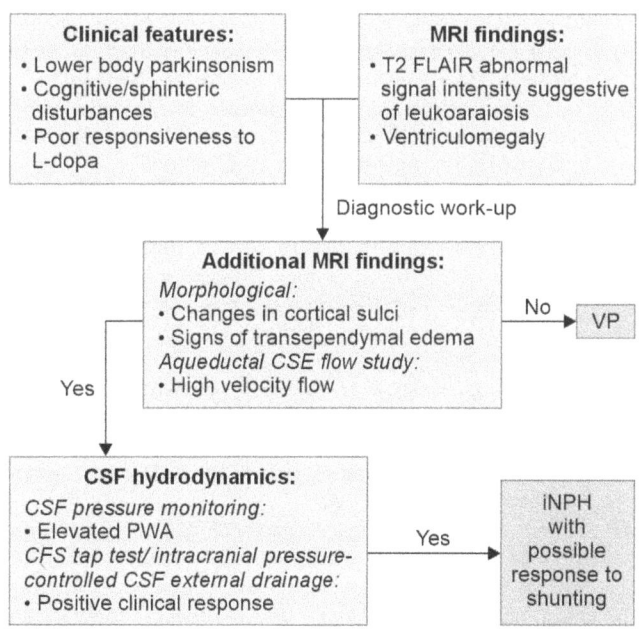

FLOWCHART 1: Differential diagnosis of VP. Diagnostic approach to a case of suspected iNPH.

(CSF: cerebrospinal fluid; iNPH: normal pressure hydrocephalus; MRI: magnetic resonance imaging; PWA: pulse wave amplitude; VP: vascular parkinsonism)

Source: Adapted with modification from: Mostile G, Nicoletti A, Zappia M. Vascular Parkinsonism: Still Looking for a Diagnosis. Front Neurol. 2018;9:411.

drainage (draining 20–30 mL of CSF by lumbar route) or tap test and CSF flow monitoring.[28] A high stroke volume across the aqueduct on MR CSF flow study generally suggests presence of NPH. The fact that even some patients with clinical and radiological features of VP could also improve after a 3-day external lumbar drainage procedure,[29] would make the issue more complicated. It is possible that VP and iNPH may be considered to be parts of a spectrum disorder which might include some cases of Alzheimer's disease (AD) as well.

CONCLUDING REMARKS

In view of the diagnostic overlaps encountered between VP and PD, VP and PSP and lastly VP and iNPH, it has been proposed recently to use, instead of the term "VP," clinical descriptors including "pseudo VP" (neurodegenerative parkinsonism with nonspecific neuroimaging signal abnormalities), "vascular pseudoparkinsonism" (e.g., akinetic mutism due to bilateral mesial frontal strokes or apathetic depression from bilateral striatal lacunar strokes), or "pseudovascular pseudoparkinsonism" (e.g., higher-level gait disorders, including iNPH).[30]

As mentioned earlier in this Commentary, there is a need for studies looking at biological biomarkers, in order to define an integrated clinical diagnosis by laboratory/technical supports. The three different diagnostic subgroups ("acute/subacute VP," "insidious VP," and "mixed neurodegenerative parkinsonism and cerebrovascular disease") concept of VP, mentioned earlier in this Commentary, has been formulated by an expert Panel in 2017 incorporating qualitative supporting information by conventional MRI and SPECT studies.[2] A prospective validation of the proposed diagnostic approach would be needed soon enough.

REFERENCES

1. Zijlmans JC, Daniel SE, Hughes AJ, Révész T, Lees AJ. Clinicopathological investigation of vascular parkinsonism, including clinical criteria for diagnosis. Mov Disord. 2004;19:630-40.
2. Rektor I, Bohnen NI, Korczyn AD, Gryb V, Kumar H, Kramberger MG, et al. An updated diagnostic approach to subtype definition of vascular parkinsonism–Recommendations from an expert working group. Parkinsonism Relat Disord. 2017;49:9-16.
3. Eide PK. Intracranial pressure parameters in idiopathic normal pressure hydrocephalus patients treated with ventriculo-peritoneal shunts. Acta Neurochir. 2006;148:21-9.
4. Giliberto C, Mostile G, Lo Fermo S, Reggio E, Sciacca G, Nicoletti A, et al. Vascular parkinsonism or idiopathic NPH? New insights from CSF pressure analysis. Neurol Sci. 2017;38:2209-12.
5. Zacharzewska-Gondek A, Gondek T, Sasiadek M, Bladowska J. Normal pressure hydrocephalus as a possible reversible cause of dementia, neuroimaging findings. Eur Psychiatry. 2017;41:S629-30.
6. Winikates J, Jankovic J. Clinical correlates of vascular parkinsonism. Arch Neurol. 1999;56:98-102.
7. Postuma RB, Berg D, Stern M, Poewe W, Olanow CW, Oertel W, et al. MDS clinical diagnostic criteria for Parkinson's disease. Mov Disord. 2015;30:1591-601.
8. Zijlmans JC, Katzenschlager R, Daniel SE, Lees AJ. The L-dopa response in vascular parkinsonism. J Neurol Neurosurg Psychiatry. 2004;75:545-7.
9. Ondo WG, Hunter C, Ferrara JM, Mostile G. Apomorphine injections: predictors of initial common adverse events and long term tolerability. Parkinsonism Relat Disord. 2012;18:619-22.
10. Vasta R, Nicoletti A, Mostile G, Dibilio V, Sciacca G, Contrafatto D, et al. Side effects induced by the acute levodopa challenge in Parkinson's Disease and atypical parkinsonisms. PLoS One. 2017;12:e0172145.
11. Miguel-Puga A, Villafuerte G, Salas-Pacheco J, Arias-Carrión O. Therapeutic interventions for vascular parkinsonism: a systematic review and metaanalysis. Front Neurol. 2017;8:481.
12. Antonini A, Vitale C, Barone P, Cilia R, Righini A, Bonuccelli U, et al. The relationship between cerebral vascular disease and parkinsonism: the VADO study. Parkinsonism Relat Disord. 2012;18:775-80.
13. Zijlmans J, Evans A, Fontes F, Katzenschlager R, Gacinovic S, Lees AJ, et al. [123I] FP-CIT SPECT study in vascular parkinsonism and Parkinson's disease. Mov Disord. 2007;22:1278-85.
14. Contrafatto D, Mostile G, Nicoletti A, Dibilio V, Raciti L, Lanzafame S, et al. [(123) I]FP-CIT-SPECT asymmetry index to differentiate Parkinson's disease from vascular parkinsonism. Acta Neurol Scand. 2012;126:12-6.
15. Contrafatto D, Mostile G, Nicoletti A, Raciti L, Luca A, Dibilio V, et al. Single photon emission computed tomography striatal asymmetry index may predict dopaminergic responsiveness in Parkinson disease. Clin Neuropharmacol. 2011;34:71-3.
16. Caproni S, Colosimo C. Movement disorders and cerebrovascular diseases: from pathophysiology to treatment. Expert Rev Neurother. 2017;17:509-19.
17. Josephs KA, Ishizawa T, Tsuboi Y, Cookson N, Dickson DW. A clinicopathological study of vascular progressive supranuclear palsy: a multiinfarct disorder presenting as progressive supranuclear palsy. Arch Neurol. 2002;59:1597-601.
18. Williams DR, Lees AJ. What features improve the accuracy of the clinical diagnosis of progressive supranuclear palsy-parkinsonism (PSP-P)? Mov Disord. 2010;25:357-62.
19. Respondek G, Höglinger GU. The phenotypic spectrum of progressive supranuclear palsy. Parkinsonism Relat Disord. 2016;22 (Suppl. 1):S34-6.
20. Dubinsky RM, Jankovic J. Progressive supranuclear palsy and a multi-infarct state. Neurology. 1987;37:570-6.
21. Williams DR, de Silva R, Paviour DC, Pittman A, Watt HC, Kilford L, et al. Characteristics of two distinct clinical phenotypes in pathologically proven progressive supranuclear palsy: Richardson's syndrome and PSP-parkinsonism. Brain. 2005;128:1247-58.

22. Williams DR, Holton JL, Strand K, Revesz T, Lees AJ. Pure akinesia with gait freezing: a third clinical phenotype of progressive supranuclear palsy. Mov Disord. 2007;22:2235-41.
23. Nicoletti G, Fera F, Condino F, Auteri W, Gallo O, Pugliese P, et al. MR imaging of middle cerebellar peduncle width: differentiation of multiple system atrophy from Parkinson disease. Radiology. 2006;239:825-30.
24. Quattrone A, Nicoletti G, Messina D, Fera F, Condino F, Pugliese P, et al. MR imaging index for differentiation of progressive supranuclear palsy from Parkinson disease and the Parkinson variant of multiple system atrophy. Radiology. 2008;246:214-21.
25. Morelli M, Arabia G, Salsone M, Novellino F, Giofrè L, Paletta R, et al. Accuracy of magnetic resonance parkinsonism index for differentiation of progressive supranuclear palsy from probable or possible Parkinson disease. Mov Disord. 2011;26:527-33.
26. Mostile G, Nicoletti A, Cicero CE, Cavallaro T, Bruno E, Dibilio V, et al. Magnetic resonance parkinsonism index in progressive supranuclear palsy and vascular parkinsonism. Neurol Sci. 2016;37:591-5.
27. Gallia GL, Rigamonti D, Williams MA. The diagnosis and treatment of idiopathic normal pressure hydrocephalus. Nat Clin Pract Neurol. 2006;2:375-81.
28. Halperin JJ, Kurlan R, Schwalb JM, Cusimano MD, Gronseth G, Gloss D. Practice guideline: idiopathic normal pressure hydrocephalus: response to shunting and predictors of response: report of the Guideline Development, Dissemination, and Implementation Subcommittee of the American Academy of Neurology. Neurology. 2015;85:2063-71.
29. Espay AJ, Narayan RK, Duker AP, Barrett ET Jr, de Courten-Myers G. Lower body parkinsonism: reconsidering the threshold for external lumbar drainage. Nat Clin Pract Neurol. 2008;4:50-5.
30. Vizcarra JA, Lang AE, Sethi KD, Espay AJ. Vascular Parkinsonism: deconstructing a syndrome. Mov Disord. 2015;30:886-94.

Alcohol and Movement Disorders

Ambar Chakravarty

CASE VIGNETTE

A 68-year-old ex-army personnel consulted the author of the preceding chapter for a few months' onset tremor of both hands which had been causing problems with his holding the teacup and in writing bank cheques. He was subsequently seen by the present Editor as well. He was found to have a 10 Hz postural and action tremor in both hands. No other body parts were involved and there was no rest tremor. His gait and other movements were normal. Family history was negative. He had no addictions but during his career in the armed forces he had tasted alcohol on some occasions. A clinical diagnosis of essential tremor (ET) was made. But before starting him on any treatment, we decided to do an alcohol challenge test. He was asked to drink a pint of beer and closely observe for any change in his tremor in the hands. He reported his experience 1 week later. In his own words (in Hindi of course)" I felt a dramatic change...all my tremors were gone...I stood up and threw my hands toward the sky...and shouted " Jai Bajrangbali".

COMMENT

This rather dramatic effect of alcohol on ET can be used as a diagnostic test in doubtful cases and is often used by patients (specially doctors—mostly surgeons) to suppress the tremors before any public interactions (in case of surgeons before entering the operation theater) and many people ultimately get addicted to alcohol. The present Editor is aware of a surgeon who ultimately succumbed to liver cirrhosis.

The alcohol responsive hyperkinetic movement disorders include[1-3] ET, isolated vocal tremor (VT), primary writing tremor (PWT), orthostatic tremor (OT), tremor in Kennedy's disease (X-linked spinal bulbar muscular atrophy), myoclonus-dystonia linked to epsilon sarcoglycan mutation (SCGE-MD), posthypoxic myoclonus (Lance–Adams syndrome, PHM), progressive myoclonic epilepsy type 1 (EPM1), adult sialidosis type I, torticollis abductor spasmodic dysphonia (ABSD), adductor spasmodic dysphonia (ADSD), ADSD in DYT-4 Dopa-responsive dystonia (DYT-5, DRD), and generalized dystonia. The exact mechanism of alcohol responsiveness is not known. It had been hypothesized that modest dosage of alcohol possess a specific and novel ability to normalize pathologic hypermetabolism of the cerebellar Purkinje cells and deep cerebellar nuclei. It had further been proposed that Purkinje cell dysfunction (either aberrant activation or abnormal synchronous firing) is the unifying feature linking these varied hyperkinetic disorders.

It is equally important to examine the other side of the coin as well, namely the adverse effects of alcohol on basal ganglionic functions. Three major clinical scenarios may occur[1-3]—withdrawal tremulous states, cerebellar system dysfunction, and hepatic-related disorders. The tremor of alcohol withdrawal resembles that of physiologic tremor which is exacerbated by anxiety. It is the most common neurologic manifestation of alcohol withdrawal, and the tremor is most discernable some 10–20 hours after cessation of drinking. Alcoholic tremor is mostly postural. The tremor is characterized by large amplitude with frequencies varying from 6 to 11 Hz. It may persist for weeks after discontinuation of alcohol consumption, though with decreased amplitude. Two types of postural tremors can be differentiated in alcoholics. The first has a frequency > 8 Hz and an alternating EMG pattern in antagonistic muscles. The other is associated with a frequency < 8 Hz and with synchronous discrete bursts of EMG activity simultaneously in antagonistic muscles. Both of these EMG patterns can be seen in patients with ET, causing diagnostic confusion. A tremulous state, which may be transient or persistent, also occurs in infants born to alcoholic mothers. The common hepatic encephalopathy may be accompanied by a

TABLE 1: Extrapyramidal dysfunction and alcoholism.

Withdrawal tremulous states	Cerebellar dysfunctions and other movement disorders	Hepatic-related dysfunction
Common alcohol withdrawal tremor	• Acute alcohol intoxications (ataxia) • *Others*: Postural tremor, Parkinsonian tremor, chorea/orolingual dyskinesias, and akathisia	*Acute*: Tremor, asterixis, and tone abnormalities
Tremor with delirium tremens	Alcoholic cerebellar degeneration—associated with cerebellar ataxia, 3-Hz leg tremor and parkinsonian tremor	*Chronic*: Choreoathetosis; dystonia, cerebellar dysfunction; tremors (may be parkinsonian); myoclonus, and gait abnormalities
Fetal alcohol withdrawal syndrome	Acute or chronic ataxia with Wernicke–Korsakoff syndrome	

flapping tremor (in essence a negative myoclonus or asterixis) and multiple other tremors and jerky movements (choreiform or myoclonic). Chronic portosystemic encephalopathy (associated with acquired hepatocerebral degeneration) is accompanied by choreoathetoid movements and persistent coarse tremor. Distinction needs to be made from Wilson disease as both may produce similar MRI features. Asterixis, is a disorder of motor control, characterized by brief irregular lapses of posture ("negative myoclonus"). Asterixis results from an episodic dysfunction within neural circuits that are normally concerned with maintenance of sustained muscle contraction. These circuits may be vulnerable to generalized neurometabolic changes associated with various disorders including cardiac, respiratory, or renal failure, chronic hemodialysis, polycythemia, and sepsis-associated encephalopathy. It be provoked by various anticonvulsant drugs, toxic doses of salicylates and levodopa, and local lesions in the CNS, particularly in the thalamus, parietal lobe, medial frontal cortex, internal capsule, or rostral midbrain. Extrapyramidal dysfunctions recorded with alcoholism are shown in **Table 1**.

REFERENCES

1. Neiman J, Lang AE, Fornazzari L, Carlen PL. Movement disorders in alcoholism: A review. Neurology. 1990;40:741-6.
2. Weir RL. Extrapyramidal dysfunctioi in alcoholism. J Nat Med Assoc. 1980;72(2):121-6.
3. Frucht SJ, Riboldi GM. Alcohol-responsive hyperkinetic movement disorders—a Mechanistic Hypothesis. Tremor Other Hyperkinet Mov. 2020;10(1):47:1-14.

CHAPTER 16

Neuropsychiatric Manifestations of Parkinson's Disease

Ambar Chakravarty

■ INTRODUCTION

James Parkinson's initial description of what would later be known as Parkinson's disease (PD) did not include any mention of neuropsychiatric features or cognitive impairments in his illustrative cases.[1] However, in the past five decades, the introduction of PD medications, such as levodopa, advancements in clinical practices, increased patient lifespan, and extensive research have shed light on the prevalence and impact of neuropsychiatric symptoms (NPSs) and nonmotor symptoms in PD patients.[2] These complications, including cognitive impairments, have been recognized as common, debilitating, associated with poor long-term outcomes, caregiver burden, and necessitating specialized management.[3]

■ NEUROPSYCHIATRIC MANIFESTATIONS

Neuropsychiatric disturbances encompass a range of conditions such as mood and anxiety disorders, fatigue, apathy, psychosis, cognitive impairments, sleep disorders, and addictive behaviors. These disturbances can arise as part of the PD pathophysiology itself or as a result of complex interactions between the disease progression, emotional responses to parkinsonism, and treatment-related side effects. They are prevalent among PD patients, with >60% experiencing one or more psychiatric symptoms during the course of their illness.[2] These symptoms significantly contribute to disability and pose considerable challenges in the management of advanced PD.[3]

This chapter aims to provide a comprehensive overview of the primary care approach to recognizing, managing, and preventing neuropsychiatric disorders associated with PD.[4,5]

Mood Disorders in Parkinson's Disease: Recognition and Management

Mood disorders, including depression, are frequently reported by individuals with PD, but they are often underrecognized. The estimated prevalence of depression in PD is approximately 40–45% in both men and women.[2] Depression can manifest at any stage of PD, and the symptoms resemble those experienced by the general population (**Box 1**).[6] However, diagnosing depression in PD patients can be challenging due to overlapping clinical features of the two conditions.

Common symptoms of depression in PD include psychomotor slowing, difficulties with concentration and sleep, reduced appetite, diminished sexual desire, and social withdrawal. Compared to individuals with depression alone, PD patients with depression tend to experience more anxiety, brooding, irritability, cognitive deficits, pessimism, and suicidal ideation (without suicidal behavior).[7] Certain depressive symptoms that favor the diagnosis in PD include early morning awakening, diurnal variation in mood over a period of >2 weeks, and pessimistic thoughts about oneself, the world, and the future.[8]

Third party interviews can provide valuable insights into the emotional state of PD patients when diagnostic uncertainty exists. While the diagnosis of depression is primarily clinical, tools such as the Beck Depression Inventory-I (a self-administered questionnaire) or the Hamilton Depression Rating Scale can be considered for screening and assessing symptom severity.[9,10]

The cause of depressive disorders in PD is believed to involve complex interactions of neurotransmitter abnormalities, mainly affecting dopamine, serotonin, and

> **BOX 1: Diagnostic criteria of depressive disorder.**
>
> - Depression is defined as a pervasive pattern of depressed mood and/or loss of interest or pleasure causing clinically significant distress or impairment in social, occupational, or other important areas of functioning
> - Depressive disorder is diagnosed if the patient has five or more of the following symptoms during the same 2-week period and they represent a change from previous functioning (and at least one of the symptoms is either depressed mood, or loss of interest or pleasure):
>   - Affective symptoms:
>   - Depressed mood: Persistent sad, anxious, or "empty" mood
>   - Markedly diminished interest or loss of pleasure in hobbies and activities that were once enjoyed, including sex
>   - Feelings of hopelessness and pessimism
>   - Feelings of worthlessness or excessive or inappropriate guilt (which may be delusional)
>   - Anxiety
>   - Recurrent thoughts of death (not just fear of dying), recurrent suicidal ideation without a specific plan, or a suicide attempt or a specific plan for committing suicide
>   - Psychomotor symptoms:
>   - Psychomotor agitation (morbid increase in action or movement) or retardation (morbid slowing of action or movement)
>   - Apathy
>   - Restlessness and irritability
>   - Cognitive symptoms:
>   - Diminished ability to think, concentrate, or remember
>   - Difficulty in making decisions and indecisiveness
>   - Physical symptoms:
>   - Decreased energy, fatigue, and being "slowed down"
>   - Insomnia, early morning awakening, or oversleeping
>   - Loss of appetite or weight loss, or overeating and weight gain
>   - Persistent physical symptoms (e.g., headaches, digestive disorders, and chronic pain) that do not respond to treatment

> **BOX 2: Management of psychosis in Parkinson's disease.**
>
> - Psychosocial support for patients and caregivers
> - Elimination of triggering factors:
>   - Infection (pneumonia, urinary tract infection, and phlebitis)
>   - Metabolic and electrolyte disturbances
>   - Depression
>   - Sleep disorders
>   - Hearing and vision defects
> - Simplification of complicated medication regimens:
>   - Lower doses of or discontinue nonessential medications [mainly drugs with anticholinergic or sedative properties (e.g., anxiolytics, anticholinergics, mirtazapine, and tricyclic antidepressants)]
> - Reduction or discontinuation of nonessential antiparkinsonian drugs (with monitoring of motor functions) in the following order:
>   - Anticholinergic
>   - Selegiline
>   - Amantadine
>   - Dopamine agonist
>   - Catechol-O-methyltransferase (COMT) inhibitor
>   - Standard levodopa
> - Addition of antipsychotic medication if psychosis is persistent and problematic
>   - Quetiapine (first line)
>   - Clozapine (with close monitoring of blood count)
> - Addition of cholinesterase inhibitor before antipsychotic drug (if the psychosis occurs in a patient with cognitive impairment or dementia and there is no risk of injury to the patient or others)

norepinephrine. Genetic factors, such as allelic variations in serotonin transporters, have also been suggested to contribute to mood disorders.[11] Additionally, reactive depression may occur at the time of PD diagnosis when patients learn that available treatments are not curative.

Optimizing dopaminergic therapy to improve motor symptoms is an essential initial step in managing depression in PD **(Box 2)**. Medications commonly used to treat PD, such as levodopa, dopamine agonists, and selegiline, are believed to have mild antidepressant effects.[12] Psychosocial support, counseling, and psychotherapy can also be beneficial, although further research is needed in this area.[13] Individualized psychosocial counseling and structured physical therapy can help patients identify and address their problems and develop effective coping strategies.

When initiating antidepressant therapy, factors such as clinical presentation, the risk of symptom deterioration without treatment, and the patient's preferences should be considered. Selective serotonin reuptake inhibitors (SSRIs), tricyclic antidepressants (TCAs), and serotonin-norepinephrine reuptake inhibitors (SNRIs) are commonly used to treat depression in PD patients.[14] SSRIs are typically the first-line treatment[15] due to their favorable risk profile, despite some reports of potential exacerbation of parkinsonian symptoms.[16] TCAs can be useful,[3] but their tolerability issues often lead to discontinuation. SNRIs have shown promise in treating depression in PD, but further clinical trials are needed to determine their efficacy.

The choice of antidepressant should be based on the drug's pharmacological profile, the patient's comorbidities, medication history, and specific symptomatology. For example, patients with anergic depression may benefit from a nonsedating or low-sedating antidepressant, while those with sleep disturbances might respond better to fluvoxamine, mirtazapine, or a TCA. In cases of prominent anxiety symptoms, paroxetine, sertraline, or venlafaxine should be considered as first-line options.

Antidepressant dosages should be initiated at low levels and gradually increased while closely monitoring vital signs, depression symptoms, compliance, side effects, and potential drug interactions. Regular follow-up visits are essential until the neuropsychiatric condition stabilizes. Factors that increase the risk of side effects include advanced age, high medication doses, multiple drugs for the same disease, and long duration of treatment. SSRI to be used cautiously in patients taking selegiline to avoid serotonin syndrome.[17]

Electroconvulsive therapy (ECT) has proven to be an effective treatment for alleviating depressive symptoms and has shown temporary improvement in motor function.[18] As a result, individuals diagnosed with PD who experience severe depression and do not respond to traditional antidepressant treatments may be suitable candidates for ECT. Additionally, repetitive transcranial magnetic stimulation (rTMS), a less invasive alternative, has demonstrated promising results.[19] However, further research is required to establish its efficacy fully.

FATIGUE AND APATHY

Difficulties in diagnosing depression arise not only from differentiating it from parkinsonism, but also from distinguishing it from apathy and fatigue syndromes. The underlying causes of apathy and fatigue are still not well understood. In contrast to the apathy observed in depression, apathy in nondepressed patients with PD is characterized by a specific lack of motivation, without experiencing anhedonia, hopelessness, or low mood. Approximately 12–16% of PD patients report experiencing apathy.[2] Fatigue is a subjective sensation characterized by an overwhelming sense of tiredness, lack of energy, or exhaustion at any given time. It has been reported by 42% of patients with PD.[20] Both apathy and fatigue significantly impact patients' quality of life.

Managing apathy and fatigue poses challenges due to limited evidence-based guidelines. However, clinical practice has shown that educating patients and caregivers about apathy and fatigue can help differentiate these symptoms from depression and laziness. Employing energy-saving principles, coaching, prompting, and maintaining good sleep hygiene can aid in performing daily activities and reduce executive dysfunctions and fatigue. Additionally, optimizing the control of PD may alleviate apathy and fatigue. While dopamine agonists or methylphenidate have been suggested as treatment options, their clinical benefits are often underwhelming or limited by side effects. In most cases, antidepressants do not significantly alleviate symptoms of apathy or fatigue and may cause unnecessary side effects.[21]

ANXIETY

Anxiety disorders are prevalent in patients with PD, affecting up to 40% of individuals. This includes various forms of anxiety such as panic disorder, generalized anxiety disorder, and phobic disorders. The incidence of anxiety disorders in PD is higher than that observed in the general population and in groups with similar physical disabilities, such as multiple sclerosis.[5,22] Somatic symptoms associated with anxiety in PD patients may include breathlessness, sweating, chest discomfort, gastralgia, restlessness, and dizziness. Additionally, patients may experience fear of institutionalization, going insane, or dying. The exact cause of anxiety disorders in PD remains unknown. It is possible that anxiety may arise as a psychological reaction to the symptoms of PD, or it may be associated with neurochemical degenerative changes that occur in the disease, resulting in progressive reductions in dopamine, serotonin, and norepinephrine levels. Severe anxiety can be observed in conjunction with the "off" phenomenon experienced by patients with motor fluctuations in the advanced stages of PD. It is worth noting that anxiety symptoms can manifest before the appearance of any motor symptoms and may serve as an early indication or risk factor for PD.[23]

Given the frequent coexistence of anxiety and depressive symptoms, a diagnosis of anxiety in PD patients should prompt a screening for depression.

Management

The optimal first-line pharmacologic treatment for anxiety in patients with PD remains unclear. Generally, the management of anxiety in these patients follows similar principles as treating anxiety in individuals without the disease. However, when a correlation exists with the "off" period, the primary focus should be on minimizing the "off" state before considering the use of psychotropic medications. It is important to educate patients about the nature of the "off" state and provide reassurance that even prolonged periods of being "off" will eventually improve. Offering psychological support, education, and counseling to promote effective coping strategies contributes to the overall well-being of the patient.

In some cases, short-term therapy with benzodiazepines or buspirone may be beneficial. Benzodiazepines with a short half-life, such as alprazolam, lorazepam, or oxazepam, are commonly prescribed. However, caution should be exercised due to the elderly population of most PD patients, as these medications may cause side effects such as oversedation, an increased risk of falls, and cognitive impairment, which may outweigh the anxiolytic benefits. Therefore, benzodiazepines should be used cautiously and for limited durations. Long-acting benzodiazepine formulations should be avoided. Buspirone, at low doses (10–40 mg/day), has been found to be well-tolerated, but higher daily doses may worsen parkinsonism.[24] Alternatively, SSRIs or venlafaxine may be effective in treating anxiety. However, many specialists prefer prescribing these agents only when depression is also present.

MOOD FLUCTUATION AND BIPOLAR DISORDER

Mood fluctuations, characterized by significant mood changes ranging from depression to hypomania occurring multiple times within a day, have been reported in approximately 7–21% of patients with PD.[25] These mood fluctuations often coincide with motor fluctuations, with patients experiencing low mood, often a mixed depressive-anxious state, during the "off" period and normal or elevated mood, including euphoria and hypomania, during the "on" phase. However, it is also possible for mood fluctuations to occur independently of evident motor fluctuations in certain patients.[25]

Bipolar disorder is considered rare in PD. Instances of manic symptoms developing during the "on" phase have been described, often associated with anticholinergic therapy or as a side effect of pallidotomy or deep brain stimulation (DBS).

The management of mood fluctuations and bipolar disorder in PD involves adjusting dopaminergic medications to minimize evident "on-off" fluctuations as a potential initial step. Since no specific treatment trials for these conditions have been conducted in PD, treatment is tailored to the individual patient's needs. It is advisable to seek a psychiatric consultation to guide the treatment approach. The use of anxiolytics and antipsychotics, such as quetiapine or clozapine, may be beneficial, depending on the individual's requirements and tolerability.

PSYCHOSIS

Psychosis is observed in approximately 20–40% of patients with PD.[26] Patients may experience various perceptual disorders, including a sense of presence, illusions, or hallucinations (visual, auditory, and tactile).[27] Visual hallucinations are more common in the evening and tend to be complex, often involving the perception of people and animals in motion (sideways passage). Initially, patients may retain insight that these hallucinations are not real, but over time, they may begin to act as if they are. Paranoid delusions, particularly pathologic jealousy (e.g., unfounded suspicions of a spouse having sexual encounters with another person), can also develop and significantly impact the patient's well-being and quality of life (**Box 2**).

Several hypotheses regarding the pathophysiology of psychosis in PD are currently being investigated. Notable risk factors that have been identified include advanced age, prolonged disease duration and severity, cognitive impairment, depression, and sleep disorders. Some studies have also explored the potential contribution of visual retinal and cortical sensory dysfunction.[27,28] The long-standing "continuum hypothesis" for drug-induced psychosis associated with antiparkinsonian medications (particularly dopaminergic and anticholinergic agents) is currently under review. According to this hypothesis, drug-induced sleep disruption leads to vivid dreams, which can eventually progress to hallucinations and delirium. However, it is worth noting that psychosis does not develop in all patients taking these medications.[26,29]

Management

Managing psychosis in PD is a challenging task due to the complexities involved. The optimization of motor function with higher doses of dopaminergic drugs can often lead to the development of psychosis, while antipsychotic medications can worsen motor symptoms. The approach to management varies depending on the severity and impact of the psychosis.[30]

When hallucinations arise without causing significant distress and insight is preserved, providing support and counseling may be sufficient. However, if the hallucinations or delusions are distressing, insight is lost, and there is a risk of harm to oneself or others, more robust interventions are necessary.

The severity of psychosis can be reduced through an effective treatment approach. Initially, any reversible causes should be identified and addressed, similar to managing delirium. This may involve lowering or discontinuing nonessential medications and simplifying the antiparkinsonian drug regimen. If simplifying the regimen leads to unacceptable motor function decline despite persistent psychosis, a second-line approach involving antipsychotic drug therapy can be considered.[31]

It is important to exercise caution when using antipsychotic agents in patients with PD due to the risk of severe antipsychotic sensitivity reactions, which can significantly reduce survival. Typical antipsychotic agents should be avoided as they worsen motor symptoms. Atypical antipsychotic agents, such as quetiapine, are preferred due to their lower likelihood of causing extrapyramidal side effects. Quetiapine is currently considered the first-line choice, with a starting dose of 12.5-25 mg/day at bedtime and a mean maintenance dose of around 75 mg/day. Clozapine is the most effective, but it is considered a second-line choice due to the risk of agranulocytosis and the need for frequent blood count monitoring.[32] Risperidone and olanzapine have been found to worsen PD and are not recommended.[33]

Recently, pimavanserin, a selective serotonin 2A (5-HT2A) receptor inverse agonist without dopamine receptor-blocking properties, has been approved by the Food and Drug Administration (FDA) for the treatment of PD psychosis.[34] It has shown positive results in clinical trials, although further research is needed to evaluate its efficacy, safety, and tolerability, especially in patients with comorbid dementia.

For patients with PD who have psychosis along with cognitive impairment or dementia but are not at risk of self-harm or harm to others, the use of a cholinesterase inhibitor may be considered before resorting to antipsychotic agents.[35]

COGNITIVE IMPAIRMENT AND DEMENTIA

Approximately 50% of patients with PD who do not have dementia experience mild cognitive impairment (MCI) when assessed using standardized cognitive tests. Cognitive impairment can manifest early in the disease and may precede the development of memory deficits. The specific types of impairments reported in the literature are diverse but primarily involve executive functioning (such as impaired planning and working memory), visuospatial abilities, attention, and language functioning.[36]

Among the nonmotor symptoms that can occur in PD, significant cognitive impairment poses the greatest challenge and concern. Initially, it was believed that around 30% of patients with PD suffered from Parkinson's disease dementia (PDD), and that the cognitive profile in PD was distinct from that of Alzheimer's disease (AD). It was thought that cognitive changes in PD primarily affected executive abilities and attention, while AD primarily affected memory and language. However, it is now recognized that cognitive impairments in PD can occur across various domains, including executive functions, memory, visuospatial abilities, attention, and language, even in patients with mild cognitive deficits or MCI.[28]

There is a point of controversy regarding the relationship between PD and dementia with Lewy bodies (DLBs) and whether the differences between them are categorical or dimensional. DLB, which is characterized by dementia along with a combination of parkinsonism, psychosis, and rapid eye movement (REM) sleep behavior disorder (RBD), is challenging to distinguish clinically and neuropathologically from PDD, except for increased AD pathology or biomarkers in DLB compared to PDD, or potentially alpha-synuclein genetic variability. There is a controversial "1-year rule" in place, where dementia preceding or occurring within 1 year of parkinsonism onset is labeled as DLB, while all other cases are diagnosed as PDD.

Prospective studies have demonstrated cognitive decline in individuals with prodromal or at-risk PD, including those with impaired olfaction, dopamine transporter deficits, or RBD. Cognitive impairments in this population may predict conversion to DLBs rather than PD.

Dementia typically occurs later in the disease process, affecting up to 30% of people with PD. NPSs are more common in Parkinson's disease patients with dementia. Currently, there are no specific criteria for diagnosing dementia in PD, so generic criteria like those in the Diagnostic and Statistical Manual of Mental Disorders, Fourth Edition (DSM-4) are applied ("dementia due to other general medical conditions"). In theory, patients with PD can develop any type of dementia, similar to the general population. Distinguishing PDD from DLB is complex and beyond the scope of this review, as their clinical courses and treatments may differ.[37]

Assessing patients for cognitive impairment can be done partially through the use of the mini-mental state examination in the office.[38] However, additional neurological and neuropsychological consultations may be helpful in further evaluating cognitive function in patients with PD. Several tests have been proposed by Camicioli and Gauthier to study cognition and neuropsychological features in PDD.[39]

The cognitive symptoms of PDD are believed to involve deficits in multiple neurotransmitter systems, including dopamine, acetylcholine, serotonin, and norepinephrine. The progressive loss of dopaminergic functioning in the substantia nigra, interference with frontal subcortical dopaminergic neurons, and the loss of cholinergic cells in the nucleus basalis of Meynert are thought to play a significant role in major cognitive impairment and PDD. The link between cortical and subcortical Lewy bodies and dementia in PD remains controversial.[40-43]

Management of PDD primarily focuses on symptomatic treatment. Exacerbating factors contributing to cognitive impairment should be addressed, such as treating infections, ensuring hydration, and addressing metabolic factors. Discontinuing nonessential medications with anticholinergic or sedative properties may be beneficial. The use of cholinesterase inhibitors, such as rivastigmine, has shown some cognitive benefit and reduction in NPSs in PDD, although further randomized trials are needed to draw definitive conclusions. Other agents such as donepezil and galantamine have shown modest cognitive benefits in small controlled studies, but more research with larger patient populations is necessary.[44-49]

SLEEP DISORDER

Sleep disorders are highly prevalent in PD, affecting a large percentage of patients, ranging from 60 to 98%.[50] These sleep disorders can arise due to PD itself, medications used for treatment, or comorbidities such as mood disorders, cognitive impairment, or pain **(Box 3)**.[30]

Sleep disorders in PD can be classified into two main categories: Dyssomnia, which includes insomnia or hypersomnia, and parasomnia.[50] Insomnia is characterized by a perception of insufficient or poor-quality sleep, leading to feelings of unrefreshed sleep. It encompasses difficulties in initiating sleep, sleep fragmentation, and early morning awakening. Various factors can contribute to insomnia in PD, such as motor manifestations of the disease (stiffness, tremor, dystonic movements, and cramps), nocturia, psychiatric disorders (depression, anxiety, and hallucinations), dementia, other sleep disorders (restless legs syndrome, periodic limb movement disorder, and obstructive sleep apnea syndrome), and certain medications.[50]

Hypersomnia refers to excessive daytime sleepiness and sleep attacks. Excessive daytime sleepiness is a common occurrence in PD, affecting 20–50% of patients, leading to significant interference with daily activities. Sleep attacks, on the other hand, are rare but defined as sudden and overwhelming sleepiness that can occur in stimulating situations such as eating, walking, or driving.[51]

Excessive daytime sleepiness in PD can result from multiple factors, including difficulties with sleep at night, the disease process itself, dopaminergic medications, other medications (such as psychotropic agents), and comorbid conditions such as depression, dementia, or sleep apnea. Sleep attacks have been associated with dopamine agonists and, occasionally, with levodopa alone.[51]

Parasomnia encompasses various signs and symptoms that occur during sleep in PD. These include vivid dreams, nocturnal hallucinosis, nightmares, night terrors, nocturnal vocalizations, sleepwalking, sleep talking, panic

> **BOX 3: Common sleep disorders in Parkinson's disease.**
>
> *Dyssomnia*:
> - Insomnia
> - Idiopathic insomnia hypnotic medication
> - Motor manifestations of Parkinson's disease (stiffness, inability to move, cramps, dystonia, and pain)
> - Adjustment of dopaminergic medication, analgesic, and use of satin sheets (to relieve stiffness and pain)
> - Nocturia: Alpha-adrenergic blocker; 5α-reductase inhibitor
> - Restless legs syndrome and periodic limb movement disorder
> - Adjustment of dopaminergic medication; anticonvulsant
> - Breathing-related disorder (obstructive sleep apnea syndrome)
> - Weight loss; CPAP
> - Hypersomnia
> - Excessive daytime sleepiness
> - Adjustment of dopaminergic medication, caffeine, methylphenidate, and modafinil
> - Sleep attacks
> - Adjustment of dopaminergic medication; modafinil
>
> *Parasomnia:*
> - Arousal disorder (vivid dreams and sleep terror disorder)
> - Adjustment of dopaminergic medication
> - Sleep–wake transition disorder (e.g., nocturnal vocalizations, sleep talking, and hypnagogic jerks)
> - Adjustment of dopaminergic medication
> - REM sleep disorder (nightmare disorder and REM behavior disorder)
> - Adjustment of dopaminergic medication; clonazepam
>
> *Sleep disorder related to psychiatric disorder:*
> - Anxiety, depression: Anxiolytic; antidepressant
> - Cognitive impairment, dementia: Cholinesterase inhibitor
> - Psychosis: Antipsychotic (quetiapine and clozapine)
>
> (CPAP: continuous positive airway pressure; REM: rapid eye movement)

attacks, and RBD. RBD is a distressing syndrome in which patients lack the normal muscle atonia associated with REM sleep, leading to acting out their dreams through physical movements such as kicking, grabbing, yelling, or falling out of bed. RBD may even precede the onset of motor symptoms in some patients with PD and can occur in up to 33% of patients.[52]

Management

The management of sleep disorders in PD requires a comprehensive approach that involves identifying and addressing the underlying factors contributing to

> **BOX 4: Sleep disorder management: Recommended sleep hygiene.**
>
> - Maximize daytime activities
> - Maximize daytime exposure to bright light
> - Minimize daytime napping
> - Avoid stimulants (caffeine, alcohol, and tobacco) and fluids near bedtime
> - Avoid heavy late-night meals
> - Practice relaxation technique before bed
> - Follow a regular sleep schedule
> - Institute and maintain a bedtime routine
> - Limit time in bed (7–8 hours per night)
> - Reserve bedroom for sleeping

disturbed sleep **(Box 4)**. Evaluating and optimizing sleep hygiene practices is an essential step **(Box 4)**. Specific sleep disorders should be investigated in clinical practice, and if necessary, further assessment in a sleep laboratory may be warranted. The effects of medications should be carefully assessed in individuals with PD experiencing disturbed sleep or excessive daytime sleepiness. Additionally, it is crucial to engage in open discussions with family members and caregivers to address and manage sleep disorders associated with PD.

ADDICTION AND RELATED DISORDERS

The primary treatment approach for PD involves the use of medications aimed at restoring cerebral dopaminergic neurotransmission. It is important to note that the dopaminergic system, which includes dopamine D2 receptors, the nucleus accumbens, and the mesolimbic pathway, plays a role in the brain's reward mechanisms and is implicated in different types of addictions.[53] Consequently, the use of dopaminergic medications can potentially contribute to the development of secondary behavioral disorders.

SUBSTANCE ABUSE AND DEPENDENCE

There is currently a lack of formal studies on substance abuse and dependence specifically in PD. However, a phenomenon known as severe dopamine addiction or levodopa misuse has been well-documented.[53] In this condition, patients exhibit a pattern of increasing dopaminergic drug consumption as psychostimulants, despite experiencing severe drug-induced dyskinesia. Along with worsening motor function, mood disorders such as drug-induced hypomania or manic psychosis may also arise. Dopaminergic therapy can be associated with other NPSs, including punding (repetitive, purposeless behaviors resembling those seen in amphetamine or cocaine addiction), drug hoarding, and drug-seeking behaviors.

Severe dopamine addiction can significantly impair occupational and social functioning. Managing this condition is challenging, but typically involves a gradual reduction of dopaminergic drug doses alongside the symptomatic treatment of psychiatric symptoms.

PATHOLOGICAL GAMBLING

Pathological gambling is a type of impulse control disorder characterized by an individual's inability to resist the urge to gamble, even in the face of significant personal, familial, or vocational consequences. It is difficult to determine the exact prevalence of this condition, but it has been observed to affect approximately 1.5% of individuals using pramipexole and around 0.3% of those using other dopamine agonists.[54]

The underlying causes of pathological gambling are not well understood. While the disorder may not be exclusive to a particular medication, it could be associated with the overall dopaminergic effect.[55] Some experts argue that the risk of developing pathological gambling is similar among patients taking ropinirole, pergolide, and pramipexole.[56] However, others suggest that the disorder is more commonly observed in individuals using pramipexole.[57]

HYPERSEXUALITY

The rekindling of sexual interest is a widely recognized side effect of dopaminergic therapy in individuals with PD.[58] However, less frequently reported are instances of hypersexuality, characterized by an incessant desire for sexual intercourse that may exhaust the partner, as well as an increase in engagement with online sex chat rooms, pornography, or prostitutes. Additionally, sexual deviations such as zoophilia[59] and transvestic fetishism[60] have been observed. These disorders often manifest in patients without a previous psychiatric history or evident cognitive impairments.[61] A recent review indicated that paraphilia accounted for 3% of all neuropsychiatric complications associated with drug treatment for PD.[62]

The cause of this compulsive behavior is not well understood, but it may be linked to either an amplified sexual drive beyond the norm or a lack of impulse control regarding sexual behavior, both of which are influenced by dopaminergic regulation. However, in certain cases, particularly when cognitive impairment is present alongside PD, sexually compulsive behaviors may be associated with a deficiency in behavioral inhibition.

MANAGEMENT

Behaviors such as gambling, hypersexuality, and sexual deviation are frequently concealed by patients and may not be readily recognized by clinicians in the context of PD. However, if left unidentified and untreated, these impulsive behaviors can lead to significant distress, conflicts within relationships, financial difficulties, and even legal issues. Therefore, it is crucial for all patients receiving dopaminergic therapy to be informed and closely monitored for the development of impulse control disorders.

These disorders often exhibit a dose-dependent relationship, and symptoms tend to diminish when the dosage of dopaminergic medication is reduced or when the therapy is discontinued. It is important to provide counseling and support not only to the patients but also to their families and caregivers in order to address the challenges associated with these behaviors.

CONCLUDING REMARKS

Neuropsychiatric complications are frequently observed in individuals with PD, leading to increased disability, reduced quality of life, and caregiver distress. Early identification of nonmotor symptoms is crucial for effective management. The pathophysiology of these complications is multifaceted, involving degenerative changes, medication effects, and emotional responses to chronic illness. Treatment can be challenging but often yields positive outcomes. A comprehensive, multidisciplinary approach is essential for both patients and caregivers.

LEARNING POINTS

- In the past two decades, our understanding of psychiatric and cognitive complications in PD has evolved to a great extent.
- Longitudinal studies have revealed higher cumulative prevalence rates than previously thought, with some disorders exceeding 50% and long-term rates of dementia and sleep disorders potentially reaching 80%.
- Nonmotor complications significantly contribute to disability, poorer quality of life, adverse outcomes, and increased caregiver burden.
- Diagnostic tools and criteria have improved, enhancing clinical management and research quality.
- Neurologically, nonmotor complications involve a complex interplay of PD pathology, other neurodegenerative disease processes, neurotransmitter system alterations, neural circuitry impairments, and genetic factors.
- Core treatments such as dopamine replacement therapy (DRT) and DBS have diverse effects on psychiatric and cognitive symptoms.
- However, treatment options remain limited, with most drugs initially developed for similar conditions in non-PD patients.

ACKNOWLEDGMENT

The author is indebted to Dr Sayan Malakar of VIMS, Kolkata, for his help in the preparation of this Chapter.

REFERENCES

1. Obeso JA, Stamelou M, Goetz CG, Poewe W, Lang AE, Weintraub D, et al. Past, present, and future of Parkinson's disease: a special essay on the 200th anniversary of the shaking palsy. Mov Disord. 2017;32:1264-310.
2. Chaudhuri K, Healy D, Schapira A. Non-motor symptoms of Parkinson's disease: diagnosis and management. Lancet Neurol. 2006;5:235-45.
3. Guttman M, Kish SJ, Furukawa Y. Current concepts in the diagnosis and management of Parkinson's disease. CMAJ. 2003;168(3):293-301.
4. Aarsland D, Larsen JP, Lim NG, et al. Range of neuropsychiatric disturbances in patients with Parkinson's disease. J Neurol Neurosurg Psychiatry. 1999;67:492-6.
5. Miyasaki JM, Shannon K, Voon V, Ravina B, Kleiner-Fisman G, Anderson K, et al. Practice Parameter: evaluation and treatment of depression, psychosis, and dementia in Parkinson disease (an evidence-based review): report of the Quality Standards Subcommittee of the American Academy of Neurology. Neurology. 2006;66:996-1002.
6. American Psychiatric Association. Diagnostic and Statistical Manual of Mental Disorders, 4th edition. Washington: American Psychiatric Association; 2001.
7. Schiffer RB, Kurlan R, Rubin A, Boer S. Evidence for atypical depression in Parkinson's disease. Am J Psychiatry. 1988; 145:1020-2.
8. Rickards H. Depression in neurological disorders: Parkinson's disease, multiple sclerosis, and stroke. J Neurol Neurosurg Psychiatry. 2005;76(Suppl 1):i48-52.
9. Leentjens AF, Verhey FR, Luijckx GJ, Troost J. The validity of the Beck Depression Inventory as a screening and diagnostic instrument for depression in patients with Parkinson's disease. Mov Disord 2000;15:1221-4.
10. Leentjens AF, Verhey FR, Lousberg R, Spitsbergen H, Wilmink FW. The validity of the Hamilton and Montgomery–Asberg depression rating scales as screening and diagnostic tools for depression in Parkinson's disease. Int J Geriatr Psychiatry. 2000;15:644-9.
11. Mossner R, Henneberg A, Schmitt A, Syagailo YV, Grässle M, Hennig T, et al. Allelic variation of serotonin transporter expression is associated with depression in Parkinson's disease. Mol Psychiatry 2001;6:350-2.
12. Maricle RA, Nutt JG, Valentine RJ, Carter JH. Dose-response relationship of levodopa with mood and anxiety in fluctuating Parkinson's disease: a double-blind, placebo-controlled study. Neurology. 1995;45:1757-60.

13. Cole K, Vaughan FL. The feasibility of using cognitive behaviour therapy for depression associated with Parkinson's disease: a literature review. Parkinsonism Relat Disord. 2005;11:269-76.
14. Weintraub D, Morales KH, Moberg PJ, Bilker WB, Balderston C, Duda JE, et al. Antidepressant studies in Parkinson's disease: a review and meta-analysis. Mov Disord. 2005;20:1161-9.
15. Richard IH, Maughn A, Kurlan R. Do serotonin reuptake inhibitor antidepressants worsen Parkinson's disease? A retrospective case series. Mov Disord. 1999;14:155-7.
16. Mendis T, Suchowersky O, Lang A, Gauthier S. Management of Parkinson's disease: a review of current and new therapies. Can J Neurol Sci. 1999;26:89-103.
17. Richard IH, Kurlan R, Tanner C, Factor S, Hubble J, Suchowersky O, et al. Serotonin syndrome and the combined use of deprenyl and an antidepressant in Parkinson's disease. Parkinson Study Group. Neurology. 1997;48:1070-7.
18. Moellentine C, Rummans T, Ahlskog JE, Harmsen WS, Suman VJ, O'Connor MK, et al. Effectiveness of ECT in patients with parkinsonism. J Neuropsychiatry Clin Neurosci. 1998;10:187-93.
19. Fregni F, Simon DK, Wu A, Pascual-Leone A. Non-invasive brain stimulation for Parkinson's disease: a systematic review and meta-analysis of the literature. J Neurol Neurosurg Psychiatry. 2005;76:1614-23.
20. Schwartz JE, Jandorf L, Krupp LB. The measurement of fatigue: a new instrument. J Psychosom Res. 1993;37:753-62.
21. Chatterjee A, Fahn S. Methylphenidate treats apathy in Parkinson's disease. J Neuropsychiatry Clin Neurosci. 2002;14:461-2.
22. Richard IH, Schiffer RB, Kurlan R. Anxiety and Parkinson's disease. J Neuropsychiatry Clin Neurosci. 1996;8:383-92.
23. Weisskopf MG, Chen H, Schwarzschild MA, Kawachi I, Ascherio A. Prospective study of phobic anxiety and risk of Parkinson's disease. Mov Disord. 2003;18:646-51.
24. Ludwig CL, Weinberger DR, Bruno G, Gillespie M, Bakker K, LeWitt PA, et al. Buspirone, Parkinson's disease, and the locus ceruleus. Clin Neuropharmacol. 1986;9:373-8.
25. Richard IH, Frank S, McDermott MP, Wang H, Justus AW, LaDonna KA, et al. The ups and downs of Parkinson disease: a prospective study of mood and anxiety fluctuations. Cogn Behav Neurol. 2004;17:201-7.
26. Papapetropoulos S, Mash DC. Psychotic symptoms in Parkinson's disease. From description to etiology. J Neurol. 2005;252:753-64.
27. Fenelon G, Mahieux F, Huon R, Ziégler M. Hallucinations in Parkinson's disease: prevalence, phenomenology and risk factors. Brain. 2000;123:733-45.
28. Holroyd S, Currie L, Wooten GF. Prospective study of hallucinations and delusions in Parkinson's disease. J Neurol Neurosurg Psychiatry. 2001;70:734-8.
29. Moskovitz C, Moses H 3rd, Klawans HL. Levodopa-induced psychosis: a kindling phenomenon. Am J Psychiatry. 1978;135:669-75.
30. Olanow CW, Watts RL, Koller WC. An algorithm (decision tree) for the management of Parkinson's disease (2001): treatment guidelines. Neurology 2001;56(Suppl 5):S1-S88.
31. Aarsland D, Perry R, Larsen JP, McKeith IG, O'Brien JT, Perry EK, et al. Neuroleptic sensitivity in Parkinson's disease and parkinsonian dementias. J Clin Psychiatry. 2005;66:633-7.
32. Fernandez HH, Trieschmann ME, Burke MA, Jacques C, Friedman JH. Long-term outcome of quetiapine use for psychosis among Parkinsonian patients. Mov Disord. 2003;18:510-4.
33. Juncos JL, Roberts VJ, Evatt ML, Jewart RD, Wood CD, Potter LS, et al. Quetiapine improves psychotic symptoms and cognition in Parkinson's disease. Mov Disord. 2004;19:29-35.
34. Friedman JH, Factor SA. Atypical antipsychotics in the treatment of drug-induced psychosis in Parkinson's disease. Mov Disord. 2000;15:201-11.
35. Poewe W. Treatment of dementia with Lewy bodies and Parkinson's disease dementia. Mov Disord. 2005;20(Suppl 12):S77-82.
36. Camicioli R, Fisher N. Progress in clinical neurosciences: Parkinson's disease with dementia and dementia with Lewy bodies. Can J Neurol Sci. 2004;31:7-21.
37. Aarsland D, Bronnick K, Ehrt U, De Deyn PP, Tekin S, Emre M, et al. Neuropsychiatric symptoms in patients with PD and dementia: Frequency, profile and associated caregiver stress. J Neurol Neurosurg Psychiatry. 2006;78:2-3.
38. Folstein MF, Folstein SE, McHugh PR. "Mini-mental state". A practical method for grading the cognitive state of patients for the clinician. J Psychiatr Res. 1975;12:189-98.
39. Camicioli R, Gauthier S. Clinical trials in Parkinson's disease dementia and dementia with Lewy bodies. Can J Neurol Sci. 2007;34(Suppl 1):S109-17.
40. Leroi I, Brandt J, Reich SG, Lyketsos CG, Grill S, Thompson R, et al. Randomized placebo-controlled trial of donepezil in cognitive impairment in Parkinson's disease. Int J Geriatr Psychiatry. 2004;19:1-8.
41. Dubois B, Pillon B. Cognitive deficits in Parkinson's disease. J Neurol. 1997;244:2-8.
42. Nakano I, Hirano A. Parkinson's disease: neuron loss in the nucleus basalis without concomitant Alzheimer's disease. Ann Neurol. 1984;15:415-8.
43. McKeith IG, Dickson DW, Lowe J, Emre M, O'Brien JT, Feldman H, et al.; Consortium on DLB. Diagnosis and management of dementia with Lewy bodies: third report of the DLB Consortium. Neurology. 2005;65:1863-72.
44. Feldman HH, Gauthier S, Chertkow H, Conn DK, Freedman M, Chris M; 2nd Canadian Conference on Antidementia Guidelines. Progress in clinical neurosciences: Canadian guidelines for the development of antidementia therapies: a conceptual summary. Can J Neurol Sci. 2006;33:6-26.
45. Maidment I, Fox C, Boustani M. Cholinesterase inhibitors for Parkinson's disease dementia. Cochrane Database Syst Rev. 2006;(1):CD004747.
46. Emre M, Aarsland D, Albanese A, Byrne EJ, Deuschl G, De Deyn PP, et al. Rivastigmine for dementia associated with Parkinson's disease. N Engl J Med. 2004;351:2509-18.
47. Aarsland D, Laake K, Larsen JP, C Janvin. Donepezil for cognitive impairment in Parkinson's disease: a randomised controlled study. J Neurol Neurosurg Psychiatry. 2002;72:708-12.
48. Ravina B, Putt M, Siderowf A, Farrar JT, Gillespie M, Crawley A, et al. Donepezil for dementia in Parkinson's disease: a randomised, double blind, placebo controlled, crossover study. J Neurol Neurosurg Psychiatry. 2005;76:934-9.
49. Aarsland D, Hutchinson M, Larsen JP. Cognitive, psychiatric and motor response to galantamine in Parkinson's disease with dementia. Int J Geriatr Psychiatry. 2003;18:937-41.
50. Adler CH, Thorpy MJ. Sleep issues in Parkinson's disease. Neurology. 2005;64(Suppl 3):S12-20.
51. Arnulf I. Excessive daytime sleepiness in parkinsonism. Sleep Med Rev. 2005;9:185-200.

52. Postuma RB, Lang AE, Massicotte-Marquez J, Montplaisir J. Potential early markers of Parkinson disease in idiopathic REM sleep behavior disorder. Neurology. 2006;66:845-51.
53. Lawrence AD, Evans AH, Lees AJ. Compulsive use of dopamine replacement therapy in Parkinson's disease: Reward systems gone awry? Lancet Neurol. 2003;2:595-604.
54. Stocchi F. Pathological gambling in Parkinson's disease. Lancet Neurol. 2005;4:590-2.
55. Morgan JC, Iyer SS, Sethi KD. Impulse control disorders and dopaminergic drugs. Arch Neurol. 2006;63:298-9.
56. Lu C, Bharmal A, Suchowersky O. Gambling and Parkinson disease. Arch Neurol. 2006;63:298.
57. Dodd ML, Klos KJ, Bower JH, Geda YE, Josephs KA, Ahlskog JE. Pathological gambling caused by drugs used to treat Parkinson disease. Arch Neurol. 2005;62:1377-81.
58. Barbeau A. L-dopa therapy in Parkinson's disease: a critical review of nine years' experience. Can Med Assoc J. 1969;101:59-68.
59. Fernandez HH, Durso R. Clozapine for dopaminergic-induced paraphilias in Parkinson's disease. Mov Disord. 1998;13:597-8.
60. Riley DE. Reversible transvestic fetishism in a man with Parkinson's disease treated with selegiline. Clin Neuropharmacol. 2002;25:234-7.
61. Klos KJ, Bower JH, Josephs KA, Matsumoto JY, Ahlskog JE. Pathological hypersexuality predominantly linked to adjuvant dopamine agonist therapy in Parkinson's disease and multiple system atrophy. Parkinsonism Relat Disord. 2005;11:381-6.
62. Cummings JL. Behavioral complications of drug treatment of Parkinson's disease. J Am Geriatr Soc. 1991;39:708-16.

COMMENTARY 13

Neural Basis of Impulsive Control Disorders

Ambar Chakravarty

INTRODUCTION

The adverse effects of the dopaminergic therapy for Parkinson's disease (PD) include pathological gambling, hypersexuality, compulsive eating, shopping, and internet using, which are grouped together as the impulse control disorders (ICDs). These disorders are also encountered in the general population at a much lower prevalence rate when they are referred to as "disorders in the impulsive–compulsive spectrum", "ICDs", or "behavioral addictions", and can be classified in the Diagnostic and Statistical Manual of Mental Disorders, Fourth Edition, Text Revision (DSM-4-TR) as ICDs, even though only pathological gambling has specified criteria.[1] These pathological behaviors share features similar to those of substance use disorders (SUD), which has led to the term "behavioral addictions", when the behaviors are characterized by a compulsive drive toward and impaired control over the behavior.

About 14% of patients with PD receiving dopaminergic medication develop some of the impulsive–compulsive disorders mentioned earlier. Such disorders essentially manifest features similar to SUDs.[2] Changes associated with addictions are mainly seen in the dopaminergic system of a mesocorticolimbic circuit, the so-called reward system, these excessive and reinforcing behaviors involve the dopaminergic "reward system", as do all substances of abuse.

Hence, it has been proposed to classify several of the ICDs as behavioral addictions in DSM-5, yet only pathological gambling has been moved to the "addictions and related disorders" section of DSM-5.[2]

THE NEUROANATOMY OF THE MESOCORTICOLIMBIC "REWARD" SYSTEM

The mesocorticolimbic circuit, the so-called reward system, comprises of the ventral striatum (VS) [comprising of the nucleus accumbens (NAcc)] **(Fig. 1)**, the orbitofrontal cortex (OFC), the anterior cingulate cortex (ACC), the amygdala, and the hippocampus.

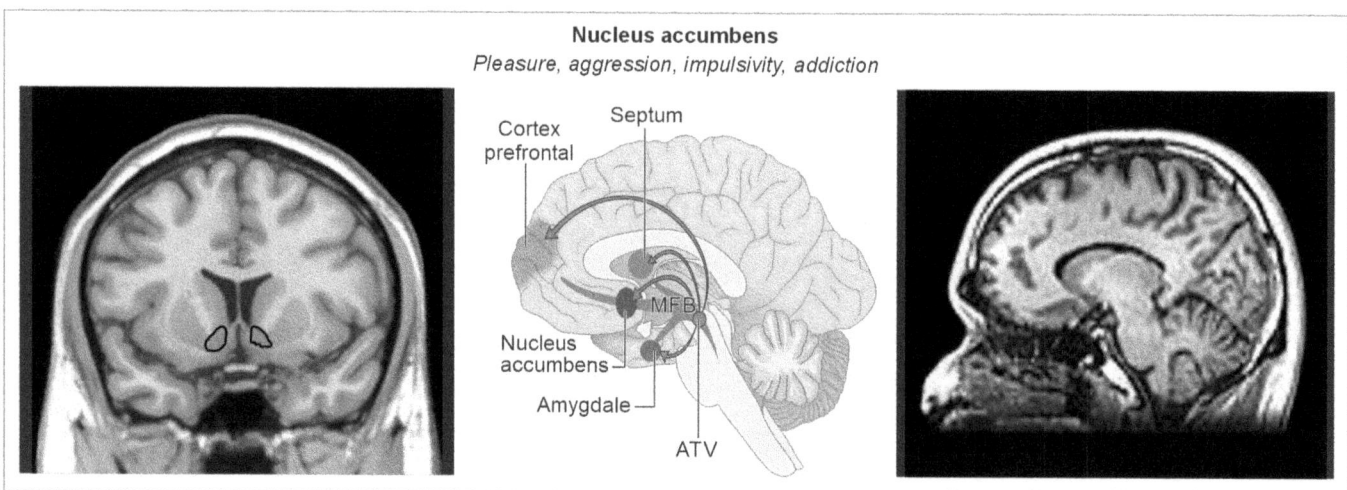

FIG. 1: Location of nucleus accumbens.
(ATV: areal tegmental ventral; MFB: medial forebrain bundle)

The amygdala and the OFC play a key role in associating reward-predicting cues with the positive emotional gains elicited by the actual reward.[3] The OFC is involved in updating the value of the reward.[4] Dopaminergic neuromodulation in the midbrain seems to enhance hippocampus-dependent long-term memory formation so that reward-related stimuli and contexts are reliably recognized in later day situations.[4] The ACC, on the other hand, is hypothesized to link rewards with actions and thus has a gating role in action selection following reward cues.[5] In a healthy brain, reward-directed behavior is adaptively controlled by inhibitory influences of the prefrontal cortex (PFC). Through the OFC and ACC, top-down influences reach mesolimbic areas again and regulate/control reward-seeking motivation.[6]

AN ALTERED SYSTEM: THE ADDICTION CIRCUITRY

Substances of abuse can be seen as having strong influence on the aforementioned circuitry. They cause a stronger release of dopamine that does not habituate as fast as with natural rewards.[4,6] Dopaminergic signals in the midbrain are thought to generate an incentive value on addictive substances and motivate appetitive behavior toward associated stimuli.[4] Heightened attribution is reflected by stronger activation of the reward system following drug associated cues (e.g., an alcoholic visualizing a bottle of beer).[7] Presumably, overactivation of the mesolimbic dopaminergic system with reduced influence of inhibitory frontal brain areas result from repeated exposure to an unconditioned stimulus.[8] The result, the efforts to control the addictive behavior gets overridden when tempted, the motivation to take the drug or carry out a behavior.

FACTORS ASSOCIATED WITH THE DEVELOPMENT OF BEHAVIORAL ADDICTIONS

Every human being possesses a reward system, but not everyone is responsive to rewards to the same degree. Quite a lot of people gamble from time to time gamble, and all of us eat, shop, or use the internet more or less frequently. But who will become addicted? **Figure 2** gives an overview of the factors that are thought to influence the genesis and development of behavioral addictions.

NEUROTRANSMITTERS

Dopamine

Currently, the contribution of neurotransmitters in behavioral and substance addictions is best understood for dopamine. It seems that preexistent, partly genetically determined, and dopaminergic abnormalities lead to pathological behaviors which in turn cause a further disbalance in the dopaminergic system. Studies focusing on the D2 receptor gene suggest that the A1 allele of the Taq1A polymorphism creates a condition that is characterized by reduced availability of D2 receptors in the striatum.[8] Nuclear imaging studies have shown that

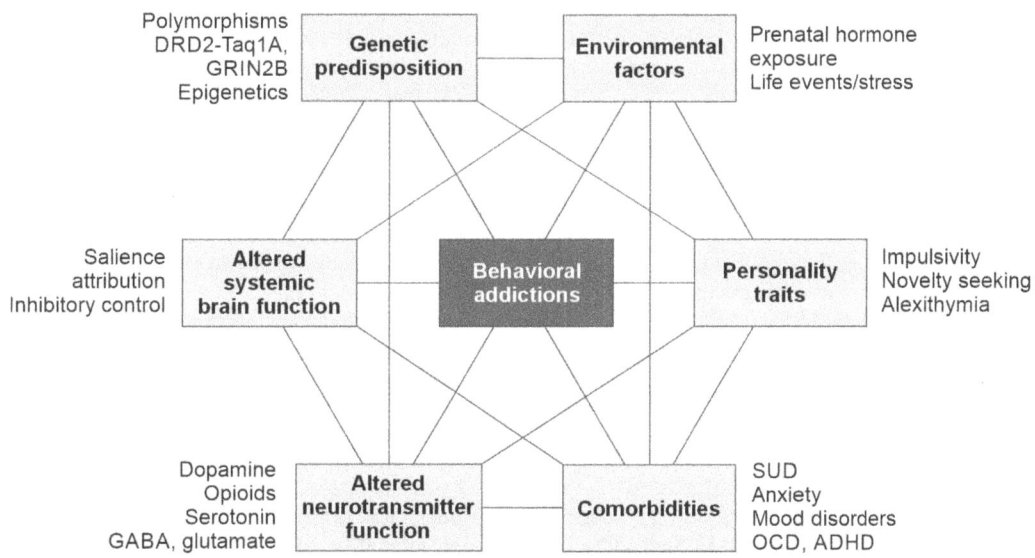

FIG. 2: Interacting factors associated with the development of behavioral addictions.
(ADHD: attention-deficit/hyperactivity disorder; OCD: obsessive–compulsive disorders; SUD substance use disorder)

pathological gamblers and people with pathological overeating or internet addiction show reduced[9] raclopride baseline binding potential in the striatum.[10-12] However, positron emission tomography (PET) studies reveal either a functional downregulation of dopamine transporters or receptors or else higher synaptic dopamine levels. This is confusing whether a basal hypodopaminergic state or a hyperdopaminergic state exists, remains unclear.

Impulsivity and disinhibition are often used synonymously when speaking of PFC-mediated top-down control. Impaired inhibition is seen in most SUDs and is associated with a hypoactive dorsal ACC and dorsolateral PFC.[13] Pathological gamblers and PD patients with ICDs also show impairments in tasks such as the stop-signal task, go/no-go paradigms, and the Stroop task that involve inhibitory control.[13-16] But there are also studies that did not find any behavioral differences between gamblers or internet addicts and controls[17-20] or PD patients with ICDs and PD controls.[21] Furthermore, findings indicate reduced activity in the ventromedial or dorsomedial PFC.[17,22] Stressing the role of dopamine, one study found that during a card game with probabilistic feedback, dopaminergic medication deactivated or inhibited brain areas implicated in impulse control like the prefrontal cortex specifically in PD patients with pathological gambling.[23] This would support the idea that the effect of dopaminergic medication may depend on different baseline dopamine levels in ICD patients and controls.[24]

Opioid antagonist therapy may be helpful in several ICDs, based on midbrain μ-opioid receptor stimulation causing inhibition of GABA and resultant dopamine release.[25-28] Regarding serotonin and ICDs, there are mixed results in relation to studies with serotoninergic medication. There is only limited evidence from preclinical trials and medication studies that glutamatergic and GABAergic medication effectively treats (behavioral) addictions.

REFERENCES

1. Task Force on DSM-IV, American Psychiatric Association. Diagnostic and Statistical Manual of Mental Disorders: Fourth Edition Text Revision (DSM-IV-TR). Washington: American Psychiatric Association; 2002.
2. Grant JE, Potenza MN, Weinstein A, Gorelick DA. Introduction to behavioral addictions. Am J Drug Alcohol Abuse. 2010;36:233-41.
3. Holden C. Psychiatry. Behavioral addictions debut in proposed DSM-V. Science. 2010;327:935.
4. Dolan RJ. The human amygdala and orbital prefrontal cortex in behavioural regulation. Philos Trans R Soc B Biol Sci. 2007; 362:787-99.
5. Everitt BJ, Robbins TW. Neural systems of reinforcement for drug addiction: from actions to habits to compulsion. Nat Neurosci. 2005;8:1481-9.
6. Goldstein RZ, Volkow ND. Dysfunction of the prefrontal cortex in addiction: neuroimaging findings and clinical implications. Nat Rev Neurosci. 2011;12:652-69.
7. Robinson TE, Berridge KC. The incentive sensitization theory of addiction: some current issues. Philos Trans R Soc B Biol Sci. 2008;363:3137-46.
8. Blum K, Gull JG, Braverman ER, Comings DE. Reward deficiency syndrome. Am Sci. 1996;84:132-45.
9. Smith KS, Berridge KC. Opioid limbic circuit for reward: interaction between hedonic hotspots of nucleus accumbens and ventral pallidum. J Neurosci. 2007;27:1594-605.
10. Steeves TDL, Miyasaki J, ZurowskiM, Lang AE, Pellecchia G, van Eimeren T, et al. Increased striatal dopamine release in parkinsonian patients with pathological gambling: a [11C] raclopride PET study. Brain. 2009;132:1376-85.
11. Wang G-J, Volkow ND, Logan J, Pappas NR, Wong CT, Zhu W, et al. Brain dopamine and obesity. Lancet. 2001;357:354-7.
12. Kim SH, Baik S-H, Park CS, Kim SJ, Choi SW, Kim SE. Reduced striatal dopamine D2 receptors in people with Internet addiction. Neuroreport. 2011;22:407-11.
13. Verdejo-García A, Lawrence AJ, Clark L. Impulsivity as a vulnerability marker for substance-use disorders: review of findings from high-risk research, problem gamblers and genetic association studies. Neurosci Biobehav Rev. 2008;32:777-810.
14. Voon V, Reynolds B, Brezing C, Gallea C, Skaljic M, Ekanayake V, et al. Impulsive choice and response in dopamine agonist-related impulse control behaviors. Psychopharmacology (Berl). 2009;207:645-59.
15. Thomsen KR, Joensson M, Lou HC, Møller A, Gross J, Kringelbach ML, et al. Altered paralimbic interaction in behavioral addiction. Proc Natl Acad Sci U S A. 2013;110(12):4744-9.
16. Forbush KT, Shaw M, Graeber MA, Hovick L, Meyer VJ, Moser DJ, et al. Neuropsychological characteristics and personality traits in pathological gambling. CNS Spectrums. 2008;13:306-15.
17. Potenza MN. An fMRI Stroop task study of ventromedial prefrontal cortical function in pathological gamblers. Am J Psychiatry. 2003;160:1990-4.
18. Lawrence AJ, Luty J, Bogdan NA, Sahakian BJ, Clark L. Impulsivity and response inhibition in alcohol dependence and problem gambling. Psychopharmacology (Berl). 2009;207:163-72.
19. Dong G, Lu Q, Zhou H, Zhao X. Impulse inhibition in people with Internet addiction disorder: electrophysiological evidence from a Go/NoGo study. Neurosci Lett. 2010;485:138-42.
20. Dong G, DeVito EE, Du X, Cui Z. Impaired inhibitory control in 'internet addiction disorder': a functional magnetic resonance imaging study. Psychiatry Res Neuroimaging. 2012;203:153-8.
21. Djamshidian A, O'Sullivan SS, Lees A, Averbeck BB. Stroop test performance in impulsive and nonimpulsive patients with Parkinson's disease. Parkinsonism Relat Disord. 2011;17:212-4.
22. De Ruiter MB, Oosterlaan J, Veltman DJ, van den Brink W, Goudriaan AE. Similar hyporesponsiveness of the dorsomedial prefrontal cortex in problem gamblers and heavy smokers during an inhibitory control task. Drug Alcohol Depend. 2012;121: 81-9.

23. van Eimeren T, Pellecchia G, Cilia R, Ballanger B, Steeves TDL, Houle S, et al. Drug-induced deactivation of inhibitory networks predicts pathological gambling in PD. Neurology. 2010;75:1711-6.
24. Cools R, Robbins TW. Chemistry of the adaptive mind. Philos Trans A Math Phys Eng Sci. 2004;362:2871-88.
25. Raymond NC, Grant JE, Kim SW, Coleman E. Treatment of compulsive sexual behaviour with naltrexone and serotonin reuptake inhibitors: two case studies. Int Clin Psychopharmacol. 2002;17:201-5.
26. Grant JE. Three cases of compulsive buying treated with naltrexone. Int J Psychiatry Clin Pract. 2003;7:223-5.
27. Grant JE, Kim SW. Medication management of pathological gambling. Minn Med. 2006;89:44-8.
28. Bosco D, Plastino M, Colica C, Bosco F, Arianna S, Vecchio A, et al. Opioid antagonist naltrexone for the treatment of pathological gambling in Parkinson disease. Clin Neuropharmacol. 2012;35:118-20.

A Note on Wilson's Disease and its Psychiatric Aspects

Ambar Chakravarty

CASE VIGNETTE

A 32-year-old sailor had been referred to the author for neurological assessment by a psychiatrist in 2011. This man was diagnosed to have bipolar disorder for which he was been treated with divalproate sodium and a selective serotonin reuptake inhibitor (SSRI). His mood improved but of late he was found to be getting slow in in motor tasking and developed tremor of his hands. These features were attributed to his developing Parkinsonian features related to divalproate therapy. The divalproate was stopped and replaced with carbamazepine. After 2 months of being off treatment with divalproate, his condition did not improve at all and if anything, his clinical condition deteriorated. This prompted a neurological referral. On examination at the present author's clinic, he was found to have symmetric parkinsonian features with tremor, rigidity, and bradykinesia. Eye examination revealed presence of a brownish ring at the limbus of both eyes. Slit lamp examination confirmed presence of Kayser-Fleischer (KF) ring. The serum ceruloplasmin level was much low and his liver enzymes were mildly raised. The diagnosis of Wilson's disease (WD) was made and he was started on a combination of D-penicillamine and zinc sulfate. His condition improved very significantly over the next 6 months. Later his psychiatric treatment could be tailed off. He continues to remain well till date. His KF rings had disappeared after about 6 years of therapy.

His younger brother, 30 years of age, was asymptomatic. A KF ring was seen in both of his eyes. The serum ceruloplasmin was low as well. This suggested the diagnosis of asymptomatic WD. He was also started on D-penicillamine which is being continued and he remains asymptomatic till this day. The KF ring had disappeared several years earlier.

Wilson's disease is a genetically determined neurometabolic disease, which can be very effectively treated in acute and chronic stages of the disease. Early diagnosis is of paramount importance as delays in treatments have much higher risk of unfavorable clinical outcomes. WD is caused by a *mutation* in the gene that encodes a copper-transporting P-type ATPase (*ATP7B*). This gene product *transports* excess copper into *bile* and thus excreted in the small bowel. The condition is inherited as *autosomal recessive* and hence both parents have to be carriers but not manifesting the disease. Over 500 ATP7B mutations have now been identified; most of these being missense mutations, small deletions/insertions in the coding region, or splice junction mutations. Rarely whole exon deletions and promoter region mutations have been found. ATP7B mutation "hot spots" vary considerably among different populations. Identification of WD remains challenging because it is a great imitator and requires a high index of suspicion for correct and timely diagnosis.[1,2]

The causes for delay in diagnosis are varied.[3-5] Walshe and Yealland[6] highlighted upon three major reasons which include underestimation of subtle early clinical features of WD (such as tremor and writer's cramp), lack of awareness among physicians/pediatricians/psychiatrists about the need to consider the possibility of WD in a given case, and lastly laboratory errors in estimation of copper and ceruloplasmin concentrations. These authors emphasized that evaluation for KF rings should be done by an experienced ophthalmologist, using a slit lamp which would differentiate KF rings from arcus senilis/juvenilis, by its position in relation to the Descemet's membrane at the limbus. It is also important to note that KF rings may not be present when illness manifests with non-neuropsychiatric features. Thus the principal causes of misdiagnosis and delayed diagnosis happen to be lack of awareness, low prevalence of disease in the community, absence of family history or history of liver disorders, comparatively late age of onset, and absence of clinical markers like KF ring. Patients presenting with behavioral problems often receive antipsychotic agents. With development of extrapyramidal symptoms with disease progression, the hallmark of WD, these are often considered as drug-related adverse event. It is also known that even after suggestive laboratory markers (like low ceruloplasmin levels), starting appropriate therapy is delayed. A number of factors may contribute which include inadequate knowledge about long-term management, nonavailability of drugs in peripheral centers, financial issues, and inappropriate counseling of patients regarding the nature of the disease and need for long continued treatment.[3]

Neurologic problems at disease onset can be seen in approximately 40–50% of patients and the rest has either hepatic or primarily psychiatric manifestations to start with. Neurologic and neuropsychiatric problems in WD are quite nonspecific and the most common clinical problems associated with early and late stages of the disease would be discussed here. Patients with neurologic symptoms may not always have any obvious hepatic symptoms. Most common neurologic abnormalities include dysarthria, dystonia, tremor, and parkinsonism. In spite of the clinical heterogeneity seen in many patients with WD, laboratory abnormalities, reflecting abnormal copper metabolism, are very specific and the diagnosis of WD essentially remains laboratory based. The clinical picture may be mimicked by several disorders affecting the basal ganglionic pathways both during the acute and chronic stages of the disease. There can be pitfalls in the standard laboratory tests used in the diagnosis. And this has necessitated the application of genetic studies for diagnostic confirmation. There again errors may occur as new sites of mutations have been described in recent times which produce phenotypically similar clinical presentations. Treatment had been standardized with use of copper chelators to induce a negative copper balance state but at times drug therapy may induce further clinical deterioration in some treated patients.

Most patients develop symptoms in adolescence to early adulthood. Neurologic symptoms generally develop approximately one decade later than hepatic presentation. The age of onset, however, may vary considerably with late disease onset noted even in the seventh and eighth decades of life, adding significant diagnostic challenge because clinical symptoms are similar to other common age-related conditions like parkinsonism. Initial signs and symptoms of WD are hepatic in approximately 40% of patients, neurologic in about 40–50%, and primarily psychiatric manifestation can be seen in about 10% of patients.[1,2] WD may be also diagnosed in presymptomatic individuals through recommended screening of siblings of affected probands or in asymptomatic individuals when routine laboratory test detects otherwise unexplained abnormalities of liver function panels. Patients presenting with liver disease may range from an asymptomatic state to life-threatening hepatic failure. Most patients with hepatic symptoms exhibit signs of chronic splenomegaly due to portal hypertension. Coombs-negative hemolytic anemia is often seen in the hepatic form of the disease.

Presentation with psychiatric symptoms is probably the most important cause of delayed diagnosis in WD because of the nonspecific nature of the symptoms.

When psychotic symptoms occur as the first manifestation of WD, both diagnostic and therapeutic challenges face the clinician. Very often such symptoms are considered to be due to schizophrenia, schizoaffective, or delusional disorder. Some guidelines suggest exclusion of WD in first episodes of psychosis.[2] Onset of WD with psychiatric symptoms often causes delay in diagnosis. Psychiatric manifestations occurring without overt hepatic or neurologic involvement may lead to misdiagnosis. A better understanding of the psychiatric presentations in WD may provide insights into the underlying mechanisms of psychiatric disorders. Psychiatric symptoms occur before concurrent with or after the diagnosis and treatment for WD. 30–40% of patients have psychiatric manifestations at the time of diagnosis, and 20% had seen a psychiatrist prior to their WD diagnosis. When psychiatric symptoms preceded neurological or hepatic involvement, the average time between the psychiatric symptoms and the diagnosis of WD was 864.3 days. The prevalence of psychiatric disorders in WD patients varies wildly (major depressive disorder, 4–47%; psychosis, 1.4–11.3%).[7] Certain gene mutations of ATP7B may correlate with specific personality traits.

LEARNING POINTS

- In the Indian subcontinent, any patient below the age of 50 years, presenting with a movement disorder, however trivial it might be, must be screened for WD. The same may be true for younger patients (<40 years) presenting with any form of psychiatric disorder as mentioned earlier.
- WD is caused by a mutation in the gene that encodes a copper-transporting P-type ATPase (*ATP7B*). This gene product transports excess copper into bile and thus excreted in the small bowel. Failure of transportation would lead to excess copper accumulation of copper in hepatocytes leading to cellular damage and liver injury in form of cirrhosis or chronic active hepatitis.
- Excess copper spill out into bloodstream and gets deposited in various organs including the brain and kidneys.
- Several non-neurological manifestations of WD occur and their early recognition is of paramount importance.

- Onset of WD with psychiatric symptoms often causes delay in diagnosis. Children presenting with behavioral and personality disorders including attention deficit hyperactivity disorders must be screened for WD.
- Also in the Indian subcontinent, assessment for proximal muscle weakness in children must include tests to exclude WD. The yield may not be very high, but early diagnosis is important.
- Seizures (both generalized and focal with secondary generalization) may be the initial presentation of WD and considering this possibility during evaluation must be kept in mind.
- Penicillamine should be started at a very small dose if used as initial therapy for WD with serial measurements of urinary copper excretion. Rapid turnover of hepatic copper may lead to excess copper deposition in brain with clinical deterioration. Deterioration may also occur with red cell deposition causing acute hemolytic crisis.
- Alternatively initial therapy may be started with oral zinc sulfate or tetrahydromolybdate and penicillamine started later when urinary copper excretion stabilizes.

REFERENCES

1. Czlonkowska A, Litwin T, Dusek P, Ferenci P, Lutsenko S, Medici V, et al. Nature Reviews Disease Primers article: Wilson disease. Nat Rev Dis Primers. 2019;4(1):21.
2. Chakravarty A. Movement disorders. In: Chakravarty A (Ed). Neurology and Internal Medicine: A Case-based Study. New Delhi: Jaypee Brothers Medical Publishers (P) Ltd.; 2021.
3. Prashanth LK, Taly AB, Sinha S, Arunodaya GR, Swamy HS. Wilson's disease: diagnostic errors and clinical implications. J Neurol Neurosurg Psychiatry. 2004;75:907-9.
4. Hedera P. Wilson's disease: A master of disguise. Parkinsonism Relat Disord. 2019;59:140-5.
5. Poujois A, Woimant F. Challenges in the diagnosis of Wilson disease. Ann Transl Med. 2019;7(Suppl 2):S67.
6. Walshe JM, Yealland M. Wilson's disease: the problem of delayed diagnosis. J Neurol Neurosurg Psychiatry. 1992;55:692-6.
7. Zimbrean PC, Schilsky ML. Psychiatric aspects of Wilson disease: a review. Gen Hosp Psychiatry. 2014;36(1):53-62.

An Overview of Headache Disorders and their Neuropsychiatric Aspects

Sanjay Prakash, Varoon Vadodaria

INTRODUCTION

Headache is one of the most common and debilitating symptoms seen in clinical practice. Unfortunately, misdiagnosis and mistreatment are common. Even common headaches such as migraine and tension-type headache (TTH) go undiagnosed for a number of years. The mean diagnostic delay for migraine is approximately 6 years, and a significant proportion of migraine sufferers undergo unnecessary surgery.[1] Similarly, it may take years for a patient with TTH to acquire an accurate diagnosis. The list of secondary headaches is extensive, further complicating the diagnosis.[2] Psychiatric disorders are also known to cause headaches. Moreover, epidemiological studies indicate that people with different primary headaches are more likely to develop psychiatric illnesses than subjects without headaches.[3,4] So, there may be bidirectional relations between headache disorders and psychiatric illness. Such patients can be difficult to diagnose and manage.

CLASSIFICATION AND EPIDEMIOLOGY OF HEADACHE DISORDERS

The Third Edition of the International Classification of Headache Disorders (ICHD-3) recognizes roughly 250 different forms of headaches. There are three main categories of headaches—(1) primary headaches, (2) secondary headaches, and (3) cranial neuropathies (**Box 1**). Migraine, TTH, and trigeminal autonomic cephalalgias (TACs) are referred to as the "big three" primary headaches, and all other main headache diseases are grouped together as "other primary headache disorders". Secondary headaches are classified in groups 5 through 12. Secondary headaches can be caused by both intracranial and extracranial structures, such as the skull, neck, eyes, nose, sinuses, ears, teeth, mouth, and other face or cervical structures.[2] Depending on the frequency of attacks, headaches can be classified as episodic or chronic. Headaches that occur <15 days a month are known as episodic headaches. Headaches occurring for 15 or more days per month for at least 3 consecutive months are called chronic daily headaches (CDH).[2]

About 90% of the population will suffer from headaches at some point in their lives.[5] The global prevalence of active headache disorders is estimated to be 52.0%. Globally, 50–75% of people between the ages of 18 and 65 years have experienced headaches in the past year. Each day, one in 16 people (15.8%) worldwide suffers from headaches.[6] Primary headaches are far more prevalent than secondary headaches. Primary headaches account for roughly 70–90% of headaches, with secondary headaches accounting for only 10–30% of the remainder. TTH is the most prevalent type of headache in the general population. However, migraine is the most common reason to visit a physician in both emergency and outpatient department (OPD) settings.[7] CDH affects 4% of the general population. Primary CDH include chronic migraine (CM), chronic TTH (CTTH), hemicrania continua (HC), and new daily persistent headache (NDPH).[8]

Approach to a Patient with Headache

In order to properly diagnose a headache, a thorough diagnostic approach is required.
- *Step 1*: A precise and thorough history
- *Step 2*: A complete neurological and physical assessment
- *Step 3*: Identify red flags in the patient's medical history and physical examinations
- *Step 4*: Investigations based on red flags
- *Step 5*: Formulate a diagnosis and identify comorbid conditions

> **BOX 1: International Classification of Headache Disorders (ICHD-3).[2]**
>
> *Primary headaches*:
> 1. Migraine
> 2. Tension-type headache (TTH)
> 3. Trigeminal autonomic cephalalgias (TACs)
>   3.1 Cluster headache (CH)
>   3.2 Paroxysmal hemicrania (PH)
>   3.3 Short-lasting unilateral neuralgiform headache attacks (SUNHA)
>   3.3.1 Short-lasting unilateral neuralgiform headache attacks with conjunctival injection and tearing (SUNCT)
>   3.3.2 Short-lasting unilateral neuralgiform headache attacks with cranial autonomic symptoms (SUNA)
>   3.4 Hemicrania continua (HC)
> 4. Other primary headache disorders:
>   4.1 Primary cough headache
>   4.2 Primary exercise headache
>   4.3 Primary headache associated with sexual activity
>   4.4 Primary thunderclap headache
>   4.5 Cold-stimulus headache
>   4.6 External-pressure headache
>   4.7 Primary stabbing headache
>   4.8 Nummular headache
>   4.9 Hypnic headache
>   4.10 New daily persistent headache (NDPH)
>
> *Secondary headache disorders*:
> 5. Headache attributed to trauma or injury to head and /or neck post-traumatic, and postcraniotomy
> 6. Headache attributed to cranial or cervical vascular disorder—temporal arteritis, carotid or vertebral artery dissection, cerebral-venous thrombosis, arteriovenous malformation, and aneurysm
> 7. Headache attributed to nonvascular intracranial disorder—intracranial neoplasia, Chiari malformation
> 8. Headache attributed to a substance or its withdrawal—alcohol-induced, medication-overuse headache (MOH)
> 9. Headache attributed to infection—meningitis or meningoencephalitis
> 10. Headache attributed to disorder of homoeostasis—headache due to arterial hypertension, hypoxia, and sleep apnea
> 11. Headache or facial pain attributed to disorder of the cranium, neck, eyes, ears, nose, sinuses, teeth, mouth, or other facial or cervical structure—cervicogenic headache, glaucoma
> 12. Headache attributed to psychiatric disorder—headache attributed to somatization disorder, psychotic disorder
>
> *Painful cranial neuropathies, other facial pains and other headaches*:
> 13. Painful cranial neuropathies and other facial pains
> 14. Other headache disorders

Step 1: History Taking in a Headache Patient[9]

History Addressing Patient Demographics

It includes age, sex, risk factors for hypercoagulable states (pregnancy, postpartum state, etc.), and associated other disorders (tuberculosis, malignancy, HIV infection, etc.). These factors aid in identifying red flags in patients.

History Addressing Headache Characteristics

It includes the *onset* of headaches, *duration* of illness, *pattern* of headache (episodic, continuous, or progressive), *site* of pain, *intensity* of pain, *character* of pain, *duration* of each attack, *and frequency* of attacks. The mode of onset and progression plays a key role in identifying the type of headache. A primary headache is characterized by recurrent episodic attacks. ICHD-3 defines the minimum number of attacks necessary for the diagnosis of primary headaches [five attacks for migraine without aura, five attacks for cluster headache (CH), and 10 attacks for TTH]. Similarly, ICHD-3 has specified the duration of attacks for a number of primary headaches—migraine lasts 4–72 hours, TTH lasts 30 minutes–7 days, and CH lasts 15–180 minutes.

History Addressing Associated Symptoms

Is there anything else wrong with you other than the headaches? It includes: (1) Constitutional symptoms—fever, weight loss, cough, breathlessness, etc., (2) suggesting intracranial pathologies (seizures, double vision, visual disturbances, gait problems, cognitive problems, etc.), (3) suggesting migrainous features (nausea, vomiting, photophobia, phonophobia, and auras), (4) cranial autonomic symptoms (lacrimation, conjunctival injection, rhinorrhea, etc.)

Step 2: Neurological and Physical Assessment

A complete physical and neurological evaluation is required for any new headaches or headaches with red flags. But in other circumstances, the examination can be limited.

- *The bare minimum examination in each patient*: Check each patient's blood pressure, fundi for papilledema, and meningeal signs even if there are no red flags. Although hypertension is not a common cause of headaches, a sudden rise in blood pressure may result in a headache. Moreover, headaches may be the only symptom of hypertension. Similarly, papilledema may be the only sign in patients with idiopathic intracranial hypertension. Neck stiffness may be the only sign of meningeal inflammation in aseptic (noninfectious) or subacute-to-chronic meningitis.
- *In the elderly*: Temporal arteritis (TA) and subacute angle closure glaucoma (SACG) can both appear with headache as the sole symptom. Therefore, temporal artery thickness as well as intraocular pressure should also be assessed in all elderly individuals who have recently developed headaches.[10]
- *Localized or side-locked headaches*: Several extracranial structures, such as neck, vessels, nose, sinuses, eyes, ears, oral-cavity, teeth, and the other facial structures may cause localized or side-locked headaches. Such patients may require extensive examination of local structures. Patients can be sent to ophthalmology, ENT, and dental departments for examinations if pains are predominantly localized to the eyes, around the nose-ear or in the oral cavity.[10]

Step 3: Identification of Red Flags

Identify red flags in the patient's medical history and physical examinations. Red flags can be:

- *Patient-specific*: It defines the epidemiological or demographic features of patients. It can be an elderly patient, a pregnant patient, a known case of tuberculosis or malignancy, human immunodeficiency virus (HIV), or a history of trauma. Any headaches in this group constitute a red flag. The prevalence of secondary headaches is about 1% in new-onset headaches in patients under the age of 50 years. After age 50, the prevalence increases significantly, reaching 6% in individuals over 50 and 12% after 75%.[11] Therefore, a new-onset headaches in a person over the age of 50 is cause for concern. The prevalence of secondary headaches varied between 30 and 40% among pregnant patients with new-onset headaches. Similarly, the prevalence of secondary headaches ranged from 30 to 70% in postpartum women with new-onset headaches. So, just having headaches during pregnancy or postpartum period is a red flag.[12]
- *Headache characteristics*: particularly pertaining to the onset, pattern, severity, and location of headaches. A sudden severe headache that peaks within 60 seconds is called thunderclap headache. Thunderclap headache is probably the most important and dangerous red flag that require urgent investigations. A new onset progressive headache may be indicative if intracranial space occupying lesions.
- *Headache triggers*: headaches triggered by Valsalva-like activities may be due to intracranial pathologies.
- *Associated symptoms or signs*: Any additional symptoms (neurological or systemic) that do not fit the migraine aura criteria should be taken seriously.

The traditional mnemonic for red flags is SNOOP4. Recently, a few additional points have been added, and it is now SNNOOP10 **(Table 1)**.[13]

Step 4: Investigations to Confirm or Rule Out Secondary Headaches

The selection of investigations is based on the presence of red flags or provisional diagnoses.[14]

- *Neuroimaging*: Investigation is typically not necessary for an isolated headache that meets the ICHD-3 criteria for either TTH or migraine. Neuroimaging is required in all suspected cases of TACs, other primary headaches, and neuralgias. All patients with red flags must have neuroimaging. In an emergency situation (a history of trauma or a sudden-onset headache), a computed tomography (CT) scan is suggested. Magnetic resonance imaging (MRI) is a preferable choice in all other circumstances.
- *Cerebrospinal fluid (CSF) examinations*: In the acute setting, CSF analysis is important to rule out infectious or inflammatory diseases in the meninges or brain parenchyma. RBCs and xanthochromia in the CSF may be signs of subarachnoid hemorrhage. In the chronic setting, CSF pressure monitoring is important to rule out idiopathic intracranial hypertension and CSF hypotension.

TABLE 1: Red flags in headache patients-mnemonics (SNNOOP10).[13]

Letter	Mnemonics (SNNOOP10)	Clinical descriptions	Secondary headaches
S	Systemic	Fever	Infection (sinus, teeth, meninges, etc.), temporal arteritis (TA), malignancy
		Weight loss	Malignancy, TA
		Cough	Carcinoma lung, tuberculosis
N	Neoplasm	History of carcinoma	Intracranial metastasis
N	Neurological	Visual disturbances	Glaucoma, optic neuritis, TA
		Cognitive, motor, sensory, or cerebellar abnormality	Intracranial pathologies (infections and malignancy)
O	Onset sudden	Peak within a few minutes	Aneurysmal rupture, cervical artery dissection, reversible cerebral vasoconstriction syndrome (RCVS)
O	Older age (>50 years)	New headache in elderly	Glaucoma, TA, malignancy, cervicogenic headache
P1	Pattern change	Recent change in pattern	Malignancy, infections
P2	Positional headache	Orthostatic, recumbent, or worsens with change in position	Low intracranial pressure (CSF leak), mass lesion, cerebral venous sinus thrombosis, and sinus pathology
P3	Precipitated by Valsalva	Coughing, sneezing, and straining	Intracranial/posterior fossa mass, Chiari malformation
P4	Papilledema	Visual symptoms	Intracranial pathologies, idiopathic intracranial hypertension
P5	Progressive	Persistent and progressive	Intracranial mass lesion, cerebral venous thrombosis (CVT)
P6	Pregnancy or puerperium	History of amenorrhea, childbirth	CVT, preeclampsia, pituitary lesion, RCVS
P7	Painful eye with autonomic features	Painful opthalmoplegia	cavernous sinus pathologies, Tolosa–Hunt syndrome; ophthalmic causes
P8	Post-traumatic	History of trauma	Subdural hematoma
P9	Pathology of the immune system	HIV, immunocompromised host	CNS infections
P10	Painkiller overuse	Overuse or new drug at onset of headache	Medication overuse headache

- *Other investigations*: Patients with red flags might require a number of tests. Erythrocyte sedimentation rate (ESR) and C-reactive protein (CRP) should be measured in all elderly individuals above the age of 50 years. ECG and Echo are advised for elderly people with vascular risk factors to rule out cardiac cephalalgia.

Step 5: Formulate the Diagnosis

Most secondary headaches are discovered through the appropriate investigations. Once the possibility of secondary headache is excluded, a diagnosis of primary headache is made. Most primary headaches are easily diagnosed if a physician is familiar with these disease entities. A few key characteristics of common primary and secondary headaches will be discussed here.

PRIMARY HEADACHES

Migraine

Migraine and TTH are the two most common primary headache disorders. **Table 2** provides a comparative view of the ICHD-3 diagnostic criteria of migraine and TTH.[2] The headache characteristics of migraine appear to be the exact opposite of TTH. However, neither migraine nor TTH has any specific symptoms, and the two conditions are commonly confused with one another. Unilateral pain, throbbing quality, severe intensity, headache aggravation by routine activities, and nausea-vomiting are suggestive of migraine. A mnemonic (DON) has been suggested to identify migraine. DON indicates disabling headache, one-day headache, and nausea during attacks.[15] There are two

TABLE 2: A comparison of diagnostic criteria of migraine and tension-type headache.[2]

	Particulars	Migraine without aura	Tension-type headache
A	Number of attacks	At least 5 attacks	At least 10 attacks
B	Attack duration	4–72 hours	30 minutes–7 days
C	Headache characteristics (Any two)		
	Location	Unilateral	Bilateral
	Quality	Pulsating	Nonpulsating
	Intensity	Moderate or severe	Mild or moderate
	Aggravation by	Routine physical activity (e.g., walking or climbing stairs)	no aggravation by routine physical activity
D	Associated symptoms	At least one of the following:	Both of the following:
		1. Nausea and/or vomiting	1. No nausea or vomiting
		2. Photophobia and phonophobia	2. No more than one of photophobia and phonophobia
E	Exclusion of other headaches	Not better accounted for by another ICHD-3 diagnosis	Not better accounted for by another ICHD-3 diagnosis

main types of migraines—(1) migraine without aura and (2) migraine with aura. Migraine with aura is distinguished by the transitory focal neurological features that primarily precede or sometimes accompany the headache. Visual and sensory are two most common auras. Other auras include speech, motor, brainstem, and retinal auras. Auras typically develop gradually, and headaches are frequently experienced afterward.[2]

Tension-type Headache

The TTH is the most common primary headache. TTH is frequently referred to as a "tension headache". The term "tension" does not, however, imply that the patient is experiencing mental tension or stress. Bilateral pain, nonthrobbing quality, mild-to-moderate intensity, no aggravation by routine activities, and absence of nausea-vomiting during attacks are suggestive of TTH.[2]

Trigeminal Autonomic Cephalalgias

The TACs are a group of four headaches that include CH, paroxysmal hemicrania (PH), short-lasting unilateral neuralgiform headache attacks (SUNHA), and HC. SUNHA includes two subtypes of headaches—(1) short-lasting unilateral neuralgiform headache with conjunctival injection and tearing (SUNCT), and (2) short-lasting unilateral neuralgiform headache attacks with cranial autonomic symptoms (SUNA). All four TACs share the following three clinical characteristics—(1) severe or very severe strictly unilateral headache in the trigeminal distribution; (2) ipsilateral cranial autonomic features in the trigeminal distribution; and (3) agitation or restlessness during attack. The TACs differ in the duration and frequency of headaches, as well as the drugs used to treat these headaches **(Table 3)**. All TACs are episodic with the exception of HC, which is characterized by continuous headaches. CH has relatively few attacks per day and the longest attack durations (15–180 minutes). PH has a mid-range attack frequency and mid-range attack duration (2–30 minutes). The shortest attack time (1–600 seconds) and maximum attack frequency are noted in SUNCT and SUNA.[2]

Other Primary Headaches

There are 10 headaches in this group. The clues for the diagnosis of most of these disorders are in their names. Most of these headache disorders have hints in their names that can help with diagnosis. A few of them are triggered by a specific precipitating factor that is specified in their titles—primary cough headache, primary exercise headache, primary headache associated with sexual activity, cold-stimulus headache, and external-pressure headache. Nummular headache, also known as coin-shaped headache, is characterized by persistent pain at a specific location on the head, typically in a rounded or coin-shaped area. A hypnic headache is a headache that occurs only during sleep. NDPH is a form of chronic daily headache that begins suddenly one day and typically does not abate.[2]

TABLE 3: A comparison of the ICHD-3 diagnostic criteria of all four TACs.[2]

Cluster headache	Paroxysmal hemicrania	SUNHA (SUNCT-SUNA)	Hemicrania continua
A. At least five attacks fulfilling criteria B–D	A. At least 20 attacks fulfilling criteria B–E	A. At least 20 attacks fulfilling criteria B–D	A. Unilateral headache fulfilling criteria B–D
B. Severe or very severe unilateral orbital, supraorbital and/or temporal pain lasting 15–180 minutes (when untreated)	B. Severe unilateral orbital, supraorbital and/or temporal pain lasting 2–30 minutes	B. Moderate or severe unilateral head pain, with orbital, supraorbital, temporal, and/or other trigeminal distribution, lasting for 1–600 seconds	B. Present for >3 months, with exacerbations of moderate or greater intensity

C. Either or both of the following:
1. At least one of the following symptoms or signs, ipsilateral to the headache:
  a. Conjunctival injection and/or lacrimation
  b. Nasal congestion and/or rhinorrhea
  c. Eyelid edema
  d. Forehead and facial sweating
  e. Miosis and/or ptosis
2. A sense of restlessness or agitation
	C. Either or both of the following:
	1. At least one of the following symptoms or signs, ipsilateral to the headache:
	  a. Conjunctival injection and/or lacrimation
	  b. Nasal congestion and/or rhinorrhea
	  c. Eyelid edema
	  d. Forehead and facial sweating
	  e. Miosis and/or ptosis
	2. A sense of restlessness or agitation
		C. At least one of the following five cranial autonomic symptoms or signs, ipsilateral to the pain:
		1. Conjunctival injection and/or lacrimation
		2. Nasal congestion and/or rhinorrhea
		3. Eyelid edema
		4. Forehead and facial sweating
		5. Miosis and/or ptosis
			C. Either or both of the following:
			1. At least one of the following symptoms or signs, ipsilateral to the headache:
			  a. Conjunctival injection and/or lacrimation
			  b. Nasal congestion and/or rhinorrhea
			  c. Eyelid edema
			  d. Forehead and facial sweating
			  e. Miosis and/or ptosis
			2. A sense of restlessness or agitation, or aggravation of the pain by movement

D. Occurring with a frequency between one every other day and 8 per day	D. Occurring with a frequency of >5 per day	D. Occurring with a frequency of at least one a day	
	E. Prevented absolutely by therapeutic doses of Indomethacin		D. Responds absolutely to therapeutic doses of indomethacin
E. Not better accounted for by another ICHD-3 diagnosis	F. Not better accounted for by another ICHD-3 diagnosis	E. Not better accounted for by another ICHD-3 diagnosis	E. Not better accounted for by another ICHD-3 diagnosis

(ICHD: International Classification of Headache Disorders; SUNA: short-lasting unilateral neuralgiform headache attacks with cranial autonomic symptoms; SUNCT: short-lasting unilateral neuralgiform headache with conjunctival injection and tearing; SUNHA: short-lasting unilateral neuralgiform headache attack; TAC: trigeminal autonomic cephalalgia)

SECONDARY HEADACHES

There are roughly 250 different forms of secondary headaches. A few secondary headaches are discussed here.

Sinus Headache

It is mentioned here to draw attention to the fact that it is a highly over diagnosed condition. It was found that >80% of patients who were given the diagnosis of "sinus headache" actually had migraine.[16] Anteriorly situated headaches (frontal headaches) with autonomic symptoms of migraine, such as rhinorrhea and nasal congestion, are incorrectly labeled as "sinus headaches".

Headache Attributed to Refractory Errors

Similar to sinus headaches, refractive errors are also a frequently over diagnosed cause of headaches. Only very high dioptric errors (greater than ± 6D) cause headaches. Eyeball pain may be present more than half of the patients with migraine. Moreover, migraine patients may have cranial autonomic features related to eye (conjunctival injection and tearing). These patients may have mild refractory errors. Headaches in such people are usually misdiagnosed as headaches due to refractory errors.[17]

Medication Overuse Headache

Medication overuse headache (MOH) is a chronic headache that occurs >15 days per month in patients who have used headache medication excessively for >3 months.[2] So, MOH happens in people who already have a headache. Such patients experience a vicious cycle of headaches, using increasing amounts of painkillers to treat them, which actually leads to nearly daily headaches. In parallel, patients develop irritability, restlessness, insomnia, generalized body pain, depression, anxiety, and memory problems. Overuse is measured in terms of treatment days per month and varies according to the type of medicine. For a simple analgesic to cause MOH, it must be taken for 15 days each month for 3 months. For ergotamine, triptan, and opioid induced MOH, the days of drug usage are ≥ 10 days per month for 3 months. Stopping the overused medication(s) is the first step in treating MOH and breaking the cycle of headaches. However, it may cause withdrawal symptoms that may include nausea, anxiety, restlessness, and abdominal discomfort or diarrhea.[18]

Headaches Attributed to or Associated with Psychiatric Disorders

Both headaches and psychiatric disorders are prevalent in the general population. Therefore, comorbidity by chance is to be expected. However, epidemiological data demonstrate a higher than predicted frequency of comorbidity between headaches and psychiatric diseases.[2] Therefore, a causal association between a psychiatric disease and a new or rapidly worsening headache may exist. The relationship could be bidirectional, with the headache causing the psychiatric problem and the psychiatric disorder causing the headache. The risk of migraine in patients with depression was three times higher than in people without depression. Migraine patients have a five times higher risk of developing depression than those without a history of headaches. Patients suffering from migraine with aura are three times more likely to suffer from bipolar illness than the overall population. On the other hand, migraines are present in around a third of bipolar disorder patients. Patients with bipolar disorder have a higher frequency of migraines, which can be as high as 55%. Depression or bipolar disorder is also a significant predictor of the chronification of migraine.[3,4]

Patients with migraine have a two-to-five times higher prevalence of anxiety problems than the general population. Patients with CM experience anxiety considerably more frequently than those with episodic migraine. Migraines occur more frequently and with greater severity in patients with obsessive-compulsive disorder (OCD).[3]

These concomitant psychiatric disorders in patients with headaches, if left untreated, might increase the risk of migraine chronification, and episodic migraine may turn into CM. Furthermore, concomitant psychiatric disorders might worsen migraine-related disability, lower quality of life, and impair treatment outcomes.[3]

Similar to migraine, bidirectional relationship between psychiatric disorders and TTH are noted. Population-based studies have shown that those with TTH are more likely to suffer from psychiatric disorders such as anxiety and depression than those without TTH.[19] The frequency and severity of TTH attacks are linked to depression and anxiety. The prevalence of anxiety or mood problems may be 3–15 times higher in patients with CTTH than in controls.[20]

The NDPH also exhibits a high prevalence of several psychiatric symptoms. All psychiatric symptoms were significantly more common in NDPH patients than in healthy controls, migraine sufferers, or those with chronic low back pain.[21] In one study from India, up to 85.5% of NDPH patients noted psychiatric symptoms.[22] In one study, anxiety and depression were more common in patients with NDPH than migraine. One of the most frequent triggers of NDPH is stressful life events.

The ICHD-3 has recognized two types of headache attributed to psychiatric disorders **(Table 4)**—(1) headache attributed to somatization disorder and (2) headache attributed to psychotic disorder. **Table 5** shows the ICHD-3 diagnostic criteria for both disorders.[2] Although the ICHD-3 recognizes headache as a symptom of somatization disorder, the Diagnostic and Statistical Manual of Mental Disorders (DSM-5) has replaced somatization disorder with a new category called somatic symptom disorder.

TABLE 4: Headache attributed to psychiatric disorder (ICHD-3).[2]

ICHD-3 code	Diseases
12	Headache attributed to psychiatric disorder
12.1	Headache attributed to somatization disorder
12.2	Headache attributed to psychotic disorder
A	Appendix
A12.3	Headache attributed to depressive disorder
A12.4	Headache attributed to separation anxiety disorder
A12.5	Headache attributed to panic disorder
A12.6	Headache attributed to specific phobia
A12.7	Headache attributed to social anxiety disorder (social phobia)
A12.8	Headache attributed to generalized anxiety disorder
A12.9	Headache attributed to post-traumatic stress disorder (PTSD)

TABLE 5: Headache attributed to psychiatric disorder (ICHD-3).[2]

	Particulars	Headache attributed to somatization disorder	Headache attributed to psychotic disorder
A	Any headache	Any headache fulfilling criterion C	Any headache fulfilling criterion C

B	A diagnosis of psychiatry disorders	A diagnosis has been made of somatization disorder. Include both of the following:
		1. A history of multiple physical symptoms beginning before age 30 years
		2. All of the following:
		  a. At least four pain symptoms
		  b. At least two gastrointestinal symptoms
		  c. At least one sexual symptom
		  d. At least one pseudo neurological symptom
			Presence of a delusion

C	Evidence of causation	At least three of the following: 1. Headache has evolved or worsened in parallel with symptoms of somatization 2. Constant or remitting headache parallels in time the fluctuation of somatic symptoms 3. Headache has remitted in parallel with remission of somatization disorder	Either or both of the following: 1. Headache has developed with or after the onset of the delusion, or led to its diagnosis 2. Headache has remitted after remission of the delusion
D	Exclusion of other diagnosis	Not better accounted for by another [International Classification of Headache Disorders (ICHD-3)] diagnosis	Not better accounted for by another ICHD-3 diagnosis

In addition to these two, seven other types of headaches related to psychiatric disorders have been discussed in the "Appendix" section **Table 4**. However, there is no strong evidence to imply a causal relationship between headaches and the disorders described in the "Appendix" section. All subtypes have the same general diagnostic criteria, as follows: (A) Any headache fulfilling criterion C; (B) psychiatric disorders have been diagnosed according to DSM-5 criteria; (C) headache occurs exclusively during given psychiatric disorder; and (D) not better accounted for by another ICHD-3 diagnosis.

MANAGEMENT

Headache management includes headache education, pharmacological management, nonpharmacological management, and surgical intervention. Pharmacological management includes treating acute attacks (abortive therapy) and preventing episodes in the future (preventive or prophylactic therapy).

Education

If patients have primary headaches, reassure them that their condition is benign. Most primary headaches are relapsing-remitting in nature. Make an attempt to persuade them to understand the relapsing-remitting nature of the primary headaches. Currently available medications can lower the frequency, severity, duration, and other disabilities, but it cannot be cured completely. Relapse can occur at any time, with no warning and without any precipitating factors. Patients must find out their headache triggers. In order to effectively manage headaches, triggers must be avoided. Patients should make lifestyle changes if they experience frequent headaches. Patients with migraine and TTH benefit significantly from adequate hydration, proper eating and sleeping habits, regular exercise, and stress reduction. Patients should be made aware of the therapeutic limitations of medications. In the beginning, a 50% decrease in attack frequency may be regarded as a good outcome. There may be a delay before the desired effects of a medication become evident. Patients may experience headache attacks despite taking regular medications.

Pharmacological Management

Migraine

Treatments for migraine include abortive and prophylactic medications **(Tables 6 and 7)**. Abortive medications should be administered as soon as the headache begins, when the headache is still mild. Simple analgesics (acetaminophen and aspirin) and nonsteroidal anti-inflammatory drugs (NSAIDs) are first-line agents for acute migraine treatment. In most comparison studies, NSAIDs are more effective than acetaminophen and

TABLE 6: Specific acute migraine treatments.

Drugs	Dose
First-line agents:	
• Simple analgesic:	
○ Acetaminophen	1,000 mg
○ Aspirin	1,000 mg
• NSAIDs:	
○ Ibuprofen	400 mg
○ Naproxen	500 mg
○ Diclofenac	100 mg
○ Ketoprofen	75 mg
Second-line agents:	
• Triptan:	
○ Almotriptan	12.5–25 mg
○ Eletriptan	20–40 mg
○ Frovatriptan	2.5–5.0 mg
○ Naratriptan	2.5–5.0 mg
○ Rizatriptan	5–15 mg
○ Sumatriptan	25–300 mg
○ Zolmitriptan	2.5–0 mg
Third-line agents:	
• Gepants	
○ Rimegepant	75 mg
○ Ubrogepant	50–200 mg
• Ditans	
○ Lasmiditan	50–200 mg

TABLE 7: Preventive therapy in migraine.

Drugs	Dose/Day
First-line agents:	
• Anticonvulsants:	
○ Topiramate	50–200 mg oral/day
• Beta-blocker:	
○ Propranolol	40–160 mg oral/day
○ Metoprolol	50–200 mg oral/day
○ Atenolol	50–200 mg oral/day
○ Bisoprolol	5–10 mg oral/day
• Angiotensin II-receptor blocker:	
○ Candesartan	16–32 mg oral/day
Second-line agents:	
• Anticonvulsants:	
○ Sodium valproate	400–1,600 mg oral/day
• Calcium antagonist:	
○ Flunarizine	5–10 mg oral/day
• Tricyclic antidepressant:	
○ Amitriptyline	10–100 mg oral/day
Third-line agents:	
• Botulinum toxin	Injection in muscles, every 4–6 months
• CGRP mAbs:	
○ Erenumab	70–140 mg, SC, monthly
○ Fremanezumab	225 mg SC, monthly
○ Galcanezumab	120 mg SC, monthly

aspirin. Triptans are second-line medications that should be taken if NSAIDs or simple analgesics are not providing adequate headache relief. A drug is considered ineffective if there is no or minimal therapeutic response in three consecutive episodes. If one triptan is useless, others may still be helpful. If all available triptans are ineffective, third-line medicines (ditans and gepants) or other medications can be used.[23,24]

Preventive medication is necessary for patients who suffer from frequent attacks (more than two per month), severe attacks, or attacks that persist for several days. It usually takes time for a preventative treatment to show results. A drug is considered ineffective if there is no or insufficient response in 2–3 months. An alternative should be sought if a therapeutic dose of an oral preventative medicine is ineffective after 2–3 months.[23]

Tension-type Headache

Like migraine, treatments for TTH include abortive and prophylactic medications. Simple analgesics (paracetamol or aspirin) or NSAIDs are the main drugs in the acute therapy of TTH. However, NSAIDs are superior to acetaminophen and aspirin in most of the comparative studies. Ibuprofen (400–800 mg) is the drug of choice for acute TTH, followed by naproxen sodium (375–825 mg) due to its lower incidence of gastric adverse effects. Some patients may respond better to the combination of analgesics with caffeine, sedatives, or tranquillizers than to NSAIDs or simple analgesics.[25]

Preventive therapy is considered in patients who suffer from frequent attacks (2–3 headache days/week). Amitriptyline is the treatment of choice for chronic or frequent episodic TTH. If amitriptyline is not well tolerated, other antidepressants such as mirtazapine, venlafaxine, doxepin, nortriptyline, protriptyline, and nortriptyline may be used. The effect of the antidepressants in the headaches of TTH is not related to the presence of depression.[25]

Trigeminal Autonomic Cephalalgias

The HC and PH respond dramatically to therapeutic doses of indomethacin. The first-line treatment for SUNCT/SUNA is lamotrigine. Acute therapy is not required for patients with PH and SUNHA, as these are short-lasting headaches. Patients with CH, on the other hand, require abortive medicines because it can last a few hours. For an acute CH attack, oxygen inhalation and subcutaneous sumatriptan are recommended. Verapamil and lithium are first-line agents for the initial preventive therapy for CH.[2,26]

Nonpharmacological Management

Nutraceuticals

Nutraceuticals are "natural" substances that are derived from food sources. The nutraceuticals found to be effective in migraine include feverfew, butterbur, vitamin B2, magnesium, coenzyme Q10, and vitamin D.[27]

Behavioral Therapy

Behavioral approaches intended to modify maladaptive behaviors and thought that could increase headaches and headache-related disabilities. It include biofeedback (BFB), relaxation therapy, cognitive behavioral therapy (CBT), mindfulness-based therapy, and acceptance and commitment therapy (ACT).[27,28]

In BFB, an individual can learn to actively control and self-regulate their physiological responses related to headaches. BFB training may be effective in a subset of patients with CM and CTTH.

Relaxation therapies include muscle group relaxation exercises to decrease sympathetic arousal and physiological responses to stress. CBT refers to psychological therapies that combine cognitive (thought-based) and behavioral (action-based) intervention components. Patients first recognize abnormal thoughts, behaviors, and reactions to stress that worsen or trigger headaches. Patients later modify their behaviors by changing their attitudes towards the relevant issues.

Mindfulness-based therapy is a modified form of CBT that incorporates mindfulness practices that include present moment awareness in a nonjudgmental way, meditation, and breathing exercises. The frequency and duration of headache attacks among CM and CTTH patients were reported to have decreased in various studies after mindfulness-based therapy.

In ACT, acceptance is considered a way to deal with negative thoughts, feelings, symptoms, or circumstances. The goal of ACT is to alter the patients' thoughts and emotions so that they no longer perceive them as "symptoms."

Noninvasive Neuromodulation

Although earlier neuromodulation treatments were invasive, various noninvasive neuromodulation techniques have lately been developed. It included transcranial magnetic stimulation (TMS), single pulse TMS (sTMS), repetitive TMS (rTMS), supraorbital nerve stimulation (SNS), transcranial direct current stimulation (tDCS), noninvasive vagal nerve stimulation (nVNS), caloric vestibular stimulation (CVS), and nonpainful remote electrical skin stimulation. The readers are encouraged to read the related article for details.[27,29]

Surgical Interventions

Botulinum toxin injection is one of the treatment options for patients with CM. However, there are several other surgical interventions that are mainly used in patients who did not respond to conventional treatment or who could not tolerate the side effects of medications.[30] Surgical interventions for various primary headaches include peripheral nerve block, ganglion block (sphenopalatine), radiofrequency ablation, neuromodulation (occipital nerve stimulation, vagus nerve stimulation, sphenopalatine ganglion stimulation, and SNS), and decompression surgery. The readers are encouraged to read the related article for details.

CONCLUDING REMARKS

There are around 18 different types of primary headaches and over 250 different types of secondary headaches. However, up to 90% of patients who go to clinics for headaches have primary headaches, especially migraine. However, a primary headache is diagnosed only after the possibility of secondary headaches has been ruled out. Red flags guide us for appropriate investigations to rule out secondary headaches. Education regarding headaches is an essential component of headache management. The majority of primary headaches respond to some specific class of drugs. An early and proper treatment is important to prevent the development of MOH.

LEARNING POINTS

- Primary headaches are more prevalent than secondary headaches in clinical practice.
- Identification of red flags through history taking and physical examinations is critical for ruling out secondary headaches.
- Primary headaches are diagnosed though ICHD-3 criteria.
- There is bidirectional relationship between psychiatric symptoms and headaches, with the headache causing the psychiatric problem and the psychiatric disorder causing the headache.
- Early intervention is necessary to prevent the chronification of primary headaches.

REFERENCES

1. Al-Hashel JY, Ahmed SF, Alroughani R, Goadsby PJ. Migraine misdiagnosis as a sinusitis, a delay that can last for many years. J Headache Pain. 2013;14:97.
2. Headache Classification Committee of the International Headache Society (IHS) The International Classification of Headache Disorders, 3rd edition. Cephalalgia. 2018;38(1):1-211.
3. Minen MT, De Dhaem OB, Van Diest AK, Kroon Van Diest A, Powers S, et al. Migraine and its psychiatric comorbidities. J Neurol Neurosurg Psychiatry. 2016;87(7):741-9.
4. Dresler T, Caratozzolo S, Guldolf K, Huhn JI, Loiacono C, Niiberg-Pikksööt T, et al. Understanding the nature of psychiatric comorbidity in migraine: A systematic review focused on interactions and treatment implications. J Headache Pain. 2019; 20(1):51.
5. Rasmussen BK, Jensen R, Schroll M, Olesen J. Epidemiology of headache in a general population—a prevalence study. J Clin Epidemiol. 1991;44:1147-57.
6. Stovner LJ, Hagen K, Linde M, Steiner TJ. The global prevalence of headache: an update, with analysis of the influences of methodological factors on prevalence estimates. J Headache Pain. 2022;23(1):34.
7. Tepper SJ, Dahlöf CG, Dowson A, Newman L, Mansbach H, Jones M, et al. Prevalence and diagnosis of migraine in patients consulting their physician with a complaint of headache: data from the Landmark Study. Headache. 2004;44(9):856-64.
8. Yancey JR, Sheridan R, Koren KG. Chronic daily headache: diagnosis and management. Am Fam Physician. 2014;89(8):642-8.
9. Ravishankar K. The art of history-taking in a headache patient. Ann Indian Acad Neurol. 2012;15(S1):S7-S14.
10. Prakash S, Rathore C. Side-locked headaches: an algorithm-based approach. J Headache Pain. 2016;17(1):1-4.
11. Goldstein JN, Camargo Jr CA, Pelletier AJ, Edlow JA. Headache in United States emergency departments: demographics, work-up and frequency of pathological diagnoses. Cephalalgia. 2006;26(6):684-90.
12. Sandoe CH, Lay C. Secondary headaches during pregnancy: when to worry. Curr Neurol Neurosci Rep. 2019;19(6):27.
13. Do TP, Remmers A, Schytz HW, Schankin C, Nelson SE, Obermann M, et al. Red and orange flags for secondary headaches in clinical practice: SNNOOP10 list. Neurology. 2019;92(3):134-44.
14. Ravishankar K. WHICH headache to investigate, WHEN, and HOW?. Headache. 2016;56(10):1685-97.
15. Prakash S, Rana K. Pitfalls in the Diagnosis of Migraine, Chronic Migraine, and Medication Overuse Headaches. In: Chakravarty A (Ed). Pitfalls in the Diagnosis of Neurological Disorders, 1st edition. Delhi: Jaypee Brothers Medical Publishers (P) Ltd.; India. 2022. pp. 75-81.
16. Lipton RB, Diamond S, Reed M, Diamond ML, Stewart WF. Migraine diagnosis and treatment: Results from the American Migraine Study II. Headache. 2001;41(7):638-45.
17. Roth Z, Pandolfo KR, Simon J, obal-Ratner J. Headache and refractive errors in children. J Pediatr Ophthalmol Strabismus. 2014;51(3):177-9.
18. Diener HC, Dodick D, Evers S, Holle D, Jensen RH, Lipton RB, et al. Pathophysiology, prevention, and treatment of medication overuse headache. Lancet Neurol. 2019;18(9):891-902.
19. Romero-Godoy R, Romero-Godoy SR, Romero-Acebal M, Gutiérrez-Bedmar M. Psychiatric comorbidity and emotional dysregulation in chronic tension-type headache: A Case-control study. J Clin Med. 2022;11(17):5090.
20. Song TJ, Cho SJ, Kim WJ, Yang KI, Yun CH, Chu MK. Anxiety and depression in tension-type headache: A population-based study. PLoS One. 2016;11(10):e0165316.
21. Peng KP, Wang SJ. Update of new daily persistent headache. Curr Pain Headache Rep. 2022;26(1):79-84.
22. Uniyal R, Paliwal VK, Tripathi A. Psychiatric comorbidity in new daily persistent headache: A cross-sectional study. Eur J Pain. 2017;21:1031-8.
23. Eigenbrodt AK, Ashina H, Khan S, Diener HC, Mitsikostas DD, Sinclair AJ, et al. Diagnosis and management of migraine in ten steps. Nat Rev Neurol. 2021;17(8):501-14.
24. Ailani J, Burch RC, Robbins MS; Board of Directors of the American Headache Society. The American Headache Society Consensus Statement: Update on integrating new migraine treatments into clinical practice. Headache. 2021;61(7):1021-39.
25. Bentivegna E, Luciani M, Paragliola V, Baldari F, Lamberti PA, Conforti G, et al. Recent advancements in tension-type headache: A narrative review. Expert Rev Neurother. 2021;21(7):793-803.
26. Nahas SJ. Cluster headache and other trigeminal autonomic cephalalgias. Continuum (Minneap Minn). 2021;27(3):633-51.
27. Grazzi L, Toppo C, D'Amico D, Leonardi M, Martelletti P, Raggi A, et al. Non-pharmacological approaches to headaches: Non-invasive neuromodulation, nutraceuticals, and behavioral approaches. Int J Environ Res Public Health. 2021;18(4):1503.
28. Bae JY, Sung HK, Kwon NY, Go HY, Kim TJ, Shin SM, et al. Cognitive behavioral therapy for migraine headache: A systematic review and meta-analysis. Medicina. 2021;58(1):44.
29. Coppola G, Magis D, Casillo F, Sebastianelli G, Abagnale C, Cioffi E, et al. Neuromodulation for chronic daily headache. Curr Pain Headache Rep. 2022;26(3):267-78.
30. Plato BM, Whitt M. Interventional Procedures in Episodic Migraine. Curr Pain Headache Rep. 2020;24(12):75.

COMMENTARY 15

A Note on Medication Overuse Headache

Ambar Chakravarty

CASE VIGNETTE

A 43-year-old lady doctor had over 20 years history of migraine without aura which had been mostly menstrual and she used to take two to three tablets of naproxen 250 mg every month which used to give her some relief. She consulted the present author in 2014 with daily headaches—pulsatile and dull band like even while on topiramate (TPM) 150 mg/day and she started taking naproxen + over the counter pain killers often in addition. TPM was changed to divalproate and in spite of warning on the risks of medication overuse headache (MOH) she continued to overuse NSAIDs + pain killers. Later naproxen was stopped and she could be managed with a combination of divalproate 1,000 mg and gabapentin 1,200 mg with only brief monthly headaches relieved with nasal zolmitriptan. She was seen again in February 2016 with daily headaches which recurred and she was taking zolmitriptan NS 2–3 times/day + frequent doses of naproxen + gabapentin 1,200 mg/day + divalproate 1,000 mg/day. She was strongly advised against frequent use of zolmitriptan + naproxen. She reported no benefit and a bilateral greater occipital nerve block was given which relieved her daily headaches for a brief period. With recurrence of daily headache after about 1 week, she was given a course of botulinum toxin, results were not very satisfactory and she reverted back to frequent compulsive use of naproxen and over-the-counter (OTC) pain killers along with gabapentin and divalproate. Counseling was started but she was crazy about getting a Cefaly device [a form of transcutaneous electrical nerve stimulation (TENS) therapy]. After she got hold of a Cefaly device, counseling was continued and the therapy was changed to divalproate and amitriptyline. Some improvement was observed and she took a European holiday and seemed very happy. However, she changed her job at least three times during this period presumably due to problems with colleagues in the hospitals. *In Mid-2017*, she was seen for daily headaches almost 24 hours for >3 weeks → daily intake of naproxen 500–1,000 mg + 2–3 OTC painkillers + Cefaly. She was advised accordingly with counseling + a short course of steroids + TPM + amitriptyline. She changed her job again and defaulted from the clinic. She came back in January 2019 with daily headaches while she had been taking 2–3 tablets of oral triptan daily. She was strongly advised against such use to which she agreed. Soon she was admitted to intensive coronary care unit (ICCU) with vasospastic angina and coronary angiography revealed a myocardial bridge. She never returned to Neurology thereafter.

DISCUSSION

The International Classification of Headache Disorders, 3rd edition (ICHD-3) headache diagnosis would be chronic migraine with MOH.

It has been known since the 1950s that an excessive use of acute medication can cause headache to worsen and that withdrawal from the overused substances can restore the headache pattern. The diagnosis of MOH was mentioned in the first edition of the ICHD-1 (1988). In this edition, the diagnosis required daily intake of a certain dose and required remission of the headache 1 month after withdrawal. In 2004 (ICHD-2), the diagnosis was changed to depend on days with intake but still depended on the headache being resolved 2 months after withdrawal. This was changed with the appendix criteria of 2006 and in ICHD-3β to be more clinically relevant and easier to apply in daily practice.[1] The MOH diagnosis can now be given before withdrawal, as it now only requires medication overuse and a preexisting headache.

THE INTERNATIONAL CLASSIFICATION OF HEADACHE DISORDERS (ICHD-3) (2018) CRITERIA FOR MEDICATION OVERUSE HEADACHE

Description

Headache occurring on 15 or more days/month in a patient with a preexisting primary headache and developing as a consequence of regular overuse of acute or symptomatic headache medication (on 10 or more or 15 or more days/month, depending on the medication) for >3 months. It usually, but not invariably, resolves after the overuse is stopped.

Diagnostic Criteria

A. Headache present on 15 or more days/month in a patient with a preexisting headache disorder.
B. Regular overuse for >3 months of 1 or more drugs that can be taken for acute and/or symptomatic treatment of headache.
   1. Ergotamine, triptans, opioids, or combination analgesics on 10 or more days/month
   2. Simple analgesics on 15 or more days/month
   3. Any combination of acute/symptomatic drugs on 10 or more days/month without overuse of any single class alone
C. Not better accounted for by any other ICHD-3 diagnosis

Risk Factors

- Of female sex
- Have lower levels of educational attainment
- Be married
- Be unemployed
- Have migraine remission during pregnancy
- Be menopausal
- Have constipation
- Not use oral contraceptives
- Have higher use of healthcare resources
- Be on polypharmacy (sedative-hypnotics, antihypertensives)

Comorbidities

- General QOL poorer in MOH patients
- MIDAS score three times higher
- Subclinical obsessive compulsive disorder as measured by the Yale-Brown scale more common in patients with MOH than in patients with episodic or chronic migraine.
- Anxiety and mood disorders are more frequent.
- Increased risk of mood disorders, anxiety, and disorders associated with the use of psychoactive substances other than analgesics in patients with MOH.
- Risk significantly more frequent even before the transformation from migraine into CM + MOH than after MOH had developed.
- Psychiatric comorbidities also seen in patients with tension-type headache (TTH) transforming to MOH.
- According to DSM-IV, the overuse of analgesics and acute migraine drugs fulfils the criteria of substance abuse disorder in two-thirds of all patients with MOH.
- High prevalence of smokers and individuals with a body-mass index of >30 among patients with MOH.
- The presence of these features might be indicative of frontal lobe dysfunction in patients with MOH (*? Cause of compulsivity to drug taking*).
- Sleeping problems are also more common in patients with MOH than in patients with episodic headache.

COMPLICATIONS OF MEDICATION OVERUSE

- Several somatic complications, most of which are caused by the side-effects of the overused drugs.
- Most of the problems in patients with MOH have been described for ergotamine overuse:
  - Sensory neuropathy
  - Slowing of central cognitive processing
  - Decreased distensibility or changes in the arterial vessel wall structure in the brain
- Impaired psychological functioning, described as distress
- Other types of drug overuse can also cause changes in the nervous system: Increased latencies of peripheral autonomic potentials
- There is no evidence to date that any analgesics without phenacetin can induce nephropathy with MOH.

Pathophysiology:[2-4] The Vicious Cycle of MOH

The Vicious cycle of MOH and pathophysiology of MOH are shown in **Figures 1 and 2**.

CONCLUDING REMARKS

Derangement in the central pain modulating system as a result of chronic medication use may increase sensitivity to pain perception and foster or reinforce MOH.

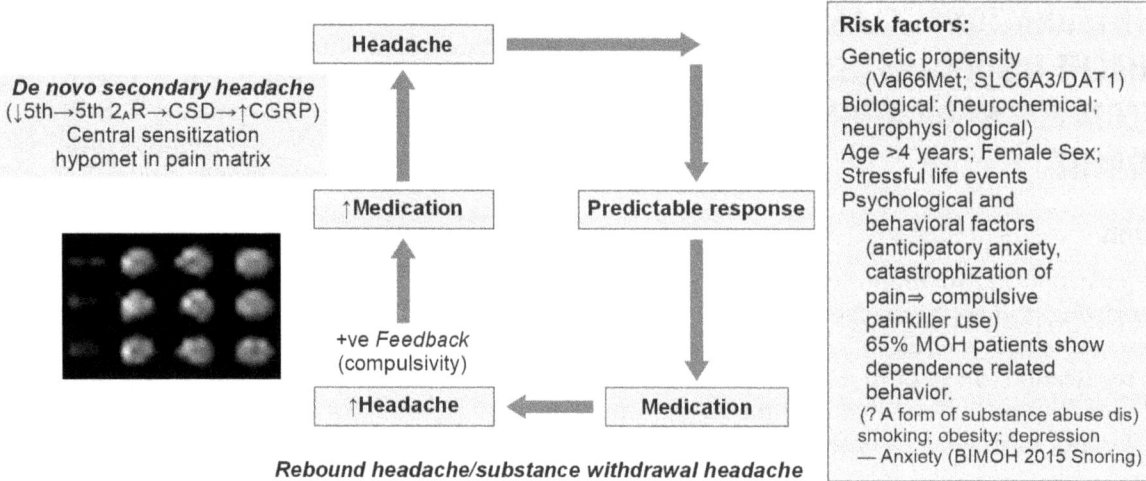

FIG. 1: Vicious cycle of medication overuse headache (MOH).
Source: Chakravarty 2016.

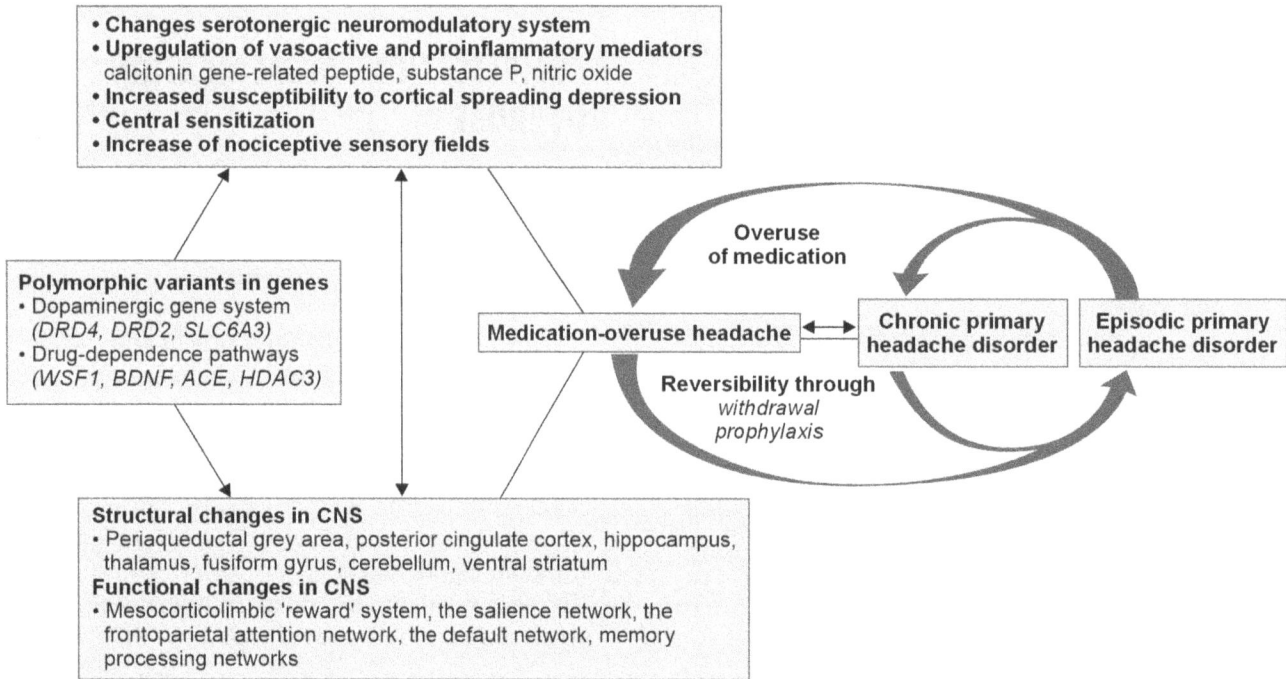

FIG. 2: Pathophysiology of medication overuse headache (MOH).
Source: Vandenbussche N, Laterza D, Lisicki M, Lloyd J, Lupi C, Tischler H, et al. Medication-overuse headache: a widely recognized entity amidst ongoing debate. J Headache Pain. 2018;19(1):50.

Management Principles[4]

- *Withdrawal treatment*: The goal of this treatment is not only to detoxify the patients and stop the chronic headache but also to improve responsiveness to acute or prophylactic drugs.
- *Withdrawal procedure*:
  - Abrupt withdrawal
  - Tapered Withdrawal: *Opioids, barbiturates, benzodiazepines*
- *Withdrawal symptoms*: Triptan (4.1d); ergot (6.7d); nonsteroidal anti-inflammatory drug NSAID (9.5d)
  - *Management*:
    - Cautious use of triptans/NSAIDs sos
    - Bridge Therapy: Short course regular NSAIDS + triptan sos
    - Corticosteroids: 7–10 days taper
- *Only withdrawal or withdrawal + prophylactics?*
  - *Prophylaxis*: Migraine or TTH?
  - Topiramate/divalproate ± amitriptyline ± BNTX

LEARNING POINTS

- Patients rarely volunteer excessive drug use.
- Think of MOH in any patient with daily or near daily headache.
- Suspect MOH when frequency or severity of any primary headache increases.
- Think of MOH even before diagnostic criteria fulfilled.
- Suspect MOH in migraine patients when headache starts developing first thing in morning.
- *Do not over diagnose MOH*: Several sinister conditions may make any primary headache worse.
- Take due notice of the underlying psychiatric state.

REFERENCES

1. Ferrari A, Baraldi C, Sternieri E. Medication overuse and chronic migraine: a critical review according to clinical Pharmacology. Expert Opin Drug Metab Toxicol. 2015;11(7): 1127-44.
2. Srikiatkhachorn A, le Grand SM, Supornsilpchai W, Storer RJ. Pathophysiology of medication overuse headache--an update. Headache. 2014;54(1):204-10.
3. Meng ID, Dodick D, Ossipov MH, Porreca F. Pathophysiology of medication overuse headache: insights and hypotheses from preclinical studies. Cephalalgia. 2011;31(7):851-60.
4. Evers S, Marziniak M. Clinical features, pathophysiology, and treatment of medication-overuse headache. Lancet Neurol. 2010;9(4):391-401.

CHAPTER 18

An Overview of Neuromuscular Diseases for the Psychiatrists

Satish V Khadilkar, Varsha A Patil

INTRODUCTION

Neuromuscular diseases (NMDs) are a heterogeneous group of disorders that arise due to damage or dysfunction of the peripheral nerves or muscles.[1] Broadly, they are differentiated depending upon the level of localization, which may range from the motor neurons (cranial or spinal), spinal nerve roots, peripheral nerves or plexuses, neuromuscular junction (NMJ), muscle, or any combination of these sites.[2] Largely, as a group of disorders, these affect the peripheral nervous system, however, involvement of the central nervous system may also be seen. The etiology can be variable ranging from inherited disorders, neurodegenerative disorders, toxins, infections, autoimmune disorders, metabolic disorders, and paraneoplastic disorders.[3] The estimated prevalence of NMDs is approximately 160 per 100,000 people worldwide; however, this is still an underestimate.[4]

COMPONENTS OF THE PERIPHERAL NERVOUS SYSTEM

The peripheral nervous system comprises the cranial nerves, spinal nerves and their roots and branches, peripheral nerves, and NMJ. The anterior horn cell, although a component of the central nervous system, is often described in the context of the motor unit. The upper motor neuron (UMN) is a motor neuron whose cell body arises from the motor cortex of the cerebrum. Its axons form the corticobulbar and corticospinal tracts. The lower motor neuron (LMN) lies in the brainstem motor nuclei and the anterior horns of the spinal cord. It directly innervates the skeletal muscles.[5]

CLINICAL PRESENTATION

The most common presenting symptom for an NMD is muscle weakness, muscle atrophy, and/or loss of sensation in the limbs, depending upon the level at which the peripheral nervous system is affected. Most disorders of the peripheral nervous system present focally or bilaterally, resulting in muscle atrophy, present with loss of sensation in the distal extremities, and diminished or absent deep tendon jerks.[1] Broadly, motor weakness may be due to affection of the UMN or LMN or a combination of the two **(Table 1)**.

The neuromuscular disorders can be broadly classified into various categories based on the site of affection in the peripheral nervous system **(Table 2)**.[6]

When the peripheral nerves are affected, the symptoms vary depending on the type of nerves involved (sensory,

TABLE 1: Clinical symptoms and signs of upper and lower motor neuron disorders.

	Upper motor neuron disorder	Lower motor neuron disorder
Clinical symptoms	• Loss of dexterity • Loss of muscle strength (mild weakness) • Spasticity • Pseudobulbar (spastic bulbar) palsy	• Loss of muscle strength (moderate-to-severe weakness) • Muscle atrophy • Muscle cramps
Signs	• Pathological hyperreflexia • Pathological reflexes (Babinski, Hoffmann sign, loss of abdominal reflexes)	• Hyporeflexia • Muscle hypotonicity or flaccidity • Fasciculations

TABLE 2: Broad categories of neuromuscular disorders.

Affected site in the peripheral nervous system	Examples	
	Inherited/Neurodegenerative	Acquired
Motor neuronopathy	• Amyotrophic lateral sclerosis (ALS) and its variants • Spinal muscular atrophy	• Infectious (poliomyelitis, West Nile virus) • Focal motor neuron disease (monomelic amyotrophy)
Sensory neuronopathy		• Autoimmune • Paraneoplastic • Toxic • Infectious
Radiculopathy		• Disk herniation • Spondylosis • Neoplasia • Hemorrhage • Abscess • Infarction • Infectious • Inflammatory • Neoplastic • Demyelinating
Plexopathy		• Neonatal trauma (Erb's palsy) • Radiation induced • Neoplastic • Entrapment • Diabetic • Hemorrhagic • Inflammatory
Neuropathy	Charcot–Marie–Tooth (CMT) disease	• Entrapment • Trauma • Mononeuritis multiplex
Neuromuscular junction disorders	*Postsynaptic*: • Congenital *Presynaptic*: • Congenital	*Postsynaptic*: • Myasthenia gravis • Toxic *Presynaptic*: • Lambert–Eaton myasthenic syndrome • Botulism • Toxic
Myopathy	• Muscular dystrophy • Congenital	• Metabolic • Acquired • Inflammatory • Toxic • Endocrine • Infectious

motor, or autonomic). The common positive sensory symptoms are prickling, searing, burning, and tight band-like sensations or paresthesia (unpleasant sensations arising spontaneously without an apparent stimulus).[7]

Negative sensory manifestations include loss or reduction of pain, temperature, or touch sensation. When the proprioceptive fibers are affected, there may be imbalance and gait disturbance. Besides, the sensory loss may be in the distribution of a peripheral nerve (mononeuropathy) or multiple nerves (polyneuropathy or mononeuritis multiplex).[1,8] When the motor nerves are affected, the patient may present with negative motor symptoms (weakness, atrophy, and walking difficulties) and/or positive motor symptoms (muscle cramps, fasciculations, myokymia, or tremors).[8] Autonomic nervous dysfunction may be evident if there are symptoms of orthostatic intolerance (lightheadedness, presyncopal symptoms, or syncope); reduced or excessive sweating; heat intolerance; and bladder, bowel, and sexual dysfunction, or gastroparesis (anorexia, early satiety, nausea, and vomiting).[9]

Disorders of the NMJ usually result in weakness, which may be worse with activity and improve with exercise. Ptosis (unilateral, often bilateral) or diplopia may be the presenting symptom in nearly two-thirds of patients. Depending on the muscles affected, the other symptoms experienced are chewing difficulty, speech disturbances, swallowing difficulty, or limb weakness.[10] Disorders of the muscles may present with positive symptoms (cramps, contractures, muscle hypertrophy, myalgias, myoglobinuria, and stiffness) or negative symptoms (exercise intolerance, fatigue, muscle atrophy, and weakness).[11]

Depending on the age group at onset, symptoms may vary, especially in children (a major group where inherited NMDs are commonly suspected).[12] The presenting complaints from parents may include floppiness or hypotonia **(Fig. 1A)**, delay in motor milestones, feeding and respiratory difficulties, abnormal gait characteristics, frequent falls, difficulty ascending stairs or arising from the floor, muscle cramps, or stiffness. Disorders such as very severe forms of spinal muscular atrophies (SMAs) or connective tissue disorders with intrauterine onset may present with poor fetal movements, severe respiratory distress at birth, or contractures (arthrogryposis).[3] Spinal deformities and respiratory insufficiency (restrictive lung disease) are common accompaniments in many congenital myopathies and muscular dystrophies **(Fig. 1B)**.[13]

The other important aspects in the clinical diagnosis of NMD are the duration of illness (acute, subacute, or chronic) and progression (static or progressive).[3,8,11]

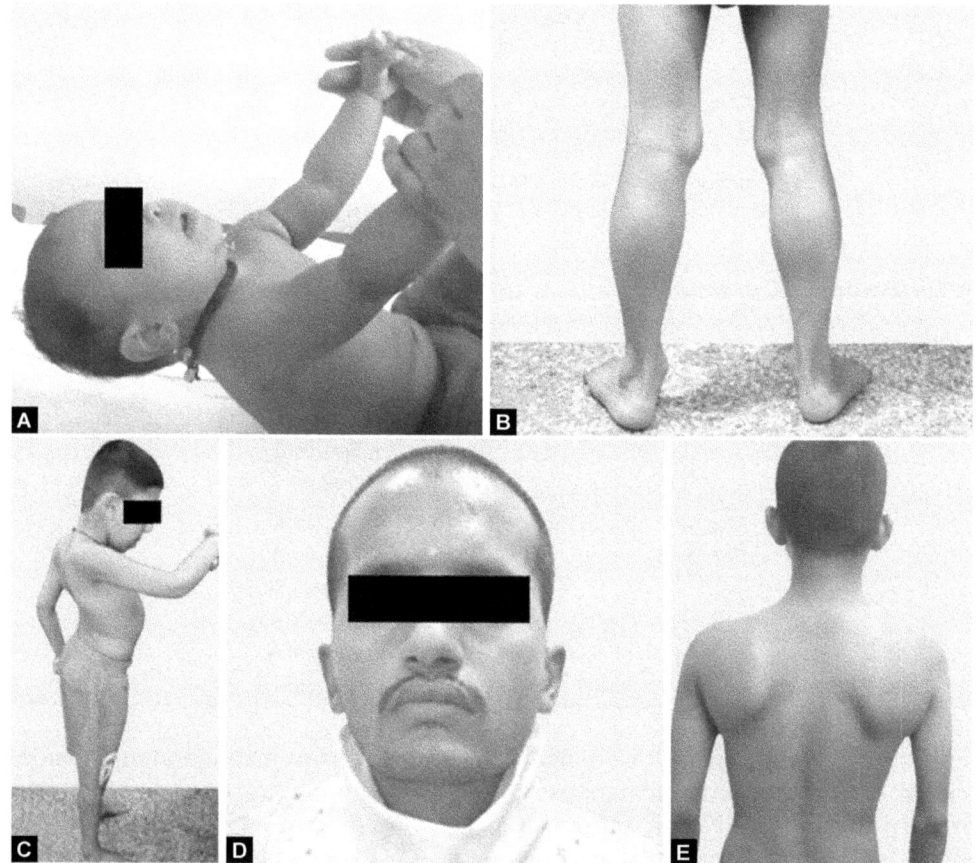

FIGS. 1A TO E: Clinical photographs depicting (A) floppy infant, (B) pseudohypertrophy of calves in a child with Duchenne muscular dystrophy, (C) spinal deformity in advanced stages of Duchenne muscular dystrophy, (D) facial features of myotonic dystrophy type 1, and (E) scapular winging in facioscapulohumeral dystrophy.

As a general rule, chronicity and slow progression point toward an inherited or a neurodegenerative disorder; whereas acute or subacute and rapidly progressing illness points toward an acquired etiology. Neurodegenerative disorders such as motor neuron disease (MND) are an exception, as certain types tend to progress fast. Similarly, the pattern of involvement may be pertinent in the case of peripheral neuropathy; "length dependent or glove and stocking" pattern points toward an inherited or toxic etiology versus a "non-length dependent" pattern points toward an acquired demyelinating etiology such as Guillain-Barré syndrome (GBS) or chronic inflammatory demyelinating polyradiculoneuropathy (CIDP).[3,8] A thorough clinical examination may point toward features such as pes cavus, kyphoscoliosis, optic atrophy, or inverted champagne bottle appearance characteristic of inherited neuropathy.[3,12] Likewise, associated rash, joint pains, ulcers, alopecia, hepatosplenomegaly, cherry red spot or retinitis pigmentosa on the fundus, and hearing loss examination may be pertinent clues for an underlying connective tissue disorder, lysosomal storage disorder, or a mitochondrial disorder. Certain types of muscular dystrophies can be identified clinically depending upon the age at presentation. The pattern of involvement may hint toward the type of myopathy **(Table 3)**.[11]

Affection of the central nervous system in the form of cognitive loss, memory loss, or behavioral disturbances is usually an exception for a typical NMD.[1] A significant intellectual impairment may, however, be seen in congenital and noncongenital myotonic muscular dystrophy type 1 (DM1), proximal myotonic myopathy (PROMM; DM2), Fukuyama congenital muscular dystrophy (CMD), phosphoglycerate kinase deficiency, some mitochondrial encephalomyelopathies, and a small proportion of cases of Duchenne muscular dystrophy (DMD).[3] Frontotemporal dementia (FTD) may present with additional affection of the anterior horn cell [bFTD with amyotrophic lateral sclerosis (ALS), c9orf72 associated FTD].[14]

The family history is very important in inherited disorders, e.g., DMD and Becker muscular dystrophy (BMD) are the most common muscular dystrophy and clearly follow an X-linked inheritance.[15] Most of the inherited myopathies or neuropathies (Charcot-Marie-Tooth disease) have an autosomal recessive inheritance; however, autosomal dominant and maternal inheritance are also well known.[8] Respiratory involvement may be seen in muscular dystrophies [DMD, BMD, limb girdle muscular dystrophy (LGMD) 2A and 2I, facioscapulohumeral dystrophy (FSHD), Emery-Dreifuss muscular dystrophy (EDMD), and myotonic dystrophy), congenital myopathies, acid maltase deficiency, centronuclear or nemaline myopathy, and mitochondrial disorders. Cardiac involvement may be seen in certain myopathies

TABLE 3: Pattern of involvement in myopathies.

Pattern of muscle weakness	Examples
Proximal limb girdle weakness	• Endocrine and toxic myopathies • Inflammatory myopathies • Limb girdle muscular dystrophies
Prominent distal weakness	• Distal myopathies • Centronuclear myopathy • Debrancher deficiency • Hereditary inclusion body myopathy • Inclusion body myositis • Myofibrillar myopathy • Myotonic dystrophy
Scapuloperoneal pattern	• FSHD • Scapuloperoneal dystrophy • Emery-Dreifuss dystrophy • LGMD 2A (calpainopathy) • Acid maltase deficiency (Pompe disease)

Extraocular muscle weakness (myopathies with ptosis or ophthalmoparesis)	• *Ptosis without ophthalmoparesis*:
	  ○ Congenital myopathies
	  ○ Nemaline myopathy
	  ○ Central core myopathy
	  ○ Desmin (myofibrillar) myopathy
	  ○ Myotonic dystrophy
	• *Ptosis with ophthalmoparesis*:
	  ○ Centronuclear myopathy
	  ○ Mitochondrial myopathy
	  ○ Multicore disease
	  ○ OPMD
	  ○ Oculopharyngodistal myopathy
	  ○ Neuromuscular junction disease (myasthenia gravis, Lambert-Eaton syndrome)

Neck extensor weakness	• Isolated neck extensor myopathy • Dermatomyositis • Polymyositis • Inclusion body myositis • Carnitine deficiency • Facioscapulohumeral dystrophy • Myotonic dystrophy • Congenital myopathy • Hyperparathyroidism
Bulbar weakness	• OPMD • LGMD type 1A (myotilinopathy) • Myasthenia gravis and Lambert-Eaton myasthenic syndrome • Inflammatory myopathy

Continued

Continued

Pattern of muscle weakness	Examples

Episodic pain, weakness, and myoglobinuria	• *Related to exercise*:
	  ○ Couch potato syndrome
	  ○ Glycogenoses (McArdle and so forth)
	  ○ Lipid disorders (CPT deficiency)
	• *Not related to exercise*:
	  ○ Central non-neuromuscular causes
	  ○ Neuroleptic malignant syndrome
	  ○ Status epilepticus
	  ○ Drugs/toxins
	  ○ Malignant hyperthermia
	  ○ Polymyositis/dermatomyositis (rarely)
	  ○ Viral/bacterial infections

Episodic weakness delayed or unrelated to exercise	• *Periodic paralysis (PP)*:
	  ○ Ca^{2+} channelopathies (hypokalemic)
	  ○ Na^{2+} channelopathies (hyperkalemic)
	  ○ Andersen–Tawil syndrome
	  ○ Secondary PP (thyrotoxicosis)
	• *Other*: Neuromuscular junction diseases

Stiffness and decreased ability to relax	• *Improves with exercise*:
	  ○ Myotonia: Na^{2+} or Cl– channelopathy
	• *Worsens with exercise/cold sensitivity*:
	  ○ Paramyotonia: Na^{2+} channelopathy
	  ○ Brody disease
	• *With fixed weakness*:
	  ○ Myotonic dystrophy (DM 1)
	  ○ Proximal myotonic myopathy (DM 2)
	  ○ Becker disease (AR Cl– channelopathy)
	• *Other*:
	  ○ Malignant hyperthermia
	  ○ Neuromyotonia
	  ○ Rippling muscle
	  ○ Stiff-person syndrome

(CPT: carnitine palmitoyltransferase; DM: myotonic dystrophy; FSHD: facioscapulohumeral dystrophy; LGMD: limb girdle muscular dystrophy; OPMD: oculopharyngeal muscular dystrophy)

such as muscular dystrophies (DMD; BMD; LGMD 1B, 2C-F, 2G), nemaline myopathy, EDMD, myotonic muscular dystrophy, polymyositis and mitochondrial disorders, acid maltase deficiency, and carnitine deficiency.[3]

DIAGNOSTIC WORKUP

The clinical localization of the level at which the peripheral nervous system is affected helps guide further investigations. The various investigations for the workup of NMD are as follows:

- *Creatine kinase (CK)*: Creatine phosphate is catalyzed to high-energy phosphates by the CK enzyme. Disorders that affect the sarcolemmal muscle membrane result in the elevation of transaminases, aldolase, and CK.[3] CK levels are significantly elevated in various muscular dystrophies. Very high values are noted in disorders such as DMD and BMD, especially in the early course of the illness.[15] Moderate elevation is noted in EDMD, LGMD, FSHD, and certain congenital muscular dystrophies. Elevated CK values (>1,000) may be seen in dystrophic myopathies (LGMD 2A-2I, LGMD 1C, and Miyoshi myopathy), immune myopathy [with anti-signal recognition particle (SRP) and anti-3-hydroxy-3-methylglutaryl-coenzyme A reductase (HMG-CoAR) antibody], paraneoplastic syndromes, acid maltase deficiency, and acute muscle injury. Other conditions with high CK values are polymyositis, dermatomyositis, acute rhabdomyolysis, malignant hyperthermia, and hypothyroidism.[3] A normal value or mildly elevated CK may be seen in certain congenital myopathies (central core disease, nemaline rod myopathy, and fiber type disproportion syndrome) and SMA.[16]

- *Lactate and pyruvate levels*: A metabolic myopathy or mitochondrial disorders may have additionally elevated lactate and pyruvate levels.[17] Lactic acidosis may be seen in mitochondrial encephalomyelopathies such as Kearne–Sayre syndrome; mitochondrial encephalomyopathy, lactic acidosis, and stroke-like episodes (MELAS); and myoclonic epilepsy with ragged red fibers (MERFF).[18]

- *Other biochemical tests*: Among the acquired causes of peripheral neuropathy, diabetes mellitus remains the most common cause followed by toxins, infections, and inflammatory disorders.[8] Depending on the probable etiology, a panel of tests to be done should include blood glucose, erythrocyte sedimentation rate (ESR), antinuclear antibodies (ANA) and ANA blot, serology for antineutrophil cytoplasmic antibody (ANCA), angiotensin-converting enzyme (ACE) (if sarcoidosis is suspected), and serology for human immunodeficiency virus (HIV) and hepatitis B and C. Certain inherited disorders such as mitochondrial disorders, peroxisomal disorders, or lysosomal storage require additional tests for very long-chain fatty acid and enzyme level assay.[8,18]

- *Electromyography and nerve conduction studies*: Electromyography and nerve conduction studies are an extremely important aid for the localization of pathology within the LMN.[3] It is very helpful in differentiating various forms of peripheral neuropathies. Depending on the pattern observed (demyelinating or axonal), the clinician can guide further tests such as genetics for a suspected CMT.[8] They are essential in diagnosis of an acquired peripheral neuropathy [acute inflammatory demyelinating polyneuropathy (AIDP) or CIDP] and MND.[1,3] Disorders of the NMJ [myasthenia gravis (MG), Lambert–Eaton myasthenic syndrome (LEMS), and congenital myasthenia] can be diagnosed based on the characteristic decremental or incremental responses.[10] The electromyography is also a helpful guide for choosing an appropriate site for a muscle biopsy.[3] Certain diagnostic patterns such as myotonia, fibrillation potentials, neuromyotonia, or after-discharges may give a clue toward disorders such as myotonic dystrophy, neuromyotonia, or other disorders affecting the ion channels.[19]
- *Muscle and nerve biopsy*: With the advent of molecular genetic testing, the role of muscle and nerve biopsy has been limited to certain selected disorders.[20] Nerve biopsies are helpful in certain autoimmune neuropathies and vasculitis.[8] Besides, they are useful in disorders such as leprosy, infiltrative disorders, and nerve tumors.[21] Muscle biopsy may be helpful in vasculitis, inflammatory myopathy, mitochondrial myopathies, and glycogen storage disorder (Pompe disease).[3]
- *Muscle and nerve imaging*: Ultrasound imaging can be used as a screening tool for certain muscle and nerve disorders.[22-24] With improvement in imaging techniques, magnetic resonance imaging (MRI) serves as a valuable noninvasive tool for various neuromuscular disorders, especially to detect the extent of involvement and progression of the disease.[25-27] Muscle imaging has been studied to detail various types of muscular dystrophies, SMA, and inflammatory myopathies.[28] The site for muscle biopsy can be identified based on the muscle imaging pattern. MR neurography has also evolved over the last few years to delineate disorders affecting the LMN, especially most useful to evaluate proximal conditions such as chronic immune sensorimotor polyradiculopathy (CISMP) and sciatic neuropathies and characterization of nerve tumors.[29]
- *Genetics*: The diagnostic paradigm of inherited NMDs has changed with advances in molecular genetic testing.[20] According to the GeneTable of Neuromuscular Disorders [http://www.musclegenetable.fr/ (last accessed June, 2023)], by January 2023, almost 658 genes had been associated with NMD.[30] Molecular diagnostic testing has reduced the need for invasive procedures such as muscle and nerve biopsy, especially in inherited NMDs.[31] However, the disadvantage remains the high cost of testing and variants of uncertain significance (VUS), which may affect the diagnosis.[20] A robust phenotype-genotype correlation is known in single gene disorders. Next-generation sequencing (NGS) helps in the diagnosis of clinically heterogeneous NMDs by examining several genes at the same time. Other options available are whole exome sequencing (WES, to analyze the entire coding portion of the genome) and whole genome sequencing (WGS).[32] Involving a geneticist early in the diagnostic algorithm may be important for inherited NMDs.[33]

TREATMENT OF NEUROMUSCULAR DISORDERS

Treatment of NMDs may be supportive or curative depending upon the nature of illness and the underlying etiology. Acquired peripheral neuropathies as a group may be amenable to treatment in the form of control of underlying disease, avoiding use of toxins (in drug induced neuropathies), and drugs for neuropathic pain.[3] Immunologically-mediated disorders such as GBS, CIDP, inflammatory myopathy, and MG may benefit from various immunotherapies such as intravenous immunoglobulins (IVIgs), plasma exchange (PLEX), steroids, and steroid-sparing agents.[3,8] Although inherited disorders may not be curable, a multidisciplinary team approach consisting of a neuromuscular specialist, physiotherapist, occupational therapist, respiratory specialist, speech and language therapist, trained nurse and social worker, with referrals to various other specialties such as cardiology, orthopedics, genetics, pulmonologist, and palliative care team, is important for comprehensive management of these patients.[20]

In the recent era, gene therapies have emerged as promising therapies for inherited disorders.[34] Gene therapies consist of a vector or delivery formulation/system containing a genetic construct engineered to express a specific transgene. Two main categories of gene transfer exist: (1) In vivo, where the genetic modification of the cell takes place inside the body, and (2) Ex vivo, where the cells are modified outside the body and then delivered back to the patient.[35] Recent advances in the treatment of SMA include disease-modifying therapies such as gene replacement therapy with onasemnogene abeparvovec-xioi (Zolgensma) to replace mutated SMN1 with normal SMN1 cDNA packaged in adenoassociated virus (AAV) vector and treatments directed at *SMN2* gene-antisense oligonucleotide, nusinersen (Spinraza) to modify splicing of the *SMN2* gene or small molecule SMN2 RNA splicing modifier, risdiplam (Evrysdi) to increase production of normal, full-length survival motor neuron (SMN) protein. Notable treatments for DMD include eteplirsen that targets exon 51, golodirsen and viltolarsen that target exon 53, and casimersen that targets exon 45.[36] The latest therapeutic development includes gene replacement therapy and involves the use of AAV vectors to deliver genes that code micro/mini-dystrophin.[34]

SPECIFIC DISORDERS

- *ALS*: It is characterized by progressive muscle weakness and atrophy associated with evidence of both UMN and LMN degeneration.[1] About 5–10% of ALS is familial; the remainder is sporadic. The most common mutations found are C9orf72 and SOD1.[37] The only approved pharmacological treatment for ALS is riluzole, which is a modifier of the neurotransmitter glutamate, known to prolong the survival by 2–3 months equating to a 9% increase in 1-year survival.[38,39] Other disorders such as poliomyelitis, West Nile virus, and Kennedy disease affect only the LMN.[1]
- *SMA*: It is a group of genetically determined (mostly autosomal recessive) disorders caused by homozygous deletion of the *SMN* gene on chromosome 5. Based on the age at onset, SMA is classified into four types: SMA type 1 (infantile SMA or Werdnig–Hoffmann syndrome), SMA type 2 (intermediate SMA), SMA type 3 (juvenile SMA or Kugelberg–Welander disease), and SMA type 4 (adult-onset SMA, pseudomyopathic SMA).[5] A very severe prenatal form of SMA (type 0 SMA) can manifest prenatally with reduced fetal movements and respiratory distress at birth. The estimated incidence of infantile and juvenile recessive SMA is 1 in 6,000 to 10,000 live births.[40] The infantile form presents as a floppy infant with hypotonia, weak cry, respiratory distress, and tongue fasciculations (in about 50%) with an alert expression. The intercostal muscles are severely weak leading to respiratory distress. The juvenile forms occur typically after 18 months of age with walking difficulty; while the SMA three and four present as a slowly progressive limb-girdle weakness. Fasciculations occur in 75% of patients. Bulbar signs, bony deformities such as scoliosis, and respiratory weakness are rare in the older forms. Progress in gene therapies have resulted in promising new drugs; however, treatment still remains palliative in severely affected forms.[5]
- *Mononeuropathy multiplex*: It is characterized by a step-wise loss of both sensory and motor function in the distribution of multiple individual peripheral nerves.[1] Electrodiagnostic studies are suggestive of an asymmetric pattern of involvement.[3,8] The classical cause for mononeuritis multiplex is vasculitis, others being diabetes, Lyme disease, Hansen disease, and lymphoma.[3] The etiological workup should include tests for systemic vasculitis, rheumatologic diseases, infectious diseases (HIV, hepatitis B and C, and Hansen disease), and diabetes. Nerve and muscle biopsies are required to diagnose vasculitic neuropathy.[41] Nerve biopsy or a combined nerve and muscle biopsy can be of a diagnostic yield of up to 75%.[42]
- *Acute peripheral polyneuropathy*: It is characterized clinically by a rapidly progressive loss of sensation and muscle strength with an absence of reflexes.[1] An acute polyneuropathy is usually indicative of GBS. It may be of various forms: Demyelinating (AIDP) or axonal [acute motor axonal neuropathy (AMAN)] or acute motor and sensory axonal neuropathy (AMSAN).[8] The electrodiagnostic studies are an important part of the diagnostic algorithm, with various patterns clearly evident in a detailed study performed in week 2 or onward.[3,8] A lumbar puncture to look for albuminocytologic dissociation (elevated protein and few or no white blood cells) is characteristic.[8] The recovery patterns vary, with axonal forms being more disabling with a poor recovery and prolonged disability. The treatment comprises IVIg or plasmapheresis and supportive care.[8]
- *Chronic sensory or sensory-motor peripheral polyneuropathy*: It is characterized clinically by a slowly progressive distal numbness (and/or distal weakness at a later stage).[1,8] The common causes of chronic peripheral neuropathy are diabetes, autoimmune (CIDP and monoclonal gammopathy), vitamin deficiencies, toxins (medications, chemotherapy drugs, and heavy metals), metabolic (uremic or hepatic), infectious (HIV and syphilis), and hereditary (Charcot–Marie–Tooth disease).[8] Electrophysiology helps in the diagnosis of patterns (acquired versus hereditary) and the extent of involvement. The other investigations include blood workup and nerve biopsy (in rare cases). Autoimmune neuropathies additionally may require antibody panels (antiganglioside antibody or anti-neurofascin antibodies) as a guide to treatment for aggressive forms or relapsing forms.[43] As a group, autoimmune neuropathies are responsive to therapies such as IVIg, steroids, and plasmapheresis as first-line therapy followed by chronic immunotherapy.[44] Toxic neuropathies may respond to the stoppage of culprit drugs or chelation (in case of heavy metal poisoning).[45] Most other peripheral neuropathies require general measures such as control of sugars, pharmacotherapy for neuropathic pain, and physiotherapy.[46]

- *Myopathies*: Myopathies are characterized clinically by progressive proximal motor weakness without sensory changes.[1] The various causes include hypothyroidism, infections, toxins/medications, autoimmunity/inflammation, and hereditary factors. Among drug-induced myopathy, the common agents noted are cholesterol-lowering agents (statins and fibrates), corticosteroids, and colchicine. The inherited causes form an important cause of muscle disorders such as muscular dystrophies, mitochondrial diseases, and metabolic myopathies (due to abnormalities in the metabolism of glycogen or lipids).[11,17,18]
    - *DMD and BMD*: The most common muscular dystrophies are mutations in the dystrophin gene that result in both DMD and BMD. The incidence of DMD is 1 per 3,500 among live born males. The prevalence in the general population is approximately 3 per 100,000.[15] The incidence of BMD is one-tenth of that of DMD. Parents notice delayed motor development, mainly delayed walking, and later repeated falls. As the disease progresses, there may occur pseudohypertrophy of the calf muscles **(Fig. 1C)** and difficulty in up squatting (Gower sign). Wheelchair dependency (by an average of 12 years of age), followed by joint contractures, leads to support for almost all activities as the disease progresses. The BMD is a milder phenotype with onset in the late first decade or even later (sometimes up to the fourth decade). Cardiac involvement in the form of dilated cardiomyopathy is more common in BMD. These children usually succumb to repeated cardiorespiratory complications during their 20s and 30s.[45] Physiotherapy is to prevent joint contractures and avoid disuse muscle atrophy and immobility-associated weight gain. Oral steroids [oral prednisone (0.75 mg/kg/day) and deflazacort (0.9 mg/kg/day)] may be beneficial in the early stages in boys with DMD. Newer therapies are still in the investigative phase.[15]
    - *LGMD*: It is an umbrella term that covers a group of genetic muscle diseases with the predominant involvement of muscles of the shoulder and hip girdle. The first description of the autosomal recessive transmission of LGMD was given by Levison in 1951.[47] With the advent of immunohistochemistry and later on genetic analysis, a more detailed analysis of subtypes of LGMD has now become possible. Dysferlinopathy, GNE myopathy, calpainopathy, and sarcoglycanopathies are common in India.[48]
    - *DM1*: This is the second most common muscular dystrophy that is characterized by muscle wasting and weakness associated with myotonia and several other systemic abnormalities.[19] It is an autosomal dominant disorder with an incidence of approximately 1 per 8,000 live births. The myopathy is caused by mutations in the gene that encodes for myotonic dystrophy protein kinase (DMPK), located on chromosome 19q13.3. In DM1, there are CTG trinucleotide repeats, which expand into the hundreds or thousands (compared to 5–30 in the normal population).[49] Typically, the disease begins in the early teens with noticeable weakness of the hands, foot drop, and neck muscle weakness. In middle age, repeated falls are common. The demonstration of myotonia is either by sharp percussion of the muscle with a reflex hammer or after firm voluntary contraction clinches the diagnosis clinically. The other features include frontal balding and hatchet face **(Fig. 1D)**; cataracts and retinal degeneration; hypogonadism and insulin resistance; reduced response to hypoxia, hypercapnia, Pickwickian syndrome, and obstructive sleep apnea; and ventricular arrhythmias, atrial arrhythmias, ectopic beats, tachyarrhythmias, cardiomyopathy, dysphagia, and constipation. They have a tendency for malignancies such as pilomatricomas, testicular malignancies, endometrial, non-Hodgkin lymphoma, and basal cell skin cancer. Congenital myotonic dystrophy occurs in infants of affected mothers. These children present with hypotonia, facial paralysis, failure to thrive, feeding difficulties, and mental retardation.[19]
- *FSHD*: The worldwide prevalence of FSHD ranges between 2.03 and 6.8 per 100,000 individuals.[50] It is the third most common dystrophy after DMD and DM1. It affects males compared to females. FSHD1 comprises 95% of the cases, while the remainder (5%) is of FSHD2 type; the clinical features remain the same.[50] The common phenotype is facial and scapular muscle weakness **(Fig. 1E)** (72–85%), usually asymmetric. The other phenotypes include face sparing, foot drop, proximal leg weakness, and distal posterior leg weakness. The prognosis is worse in patients with younger age at onset. The various systemic features include sensorineural hearing loss, Coats disease, retinal telangiectasia and detachment, hypertension, arrhythmia or conduction block, mental retardation, and epilepsy.
- *Congenital muscular dystrophy*: These are a heterogeneous group of disorders that occur due to disruption of components of the muscle extracellular matrix and its interaction with the sarcolemmal membrane. The inheritance is largely autosomal recessive, except for

certain disorders of collagen 6, which may be inherited dominantly.[16] The broad categories include LAMA2-related (merosin deficient) disorders, collagen 6-associated disorders, α-dystroglycanopathies, and laminopathies. The LAMA2-related CMDs are the most common; these have normal intelligence with severe disability and are often nonambulatory. The collagen 6-related disorders include the milder form (Bethlem myopathy) or the severe form (Ullrich myopathy) and have characteristic joint hyperlaxity and a tendency for keloid formation. Mental retardation and seizures with MRI brain abnormalities such as cobblestone lissencephaly may be seen in severe forms of α-dystroglycanopathies.

- *Disorders of the NMJ*: These comprise disorders that are immune-mediated or genetic (congenital myasthenia) disorders with characteristic fluctuating weakness, ptosis, and limb girdle weakness due to antibody-mediated damage at the NMJ.[10] Acquired MG is the most common primary disorder of NMJ. It may begin at any age from infancy to very old age, with two distinct peaks. The weakness remains restricted to the ocular muscles in approximately 10–15% of cases; it may progress to a generalized form in the rest.[51] The autoantibodies associated with acquired MG include antiacetylcholine receptor (AChR) antibodies (80–85%), antimuscle specific kinase (MuSK) antibodies (10%), and rarely antiagrin and antilipoprotein receptor-related protein 4 (LRP4) antibodies may be seen.[52-54] It is often associated with other immune-mediated diseases, especially hyperthyroidism and rheumatoid arthritis. The mainstay of treatment for MG is steroids and steroid-sparing agents (azathioprine, tacrolimus, and mycophenolate mofetil). In severe cases (myasthenic crisis), therapies such as IVIg and PLEX are useful.[10] Thymectomy may be done in indicated cases, especially when associated with a thymoma.[55] Congenital myasthenic syndrome (CMS) are largely autosomal recessive disorders that affect the NMJ, except the slow-channel syndrome, which has an autosomal dominant inheritance. Currently, 35 causative genes are found, with the most common causative genes being *CHAT, COLQ, RAPSN, CHRNE, DOK7,* and *GFPT1*.[56] The diagnosis of CMS is suggested by the clinical features and the response to cholinesterase inhibitors, or findings on standard electrodiagnostic studies.[57] Determination of the specific genetic or physiologic defect requires genetic studies or specialized morphological and electrophysiological studies on muscle tissue. LEMS results from an immune-mediated attack against the P/Q type voltage-gated calcium channels (VGCC) on presynaptic cholinergic nerve terminals at the NMJ and in autonomic ganglia.[58] The symptoms usually begin after the age of 40 years, with equal affection for males and females. Most patients report gradual onset of lower extremity weakness, dry mouth, erectile dysfunction, postural hypotension, constipation, and dry eyes. Ocular and bulbar symptoms are generally not prominent. Approximately one-half of patients have an underlying malignancy, the most common being small-cell lung cancer (80%). The other disorders affecting the NMJ are toxins such as botulinum toxin and envenomation.[10]

- *Inflammatory myopathies*: These are often characterized by acute/subacute onset progressive weakness of proximal (limb girdle type weakness) with rash or joint pains or other features of a rheumatological disorder.[1,3] Inflammatory myopathy occurs in three forms: Polymyositis, dermatomyositis, and inclusion body myositis. Polymyositis and dermatomyositis both respond well to immunosuppressive treatments.[59] The mainstay of treatment for polymyositis and dermatomyositis is steroids, though often in conjunction with methotrexate or other steroid-sparing immunosuppressive agents. In severe forms, IVIg may be given as the first line therapy.[3,59]

CHRONIC DISABILITY AND BURDEN ON THE QUALITY OF LIFE

The quality of life and well-being in these patients are affected due to various patient- and caregiver-related factors and the ongoing chronic disability.[60] Besides, markedly low scores on self-reported health-related quality of life (HRQOL) scales, a significant caregiver burden is a frequent observation, especially when the patients tend to become wheelchair bound.[61] The major factors affecting the care of such patients include emotional burden on the carer, physical burnout, reorganization of the social life and family dynamics, and sometimes social stigma in certain disorders, e.g., DMD.[35,62-64] A large study focusing on the psychosocial factors affecting the care of patients with NMDs found that a majority of caregivers (70.7%) suffer from a certain level of caregiver burden.[61] The factors observed were psychosocial characteristics of the person with NMD, the age at diagnosis, and at what age wheelchair use began. In the Indian context, many social and cultural norms further play a role in patient care. For example, a strong desire for a normal male child, taboos, and cultural beliefs may lead to multiple children with disability. This has been well demonstrated in a review on DMD by Nadkarni et al.,[62] where the authors have seen up to six boys with DMD in a family. Besides, patients and carers tend to opt for alternative medical systems such as Ayurveda, Unani, and Homeopathic, or other local folk remedies, when allopathy does not seem to find a cure for inherited NMDs.[62]

PSYCHIATRIC ISSUES IN NEUROMUSCULAR DISORDERS

A majority of NMDs lead to immobility in the due course of illness.[3] This is a common occurrence in disorders such as ALS, muscular dystrophies, congenital muscular dystrophies, and occasionally in severe forms of neuropathies. Poor self-image and mild-to-moderate depression occur in such patients.[65] Besides, the incurable nature of the illness or associated morbidities (respiratory or cardiac involvement) in certain disorders leads to a sense of alienation, profound isolation, and mood disturbances.[66,67] A Japanese study on BMD patients found that 21% of patients had psychiatric diseases and 24% had mental problems.[68] Schizophrenia and neurosis were more frequent in their study participants than in the general population.[68] Physical handicap or bullying may influence their mental state, as many children with BMD have high-trait anxiety. In addition to depression and anxiety, neurodevelopmental disorders such as autistic spectrum disorders and attention-deficit/hyperactive disorders have been reported in DMD, BMD, and myotonic DM1.[69-71] Mitochondrial disorders such as MELAS may have psychiatric symptoms as a part of the primary neurological syndrome.[72] Patients with acquired disorders such as MG or GBS where the life expectancy may not be affected have a high level of stress and anxiety, depending upon the personality trait.[73] Fatigue has been an under-recognized aspect of long-standing NMDs. Fatigue may be peripheral in origin (local effect on muscle function) or central fatigue (result of central feedback of the pathological peripheral nervous system affection).[74] Although distressing to the patient, it may at times be helpful as further tissue damage is prevented by ongoing physical activity.[75] Psychopharmacological treatments are helpful in management of various psychiatric illnesses in patients with NMD.[76]

CONCLUDING REMARKS

As a group of disorders, NMDs are a heterogeneous group with long-term disability and significant affection of QOL occurs as the disease progresses. A multidisciplinary approach to the care of such patients is the key to a good patient–clinician relationship. With advances in molecular genetics and newer therapies including gene therapies, a window of opportunity for treatability has opened for the once thought incurable NMDs.

LEARNING POINTS

- Neuromuscular disorders are a heterogeneous group of disorders that affect the peripheral nervous system.
- A multidisciplinary approach will help in the comprehensive care of patients with neuromuscular disorders.
- DMD and BMD are the most common muscular dystrophies followed by myotonic muscular dystrophy and FSHD.
- The common causes of chronic peripheral neuropathy are diabetes, autoimmune, vitamin deficiencies, toxins, metabolic, infectious, and hereditary (Charcot–Marie–Tooth disease).
- A pattern recognition approach coupled with relevant investigations helps in the diagnosis of these disorders. Advances in molecular genetics have opened new avenues for noninvasive diagnostics and gene therapies.
- The quality of life and well-being in these patients are affected due to various patient- and caregiver-related factors and the ongoing chronic disability.

REFERENCES

1. Morrison BM. Neuromuscular diseases. Semin Neurol. 2016;36(5): 409-18.
2. Morrison BM, Griffin JW. Neuromuscular diseases. In: Irani DN (Ed). Cerebrospinal Fluid in Clinical Practice. US: WB Saunders; 2009. pp. 121-6.
3. McDonald CM. Clinical approach to the diagnostic evaluation of hereditary and acquired neuromuscular diseases. Phys Med Rehabil Clin N Am. 2012;23(3):495-563.
4. Deenen JC, Horlings CG, Verschuuren JJ, Verbeek AL, van Engelen BG. The epidemiology of neuromuscular disorders: A comprehensive overview of the literature. J Neuromuscul Dis. 2015;2(1):73-85.
5. Quinn C, Elman L. Amyotrophic lateral sclerosis and other motor neuron diseases. Continuum (Minneap Minn). 2020;26(5): 1323-47.
6. Preston DC, Shapiro BR. Approach to nerve conduction studies and electromyography. In: Preston DC, Shapiro BE (Eds). Electromyography and Neuromuscular Disorders, 3rd edition. US: WB Saunders; 2013. pp. 1-7.
7. London ZN. A structured approach to the diagnosis of peripheral nervous system disorders. Continuum (Minneap Minn). 2020;26(5):1130-60.
8. Siao P, Kaku M. A clinician's approach to peripheral neuropathy. Semin Neurol. 2019;39(5):519-30.

9. Cheshire WP Jr. Autonomic history, examination, and laboratory evaluation. Continuum (Minneap Minn). 2020;26(1):25-43.
10. Pasnoor M, Dimachkie MM. Approach to muscle and neuromuscular junction disorders. Continuum (Minneap Minn). 2019;25(6):1536-63.
11. Barohn RJ, Dimachkie MM, Jackson CE. A pattern recognition approach to patients with a suspected myopathy. Neurol Clin. 2014;32(3):569-93.
12. Mary P, Servais L, Vialle R. Neuromuscular diseases: Diagnosis and management. Orthop Traumatol Surg Res. 2018;104(1S):S89-95.
13. Voulgaris A, Antoniadou M, Agrafiotis M, Steiropoulos P. Respiratory involvement in patients with neuromuscular diseases: A narrative review. Pulm Med. 2019;2019:2734054.
14. Portet F, Cadilhac C, Touchon J, Camu W. Cognitive impairment in motor neuron disease with bulbar onset. Amyotroph Lateral Scler Other Motor Neuron Disord. 2001;2(1):23-9.
15. Bushby K, Finkel R, Birnkrant DJ, Case LE, Clemens PR, Cripe L, et al; DMD Care Considerations Working Group. Diagnosis and management of Duchenne muscular dystrophy, part 1: diagnosis, and pharmacological and psychosocial management. Lancet Neurol. 2010;9(1):77-93.
16. Butterfield RJ. Congenital muscular dystrophy and congenital myopathy. Continuum (Minneap Minn). 2019;25(6):1640-61.
17. Lilleker JB, Keh YS, Roncaroli F, Sharma R, Roberts M. Metabolic myopathies: a practical approach. Pract Neurol. 2018;18(1):14-26.
18. Rahman S, Hanna MG. Diagnosis and therapy in neuromuscular disorders: diagnosis and new treatments in mitochondrial diseases. J Neurol Neurosurg Psychiatry. 2009;80(9):943-53.
19. Miller TM. Differential diagnosis of myotonic disorders. Muscle Nerve. 2008;37(3):293-9.
20. Paganoni S, Nicholson K, Leigh F, Swoboda K, Chad D, Drake K, et al. Developing multidisciplinary clinics for neuromuscular care and research. Muscle Nerve. 2017;56(5):848-58.
21. Khadilkar SV, Yadav RS, Soni G. A practical approach to enlargement of nerves, plexuses and roots. Pract Neurol. 2015;15(2):105-15.
22. Heckmatt JZ, Pier N, Dubowitz V. Real-time ultrasound imaging of muscles. Muscle Nerve. 1988;11(1):56-65.
23. Zaidman CM, Connolly AM, Malkus EC, Florence JM, Pestronk A. Quantitative ultrasound using backscatter analysis in Duchenne and Becker muscular dystrophy. Neuromuscul Disord. 2010;20(12):805-9.
24. Heckmatt JZ, Dubowitz V. Ultrasound imaging and directed needle biopsy in the diagnosis of selective involvement in neuromuscular disease. J Child Neurol. 1987;2(3):205-13.
25. Finanger EL, Russman B, Forbes SC, Roonney WD, Walter GA, Vandenborne K. Use of skeletal muscle MRI in diagnosis and monitoring disease progression in Duchenne muscular dystrophy. Phys Med Rehabil Clin N Am. 2012;23(1):1-10.
26. Liu GC, Jong YJ, Chiang CH, Jaw TS. Duchenne muscular dystrophy: MR grading system with functional correlation. Radiology. 1993;186(2):475-80.
27. Tomasová Studynková J, Charvát F, Jarosová K, Vencovsky J. The role of MRI in the assessment of polymyositis and dermatomyositis. Rheumatology (Oxford). 2007;46(7):1174-9.
28. Fischer D, Bonati U, Wattjes MP. Recent developments in muscle imaging of neuromuscular disorders. Curr Opin Neurol. 2016;29(5):614-20.
29. Khadilkar S, Deshmukh ND, Shah NH, Jaggi S, Mansukhani KA, Patel B, et al. Optimizing Investigations for Evaluation of Enlargements of the Roots, Plexuses and Nerves: A Study of 133 Patients. Ann Indian Acad Neurol. 2020;23(5):666-73.
30. Benarroch L, Bonne G, Rivier F, Hamroun D. The 2023 version of the gene table of neuromuscular disorders. Neuromuscul Disord. 2023;33(1):76-117.
31. Kassardjian CD, Amato AA, Boon AJ, Childers MK, Klein CJ. The utility of genetic testing in neuromuscular disease: a consensus statement from the AANEM on the clinical utility of genetic testing in diagnosis of neuromuscular disease. Muscle Nerve. 2016;54(6):1007-9.
32. Warman Chardon J, Beaulieu C, Hartley T, Boycott KM, Dyment DA. Axons to exons: the molecular diagnosis of rare neurological diseases by next-generation sequencing. Curr Neurol Neurosci Rep. 2015;15(9):64.
33. Su X, Kang PB, Russell JA, Simmons Z. Ethical issues in the evaluation of adults with suspected genetic neuromuscular disorders. Muscle Nerve. 2016;54(6):997-1006.
34. Scoto M, Finkel R, Mercuri E, Muntoni F. Genetic therapies for inherited neuromuscular disorders. Lancet Child Adolesc Health. 2018;2(8):600-9.
35. Landfeldt E. Gene therapy for neuromuscular diseases: Health economic challenges and future perspectives. J Neuromuscul Dis. 2022;9(6):675-88.
36. Mendonça RH, Zanoteli E. Gene therapy in neuromuscular disorders. Arq Neuropsiquiatr. 2022;80(5 Suppl 1):249-56.
37. Renton AE, Chiò A, Traynor BJ. State of play in amyotrophic lateral sclerosis genetics. Nat Neurosci. 2014;17(1):17-23.
38. Bensimon G, Lacomblez L, Meininger V; ALS/Riluzole Study Group. A controlled trial of riluzole in amyotrophic lateral sclerosis. N Engl J Med. 1994;330(9):585-91.
39. Rooney J, Byrne S, Heverin M, Tobin K, Dick A, Donaghy C, et al. A multidisciplinary clinic approach improves survival in ALS: a comparative study of ALS in Ireland and Northern Ireland. J Neurol Neurosurg Psychiatry. 2015;86(5):496-501.
40. Sangaré M, Hendrickson B, Sango HA, Chen K, Nofziger J, Amara A, et al. Genetics of low spinal muscular atrophy carrier frequency in sub-Saharan Africa. Ann Neurol. 2014;75(4):525-32.
41. Vrancken AF, Gathier CS, Cats EA, Notermans NC, Collins MP. The additional yield of combined nerve/muscle biopsy in vasculitic neuropathy. Eur J Neurol. 2011;18(1):49-58.
42. Nunokawa T, Yokogawa N, Shimada K, Enatsu K, Sugii S. The use of muscle biopsy in the diagnosis of systemic vasculitis affecting small to medium-sized vessels: a prospective evaluation in Japan. Scand J Rheumatol. 2016;45(3):210-4.
43. Uncini A. Autoimmune nodo-paranodopathies 10 years later: Clinical features, pathophysiology and treatment. J Peripher Nerv Syst. 2023;28(Suppl 3):S23-S35.
44. Nobile-Orazio E, Gallia F. Update on the treatment of chronic inflammatory demyelinating polyradiculoneuropathy. Curr Opin Neurol. 2015;28(5):480-5.
45. Darras BT, Menache-Stroninki CC, Hinton V, Kunkel LM. Dystrophinopathies. In: Darras BT, Jones HR Jr, Ryan MM, De Vivo DC (Eds). Neuromuscular Disorders of Infancy, Childhood and Adolescence: A Clinician's Approach, 2nd edition. San Diego: Academic Press; 2015. p. 551.
46. Staff NP. Peripheral neuropathies due to vitamin and mineral deficiencies, toxins, and medications. Continuum (Minneap Minn). 2020;26(5):1280-98.

47. Levison H. Dystrophia musculorum progressiva; clinical and diagnostic criteria, inheritance. Acta Psychiatr Neurol Scand Suppl. 1951;76:1-176.
48. Khadilkar SV, Faldu HD, Patil SB, Singh R. Limb-girdle muscular dystrophies in India: A Review. Ann Indian Acad Neurol. 2017;20(2):87-95.
49. Hamel JI. Myotonic dystrophy. Continuum (Minneap Minn). 2022;28(6):1715-34.
50. Tawil R, Van Der Maarel SM. Facioscapulohumeral muscular dystrophy. Muscle Nerve. 2006;34(1):1-15.
51. Meriggioli MN, Sanders DB. Muscle autoantibodies in myasthenia gravis: beyond diagnosis? Expert Rev Clin Immunol. 2012;8(5):427-38.
52. Leite MI, Jacob S, Viegas S, Cossins J, Clover L, Morgan BP, et al. IgG1 antibodies to acetylcholine receptors in 'seronegative' myasthenia gravis. Brain. 2008;131(Pt 7):1940-52.
53. Zhang B, Xiong WC, Mei L. Get ready to Wnt: prepatterning in neuromuscular junction formation. Dev Cell. 2009;16(3):325-7.
54. Shen C, Lu Y, Zhang B, Figueiredo D, Bean J, Jung J, et al. Antibodies against low-density lipoprotein receptor-related protein 4 induce myasthenia gravis. J Clin Invest. 2013;123(12): 5190-202.
55. Hehir MK 2nd, Li Y. Diagnosis and management of myasthenia gravis. Continuum (Minneap Minn). 2022;28(6):1615-42.
56. Ohno K, Ohkawara B, Shen XM, Selcen D, Engel AG. Clinical and pathological features of congenital myasthenic syndromes caused by 35 genes-A comprehensive review. Int J Mol Sci. 2023;24(4):3730.
57. Finsterer J. Congenital myasthenic syndromes. Orphanet J Rare Dis. 2019;14(1):57.
58. Kesner VG, Oh SJ, Dimachkie MM, Barohn RJ. Lambert–Eaton myasthenic syndrome. Neurol Clin. 2018;36(2):379-94.
59. Manousakis G. Inflammatory myopathies. Continuum (Minneap Minn). 2022;28(6):1643-62.
60. Walklet E, Muse K, Meyrick J, Moss T. Do psychosocial interventions improve quality of life and wellbeing in adults with neuromuscular disorders? A systematic review and narrative synthesis. J Neuromuscul Dis. 2016;3(3):347-62.
61. Pousada T, Groba B, Nieto-Riveiro L, Pazos A, Díez E, Pereira J. Determining the burden of the family caregivers of people with neuromuscular diseases who use a wheelchair. Medicine (Baltimore). 2018;97(24):e11039.
62. Nadkarni JJ, Dastur RS, Viswanathan V, Gaitonde PS, Khadilkar SV. Duchenne and Becker muscular dystrophies: an Indian update on genetics and rehabilitation. Neurol India. 2008;56(3):248-53.
63. Pangalila RF, van den Bos GA, Stam HJ, van Exel NJ, Brouwer WB, Roebroeck ME. Subjective caregiver burden of parents of adults with Duchenne muscular dystrophy. Disabil Rehabil. 2012;34(12):988-96.
64. Carnevale FA, Alexander E, Davis M, Rennick J, Troini R. Daily living with distress and enrichment: the moral experience of families with ventilator-assisted children at home. Pediatrics. 2006;117(1):e48-60.
65. Vuillerot C, Hodgkinson I, Bissery A, Schott-Pethelaz AM, Iwaz J, Ecochard R, et al. Self-perception of quality of life by adolescents with neuromuscular diseases. J Adolesc Health. 2010;46(1): 70-6.
66. Oldford L, Hanson N, Ross I, Croken E, Bleau L. Exploring the psychosocial impact of simple robotic assistive technology on adolescents with neuromuscular disease. J Rehabil Assist Technol Eng. 2022;9:20556683221087522.
67. Graham CD, Simmons Z, Stuart SR, Rose MR. The potential of psychological interventions to improve quality of life and mood in muscle disorders. Muscle Nerve. 2015;52(1):131-6.
68. Mori-Yoshimura M, Mizuno Y, Yoshida S, Ishihara N, Minami N, Morimoto E, et al. Psychiatric and neurodevelopmental aspects of Becker muscular dystrophy. Neuromuscul Disord. 2019;29(12): 930-9.
69. Darmahkasih AJ, Rybalsky I, Tian C, Shellenbarger KC, Horn PS, Lambert JT, et al. Neurodevelopmental, behavioral, and emotional symptoms common in Duchenne muscular dystrophy. Muscle Nerve. 2020;61(4):466-74.
70. Lambert JT, Darmahkasih AJ, Horn PS, Rybalsky I, Shellenbarger KC, Tian C, et al. Neurodevelopmental, behavioral, and emotional symptoms in Becker muscular dystrophy. Muscle Nerve. 2020;61(2):156-62.
71. van der Velden BG, Okkersen K, Kessels RP, Groenewoud J, van Engelen B, Knoop H, et al. Affective symptoms and apathy in myotonic dystrophy type 1 a systematic review and meta-analysis. J Affect Disord. 2019;250:260-9.
72. Anglin RE, Garside SL, Tarnopolsky MA, Mazurek MF, Rosebush PI. The psychiatric manifestations of mitochondrial disorders: a case and review of the literature. J Clin Psychiatry. 2012;73(4):506-12.
73. Bogdan A, Barnett C, Ali A, AlQwaifly M, Abraham A, Mannan S, et al. Prospective study of stress, depression and personality in myasthenia gravis relapses. BMC Neurol. 2020;20(1):261.
74. de Vries JM, Hagemans ML, Bussmann JB, van der Ploeg AT, van Doorn PA. Fatigue in neuromuscular disorders: focus on Guillain-Barré syndrome and Pompe disease. Cell Mol Life Sci. 2010;67(5):701-13.
75. Torri F, Lopriore P, Montano V, Siciliano G, Mancuso M, Ricci G. Pathophysiology and Management of Fatigue in Neuromuscular Diseases. Int J Mol Sci. 2023;24(5):5005.
76. Brusa C, Gadaleta G, D'Alessandro R, Urbano G, Vacchetti M, Davico C, et al. Psychopharmacological treatments for mental disorders in patients with neuromuscular diseases: A scoping review. Brain Sci. 2022;12(2):176.

CHAPTER 19

Chronic Pain and Chronic Fatigue: A Diagnostic and Therapeutic Challenge

Satish V Khadilkar, Hiral Halani

INTRODUCTION

The profound change in the perspectives of chronic pain solidifies Michael Cousins' assertion that chronic pain will be regarded as the disease of 21st century.[1] Chronic pain and chronic fatigue are prevalent and multifaceted issues that significantly impact the individual and society. The global burden of chronic pain and related disorders has seen a noticeable increase and is one of the leading contributors to disability as reported in the Global Burden of Disease study.[2] Additionally, the most frequent causes of years lived with disability (YLD) were found to be chronic low backache, depression, neck pain, migraine, and osteoarthritis (OA).[3] Various epidemiological studies have shown the prevalence of chronic pain to be as high as 40% and a meta-analysis from low- and middle-income countries (LMICs) also has revealed similar estimates of (~34%) persistent pain in the community.[4] These conditions can manifest either as coexisting symptoms of the underlying disease or as independent disorders in their own rights. A myriad of chronic diseases including musculoskeletal, neuropathic, rheumatological, visceral, and oncological conditions have pain and fatigue as prominent manifestations that are not amenable to the standard treatment modalities. The current conceptualization of chronic pain as a very complex central nervous system (CNS) state of aberrant sensitization both peripherally and centrally affecting different cortical and subcortical regions has revolutionized our understanding and unfolded the novel therapeutic aspects. Chronic fatigue syndrome (CFS) is another underrecognized cause of significant morbidity and disability in adult population. Its importance is being increasingly realized particularly in the post-COVID-19 pandemic era. This chapter focuses on the definitions and mechanisms for chronic pain and fatigue, their common presentations and associations, as well as the approach to their management.

CHRONIC PAIN: DEFINITION AND CLASSIFICATION

The International Association for the Study of Pain (IASP) defines the pain as "an unpleasant sensory and emotional experience associated with actual or potential tissue damage."[4] Acute pain was described by Sherrington as "the psychical adjunct of an imperative, protective reflex." Unlike acute pain, which has a protective value in order to avoid noxious stimuli and promote healing and recovery, chronic pain has no apparent biological value. This was decorously stated by John J Bonica, the founding father of pain medicine, in 1953, "Pain becomes pathologic when, if persisting, loses its biologic damage signaling function and, with its devastating psychophysiologic consequences, becomes a destructive force hard to manage with traditional therapeutic means."[5] The chronicity denotes the persistence of pain beyond the normal tissue healing time; the temporal criterion added by the IASP is the pain that lasts or recurs for >3 months. The IASP distinguishes two broad categories of chronic pain: Chronic primary pain that cannot be better accounted for by any other pain condition and chronic secondary pain syndromes that are linked to other diseases as underlying cause, for which pain may initially be regarded as a symptom and later on, the pain continues beyond the successful treatment of the underlying condition. Both the primary and secondary pain syndromes are further subcategorized under several heads and some degree of overlap can be present between these two categories **(Flowchart 1)**.

PATHOPHYSIOLOGY OF CHRONIC PAIN

Chronic pain emerges as a consequence of the maladaptive nociceptive pathways in certain chronic pathological states. Chronic exposure to inflammatory mediators or

Chronic Musculoskeletal Pain

The Pain Task Force (IASP) defines chronic primary musculoskeletal pain (CPMP) as "chronic pain in the muscles, bones, joints, or tendons that is characterized by significant emotional distress (i.e., anxiety, anger, frustration, and depressed mood) or functional disability."[15] This is one of the leading contributors to disability worldwide and carries a large socioeconomic impact. The most prevalent forms are chronic low backache being extremely common (~30–40% of adults) followed by others such as neck pain, OA, RA, and posttraumatic pain.[16] Symptomatically, it can have various components such as inflammatory pain, somatic pain (arising from the skin/subcutaneous tissues/muscles), bone pain as well as a neuropathic component.

The low backache for its outstandingly high prevalence in mid to late adulthood needs specific mention here. These patients are often encountered by physicians, orthopedics, physiotherapists, psychiatrists, or neurologists in outpatient clinics **(Table 2)**.

Chronic Neuropathic Pain

The IASP defines neuropathic pain as "pain initiated or caused by a primary lesion or dysfunction in the nervous system."[4] Clinically there can be negative symptoms such as loss of sensation (e.g., numbness) or positive symptoms such as hyperalgesia (increased response to painful stimulus), allodynia (painful response to a nonpainful stimuli), and paresthesia (abnormal spontaneous sensations such as tingling and burning). It is useful to divide them into peripheral and central neuropathic types for both have distinct anatomic site of lesion, clinical manifestations, and pathophysiology of pain **(Table 3 and Flowchart 2)**.

Fibromyalgia

Fibromyalgia is a frequent cause of chronic widespread pain with a prevalence of 2–3% in general population.[24] In addition to pain, there exists a complex polysymptomatology comprising fatigue,[25,26] sleep disturbances, and autonomic, somatic, and psychiatric features **(Fig. 1)**. The pathophysiology is still obscure but various factors such as genetic predisposition, stressful life events, peripheral neuroinflammation along with central maladaptive coping mechanisms together produce a set of neuromorphological modifications ("nociplastic pain") and pain dysperception. The recommended treatment strategies include psychotherapy and pharmacological and nonpharmacological therapies as shown in **Figure 2**.

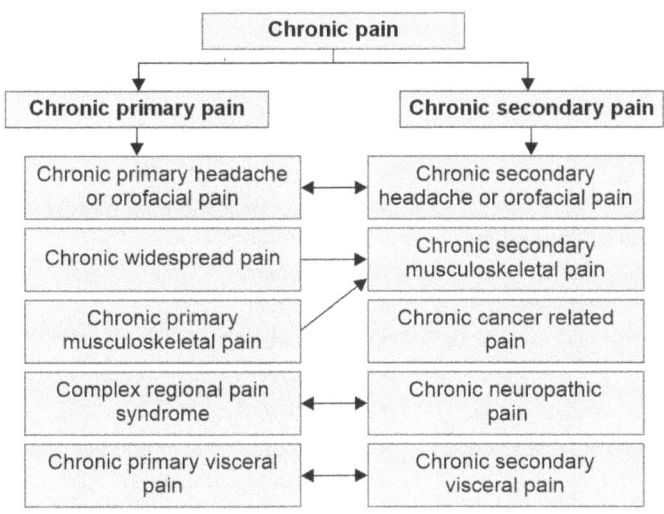

FLOWCHART 1: The International Association for the Study of Pain (IASP) classification of pain.

any other noxious stimuli leads to reduction in threshold and heightened responsiveness of peripheral terminals, a phenomenon known as peripheral sensitization. The central pain pathways project from the dorsal root ganglion (DRG) to the thalamus and somatosensory cortices and various other regions involved in affective pain experience including basal ganglia, cingulate gyrus, insula, hypothalamus, amygdala, and prefrontal cortex (PFC).[6] The emergence of centralized pain, decoupled from the peripheral stimuli, occurs due to a disequilibrium in these pain processing pathways. "Central sensitization" refers to the enhanced functional status of the neuronal circuits in the nociceptive pathways caused by various mechanisms such as membrane hyperexcitability, synaptic efficacy, and resultant recruitment of subthreshold inputs and alteration in the receptive field properties, neurochemical changes, as well as contribution from non-neuronal cells (immune cells, glial cells, etc.).[7] Pain research has shown that most of the chronic pain states, e.g., in OA, low back pain (LBP), irritable bowel syndrome (IBS), neuropathies, fibromyalgia, and others are in fact "mixed pain states" with variable contributions from central and peripheral elements of pain.[8,9]

We shall now discuss several common varieties of chronic pain encountered in routine practice, namely chronic headaches, musculoskeletal pain, various types of neuropathic pain, and visceral pain. **Table 1** provides an overview of prevalent types of headache and orofacial pain including their clinical hallmarks and available treatment options.

TABLE 1: Chronic headache and orofacial pain.[10-14]

Type of the headache	Clinical diagnosis	Treatment options
Acute migraine	At least five attacks of moderate or severe intensity headache lasting for 4–72 hours • Pulsating • Usually unilateral, but can be bilateral • Aggravated by activities such as walking and climbing stairs, causing avoidance • Associated with nausea and/or vomiting, photophobia, and phonophobia	• Paracetamol • NSAIDs • Triptans • Adjunct medications for nausea and vomiting *For prevention*: • Propranolol • Topiramate • Flunarizine • Amitriptyline
Chronic migraine	Headache (tension type-like or migraine-like) on at least 15 days/month for >3 months	• CGRP monoclonal antibodies • Vagus nerve stimulation • Botulinum toxin
Tension-type headache	• Pressing (nonpulsating) quality • Mild or moderate intensity • Bilateral • No nausea or vomiting • Photophobia and phonophobia are absent or only one is present	• Paracetamol • NSAIDs
Trigeminal autonomic cephalalgia	• Hallmark is severe unilateral orbital, supraorbital, and/or temporal pain • Pain attacks accompanied by at least one of ipsilateral autonomic signs or symptoms (conjunctival injection and/or lacrimation, nasal congestion and/or rhinorrhea, eyelid edema, forehead and facial sweating, and miosis and/or ptosis) The duration and frequency of pain attacks differ in various types as follows: • Cluster headache (15–180 minutes, periodicity) • Paroxysmal hemicrania (2–30 minutes) • SUNCT/SUNA (short-lasting for few seconds) • Hemicrania continua (continuous)	• High-flow oxygen therapy and triptans for cluster headache • Indomethacin response in paroxysmal hemicrania and hemicrania continua Drugs for prevention vary: • Verapamil • Topiramate • Lithium • Lamotrigine
Trigeminal neuralgia	• At least 3 attacks of unilateral facial pain occurring in ≥1 divisions of the trigeminal nerve with no radiation beyond trigeminal distribution • Recurring in paroxysmal attacks lasting from a fraction of a second to 2 minutes • Severe, electric shock like shooting, stabbing, or sharp in quality • Precipitated by innocuous stimuli to the affected side of the face • No clinically evident neurologic deficit	• Carbamazepine • Oxcarbazepine • Gabapentin • Pregabalin • Clonazepam • Baclofen
Glossopharyngeal neuralgia	• Unilateral paroxysmal attacks of facial pain lasting from a fraction of a second to 2 minutes • Distribution within the posterior part of the tongue, tonsillar fossa, pharynx, or beneath the angle of the lower jaw and/or in the ear • Sharp, stabbing, and severe, stereotyped • Precipitated by swallowing, chewing, talking, coughing, and/or yawning • There is no clinically evident neurologic deficit	• Carbamazepine • Gabapentin • Duloxetine • Clonazepam

Continued

Continued

Type of the headache	Clinical diagnosis	Treatment options
Temporomandibular pain disorder	• Clinical evidence of a painful pathology affecting elements of the temporomandibular joint(s), muscles of mastication, and/or associated structures on one or both sides • Headache has developed in temporal relation to the onset of TMJ disorder, or led to its discovery • Jaw motion, jaw function (e.g., chewing) and/or jaw parafunction (e.g., bruxism) and palpation	• NSAIDs • Muscle relaxants • Tricyclic antidepressants
Atypical facial pain	• Persistent idiopathic facial pain • Does not fit classic presentation of any neuralgia • Long duration, unilateral, deep, and poorly localized • No autonomic symptoms and no sensory loss	• Amitriptyline • Duloxetine • Pregabalin • Gabapentin

Red flags for secondary headaches: SNOOP (needs further investigations such as imaging and lumbar puncture to find the cause and treat accordingly)
- *S: S*ystemic symptoms—fever, malignancy, immunocompromised, and pregnancy
- *N: N*eurologic deficits—papilledema, focal deficits, impairment of alertness, or cognition
- *O: O*nset sudden or new thunderclap headache—peaks in 1 minute—worst headache ever
- *O: O*lder onset age >50 years
- *P: P*attern change—positional
- *P: P*rovocation—pain induced by bending, lifting, cough, or Valsalva

(CGRP: calcitonin gene-related peptide; NSAID: nonsteroidal anti-inflammatory drug; SUNCT: short-lasting unilateral neuralgiform headache attacks with conjunctival injection and tearing; SUNA: short-lasting unilateral neuralgiform headache attacks with cranial autonomic symptoms; TMJ: temporomandibular joint)

TABLE 2: Low backache: Guide to clinical diagnosis and management.[5,17,18]

Source of pain
Axial lumbosacral: • *Discogenic pain*: Pain in the center of lower back with minimal radiation or to the buttocks or thighs, pain improves with standing and lying flat and may be reduced with extension and worsen with sitting, driving, lumbar flexion, bending, twisting, and Valsalva maneuver • *Facet joint pain*: Deep and aching sensation (unilateral or bilateral), occasional radiation to one or both buttocks, groins, and/or thighs, but typically stops above the knee, provoked by lateral rotation and back extension • *Sacroiliac joint pain*: Sharp, stabbing pain, radiates from the hips and pelvis up to the lower back and thighs. Pain is worse on standing or walking • *Radicular pain*: Travels into an extremity along a dermatomal distribution secondary to nerve or dorsal root ganglion irritation • *Referred pain*: Spreads to a region remote from its source but along a nondermatomal trajectory
Temporal division
Acute (<4 weeks)   Subacute (4–12 weeks)   Chronic (>12 weeks)
Etiology: • Degenerative disease—lumbar spondylosis and spondylolisthesis • Herniated disc • Spinal stenosis • Inflammatory arthritis, e.g., ankylosing spondylitis; infectious, e.g., osteomyelitis • Neoplastic—spinal cord tumor or metastasis • Osteoporosis

Continued

Continued

Physical examination:

Inspection: Posture, symmetry, and curvature of spine; any signs of trauma, skin discoloration, and signs of spinal dysgraphism (e.g., hairy patches); range of movements (forward and lateral bending, extension—note for any pain or limitation of motion)

Palpation: Of spinous processes for any localized tenderness/tumor/abscess, etc.

- Distal arterial pulsation

Neurological examination:
- Motor—strength of muscles;
- Sensory—any hypo or hyperesthesia in dermatomal distribution; deep tendon reflexes (especially knee and ankle jerks—lost in respective nerve or root lesions); any upper motor neuron signs such as positive Babinski sign, any evidence of wasting

Specific tests:
- *SLR test*: With the patient lying supine, raise the leg with knee extended—reproduction of the radicular pain usually occurs between 30° and 70° of elevation in case of lower lumbar radiculopathy
- *Bragard test*: While performing the SLR, bringing the foot into dorsiflexion reproduces the radicular pain
- *Neri's test*: While performing the SLR, asking the patient to flex the neck reproduces the pain
- *Patrick test*: With the patient in a supine position, the examiner should passively flex, abduct, and externally rotate the hip. Pain in the groin area suggests hip pathology, while pain in the back suggests sacroiliac joint pathology

"Red flags" (Possible indicators of serious spinal pathology and needs further investigations)
- Thoracic pain
- Fever and unexplained weight loss
- Bladder or bowel dysfunction
- History of malignancy, recent trauma, osteoporosis
- Progressive neurological deficit
- Disturbed gait, saddle anesthesia
- Age of onset <20 or >55 years

"Yellow flags" (Possible indicators of long-term chronicity and disability and needs multidisciplinary management)
- High levels of pain and disability
- Obesity
- Smoking
- Low education level
- Depression, anxiety, and somatization
- Job dissatisfaction
- Monotonous tasks

Management
- *NSAIDs*: Lowest effective dose for shortest duration possible is recommended
- *Skeletal muscle relaxants*: Short-term (~2 weeks) course effective for acute LBP
- *TCAs*, e.g., amitriptyline; *SNRIs*, e.g., duloxetine and venlafaxine
- *Antiepileptics*: Gabapentin and topiramate
- *Physiotherapy*: Stretching and strengthening exercises for pain relief and functional gains

Invasive procedures:
- Epidural steroid injections for lumbar radicular pain and spinal stenosis
- Intraarticular steroid injections for sacroiliac joint disease
- *Psychological interventions*: CBT

(CBT: cognitive behavioral therapy; LBP: low back pain; NSAID: nonsteroidal anti-inflammatory drug; SLR: straight leg raise; SNRI: serotonin and norepinephrine reuptake inhibitor; TCA: tricyclic antidepressant)

Chronic Visceral Pain

Chronic visceral pain is commonly encountered in medical practice and is associated with neurovegetative signs and emotional reactions. True visceral pain is a vague and poorly defined pain usually perceived in the midline at the lower sternum or upper abdomen. Visceral pain is often associated with marked autonomic phenomena, including pallor, profuse sweating, nausea, gastrointestinal (GI) disturbances and changes in body temperature, blood pressure, and heart rate. The viscerosomatic convergence of afferents in the CNS accounts for the "Referred pain" to the somatic structures,

TABLE 3: Characteristics of central and peripheral neuropathic pain.[19,20]

Neurological disorder	Prevalence of chronic pain	Clinical characteristics	Pathophysiology of chronic pain
Poststroke pain	8–14% of all stroke patients (thalamic strokes particularly)	Variety of aching, dull, and throbbing to sharp, shooting or burning pain	• Central neuropathic pain • Complex regional pain syndrome • Spasticity-related pain • Joint subluxation
Neuromuscular disorders: ALS	15% (Variable prevalence)	Arms > other parts no specific pattern	• Neuropathic pain • Pain from spasticity or cramps • Nociceptive pain—progression of muscle weakness and atrophy, prolonged immobility
Myopathies	~60%	Muscle cramps, spasms, diffuse or focal myalgia	Muscular pain, myofascial pain syndromes, fibromyalgia, inflammatory or necrotic activity in myositis, endocrine factors such as osteomalacia and hypocalcemia
Neuropathies of various etiologies	~40–50%	Moderate-to-severe pain paresthesia, numbness, sharp shooting or radiating pains	Altered peripheral and central nociception, DRG and root involvement, small fiber neuropathies, and sodium channel hyperexcitability
Spinal cord injury	60%	• Back pain—band-like sensation or pressure over neck or back • Associated numbness, tingling sensation in hands and feet	Neuropathic and nociceptive type pain, spasticity related pain
Multiple sclerosis	50–86%	Extremity pain, trigeminal neuralgia, Lhermitte's sign, tonic spasms, and back pain and headache	• Central neuropathic pain • CRPS, neuritic pain, radicular pain
Degenerative disease process: Parkinson disease	40–60%	Musculoskeletal, dystonic, radicular, and central neuropathic	Disruption of peripheral nociception and alterations in central pain threshold/processing, dopaminergic deficiency
Alzheimer's disease	40–50%	Musculoskeletal pain + other	• Abnormalities of the noradrenergic system in the locus coeruleus • Activation of microglia in frontal cortex • Increased central neuroinflammation

(ALS: amyotrophic lateral sclerosis; CRPS: complex regional pain syndrome; DRG: dorsal root ganglion)

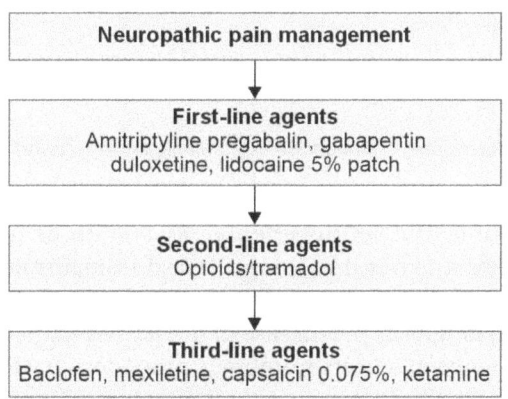

FLOWCHART 2: Management of neuropathic pain.[1,21-23]

producing secondary hyperalgesia of superficial and deep body wall tissues. Referred pain is a sharp and better localized pain and is less likely to be accompanied by autonomic signs. The functional gastrointestinal disorders (FGIDs) are one of the most common forms of visceral pains. IBS is one FGID characterized by abdominal pain and altered bowel habits. Other common conditions are dysmenorrhea in females, urinary colicky pain, and cancer-related pain. The available treatment options are nonsteroidal anti-inflammatory drugs (NSAIDs), opioids, and serotonergic compounds, and some evidence exists for use of pregabalin. Psychological interventions such as cognitive behavioral therapy (CBT) can be useful.[29-31]

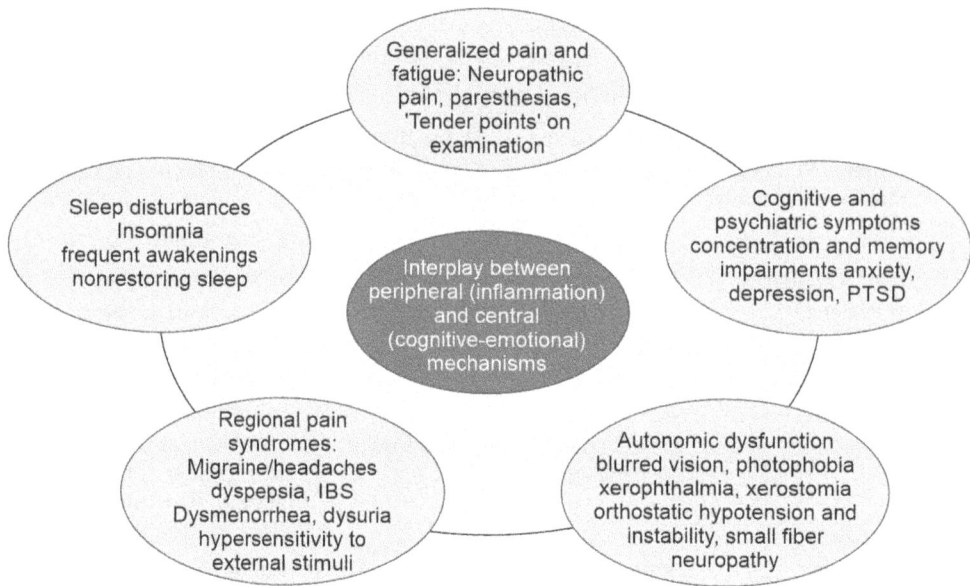

FIG. 1: Complex symptomatology of fibromyalgia.[27]
(IBS: irritable bowel syndrome; PTSD: post-traumatic stress disorder)

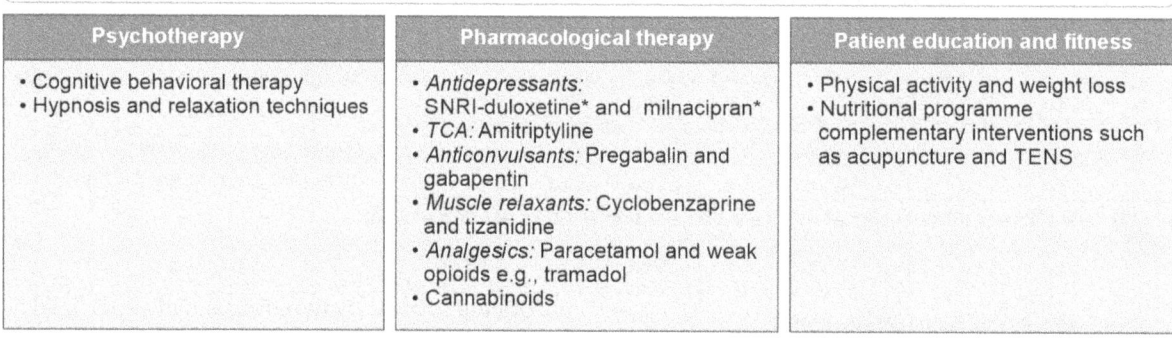

*The US Food and Drug Administration (FDA)-approved drugs.

FIG. 2: Diagnosis and management of fibromyalgia.[27,28]
(SNRI: serotonin and norepinephrine reuptake inhibitor; TENS: transcutaneous electrical nerve stimulation; TCA: tricyclic antidepressant)

Fatigue

Over the span of last few centuries, significant evolution in the experiences of fatigue becomes apparent. One would be surprised to know that fatigue as a medical entity was nearly nonexistent till 1800s'. In the earlier epochs, fatigue was regarded as an inherent facet of life; the acceptance of the demands and sensations tied to work kept it devoid of any heightened concern. It was following Beard's (1869) description of "Neuroasthenia" as a state of nervous system exhaustion that the profound transformation in perception of fatigue was witnessed. By 1900, Rabinbach declared fatigue as the disease of modern age and a direct consequence of society's embrace of modernity. This was driven by multiple factors including industrial revolution, shifts in the perception of work-life dynamics, as well as the evolving norms and lifestyles of society at large.[32,33] This perceptual shift underlies our current understanding of fatigue as a negative, even aversive state of depletion of bodily and mental energies.

Fatigue is a very common and nonspecific symptom associated with numerous health conditions. It is frequently reported in association with chronic inflammatory diseases, infections, and various cardiac, neurological and psychiatric disorders, or often related to unhealthy lifestyle habits **(Flowchart 3)**. It can be variously described as a subjective sense of tiredness, feeling of exhaustion, or difficulty in sustaining voluntary motor or cognitive tasks. Pathophysiologically, fatigue can be understood at two different levels: Cognitive or perceptual and physical or motor.

Concept of peripheral versus central fatigue:[34] Peripheral fatigue is defined as the inability to sustain a specified force or work rate because of physical limitations of the muscles, nerves, or cardiovascular system but little loss of endurance in mental tasks; thus, peripheral fatigue is associated with physical but not mental fatigue. On the other hand, central fatigue is the failure to initiate and/or sustain attentional tasks and physical activities requiring self-motivation (as opposed to external stimulation).[35] Anatomically, peripheral fatigue is ascribed to changes at or distal to the neuromuscular junction whereas central fatigue originates in the CNS (at the level of upper motor neurone and above).[36]

Chronic Fatigue Syndrome/Myalgic Encephalomyelitis

Chronic fatigue has long been acknowledged as a central feature of melancholic disorders and neurasthenia. Later in the mid-to-late 20th century, its meaning was rediscovered

History:
- First identify what is meant by "Fatigue" for the patient and try to classify into peripheral versus central fatigue; acute versus chronic; whenever possible
- *Impact on function*: Measurement of performance decrement (motor and/or cognitive) using standard questionnaires and scales e.g., Fatigue impact scale (FIS), Fatigue symptom inventory (FSI)[33,44]
- Contributing Medical comorbidities, if any
- *Associated symptoms*: Somatic and psychological
- *Social and occupational history*: Diet and lifestyle; addictions such as alcohol; sleep-duration, quality, snoring etc., work related issues—shift work/stress

Red flags:
Recent onset fatigue in previously healthy person, unintentional weight loss, cardiorespiratory dysfunction, neurological deficit on examination

Physical examination:
- General examination: For pallor, odema, lymphadenopathy. Dyspnea on exertion or other systemic signs
- Neurological examination: Motor bulk, strength, and tone assessment, stretch reflexes, check for fatigability for neuromuscular junction disorders, cognitive impairment if any

Laboratory investigations:
Hemogram, blood sugar, liver and renal function tests, thyroid profile, tests for infections, wherever relevant

Further tests:
ESR, CRP, Ferritin, HIV, ANA, RA, CPK, NCV EMG, viral serologies, etc., as directed from the history

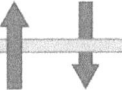

Cause identified: Manage accordingly
- *Pharmacological therapies*: Address cardiorespiratory issues, antidepressants (SSRI/SNRI) and anxiolytics, disease-specific therapy (e.g., MS)
- *Psychosocial interventions*: CBT, counseling, sleep hygiene
- Exercise therapy, endurance training to counteract deconditioning
- *Lifestyle advice as appropriate*: Weight loss and nutrition optimization

Chronic fatigue (i.e., lasting for >3–6 months):
- *Postinfectious fatigue syndrome*: Fatigue lasting for >3 months following an acute infection
- Cancer related fatigue
- ME/CFS
- Unexplained fatigue
- Look for possibility of somatic symptom disorder

FLOWCHART 3: Diagnostic approach to a patient with chronic fatigue.
(ANA: antinuclear antibody; CBT: cognitive behavioral therapy; CFS: chronic fatigue syndrome; CPK: creatine phosphokinase; CRP: C-reactive protein; ESR: erythrocyte sedimentation rate; HIV: human immunodeficiency virus; ME: myalgic encephalomyelitis; MS: multiple sclerosis; NCV EMG: nerve conduction velocity electromyography; RA: rheumatoid arthritis; SNRI: serotonin and norepinephrine reuptake inhibitor; SSRI: selective serotonin reuptake inhibitor)

in clinical context during outbreaks of widespread flu-like illness. This was the time when the term CFS was medically accepted by the United States Centers for Disease Control and Prevention (CDC) report.[37] Since then, the diagnostic criteria for CFS have been revised a few times, the National Academy of Medicine criteria 2015 remain the most widely used in clinical practice **(Box 1)**. The other available criteria are Modified CDC-1994 criteria and Canadian Consensus criteria, used mainly in secondary or tertiary care centers and for research purposes.[38,39]

Chronic fatigue syndrome/myalgic encephalomyelitis represents a debilitating condition with a global prevalence ranging from 0.3 to 0.8%.[40,41] This syndrome often eludes diagnosis for extended periods due to its diverse multisystemic manifestations, unremarkable results in routine laboratory tests, limited responsiveness to conventional therapies, and, additionally, a lack of awareness among medical practitioners. CFS is most frequently reported within the age range of 30 to 50 years, with a predilection for women (2–3:1 ratio).[39] The clinical hallmarks are profound fatigue and a lack of energy, which worsen after engaging in mental or physical activities, or when exposed to stress. Other notable features encompass disrupted sleep patterns, reported cognitive impairments, and autonomic irregularities such as postural hypotension or postural tachycardia syndrome (POTS). Furthermore, there may be concurrent indications of IBS, musculoskeletal pain, heightened allergic sensitivities, and emotional instability, anxiety, or depression. The neurological examination is usually normal. Muscle fatiguability has been demonstrated using the hand grip strength in patients with CFS.[38] The signs of dysautonomia, sensory hyperexcitability in form of allodynia, hyperalgesia, and subtle gait instabilities can be found occasionally **(Table 4)**.

Table 5 outlines the various treatment options available for CFS/ME.

BORDERLANDS OF CHRONIC PAIN AND FATIGUE AND MENTAL HEALTH DISORDERS

Epidemiologic evidence highlights a strong association between chronic pain and fatigue disorders and various mental health conditions, such as depression, anxiety, and substance abuse. Notably, two large population-based

---

BOX 1: The 2015 National Academy of Medicine diagnostic criteria for myalgic encephalomyelitis/chronic fatigue syndrome (ME/CFS).[42,43]

- *Required symptoms*:
  - Substantial reduction or impairment in the ability to engage in preillness levels of activity (occupational, educational, social, or personal life) with profound fatigue of new onset, which is present for at least 6 months, is not explained by ongoing or unusual excessive exertion, and is not substantially relieved by rest
  - Postexertional malaise* (PEM)
  - Unrefreshing sleep*
- *At least one of the following*:
  - Cognitive impairment*
  - Orthostatic intolerance

*Frequency and severity of symptoms should be assessed. The diagnosis of ME/CFS systemic exertion intolerance disease (SEID) should be questioned if patients do not have these symptoms at least half of the time with moderate, substantial, or severe intensity.

TABLE 4: Medical disorders with fatigue as a prominent feature.

Medical disorders with fatigue as a prominent feature	Comorbid conditions seen in CFS
Chronic infections: Hepatitis, tuberculosis, HIV/AIDS	Fibromyalgia
Cardiorespiratory diseases such as COPD, heart failure, or renal failure	Restless leg syndrome
Endocrine disorders: Thyroid disorders, diabetes mellitus, Addison or Cushing syndrome	Migraine- and tension-type headaches
Chronic inflammatory disorders: Rheumatoid arthritis, systemic lupus erythematosus, polymyositis, Sjögren syndrome, inflammatory bowel disease	Myofascial pain syndrome, small fiber neuropathy
Neurological disorders: Multiple sclerosis, myasthenia gravis, Parkinson disease, Alzheimer's disease, and stroke	Irritable bowel syndrome
Malignancy	Food intolerances and atopic conditions
Post-traumatic, postsurgical, postconcussion syndrome, post-ICU syndrome	Chronic pelvic pain, endometriosis
Psychiatric disorders: Bipolar disorder, anxiety, depression, anorexia, and bulimia	
Sleep disorders, e.g., OSA	
Lifestyle-related: Excessive consumption/abuse of alcohol or other substances	

(AIDS: acquired immunodeficiency syndrome; CFS: chronic fatigue syndrome; COPD: chronic pulmonary disease; HIV: human immunodeficiency virus; ICU: intensive care unit; OSA: obstructive sleep apnea)

studies have revealed a bidirectional relationship between depression rates and chronic pain, particularly in cases of chronic spinal pain.[2,44] Likewise, the prevalence of anxiety disorders looms high, ranging from 30 to 50% among patients grappling with chronic pain conditions such as fibromyalgia, CFS, IBS, and migraines.[1] Intriguingly, these patients might also exhibit borderline personality traits and a heightened disposition toward neuroticism. Even more concerning is that individuals seeking treatment for chronic pain often report elevated rates of suicidal ideations, necessitating diligent attention and a referral to a mental health professional. The functional neuroimaging studies further support such an intricate relationship. The key areas involved in the emotional processing of stimuli such as the anterior cingulate cortex (ACC) and PFC show alterations in various chronic pain related condition.[2] Evidently, these findings probably reflect the presence of shared neurobiological mechanisms that underlie chronic pain, fatigue, and various psychiatric disorders **(Fig. 3)**. This reinforces the utility of psychological interventions

TABLE 5: Management of chronic fatigue syndrome.

Nonpharmacological therapies	Pharmacological therapies
Relaxation, meditation/mindfulness	*Analgesics*: PCM
Physiotherapy, acupuncture, and acupressure	TCAs, SSRIs
Sleep hygiene	Gabapentin, pregabalin
Autonomic dysfunction: Stockings, increase in salt and water intake (>2 L/day) or rehydration solutions, drinking frequently, and postural maneuvers	Antiallergics/anti-inflammatory drugs
Diet—healthy and balanced diet, anti-inflammatory diet, reduced CH intake, adequate fluid intake, increase PUFA, omega-3 fatty acids, and proteins	• Autonomic dysfunction • Fludrocortisone, SSRI, midodrine, ivabradine, and pyridostigmine
Support measures: "Pacing" and activity management to work with the "energy envelope," adaptation strategies, occupational therapies, and education and counseling	Supplements: • Iron (if low ferritin) • Vitamin B12, B2, B6, D, and C • Co-Q, antioxidants • Omega-3/-6 FA • Alpha-lipoic acid • Carnitine and magnesium

(CH: carbohydrate; FA: fatty acid; PCM: paracetamol; PUFA: polyunsaturated fatty acid; SSRI: selective serotonin reuptake inhibitor; TCA: tricyclic antidepressant)

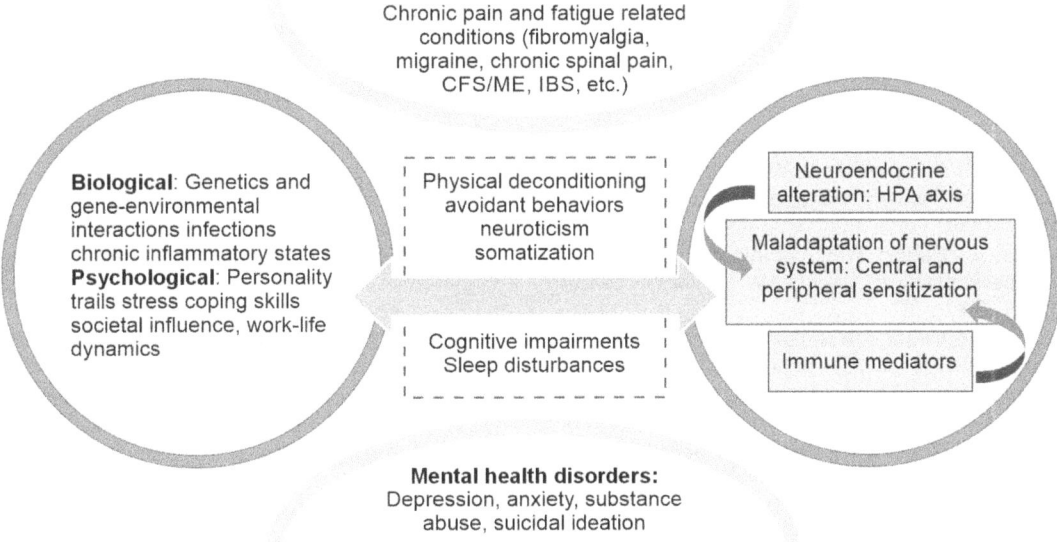

FIG. 3: Borderlands of chronic pain and fatigue and mental health disorders.
(CFS: chronic fatigue syndrome; HPA: hypothalamic-pituitary-adrenal; IBS: irritable bowel syndrome; ME: myalgic encephalomyelitis)

> **BOX 2: Nonpharmacological interventions for chronic pain and fatigue-related disorders.**
>
> - *Psychological interventions*:
>   - Cognitive behavioral therapy (CBT): A psychosocial intervention focused on challenging and changing maladaptive cognitive distortions and behaviors, improving emotional regulation, and the development of personal coping strategies
>   - Mindfulness therapy: A subtype of CBT defined as moment-to-moment awareness of one's experience without judgment
>   - Acceptance and commitment therapy (ACT): Contextually focused psychotherapy that aims to increase patients' ability to engage in values-based, positive behaviors
>   - Biofeedback: A process whereby electronic monitoring of a normally automatic bodily function is used to train someone to acquire voluntary control of that function
> - *Physiological treatment*:
>   - Exercises and physiotherapy, massage: For the purpose of improving function in the nervous, muscular, and circulatory systems; strength, balance, and flexibility training
>   - Yoga: Breathing exercises, meditation, and assuming various bodily postures to improve physical and mental well-being
> - *Complementary and alternative modalities*:
>   - Acupuncture: Relieving pain by inserting needles along specific pathways or meridian
>   - Chiropractic: A system of integrative medicine based on the diagnosis and manipulative treatment of misalignments of joints, especially in the spine, which are thought to cause other disorders by affecting nerves, muscles, and organs
>   - Music: Clinical use of musical interventions to improve quality of life
>   - TENS: Placement of small electrodes to deliver electrical impulses across the skin to relieve pain

in management of chronic pain and fatigue. Various nonpharmacological interventions for such chronic disorders are briefly discussed in **Box 2**

CONCLUDING REMARKS

In conclusion, chronic pain and chronic fatigue are complex and multifaceted issues with significant impacts on both individuals and society. The prevalence of these chronic debilitating conditions is on the rise globally and is a leading contributor to disability. The pathophysiology involves intricate interactions between peripheral and central mechanisms, further complicated by various internal and external influences. Additionally, they often intersect with mental health disorders, such as depression, anxiety, and substance abuse. The bidirectional relationship between these conditions underscores the need for comprehensive assessment and holistic management that addresses both physical and psychological aspects. A multidisciplinary approach involving psychological interventions and pharmacological treatments along with rehabilitation therapies play a crucial role in the overall well-being of patients.

REFERENCES

1. Guven Kose S, Kose HC, Celikel F, Tulgar S, De Cassai A, Akkaya OT, et al. Chronic pain: An update of clinical practices and advances in chronic pain management. Eurasian J Med. 2022;54(Suppl1):57-61.
2. Cohen SP, Vase L, Hooten WM. Chronic pain: an update on burden, best practices, and new advances. Lancet. 2021;397(10289):2082-97.
3. Nicol V, Verdaguer C, Daste C, Bisseriex H, Lapeyre É, Lefèvre-Colau MM, et al. Chronic low back pain: A narrative review of recent international guidelines for diagnosis and conservative treatment. J Clin Med. 2023;12(4).
4. Treede RD, Rief W, Barke A, Aziz Q, Bennett MI, Benoliel R, et al. Chronic pain as a symptom or a disease: The IASP Classification of Chronic Pain for the International Classification of Diseases (ICD-11). Pain. 2019;160(1):19-27.
5. Samanta jo, Kendall J, Samanta A. 10-minute consultation: Chronic low back pain. BMJ. 2003;326(7388):535.
6. Woolf CJ, Doubell TP. The pathophysiology of chronic pain--increased sensitivity to low threshold A beta-fibre inputs. Curr Opin Neurobiol. 1994;4(4):525-34.
7. Woolf CJ, Shortland P, Sivilotti LG. Sensitization of high mechanothreshold superficial dorsal horn and flexor motor neurones following chemosensitive primary afferent activation. Pain. 1994;58(2):141-55.
8. Cervero F, Laird JMA. Mechanisms of touch-evoked pain (allodynia): A new model. Pain. 1996;68(1):13-23.
9. Sillevis R, Trincado G, Shamus E. The immediate effect of a single session of pain neuroscience education on pain and the autonomic nervous system in subjects with persistent pain, a pilot study. Peer J. 2021;9:e11543.
10. Mathew PG, Garza I. Headache. Semin Neurol. 2011;31(1):5-17.
11. Olesen J. Headache Classification Committee of the International Headache Society (IHS) The International Classification of Headache Disorders, 3rd edition. Cephalalgia. 2018;38(1):1-211.

12. Do TP, Remmers A, Schytz HW, Schankin C, Nelson SE, Obermann M, et al. Red and orange flags for secondary headaches in clinical practice: SNNOOP10 list. Neurology. 2019;92(3):134-44.
13. Robbins MS, Dodick DW. Diagnosing secondary and primary headache disorders. Continuum (Minneap Minn). 2021;27(3):572-85.
14. Dodick DW. Pearls: Headache. Semin Neurol. 2010;30(1):74-81.
15. El-Tallawy SN, Nalamasu R, Salem GI, LeQuang JAK, Pergolizzi JV, Christo PJ. Management of musculoskeletal pain: An update with emphasis on chronic musculoskeletal pain. Pain Ther. 2021;10(1):181.
16. Airaksinen O, Brox JI, Cedraschi C, Hildebrandt J, Klaber-Moffett J, Kovacs F, et al. Chapter 4: European guidelines for the management of chronic nonspecific low back pain. Eur Spine J. 2006;15(Suppl 2):S192-300.
17. Nguyen C, Lefèvre-Colau MM, Kennedy DJ, Schneider BJ, Rannou F. Low back pain. The Lancet. 2018;392(10164):2547.
18. Urits I, Burshtein A, Sharma M, Testa L, Gold PA, Orhurhu V, et al. Low back pain, a comprehensive review: Pathophysiology, diagnosis, and treatment. Curr Pain Headache Rep. 2019;23(3).
19. Failde I, Dueñas M, Ribera MV, Gálvez R, Mico JA, Salazar A, et al. Prevalence of central and peripheral neuropathic pain in patients attending pain clinics in Spain: factors related to intensity of pain and quality of life. J Pain Res. 2018;11:1835.
20. Szok D, Tajti J, Nyári A, Vécsei L. Therapeutic approaches for peripheral and central neuropathic pain. Behav Neurol. 2019;2019:8685954.
21. Nishikawa N, Nomoto M. Management of neuropathic pain. J Gen Fam Med. 2017;18(2):56.
22. Bates D, Carsten Schultheis B, Hanes MC, Jolly SM, Chakravarthy KV, Deer TR, et al. A comprehensive algorithm for management of neuropathic pain. Pain Med. 2019;20(Suppl 1):S2-S12.
23. Gatchel RJ, McGeary DD, McGeary CA, Lippe B. Interdisciplinary chronic pain management. Am Psychol. 2014;69(2):119-30.
24. Clauw DJ. Fibromyalgia: A clinical review. JAMA. 2014;311(15):1547-55.
25. Gyorfi M, Rupp A, Abd-Elsayed A. Fibromyalgia pathophysiology. Biomedicines. 2022;10(12):3070.
26. Bair MJ, Krebs EE. In the clinic®: fibromyalgia. Ann Intern Med. 2020;172(5):ITC33-48.
27. Sarzi-Puttini P, Giorgi V, Marotto D, Atzeni F. Fibromyalgia: an update on clinical characteristics, aetiopathogenesis and treatment. Nat Rev Rheumatol. 2020;16(11):645-60.
28. Chinn S, Caldwell W, Gritsenko K. Fibromyalgia pathogenesis and treatment options update. Curr Pain Headache Rep. 2016;20(4):1-10.
29. Greenwood-Van Meerveld B, Johnson AC. Stress-induced chronic visceral pain of gastrointestinal origin. Front Syst Neurosci. 2017;11:315805.
30. Moloney RD, O'Mahony SM, Dinan TG, Cryan JF. Stress-induced visceral pain: Toward animal models of irritable-bowel syndrome and associated comorbidities. Front Psychiatry. 2015;6:15.
31. Holzer P, Farzi A, Hassan AM, Zenz G, Jacan A, Reichmann F. Visceral inflammation and immune activation stress the brain. Front Immunol. 2017;8:1613.
32. Murtagh J. Fatigue--a general diagnostic approach. Aust Fam Physician. 2003;32(11):873-6.
33. Hockey R. The Psychology of Fatigue: Work, Effort and Control. UK: Cambridge University Press; 2011. pp. 1-272.
34. Leavitt VM, DeLuca J. Central fatigue: issues related to cognition, mood and behavior, and psychiatric diagnoses. PM R. 2010;2(5):332-7.
35. Chaudhuri A, Behan PO. Fatigue and basal ganglia. J Neurol Sci. 2000;179(1-2):34-42.
36. Wilson J, Morgan S, Magin PJ, van Driel ML. Fatigue--a rational approach to investigation. Aust Fam Physician. 2014;43(7):457-61.
37. Bryan CS. The chronic fatigue syndrome: caveat emptor. JSC Med Assoc. 1992;88(2):79-81.
38. Plioplys AV, Plioplys S, Davis IV JS. Meeting the frustrations of chronic fatigue syndrome. Hosp Pract. 1997;32(6).
39. Working Group of the Royal Australasian College of Physicians. Chronic fatigue syndrome. Clinical practice guidelines--2002. Med J Aust. 2002;176(S9):S17-S55.
40. Sharpe M, Chalder T, White PD. Evidence-based care for people with chronic fatigue syndrome and myalgic encephalomyelitis. J Gen Intern Med. 2022;37(2):449-52.
41. Menting J, Tack CJ, Bleijenberg G, Donders R, Fortuyn HAD, Fransen J, et al. Is fatigue a disease-specific or generic symptom in chronic medical conditions? Health Psychol. 2018;37(6):530-43.
42. Bateman L, Bested AC, Bonilla HF, Chheda BV, Chu L, Curtin JM, et al. Myalgic encephalomyelitis/chronic fatigue syndrome: Essentials of diagnosis and management. Mayo Clin Proc. 2021;96(11):2861-78.
43. Nacul L, Authier FJ, Scheibenbogen C, Lorusso L, Helland IB, Martin JA, et al. European Network on Myalgic Encephalomyelitis/Chronic Fatigue Syndrome (EUROMENE): Expert Consensus on the Diagnosis, Service Provision, and Care of People with ME/CFS in Europe. Medicina (Kaunas). 2021;57(5).
44. Nieto FR, Vuckovic SM, Prostran MS. Editorial: Mechanisms and New Targets for the Treatment of Chronic Pain. Front Pharmacol. 2020;11:600037.

CHAPTER 20

Neuropsychiatric Manifestations of Demyelinating Disorders

Parthvi Ravat, Santosh Sriram Andugulapati, Sangeeta Ravat, Mayur Thakkar

■ INTRODUCTION

Psychiatric symptoms are commonly encountered in clinical neurological practice. While in many cases they occur secondary to the neurological disease, in certain situations they are an integral part of the clinical syndrome, e.g., anti-N-methyl-D-aspartate (NMDA) receptor encephalitis, frontotemporal dementia, etc. In some cases, they may be the sole manifestation of the disease. Understanding these intricacies is important for diagnosis and appropriate management, particularly in diseases such as demyelinating disorders of the central nervous system (CNS), which have a protracted course.

Diseases affecting the CNS myelin can be classified as dysmyelinating or demyelinating based on the presence of a primary biochemical abnormality in myelin or damage due to other process, respectively. Damage to normal myelin (demyelination) can occur due to infectious, immune, toxic, metabolic, and vascular process. This current chapter will focus on neuropsychiatric aspects of immune-mediated demyelination diseases of CNS.

The well-known immune-mediated demyelinating disorders are multiple sclerosis (MS), acute disseminated encephalomyelitis (ADEM), neuromyelitis optica spectrum disorders (NMOSDs), and myelin oligodendrocyte glycoprotein-associated disorders. It is important to understand the psychiatric manifestations in these diseases as they occur at a higher rate and can adversely affect patient care.

■ MULTIPLE SCLEROSIS

Multiple sclerosis is an inflammatory demyelinating disease of the CNS with a complex pathophysiology. Although this disease was reported hundreds of years ago, treatment options were limited until the past few decades. The prevalence of MS in the adult population of United States was estimated to be 309 per 100,000 population in 2010, and it is considered the most common nontraumatic disabling neurological condition in young adults **(Flowchart 1)**.[1]

The prevalence in India has been reported variably by many authors but is considered much lower than the United States. A recent meta-analysis of epidemiology of MS in Asia–Oceania region estimates a total prevalence of 37.89 per 100,000 population with higher prevalence in Oceania countries than Asian countries and lowest prevalence in southeast Asia.[2]

Pathophysiology

The pathophysiology of MS is complex, and a detailed discussion is beyond the scope of this chapter. The central thematic in the pathogenesis of MS is autoimmunity. Normally, autoreactive immune cells are deleted during development through tolerance mechanisms in the thymus (T cells) and bone marrow (B cells). When these central mechanisms of tolerance fail, some autoreactive cells are released into the peripheral circulation, which are kept in peripheral tolerance mechanisms such as regulatory T cells. A complex interplay of genetic and environmental factors leads to activation of these autoreactive cells, which lead to disease. The T-cell subsets implicated in MS are CD8+ T cells and CD4+ helper T cells Th1 and Th17.[3] Recently, the role of B cells has been increasingly recognized in MS having major implications on the therapeutic landscape. B cells produce proinflammatory cytokines such as interleukin-6 (IL-6), tumor necrosis factor-alpha (TNF-α), and granulocyte-monocyte colony-stimulating factor, which play an important role in the pathogenesis of MS.[4]

Risk Factors

- *Genetics*: HLA-DRB1*15:01 is associated with an increased risk, whereas HLA-A*02 is associated with a decreased risk of MS, respectively.[5]

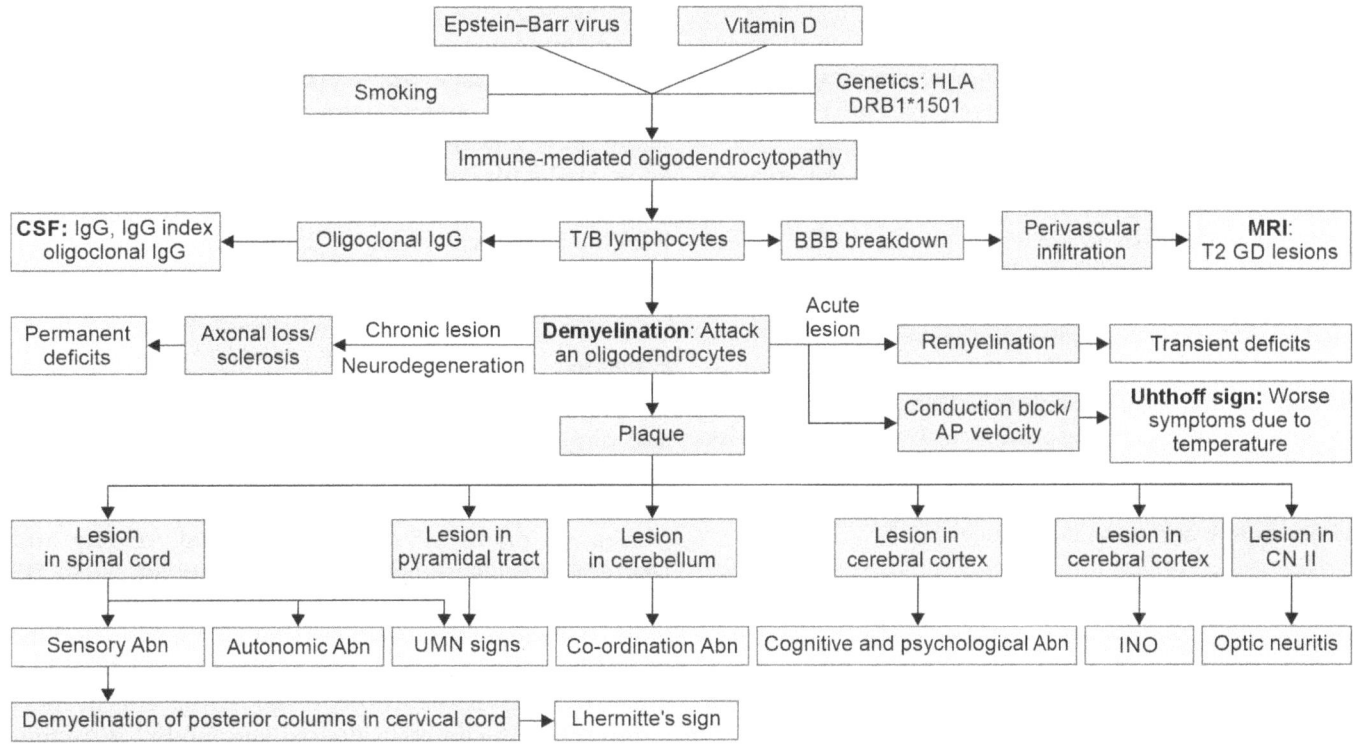

FLOWCHART 1: Overview of multiple sclerosis.
(Abn: abnormality; AP: action potential; BBB: blood–brain barrier; CSF: cerebrospinal fluid; CN: cranial nerve; Gd: gadolinium; INO: intranuclear ophthalmoplegia; MLF: median longitudinal fasciculus; MRI: magnetic resonance imaging; UMN: upper motor neuron)

- *Epstein-Barr virus (EBV)*: Many studies have consistently shown that EBV antibody seropositivity is associated with MS.[6]
- *Vitamin D*: It is proposed that vitamin D enhances immune tolerance and pathogen elimination, thus decreasing the risk of MS.[7]
- *Smoking*: It is associated with an increased risk of MS and the risk of conversion of clinically isolated syndrome to clinically definite MS.[8]
- *Obesity*: Obesity has been associated with an increased risk of MS in both adults and children, particularly in females.[9]
- *Microbiome*: Some species of Bacteroides produce short chain fatty acids that increase regulatory T-cells, which suppress autoreactive immune cells.[10]

Clinical Features

Multiple sclerosis involves white matter tracts of CNS in many locations producing a variety of clinical syndromes. There is a heterogeneity in the age of onset, initial manifestations, free quench and severity of relapse, and progression of disease. The characteristic demyelinating localizations are optic neuritis (ON), brainstem, and spinal cord. This section will focus on the neuropsychiatric manifestations of MS.

Psychiatric Disorders and Multiple Sclerosis

Psychiatric symptoms are common in people with MS.[11] Observations on neuropsychiatric manifestations in MS were made by Charcot way back in the nineteenth century in his detailed clinicopathological description of "Sclerose en Plaques."[12] Neuropsychiatric abnormalities have been reported in up to 60% of patients with MS and cause significant morbidity.[13] Psychiatric symptoms in MS usually present after the neurological diagnosis. However, psychiatric symptoms as part of first clinical presentation are reported in 2.3% and psychiatric symptoms alone as the initial presentation in 0.2–2% cases.[14] There is a significant overlap between the psychiatric symptoms and symptoms of MS such as fatigue, insomnia, and cognitive problems, which makes evaluation further difficult.

Depression and Major Depressive Disorder

Depression is the most common psychiatric disorder associated with MS with an annual prevalence rate of 15% to up to 25% in people aged 18–45 years. This is about five times the rate observed in general population.[15] Almost 50% patients with MS experience a significant depressive episode in their lifetime.[16,17] In the Diagnostic and Statistical Manual of Mental Disorders, Fifth edition (DSM-5), it is included in depressive disorders due to another medical illness category. There is no significant genetic predisposition for major depressive disorder (MDD) in MS as higher incidence of depression is not observed among first-degree relatives of depressed patients with MS.[13]

The common symptoms of depression are pervasive low mood, fatigue, irritability, and insomnia. Apathy, guilt, and worthlessness are less common in MS.[17] These symptoms are more common in the first year of diagnosis but can occur at any stage of MS.[12] The incidence of suicide is 7.5 times higher than the general population and also significantly higher than people experiencing other chronic neurological conditions.[13] Depressive symptoms are one of the factors associated with suicide. The risk factors for parasuicide are young age of onset, male gender, initial 5 years of illness, social isolation, recent functional deterioration, and substance abuse.[13,17,18]

Etiological Factors for Depression in MS

The relation between MS and depression is complex and multifactorial. Hypothalamic-pituitary-adrenal axis dysfunction, brain lesions, medications, and psychosocial factors have been implicated. Hypothalamic-pituitary-adrenal axis dysfunction is evident by elevated evening cortisol levels even in the early stages of illness.[19] About 50% of patients with MS and MDD have an abnormal dexamethasone suppression test, which is also seen in patients with isolated MDD.[19] Failure of cortisol suppression is also associated with an increased number of enhancing lesions.

The relation between brain lesions and neuropsychiatric manifestations of MS is variable. Some studies have reported that a higher lesion load in the frontal, temporal, and limbic system is associated with depression in MS. Brain lesions in areas connected to basifrontal and limbic system disrupt limbic pathways, which increase the risk of MDD. This has been demonstrated with diffusion tensor imaging and connectome analysis as abnormalities in white matter connectivity and regional integration in several regions including the hippocampus and amygdala. Magnetic resonance imaging (MRI) studies showed cortical atrophy particularly in the frontal and parietal lobes is associated with comorbid depression in MS.[13]

Corticosteroids are commonly used in treatment of MS relapses. Both their use and sudden withdrawal are known to increase the risk of mood disorders. Other drugs used for symptomatic management such as dantrolene and baclofen are also known to cause mood disorders. Among the disease-modifying therapies (DMTs), there are reports of increase in depression with treatment with beta-interferon, particularly in first 2–6 months. However, no significant association was established in subsequent studies and the increase seemed to be related to pretreatment levels of depression.[12]

Psychosocial factors play an important role in MDD and MS. Low socioeconomic status, severe physical disability, inadequate coping, and adjustment mechanisms are associated with a higher rate of depression.[13] Cognitive reframing—active attempt to acquire new perspectives—is related to lower levels of depression. While escape avoidance and emotional respite are associated with higher levels of depression.[20]

Evaluation

As there is an overlap between the MS symptoms and depressive symptoms, the American Academy of Neurology proposed Beck Depression Inventory-II and a two-question screen may be effective in the assessment of depression in MS.[12,21] The Hospital Anxiety and Depression Scale is another validated tool for use in MS patients with MDD.[13] Apart from clinician administered tools, self-report tools are also available for evaluations but their utility is limited. Standardized tools should be preferred for assessment of depression so that effectiveness of intervention can be evaluated and modify treatment accordingly.

Management

Treatment of depression should be individualized and should involve pharmacological and psychotherapeutic measures. The major aspect in the selection of treatment strategies for MDD in MS is the side effect profile of the drug, particularly on the motor and bladder functions. Pharmaceutical agents have demonstrated benefit in these patients, particularly selective serotonin reuptake inhibitors (SSRIs), because of their better tolerability and side effect profile. There is evidence that SSRIs can reduce axonal degeneration by inducing glycogenolysis in the axons.[22] Other alternatives include tricyclic antidepressants for depression and pain or bladder dysfunction and selective serotonin and noradrenergic reuptake inhibitors (SNRIs) for depression and comorbid pain and bupropion for reducing risk of sexual dysfunction in depression.[13] Mirtazapine, due to inhibition of proinflammatory cytokines and low incidence of sexual dysfunction, is also a good alternative in selected patients.

Cognitive behavioral therapy (CBT) is an effective strategy in mild-to-moderates cases coupled with pharmacological intervention.[23] Exercise and management of MS-related symptoms such as fatigue and disability also improve mood symptoms. Electroconvulsive therapy is found to be effective in intractable depressive episodes with minimal neurological deterioration.[24]

Bipolar Affective Disorder

Bipolar disorder is also well known in MS. The prevalence of bipolar affective disorder (BPAD) is 0.3–2.4%, which is almost twice the rate observed in general population.[25] Some studies have reported a higher rate. This increased rate can be attributed partly to the drugs used in MS. Up to one-third of patients experience a corticosteroid or antidepressant-induced manic episode.[26,27] Baclofen, dantrolene, and tizanidine are also implicated in hypomanic episodes. These drug-induced manic episodes are dose dependent and occur early in the treatment. Nonmedication manic symptoms also occur in MS. Some symptoms are present throughout the illness, e.g., impulsivity and emotional lability.

Evaluation

The common manic symptoms are rapid speech, impulsivity, psychomotor agitation, and insomnia.[13] The Mood Disorder Questionnaire (MDQ), although not validated in MS, is widely used to screen for bipolar disorder. It is a self-reported questionnaire to screen for lifetime history of symptoms related to BPAD. When the symptoms are subtle, the hypomania checklist (HCL-32) is a reliable tool, but it is not validated in patients with MS.[11] Patient with BPAD should also be evaluated for substance abuse. There are no specific brain MRI markers for bipolar disorder in MS and very few studies compared the MRI abnormalities of bipolar disorder in general population and in people with MS.

Management

Due to lack of specific data, the same strategies applicable to managing BPAD in general population are applied to patients with comorbid MS. Lithium has mood stabilizing properties and also potential disease-modifying effect in MS.[28] However, it may exacerbate MS-related bladder dysfunction and also cause polyuria. Corticosteroid-induced mania can be managed by olanzapine or lithium without discontinuing steroids.

Psychosis

Symptoms of psychosis are 2–3 times more common in people with MS than in general population[29] with >90% having symptoms of MS prior to the onset of psychosis. However, this does not translate into an increased diagnosis of schizophrenia as noted in a recent study where there was a decreased risk of schizophrenia in people with MS.[30]

Psychotic symptoms include hallucinations, delusions (paranoid), grandiosity, sleep disturbance, and blunted affect. Steroid-induced psychosis may be associated with grandiose or erotomanic delusions.[31] There are no MRI or neuropathological studies that define the lesions or processes underlying psychosis in MS.

Management

The management of psychosis in MS is in line with the general population. However, drug adverse effects should be considered when selecting an antipsychotic. Low dose, atypical antipsychotics are preferred in view of their safety with regard to extrapyramidal syndrome. Risperidone and quetiapine have demonstrated disease-modifying effects in experimental autoimmune encephalomyelitis mouse models.

Anxiety Disorders

The prevalence of anxiety syndromes is 35.6% in MS with a peak prevalence between 45 and 59 years.[11] Anxiety is more common in females with MS and at the time of diagnosis. MS diagnosis is a risk factor to develop anxiety. Anxiety frequently occurs with depression. Generalized anxiety disorder is seen in 19% patient while others such as panic disorder, obsessive compulsive disorder, and social anxiety disorder are not uncommon. "Self-injection anxiety" is a phenomenon seen in patients with MS who use self-injectable DMTs. Patients with this condition are unable to administer DMT such as interferon beta-1a due to phobia leading to noncompliance. CBT helps reduce anxiety and improves self-efficacy.

Evaluation and Management

Many scales have been validated for evaluating anxiety in MS, including Hamilton Anxiety Rating Scale and Beck Anxiety Inventory. There is limited data available about managing anxiety in MS. SSRIs are considered first-line treatments. Venlafaxine, buspirone, pregabalin, and beta-blockers are options in patients not responding to SSRIs. Benzodiazepines can be used for severe acute anxiety. CBT is a nonpharmacological alternative.

NEUROMYELITIS OPTICA SPECTRUM DISORDERS

Neuromyelitis optica is an immune-mediated neurological disorder due to antibodies against aquaporin-4 antigen (AQP4). The phrase "neuromyelitis optica" was coined by Eugene Devic. However, the terms neuromyelitis optica (NMO) and NMOSDs were unified in the international consensus criteria for NMOSD.[32]

Pathophysiology

Aquaporin-4 antibodies target AQP4, a transmembrane protein which facilitates water transport in the CNS.

These AQP4 antigens are expressed at the foot processes of astrocyte at the blood-brain barrier. The presence of autoantibodies against AQP4 leads to CNS degeneration, including increased neuroinflammation and disruption of distinct neurogenic processes, such as death of astrocytes, loss of hippocampal neurons, and necrosis of gray and white matter.[33] Some of these disruptions are similar to what is often observed in animal models of depression.[34] This has been hypothesized to be the result of direct demyelination of CNS structures and the unpredictable and progressive nature of the clinical course.[35] However, on imaging correlation, the areas of organic depression in the brain are spared in NMO.[36] Hence, the pathophysiology of depression in NMO is not well understood and needs more studies.

Psychiatric Disorders in Neuromyelitis Optica Spectrum Disorders

Classically, NMOSD includes one of the core clinical characteristics of ON, transverse myelitis, area postrema syndrome, brainstem syndrome, diencephalic involvement, with or without aquaporin 4 antibody positivity.

Psychiatric symptoms are considered unusual in NMOSDs. Although the initial description and distinction of NMO from MS was made in 2004, the first description of psychiatric symptoms were noted in 2010.[37] Since then, only sporadic case reports of psychiatric disorders in NMO and its association with mood disorders, psychosis, and significant cognitive impairment have been reported.[38] The real-world prevalence of psychiatric disorders is difficult to determine in NMOSDs. Patients with NMOSD experience psychiatric symptoms such as depression, anxiety, pain, and lower quality of life (QOL) than general population.[39-41]

Patients with NMO have a high prevalence of moderate-to-severe depression as well as suicidal ideation comparable to that of patients with MS. Previously diagnosed psychiatric comorbidities such as depression, panic attacks, and insomnia are more common in NMO then in MS.[35] Despite these factors, no significant difference was noted in QOL and depression between patients with MS and NMO.[39] Although not progressive, the natural history of NMO is long-standing, and longer disease duration has been found to be associated with higher levels of hopelessness, agoraphobia, and somatization.[35]

Management

Guidelines for the management of psychiatric disorders in NMOSDs are currently unavailable. Symptomatic management should be done on similar lines to patients with these disorders, without NMOSD.

MYELIN OLIGODENDROCYTE GLYCOPROTEIN-ASSOCIATED DISEASE

Myelin oligodendrocyte glycoprotein-associated disease (MOGAD) is an autoimmune demyelinating disorder, distinct from NMOSD, due to a different immunopathogenesis mediated by anti-MOG antibodies. The disease course is either monophasic or relapsing episodes of ON, transverse myelitis, ADEM, brainstem symptoms, and less frequently, cortical involvement with seizures.[32,39,40,41]

Pain is a common symptom in MOGAD. It is due to ON-related headache or periorbital pain, neuropathic pain including radicular pain, and musculoskeletal pain, which have been described anecdotally. These symptoms can severely affect the patient's mental well-being.[4,12,14-17] A systematic analysis of pain syndromes and depression in MOGAD and their impact on QOL in adult patients in Germany showed that pain and depression are highly prevalent in the spectrum of MOGAD.[42] These conditions strongly reduce QOL and ADL and are insufficiently controlled in clinical practice. Higher awareness of severely disabling neuropathic pain is of particular importance.

Management of psychiatric manifestations in MOGAD is similar to general population with particular consideration of drug interactions and adverse effects.

ACUTE DISSEMINATED ENCEPHALOMYELITIS

Acute disseminated encephalomyelitis commonly is a postinfectious syndrome with an identifiable trigger in up to 50% cases. It can occur at any age but much more common in children. Recurrent episodes of ADEM have been reported with anti-MOG antibodies. Clinical manifestations are heterogeneous. Irritability and mood disorders can be a presenting feature along with confusion and altered consciousness. Aggressiveness, auditory hallucinations, and delusions resembling schizophrenia have been reported to occur later in the disease course. Depression as a disease manifestation is rare. Management of psychiatric manifestations in ADEM is symptomatic.

CENTRAL PONTINE MYELINOLYSIS

Central pontine myelinolysis (CPM) is a neurological disorder associated with demyelinating lesions in the pons usually caused by electrolyte imbalance, especially rapid correction of severe hyponatremia. Besides neurological symptoms such as acute quadriplegia, dysarthria, dysphagia, and sometime loss of consciousness; CPM may also present with neuropsychiatric symptoms such as personality changes, inappropriate affect, emotional lability, disinhibition, catatonia, psychosis, and delirium, as described in some reports.[43,44] The symptoms resolve quickly along with the resolution of neurological symptoms. There are case reports on use of antipsychotics to achieve symptomatic remission in such cases.[45]

Neuroimaging

The correlation between MRI lesions of demyelinating diseases and psychiatric symptoms is complex and multifactorial. MRI findings should be interpreted in conjunction with clinical evaluation, patient history, and other diagnostic assessments. The presence of lesions on MRI does not necessarily indicate a direct causal relationship with psychiatric symptoms, however, some correlation has been reported (**Fig. 1**).

DIAGNOSTIC CONSIDERATIONS AND ASSESSMENT TOOLS

Challenges and Pitfalls

Evaluating psychiatric features in demyelinating disorders can present several challenges and pitfalls. Some of the key considerations include:

- *Overlapping symptoms*: Psychiatric symptoms such as depression, anxiety, etc., can be present in various neurological conditions. Distinguishing whether these symptoms are directly related to the demyelinating disorder or are independent comorbidities can be challenging. This requires a comprehensive evaluation, including clinical interviews, observation, and integration of neuroimaging findings.
- *Heterogeneity*: Demyelinating disorders encompass a range of conditions. Each disorder may have distinct patterns of psychiatric features, making it essential to consider the specific diagnosis. A comprehensive knowledge of all the psychiatric features of demyelinating disorders is required.
- *Temporal changes*: Psychiatric symptoms in demyelinating disorders can fluctuate over time, influenced by disease activity, relapses, and treatment effects. Longitudinal monitoring of symptoms is imperative.
- *Subjectivity and bias*: Assessing psychiatric symptoms relies heavily on patient self-report and clinical judgment, which can introduce subjectivity and potential bias. Validated assessment tools should be used where available.
- *Lack of standardized assessment tools*: Although various psychiatric rating scales and neuropsychological tests exist, there is no universally accepted tool for assessing psychiatric features in demyelinating disorders.
- *Treatment-related issues*: Antipsychotic medications may interact with DMTs used to manage the demyelinating disorder. In addition, cognitive and extrapyramidal side effects of antipsychotic medications may adversely affect the outcomes.

To navigate these challenges, a comprehensive, interdisciplinary approach involving neurologists, psychiatrists, neuropsychologists, and physiotherapist is required. A thorough evaluation should integrate clinical history, detailed neurological examination, neuroimaging findings, cognitive assessments, psychiatric rating scales, and longitudinal monitoring to improve diagnostic accuracy and guide treatment decisions.

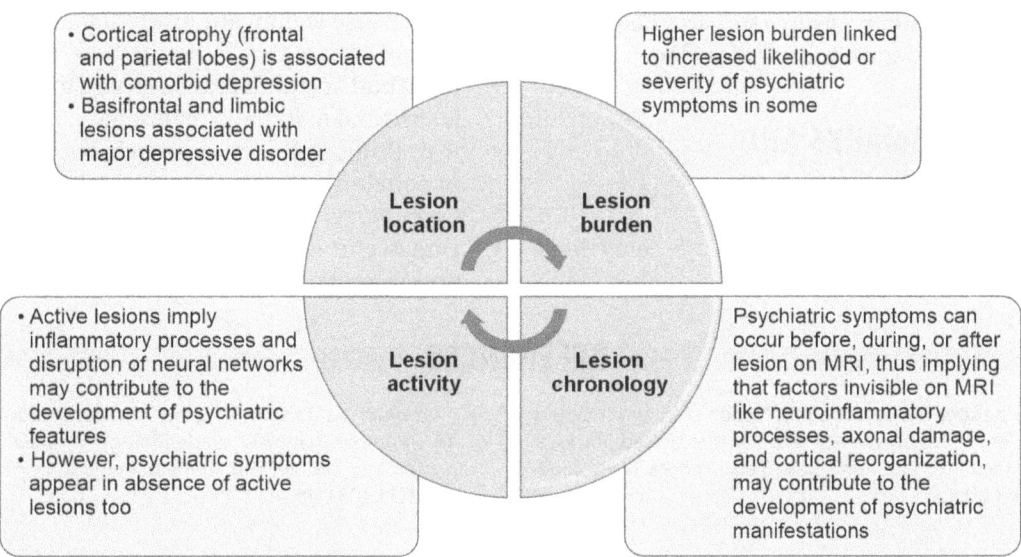

FIG. 1: Magnetic resonance imaging (MRI) factors that might affect psychiatric manifestation in demyelinating disorders.

Utilizing Psychiatric Rating Scales

Psychiatric rating scales provide standardized methods for assessing and quantifying symptoms, aiding in diagnostic clarification, monitoring treatment response, and tracking symptom severity over time. The most important step is to select the appropriate rating scale specifically designed to assess the target symptoms or domains of interest. Some have been enlisted in **Table 1**.

These scales also help in monitoring symptom severity. It is vital to administer rating scales at regular intervals to track changes over time. This longitudinal assessment helps in evaluating treatment response, identifying symptom exacerbation or remissions, and adjusting treatment plans accordingly.

A comparison to normative data is available if standardized scales are used making the assessment more objective. Rating scales can also aid in identifying specific symptom domains that require targeted intervention. By quantifying symptom severity, rating scales assist in prioritizing treatment goals and selecting appropriate interventions tailored to the patient's needs.

Nonpharmacological Management

Besides pharmacological interventions such as mood stabilizers and antidepressants, antipsychotics, anxiolytics as well as DMTs for the demyelinating disorder, few other treatment modalities are important.

These include psychotherapy and psychosocial interventions such as CBT, supportive psychotherapy, coping strategies, and stress reduction techniques.

A robust rehabilitation program will also help the patient stay active and avoid complications such as spasticity and bed sores in MS or other demyelination disorders when the patient loses ambulation. Supportive care and patient education measures can also help in the overall management of demyelinating disorders.

CONCLUDING REMARKS AND LEARNING POINTS

- Psychiatric disorders are common in CNS demyelinating disorders.

TABLE 1: Various scales used in studies for analysis of psychiatric features in demyelination disorders.

Scale	Comment
Beck Depression Inventory (BDI)	A self-reported scale widely used to assess the severity of depressive symptoms
Hamilton Rating Scale for Depression (HAM-D)	A clinician-administered scale that assesses the severity of depressive symptoms
Beck Anxiety Inventory (BAI)	A self-report scale used to measure the severity of anxiety symptoms
Hamilton Rating Scale for Anxiety (HAM-A)	A clinician-administered scale that assesses the severity of anxiety symptoms
Positive and Negative Syndrome Scale (PANSS)	A scale primarily used in schizophrenia research but can also be applied to assess psychotic symptoms in demyelinating disorders
Neuropsychiatric Inventory (NPI)	A scale commonly used to assess neuropsychiatric symptoms in various neurological disorders, including those with demyelination
Brief Psychiatric Rating Scale (BPRS)	A widely used scale that evaluates the severity of various psychiatric symptoms, including positive and negative symptoms, in multiple psychiatric disorders. While rating scales provide quantitative data, they should be used in conjunction with clinical interview and observations. These qualitative aspects provide contextual information and insights into the patient's symptoms and experiences

- They cause significant morbidity and adversely affect QOL of patients.
- Early and accurate diagnosis using standardized tools is essential to initiate treatment.
- A multidisciplinary approach is important in terms of collaboration between neurology, psychiatry, and psychology.
- Due to chronic nature of the illness, long-term follow-up is essential.

REFERENCES

1. Wallin MT, Culpepper WJ, Campbell JD, Nelson LM, Langer-Gould A, Marrie RA, et al. The prevalence of MS in the United States: a population-based estimate using health claims data. Neurology. 2019;92(10):e1029-40.
2. Forouhari A, Taheri G, Salari M, Moosazadeh M, Etemadifar M. Multiple sclerosis epidemiology in Asia and Oceania; A systematic review and meta-analysis. Mult Scler Relat Disord. 2021;54:103119.

3. Dendrou CA, Fugger L, Friese MA. Immunopathology of multiple sclerosis. Nat Rev Immunol. 2015;15(9):545-58.
4. Comi G, Bar-Or A, Lassmann H, Uccelli A, Hartung HP, Montalban X, et al. Role of B cells in multiple sclerosis and related disorders. Ann Neurol. 2021;89(1):13-23.
5. Waubant E, Lucas R, Mowry E, Graves J, Olsson T, Alfredsson L, et al. Environmental and genetic risk factors for MS: an integrated review. Ann Clin Transl Neurol. 2019;6(9):1905-22.
6. Belbasis L, Bellou V, Evangelou E, Ioannidis JP, Tzoulaki I. Environmental risk factors and multiple sclerosis: an umbrella review of systematic reviews and meta-analyses. Lacet Neurol. 2015;14(3):263-73.
7. Yeh W, Gresle M, Jokubaitis V, Stankovich J, van der Walt A, Butzkueven H. Immunoregulatory effects and therapeutic potential of vitamin D in multiple sclerosis. Br J Pharmacol. 2020;177(18):4113-33.
8. Hawkes C. Smoking is a risk factor for multiple sclerosis: a metanalysis. Mult Scler. 2007;13(5):610-5.
9. Liu Z, Zhang T, Yu J, Liu YL, Qi SF, Zhao JJ, et al. Excess body weight during childhood and adolescence is associated with the risk of multiple sclerosis: a metaanalysis. Neuroepidemiology. 2016;47(2):103-8.
10. Mowry EM, Glenn JD. The dynamics of the gut microbiome in multiple sclerosis in relation to disease. Neurol Clin 2018; 36(1):185-96.
11. Sparaco M, Lavorgna L, Bonavita S. Psychiatric disorders in multiple sclerosis. J Neurol. 2021;268(1):45-60.
12. Silveira C, Guedes R, Maia D, Curral R, Coelho R. Neuropsychiatric symptoms of multiple sclerosis: state of the art. Psychiatry Investig. 2019;16(12):877-88.
13. Murphy R, O'Donoghue S, Counihan T, McDonald C, Calabresi PA, Ahmed MA, et al. Neuropsychiatric syndromes of multiple sclerosis. J Neurol Neurosurg Psychiatry. 2017;88(8):697-708.
14. Lo Fermo S, Barone R, Patti F, Laisa P, Cavallaro TL, Nicoletti A, et al. Outcome of psychiatric symptoms presenting at onset of multiple sclerosis: a retrospective study. Mult Scler. 2010; 16(6):742-8.
15. Patten SB, Beck CA, Williams JV, Barbui C, Metz LM. Major depression in multiple sclerosis: a population-based perspective. Neurology. 2003;61(11):1524-7.
16. Minden SL, Schiffer RB. Affective disorders in multiple sclerosis review and recommendations for clinical research. Arch Neurol. 1990;47(1):98-104.
17. Feinstein A. The neuropsychiatry of multiple sclerosis. Can J Psychiatry. 2004;49(3):157-63.
18. Jefferies K. The neuropsychiatry of multiple sclerosis. Adv Psychiatr Treat. 2006;12(3):214-20.
19. Kern S, Schultheiss T, Schneider H, Schrempf W, Reichmann H, Ziemssen T. Circadian cortisol, depressive symptoms and neurological impairment in early multiple sclerosis. Psychoneuroendocrinology. 2011;36(10):1505-12.
20. Mohr DC, Goodkin DE, Likosky W, Gatto N, Baumann KA, Rudick RA. Treatment of depression improves adherence to interferon beta-1b therapy for multiple sclerosis. Arch Neurol. 1997;54(5):531-3.
21. Minden SL, Feinstein A, Kalb RC, Miller D, Mohr DC, Patten SB, et al; Guideline Development Subcommittee of the American Academy of Neurology. Evidence-based guideline: assessment and management of psychiatric disorders in individuals with MS: report of the Guideline Development Subcommittee of the American Academy of Neurology. Neurology. 2014;82(2):174-81.
22. Sijens PE, Mostert JP, Irwan R, Potze JH, Oudkerk M, De Keyser J. Impact of fluoxetine on the human brain in multiple sclerosis as quantified by proton magnetic resonance spectroscopy and diffusion tensor imaging. Psychiatry Res. 2008;164(3):274-82.
23. Hind D, Cotter J, Thake A, Bradburn M, Cooper C, Isaac C, et al. Cognitive behavioural therapy for the treatment of depression in people with multiple sclerosis: a systematic review and meta-analysis. BMC Psychiatry. 2014;14:5.
24. Steen K, Narang P, Lippmann S. Electroconvulsive therapy in multiple sclerosis. Innov Clin Neurosci. 2015;12(7-8):28-30.
25. Carta MG, Moro MF, Lorefice L, Trincas G, Cocco E, Del Giudice E, et al. The risk of bipolar disorders in multiple sclerosis. J Affect Disord. 2014;155:255-60.
26. Bhangle SD, Kramer N, Rosenstein ED. Corticosteroid-induced neuropsychiatric disorders: review and contrast with neuropsychiatric lupus. Rheumatol Int. 2013;33:1923-32.
27. Baldessarini RJ, Faedda GL, Offidani E, Vázquez GH, Marangoni C, Serra G, et al. Antidepressant-associated mood-switching and transition from unipolar major depression to bipolar disorder: a review. J Affect Disord. 2013;148(1):129-35.
28. Chiu C-T, Chuang D-M. Molecular actions and therapeutic potential of lithium in and clinical studies of CNS disorders. Pharmacol Ther. 2010;128(2):281-304.
29. Politte LC, Huffman JC, Stern TA. Neuropsychiatric manifestations of multiple sclerosis. Primary care companion to the Journal of clinical psychiatry. 2008;10(4):318.
30. Johansson V, Lundholm C, Hillert J, Masterman T, Lichtenstein P, Landén M, et al. Multiple sclerosis and psychiatric disorders: comorbidity and sibling risk in a nationwide Swedish cohort. Mult Scler. 2014;20(14):1881-91.
31. Kosmidis MH, Giannakou M, Messinis L, Papathanasopoulos P. Psychotic features associated with multiple sclerosis. Int Rev Psychiatry. 2010;22(1):55-66.
32. Wingerchuk DM, Banwell B, Bennett JL, Cabre P, Carroll W, Chitnis T, et al; International Panel for NMO Diagnosis. International consensus diagnostic criteria for neuromyelitis optica spectrum disorders. Neurology. 2015;85(2):177-89.
33. Genel O, Pariante CM, Borsini A. The role of AQP4 in the pathogenesis of depression, and possible related mechanisms. Brain Behav Immun. 2021;98:366-77.
34. Price RB, Duman R. Neuroplasticity in cognitive and psychological mechanisms of depression: an integrative model. Mol Psychiatry. 2020;25(3):530-43.
35. Shin JS, Kwon YN, Choi Y, Lee JY, Lee YI, Hwang JH, Choi SH, Kim SM. Comparison of psychiatric disturbances in patients with multiple sclerosis and neuromyelitis optica. Medicine (Baltimore). 2019;98(38):e17184.
36. Kim HJ, Paul F, Lana-Peixoto MA, Tenembaum S, Asgari N, Palace J, et al; Guthy-Jackson Charitable Foundation NMO International Clinical Consortium & Biorepository. MRI characteristics of neuromyelitis optica spectrum disorder: an international update. Neurology. 2015;84(11):1165-73.
37. Woolley J, Douglas VC, Cree BAC. Neuromyelitis optica, psychiatric symptoms and primary polydipsia: a case report. Gen Hosp Psychiatry. 2010;32:648.e5-648.e8.
38. Fernández VC, Alonso N, Melamud L, Villa AM. Psychiatric comorbidities and suicidality among patients with neuromyelitis optica spectrum disorders in Argentina. Mult Scler Relat Disord. 2018;19:40-3.
39. Chanson JB, Zéphir H, Collongues N, Outteryck O, Blanc F, Fleury M, et al. Evaluation of health-related quality of life,

fatigue and depression in neuromyelitis optica. Eur J Neurol. 2011;18(6):836-41.
40. Amato MP, Ponziani G, Rossi F, Liedl CL, Stefanile C, Rossi L. Quality of life in multiple sclerosis: the impact of depression, fatigue and disability. Mult Scler. 2001;7(5):340-4.
41. Jones KH, Ford DV, Jones PA, John A, Middleton RM, Lockhart-Jones H, et al. How People with Multiple Sclerosis Rate Their Quality of Life: An EQ-5D Survey via the UK MS Register. PLoS One. 2013;8.
42. Asseyer S, Henke E, Trebst C, Hümmert MW, Wildemann B, Jarius S, et al. Pain, depression, and quality of life in adults with MOG-antibody-associated disease. Eur J Neurol. 2021;28(5):1645-58.
43. Balhara YS, Gupta R, Sagar R. Acute psychosis with a favorable outcome as a complication of central pontine/extrapontine myelinolysis in a middle aged man. J Midlife Health. 2012;3(2):103-5.
44. Mattoo SK, Biswas P, Sahoo M, Grover S. Catatonic syndrome in central pontine/extrapontine myelinolysis: A case report. Prog Neuropsychopharmacol Biol Psychiatry. 2008;32(5):1344-6.
45. Patil V, Gupta R, Singh S, Goyal A, Deb K. Central pontine/extrapontine myelinolysis presenting with manic and catatonic symptoms. Indian J Psychol Med. 2019;41(5):491-3.

CHAPTER 21

Neuropsychiatric Aspects of Autoimmune Encephalitis

Rahul Kulkarni, Rishikesh Deshpande, Shripad Pujari

■ INTRODUCTION

Autoimmune encephalitis is a group of relatively newly described disorders, characterized by encephalopathy, seizures, movement disorders, and variety of neuropsychiatric manifestations. It is a rare condition, with a cumulative incidence of 0.8 per 100,00 person-years.[1] These conditions are antibody-mediated and respond to immune treatment. Over last two decades, many syndromes have been described. Due to a wide variety of neurological, neuropsychiatric and psychiatric manifestations which may overlap with more common neurological and psychiatric syndromes, early diagnosis of these disorders is challenging. If untreated, they lead to significant morbidity and mortality.

■ HISTORICAL ASPECTS

Although encephalitis is traditionally believed to be caused by infections, there are noninfectious causes of encephalitis. First case of presumed paraneoplastic encephalitis with psychiatric features was described by Oppenheim in 1888.[2] He described a 54-year-old woman with neuropsychiatric symptomatology along with a prominent mood dysfunction in addition to other brain dysfunctions such as aphasia and agnosia. Her autopsy revealed gastric cancer, but no abnormalities were observed in brain tissue. He postulated that the tumor could be the cause of focal neurological symptoms. About 80 years later, Brierley[3] described three patients with limbic encephalitis comprising psychiatric features such as memory impairment, depressive syndrome, behavioral abnormalities, and anxiety in addition to seizures and disturbed consciousness. The term "limbic encephalitis" was named nearly a decade later by Corsellis et al.[4]

In 2003, Dalmau et al.[5] described a young girl with acute onset behavioral changes with rapid worsening, prolonged unconsciousness, and central hypoventilation who had ovarian teratoma. She had responded to empirical immunotherapy and later found to have antibodies against N-methyl-D-aspartate receptor (NMDAR). Thereafter a large number of autoimmune encephalitis disorders are been described having antibodies against neuronal surface antigens or synaptic proteins, variable neurological and psychiatric manifestations, and response to immunotherapies.

In this chapter, we describe the neuropsychiatric manifestations of autoimmune encephalitis.

■ FEATURES

There is overlap between limbic, autoimmune, and paraneoplastic encephalitis. Classic limbic encephalitis presents with subacute confusion, depression, irritability, short-term memory loss, and seizures suggestive of medial temporal lobe dysfunction and is usually associated with magnetic resonance imaging (MRI) abnormalities in the medial temporal lobes without clinical or radiologic evidence of other areas of brain involvement. It is caused by infections, autoimmune, or paraneoplastic disorders.

Autoimmune encephalitis is caused by antibody-mediated inflammation of brain directed against synaptic proteins or cell surface antigens. By contrast, paraneoplastic encephalitis occurs in a cancer patient as a remote manifestation of cancer due to antibodies against intracellular cytoplasmic or nuclear antigens. The main differences between two are mentioned in **Table 1**.

Autoimmune encephalitis usually has a subacute onset though a more acute presentation is known. The common features include mental change, encephalopathy, or psychiatric manifestations. Depending on the target antigen and disorder, there are additional features. Graus et al.[6] had described diagnostic criteria for possible and definite autoimmune encephalitis (**Box 1**). Common autoimmune encephalitis and their salient manifestations are described in **Table 2**.

N-methyl-D-aspartate Receptor Encephalitis

The NMDAR encephalitis is the most prevalent autoimmune encephalitis syndrome.[7] It is more common in females (M:F = 4:1) with usual age of onset 25–35 years.[7] The antibodies against NR1 subunit of NMDA receptor are associated with ovarian teratoma and rarely other tumors. Viral encephalitis, especially herpes simplex virus (HSV) encephalitis can at times trigger the antibody production leading to subsequent development of autoimmune encephalitis is some patients. The syndrome has five

BOX 1: Diagnostic criteria for autoimmune encephalitis.

Possible autoimmune encephalitis: When all three of the following criteria have been met: Subacute onset (rapid progression of <3 months) of working memory deficits (short-term memory loss), altered mental status, and/or psychiatric symptoms
- At least one of the following:
  - New focal central nervous system findings
  - Seizures not explained by a previously known seizure disorder
  - CSF pleocytosis (white blood cell count of >5 cells/mm^3)
  - MRI features suggestive of encephalitis
- Reasonable exclusion of alternative causes

Definite autoimmune encephalitis: When all four of the following criteria have been met:
1. Subacute onset (rapid progression of <3 months) of working memory deficits, seizures, and/or psychiatric symptoms suggesting involvement of the limbic system
2. Bilateral brain abnormalities on T2-weighted FLAIR MRI highly restricted to the mesial temporal lobes
3. At least one of the following:
   - CSF pleocytosis (white blood cell count of >5 cells/mm^3)
   - EEG with epileptic or slow-wave activity involving the temporal lobes
4. Reasonable exclusion of alternative causes

(CSF: cerebrospinal fluid; EEG: electroencephalogram; FLAIR: fluid-attenuated inversion recovery; MRI: magnetic resonance imaging)

TABLE 1: Autoimmune versus paraneoplastic encephalitis.

	Autoimmune encephalitis	Paraneoplastic encephalitis
Antigen	Cell surface	Intracellular
Antibody response	B cell mediated	T cell mediated
Association with cancer	Weak	Strong
Psychiatric symptoms	More common	Less common
Response to immunotherapy	Good	Poor

TABLE 2: Salient features of autoimmune encephalitis.

Antigen	Main syndrome	Neurological features	Psychiatric features
NMDAR	NMDAR encephalitis	Seizures, language dysfunction, movement disorder, seizures, hypoventilation, and autonomic instability	Psychosis, catatonia, mood dysfunction, coexisting psychotic, and depressive features
LGI1	Limbic encephalitis	Classic limbic encephalitis, hyponatremia, and faciobrachial dystonic seizures	Confusion, personality changes, and hallucinations
CASPR2	Morvan syndrome and limbic encephalitis	Encephalitis, peripheral nerve hyperexcitability, autonomic dysfunction, hyperhidrosis, and insomnia, neuropathic pain	Confusion, personality changes, and hallucinations
AMPAR	Limbic encephalitis	Classic limbic encephalitis and seizures	Confusion, agitation, psychosis, and affective symptoms
GABAAR	Encephalitis with cortical-subcortical lesions	Seizures and multifocal brain lesions on imaging	Varied symptoms of encephalopathy and cognitive dysfunction
GABABR	Limbic encephalitis	Classic limbic encephalitis	Rapidly progressive dementia and behavioral changes

Continued

Continued

Antigen	Main syndrome	Neurological features	Psychiatric features
DPPX	Encephalitis and PERM	Tremors, myoclonus, seizures, transient hypersomnia, and diarrhea	Disorientation, agitation, and hallucinations
IgLON5	Sleep disorder and brainstem syndrome	Gait instability, bulbar palsy, movement disorders, sleep disorders, and neuromuscular symptoms	Cognitive impairment
GAD65	Stiff person syndrome and cerebellar ataxia	Temporal lobe epilepsy, ataxia, stiff person syndrome, and endocrinopathy	Mood disorder and cognitive impairment
GlycinR	PERM and stiff person syndrome	Seizures, trismus, and neurogenic pruritus, and atypical stiff person syndrome	Alterations of behavior and sleep
mGluR5	Cerebellar ataxia and limbic encephalitis	Ataxia and progressive memory complaints	Personality changes, behavioral issues, and Ophelia syndrome (inadvertent set of motion of events that culminate in self-inflicted harm)
D2R	Basal ganglia encephalitis	Dystonia, chorea, oculogyric crisis, parkinsonism, and seizures	Mutism and somnolence
Neurexin-3α	Encephalitis	Prodrome with fever and diarrhea, seizures, myoclonic jerks, orofacial dyskinesia, and central hypoventilation	Disorientation and confusion

(AMPAR: α-amino-3-hydroxy-5-methyl-4-isoxazolepropionic acid receptor; CASPR2: contactin-associated protein 2; DPPX: dipeptidyl aminopeptidase-like protein 6; D2R: dopamine-2-receptor; GABAAR: gamma-amino-butyric acid protein A receptor; GABABR: gamma-amino-butyric acid protein B receptor; GAD65: glutamic acid decarboxylase 65; GlycinR: glycine receptor; IgLON5: immunoglobulin-like cell adhesion molecule 5; LGI1: leucine rich glioma inactivated protein 1; mGluR5: metabotropic glutamate receptor 5; NMDAR: N-methyl-D-aspartate receptor; PERM: progressive encephalomyelitis with rigidity and myoclonus)

phases; prodromal phase, psychotic phase, unresponsive phase, hyperkinetic phase, and recovery phase.[8]

Case: A 25-year-old, previously healthy, lady developed upper respiratory infection. About 2 weeks later, she started having abnormal thoughts and auditory hallucinations. Over next 4–5 days, she became drowsy and required admission to intensive care unit (ICU). She subsequently developed clonic jerks of either limbs, orolingual dyskinetic movements, and hypoventilation requiring mechanical ventilation. Her reports showed cerebrospinal fluid (CSF) pleocytosis of 10 cells, normal MRI brain and NMDAR antibody was found in serum. Her electroencephalography (EEG) showed generalized slowing with superimposed fast beta activity (extreme delta brush) **(Fig. 1)**. Ultrasonography and computed tomography (CT) scan of abdomen and pelvis did not show any ovarian tumor. She was treated with antiseizure medicines, methylprednisolone, plasma exchange, and later with rituximab. She required prolonged hospital stay and made gradual recovery over 2 months. Her subsequent CT scan of pelvis 6 months later revealed an ovarian tumor which was removed laparoscopically and turned out to be a teratoma. She made complete recovery over 9–12 months.

Prodromal phase consists of headache, fever, nausea, vomiting, diarrhea, or upper respiratory tract symptoms. Within few weeks (<3 months), complex neuropsychiatric features develop. The onset is abrupt and progression is more rapid than a primary psychiatric disorder requiring admission to hospital. The psychiatric symptoms often precede the appearance of neurologic symptoms in adults while in children, seizures, and movement disorders are often the presenting features.[7]

Various positive and negative psychiatric symptoms have been described with NMDAR encephalitis and in a patient, the symptoms can change over course of illness. Patient can develop auditory and visual hallucinations, delusions, schizoaffective episodes, psychosis, depression, mania, affective disorder, amnesia, and agitation with no prior psychiatric history with rapid progression.[7,9] Other neuropsychiatric symptoms seen in NMDAR encephalitis include apathy, anxiety, fluctuating sensorium, bizarre behaviors, hypersexuality, wandering, aphasia, amnesia, apraxia, sleep-wake cycle disruption, aggression, homicidal ideation, and catatonia.[7,9-12]

In a study of 108 patients, 104 (95%) developed psychiatric features during the course of illness[13] that included aggression (40%), depression (26%), catatonia (14%),

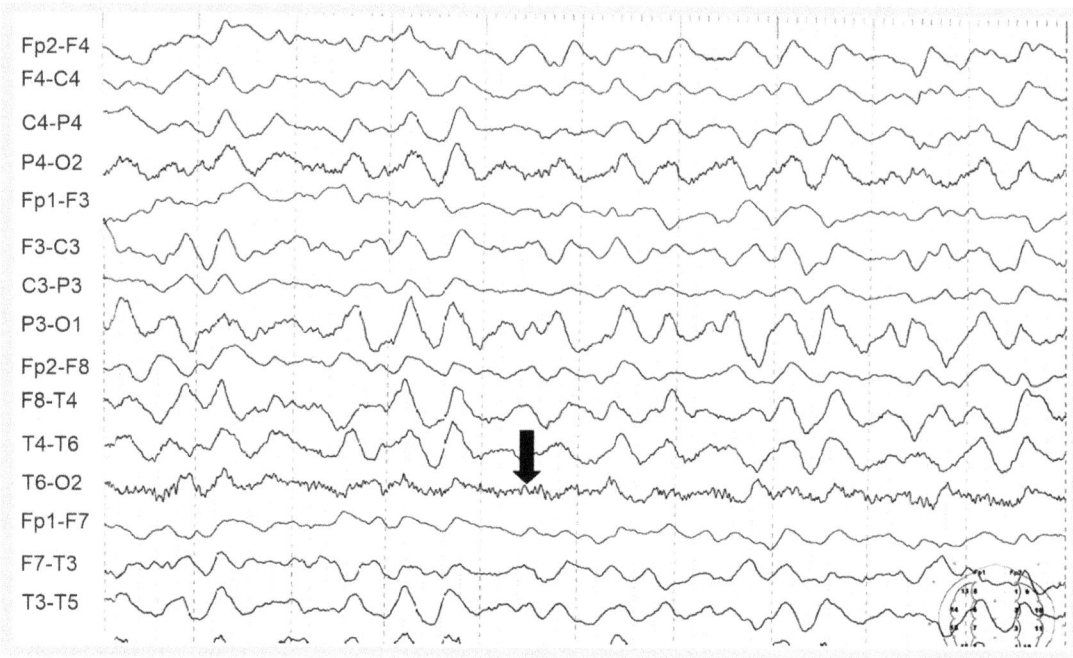

FIG. 1: Electroencephalogram (EEG) of a case of N-methyl-D-aspartate receptor (NMDAR) encephalitis showing generalized slowing with superimposed fast activity (extreme delta brush).

anxiety (24%), psychosis (50%), mania (62%), suicidal ideation (10%), and insomnia (26%). Isolated psychiatric symptoms are also rarely described. In 571 patients, 23 (4%) developed delusional thinking (74%), mood disturbances (70%, usually manic), and aggression (57%).[14]

Features that differentiate NMDAR encephalitis from a primary psychiatric illness are abrupt onset, rapid progression, multiple symptoms, a combined mood-psychosis syndrome, intolerance to neuroleptics, and concomitant-associated neurological symptoms.

Following the psychotic phase, patients rapidly develop alteration in consciousness and become mute with reduced motor movements. Most of them also develop various movement disorders the most classic being orolingual dyskinesia. Some of the movement disorders are so bizarre that these cannot be classified into any know phenotype. Seizures, and sometime status epilepticus, also develop during the course of illness more so in children. Autonomic dysfunction including labile hypertension, central hypoventilation, cardiac arrhythmia, and temperature abnormalities develop subsequently. Usually, these patients require longer stay in hospital needing ventilatory support, may develop secondary medical complications, and may recover gradually after immunotherapy.

Once suspected, the diagnosis is achieved by doing testing for NMDAR antibody with higher positivity rates in CSF than serum.[7] Routine CSF may show raised proteins and cellularity. MRI brain may be normal and may show T2/fluid-attenuated inversion recovery (FLAIR) hyperintensities, more often in hippocampus. EEG shows focal or more often generalized slowing. A pathognomonic pattern, superimposed fast beta activity over slow delta activity, called "extreme delta brush" is seen in NMDAR encephalitis **(Fig. 1)**.[7] As mentioned earlier, association with ovarian teratoma is well known and once a diagnosis is achieved, investigations are carried out to look for a tumor. Positron emission tomography (PET) scan often fail to detect these tumors which are not hypermetabolic; transvaginal ultrasonography, CT scan, or MRI are investigations of choice. In some cases, the tumor may not be apparent immediately and 6 monthly tumor surveillance is carried out for at least 4 years following a diagnosis.[7,15,16]

Leucine Rich Glioma Inactivated Protein 1 Encephalitis

Limbic encephalitis and presence of voltage-gated potassium channel (VGKC) antibodies were described in 2001 by Buckley at al.[17] It was later discovered that antibodies are not against potassium channels, but to their associated proteins; namely LGI1 and contactin-associated protein 2 (CASPR2) and two distinct syndromes were described.[18]

Leucine rich glioma inactivated protein 1 encephalitis typically presents in adult males of >60 years with subacute onset of memory loss, seizures, and psychiatric features suggestive of limbic encephalitis, hyponatremia, and unusual dystonic seizures involving face and upper limbs called faciobrachial dystonic seizures. If untreated, these patients can develop dementia. About 10% patients have underlying tumors such as thymoma and lung cancer.[19]

Various neuropsychiatric features have been described with LGI1 encephalitis which include apathy, disinhibition, psychosis, mood symptoms, irritability, visual hallucinations, personality changes, depressive syndrome, anxiety, and insomnia.[20] In a review of 485 cases of LGI1 encephalitis, 28% had emotionalist ability deficits, 22% aberrant motor behaviors, 13% apathy, 10% hallucinations, 8% mental disorders, 7% agitation, 6% delusions, 5% disinhibition, 4% anxiety, 3% depression, and 5% personality changes.[21] It is important to diagnose this disease early, as it is treated with immunotherapy with good response and if untreated, can lead to frontotemporal like dementia.[20]

CASPR2 Encephalitis

CASPR2 antibodies are identified as a part of VGKC-complex and often coexist with LGI1 antibodies. CASPR2 antibody associated diseases include peripheral nerve hyperexcitability presenting with neuromyotonia, encephalitic syndrome, and Morvan's syndrome that presents with neuromyotonia and additional neuropathic pain, hyperhidrosis, sleep disturbances, and mental change. In a large series, most common manifestation was limbic encephalitis in 42% patients.[22] The neuropsychiatric features included amnesia, behavioral disorders, hallucinations, psychosis, and insomnia.

Alpha-amino-3-hydroxy-5-methyl-4-isoxazolepropionic Acid Encephalitis

It typically presents in elderly with limbic encephalitis and has frequent association with tumors. Neuropsychiatric features include behavioral abnormalities including agitation and lethargy, short-term memory dysfunction, confabulation, disorientation, hallucinations, and insomnia.[23] A lady with rapid cycling bipolar symptoms has also been described.[24]

Gamma-amino-butyric Acid A Receptor Encephalitis

Gamma-amino-butyric acid A receptor (GABAAR) encephalitis is rare autoimmune encephalitic syndrome that presented with seizures, altered mental status, behavioral abnormalities, cognitive impairment, movement disorders, and is characterized by multifocal cortical and subcortical T2/FLAIR hyperintense lesions on MRI.[25]

Gamma-amino-butyric Acid B Receptor Encephalitis

Gamma-amino-butyric acid B receptor (GABABR) encephalitis is a type of limbic encephalitis where seizures are the most prominent feature. The average age of onset was 52 years in one series with relatively sudden onset.[26] Features include frequent epileptic seizures, cognitive dysfunction, episodic memory dysfunction, confusion, behavioral disorders, agitation, catatonic features, echolalia, and mutism.[26,27]

Glutamic Acid Decarboxylase 65 Encephalitis

Autoantibodies against glutamic acid decarboxylase 65 (GAD65) have been linked to diabetes mellitus type 1 (DM1) and various neurological syndromes including stiff-person syndrome, cerebellar ataxia, epilepsy, and limbic encephalitis. GAD65 encephalitis presents with seizures (97%), memory impairment (56%), and psychiatric features (28%) including depression and behavior or personality changes.[28] Mood dysfunction is also seen in some cases.[29]

The neuropsychiatric manifestations of other less common autoimmune encephalitis are described in **Table 2**.

Paraneoplastic Encephalitis

Paraneoplastic neurological syndromes present with variable neurological features with limbic encephalitis, seizures, retinopathy, myelopathy, and neuropathy. **Table 3** describes the paraneoplastic encephalitis syndromes.

Autoimmune Psychosis

Some of the patients presenting with epilepsy or psychosis have underlying autoimmune process as a cause of these disorders. These patients may not get other classic features of autoimmune encephalitis. These are now termed as autoimmune epilepsy[30] and autoimmune psychosis,[31] respectively.

Autoimmune psychosis is a newly coined term. It is believed that a proportion of cases of new onset psychosis have underlying immune-mediated cause and all of these may not have all manifestations of an autoimmune encephalitis syndrome. They are believed to have a milder phenotype or forme fruste of autoimmune encephalitis. Recently criteria have been proposed for diagnosis of these psychoses **(Box 2)**.[31] These patients should be investigated like other autoimmune encephalitis patients and treated with immunotherapy.

TABLE 3: Features of paraneoplastic encephalitis.

Antibody	Underlying malignancy	Neurological syndrome	Psychiatric features
Anti-Hu	Small cell lung	Encephalomyelitis	Memory impairment, change in personality, depression, anxiety, and hallucinations
Anti-CV2/CRMP5	Thymoma, small cell lung	Ataxia, chorea, Eaton–Lambert myasthenic syndrome, and movement disorders	Catatonic behavior, mutism, amnesia, cognitive impairment, disorientation, depressive, psychotic episodes, and OCD
Adenylate kinase 5 antibody	Lung	Limbic encephalitis	Memory deficit, personality changes, behavioral symptoms, agitation, aggression, mood disturbance, depressive syndrome, and anxiety
Anti-Yo	Ovary	Subacute cerebellar ataxia	Schizoaffective disorder, mood dysfunction, and psychosis
Anti-Ma2	Testis	Limbic encephalitis	OCD, delirium, depression, personality changes, amnesia, behavioral changes, and lethargy
Anti-SOX1	Lung	Limbic encephalitis	Cognitive impairment
Anti-Ri	Breast and gynecological malignancy	Subacute onset cerebellar ataxia	Personality changes

(CRMP5: collapsin response mediator protein 5; OCD: obsessive compulsive disorder; SOX1: sry-like high mobility group box 1)

BOX 2: Proposed diagnostic criteria for autoimmune psychosis.[31]

Possible autoimmune psychosis

Abrupt onset (rapid progression of <3 months) psychotic symptoms with at least one of the following:
1. Currently or recently diagnosed with a tumor
2. Movement disorder (catatonia or dyskinesia)
3. Adverse response to antipsychotics
4. Severe or disproportionate cognitive dysfunction
5. A decreased level of consciousness
6. The occurrence of seizures that are not explained by a previously known seizure disorder
7. A clinically significant autonomic dysfunction

Possible autoimmune psychosis should be investigated with EEG, MRI, serum autoantibodies, and CSF analysis

Probable autoimmune psychosis

Abrupt onset (rapid progression of <3 months) psychotic symptoms with at least one of the seven clinical criteria listed above for possible autoimmune psychosis and at least one of the following:
- CSF pleocytosis of >5 white blood cells per μL
- Bilateral brain abnormalities on T2-weighted fluid-attenuated inversion recovery MRI highly restricted to the medial temporal lobes

Or two of the following:
- Abnormal EEG
- CSF oligoclonal bands or increased IgG index
- The presence of a serum anti-neuronal antibody

Definite autoimmune psychosis

The patient must meet the criteria for probable autoimmune psychosis and presence of antineuronal antibodies in CSF

(CSF: cerebrospinal fluid; EEG: electroencephalogram; MRI: magnetic resonance imaging)

Seronegative Autoimmune Encephalitis

Although many autoimmune encephalitic syndromes have been described, a large number of cases of suspected autoimmune encephalitis have no identifiable pathogenic antibodies even on repeated testing. Subacute onset, combination of seizures, cognitive and psychiatric symptoms, CSF and MRI abnormalities, and response to immunotherapy help for the diagnosis of this syndrome.[32] Most of these patients present with limbic encephalitic syndrome and are diagnosed on basis of Graus et al. criteria **(Box 1)**.[6] These criteria have been recently validated in a large cohort of patients.[33]

Other systemic autoimmune diseases like systemic lupus erythematosus are well known to have neuropsychiatric manifestations. Autoimmune diseases involving nervous system like neuromyelitis optica can sometimes develop neuropsychiatric symptoms like cognitive impairment, symptomatic narcolepsy.

When to Suspect an Autoimmune Encephalitis?

Since the manifestations are diverse and overlapping, diagnosis of these disorders is challenging. In a patient presenting with psychiatric feature, presence of one or some of the following features would raise a possibility of autoimmune encephalitis:[34]
- Rapid progression of psychosis
- Headache
- Epileptic seizures
- Faciobrachial dystonic seizures (LGI1)
- Decreased level of consciousness
- Abnormal postures or movements (orofacial and limbs dyskinesia)
- Catatonia

- Focal neurological deficits
- Speech disturbance (dysarthria and aphasia)
- Suspicion of underlying malignancy
- Presence of other autoimmune diseases
- Hyponatremia
- MRI abnormalities (medial temporal hyperintensities, atrophy pattern)
- Abnormal CSF
- EEG abnormalities (slowing, extreme delta brush, and epileptiform activity)

Misdiagnosis of Autoimmune Encephalitis

Although autoimmune encephalitis is increasingly diagnostic consideration with subacute onset cognitive, psychiatric symptoms and seizures due to greater awareness among clinicians, the disease is still rare. Differential diagnosis includes functional neurological disorders, primary psychiatric disease, neurodegenerative disorders, toxic/metabolic encephalopathies, and neoplasms which are more common diseases. Thus, there is a chance of misdiagnosing a patient as autoimmune encephalitis. In a study of 107 patients of suspected autoimmune encephalitis,[35] correct diagnoses included functional neurologic disorder (25%), neurodegenerative disease (20.5%), primary psychiatric disease (18%), cognitive deficits from comorbidities (10%), cerebral neoplasm (19.5%), and other (17%). The diagnostic errors occurred due to overinterpretation of a nonspecific positive antibody result, misinterpretation of nonspecific symptoms as neurologic, functional neurologic features mistaken for true neurologic symptoms, psychiatric manifestations thought to be from autoimmune encephalitis and failure to accept a psychiatric diagnosis, and misinterpretation of imaging and CSF findings.

Box 3 mentions the red flags for a diagnosis of autoimmune encephalitis. Presence of any one these should raise a suspicion about diagnosis of autoimmune encephalitis. Thus, it is important to rule out all alternate causes while diagnosing autoimmune encephalitis.

PATHOLOGY AND PATHOPHYSIOLOGY

As mentioned earlier, antibody-mediated neurological disorders are classified into two broad categories, paraneoplastic and autoimmune, based on the presence or absence of an underlying malignancy. Paraneoplastic syndromes develop in a cancer, when common antigens shared by tumor cells and native neuronal cells result in an antibody-mediated attack on neuronal structures. The antibodies target intracellular onconeural antigens using cytotoxic T-cell mechanisms. These antibodies are less

> **BOX 3: Red flags in autoimmune encephalitis diagnosis.**
>
> *Clinical*
> - Insidious onset
> - Multiple comorbidities that cause cognitive deficits such as polypharmacy chronic pain, fibromyalgia, and sleep disorders
> - Examination results consistent with functional neurologic disorder
> - Features of mitochondrial disease present
>
> *Tests*
> - Normal neuropsychological test result
> - Normal MRI brain
> - Progressive atrophy without signal abnormalities or enhancement
> - Lesion(s) continuing to expand despite immunotherapy
> - Noninflammatory CSF
>
> *Serology*
> - Thyroid peroxidase antibodies of any titer
> - Low titer–positive GAD65 antibodies
> - Voltage-gated potassium channel complex antibodies negative for LGI1/CASPR2
> - Low-titer antibody positives by older generation techniques
> - Isolated serum NMDAR antibody negative in CSF
> - Immunoblot or line blot antibody positivity in isolation
> - Low titer positive CASPR2 antibodies
> - Antibody detection in noncertified laboratories
>
> (CASPR2: contactin-associated protein 2; CSF: cerebrospinal fluid; LGI1: leucine rich glioma inactivated protein 1; MRI: magnetic resonance imaging; NMDAR: N-methyl-D-aspartate receptor)

specific clinical markers of paraneoplastic syndromes and can also be seen in patients with cancer without features of paraneoplastic syndromes.

By contrast, autoimmune encephalitis is causes by antibodies that target cell-surface neuronal antigens, using humoral immune mechanisms of neurotoxicity. The antibodies also represent a more specific clinical marker of disease, with reduction in serum antibody titers following treatment. These antibodies often target synaptic proteins, causing downregulation of receptors, altered synaptic transmission, but relatively little neuronal death. Antibodies causing autoimmune encephalitis play a direct role in disease pathogenesis. This has been most clearly demonstrated for antibodies directed against NMDAR. In vitro studies on rat model confirm a direct role for antibodies in the pathogenesis of NMDAR encephalitis.[36]

Antibody production is triggered by underlying tumor, although the frequency of this association is clearly lower. Examples include ovarian teratoma in NMDAR encephalitis, lung cancer with GABABR limbic encephalitis, and thymoma in CASPR2. Antibodies also develop following a viral infection, most common example being NMDAR encephalitis after HSV encephalitis. Recently, antibodies development following use of class of drugs called immune checkpoint inhibitors has been seen.[37] However, in many cases, no clear etiology is identified.

Human leukocyte antigen (HLA) is the genetic factor related to autoimmunity and several autoimmune encephalitides were associated with HLA haplotypes. LGI1 encephalitis, CASPR2 syndrome, GAD65 encephalitis, and immunoglobulin-like cell adhesion molecule 5 (IgLON5) have been associated with certain HLA allele suggesting a genetic predisposition in autoimmune encephalitis.[37]

INVESTIGATIONS

Investigations are carried out to diagnose the autoimmune process, a particular syndrome and rule out alternative causes. The investigations would vary from patient to patient.

Most of the patients undergo MRI brain. Various MRI abnormalities described are unilateral or bilateral hippocampal or mesial temporal hyperintensities (limbic encephalitis) **(Fig. 2)**, cortical and subcortical hyperintensities (GABAAR encephalitis), mild atrophy, or nonspecific lesions. MRI can be normal at times. PET scan shows medial temporal hypermetabolism in limbic encephalitic syndromes.

Electroencephalogram abnormalities include focal or diffuse slow activity, epileptiform discharges or extreme

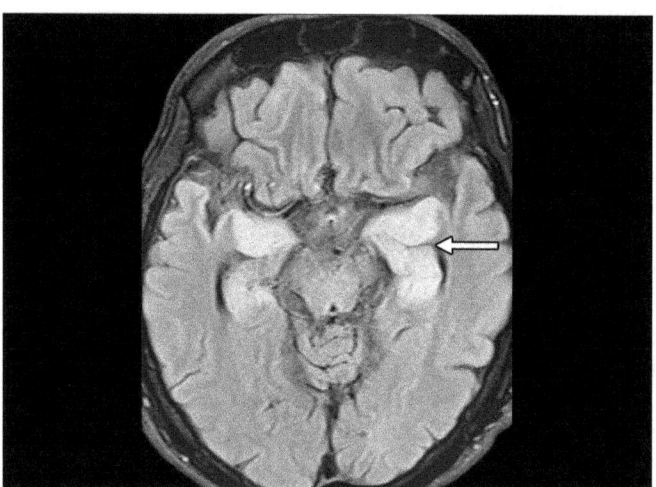

FIG. 2: Axial fluid-attenuated inversion recovery (FLAIR) MRI brain showing bilateral mesial temporal hyperintensities in a case of leucine rich glioma inactivated protein 1 (LGI1) encephalitis.

delta brush pattern (NMDAR encephalitis) **(Fig. 1)**. CSF is usually abnormal and has pleocytosis suggestive of inflammatory process and also has elevated proteins and oligoclonal bands.

Detecting antibody is often considered gold standard for diagnosis of autoimmune encephalitis. Most of the antibodies are detected in serum as well as in CSF. NMDAR antibody particularly has higher detection rates in CSF than serum and simultaneous serum and CSF testing should be done.[7] Standard laboratory and cell-based assay reduce chances of false negative tests.[35]

Since many autoimmune encephalitis have associated tumors, a systemic workup for tumor is required in all patients. Whole body PET CT to look for malignancy, transvaginal ultrasonography, and CT or MRI of pelvis are needed for detecting ovarian teratoma. In a male with NMDAR encephalitis, CT/MRI of chest, abdomen and testis are done to detect an underlying teratoma.

MANAGEMENT

Detail management of autoimmune encephalitis is beyond scope of this chapter. The basic principles of management include early initiation of immunotherapy with intravenous methylprednisolone, plasma exchange, intravenous immunoglobulin, or combination.[38] In LGI1 encephalitis, oral prednisolone is usually sufficient. Second-line agents rituximab or cyclophosphamide are initiated if the response to first-line therapy is inadequate or if a protracted course is expected, such as in NMDAR encephalitis. The treatment regimen is tailored as per clinical response to therapy. Most of the patients usually need maintenance immunosuppressive therapies to facilitate eventual cessation of first-line treatment and prevent relapses. Commonly used drugs for maintenance are rituximab, azathioprine, and mycophenolate mofetil.

Treatment of the underlying neoplasm in these cases can result in clinical improvement, especially in NMDAR encephalitis where early resection of an ovarian teratoma can result in rapid recovery. Additional symptomatic drugs such as antiseizure medications, antipsychotics, antidepressants, and anxiolytics are used as per the symptoms.

CONCLUDING REMARKS

Autoimmune encephalitis is a subacute illness with cognitive, psychiatric symptoms, seizures, and other neurological symptoms. Rapid progression, multiple symptoms, and associated neurological symptoms help a psychiatrist to diagnose it. High degree of clinical suspicion is needed even in isolated psychiatric symptoms. It is critical that a psychiatrist recognizes immune-mediated etiologies early in the course of illness as treatment delay can result in poorer outcome. Once diagnosis is achieved, effort must be made to find out associated tumor. The mainstay of treatment includes immunotherapy while the response to symptomatic drugs is often poor. With expansion of knowledge, newer autoimmune encephalitic syndromes with novel features have been described and one must try to remain updated about this exciting field of neuropsychiatry.

LEARNING POINTS

- Suspect autoimmune encephalitis as a cause of underlying psychiatric illness, if patient has subacute onset, rapid progression, and concomitant neurological symptoms.
- Autoimmune encephalitis can present with multiple psychiatric symptoms which may vary from patient to patient and in one patient through the course of illness.
- Autoimmune psychosis needs high degree of clinic suspicion and the proposed diagnostic criteria will aid in reaching a diagnosis.
- Presence of headache, seizures, underlying systemic disease (connective tissue disease), abnormal MRI, and suspicion of underlying malignancy points toward autoimmune rather than pure psychiatric disease.
- Evaluation of these diseases should include workup to look for an underlying tumor.
- Treatment is often multidisciplinary and immunotherapy is mainstay of treatment. Many patients require ICU admission and long hospital stay.
- Be aware of red flags of autoimmune encephalitis to avoid a misdiagnosis.
- These disorders should not be confused with paraneoplastic encephalitis where association with cancer is stronger and has poorer response to therapies.

REFERENCES

1. Dubey D, Pittock SJ, Kelly CR, McKeon A, Lopez-Chiriboga AS, Lennon VA, et al. Autoimmune encephalitis epidemiology and a comparison to infectious encephalitis. Ann Neurol. 2018;83(1):166-77.
2. Schulz P, Prüss H. "Hirnsymptome bei Carcinomatose"—Hermann Oppenheim and an Early Description of a Paraneoplastic Neurological Syndrome. J Hist Neurosci. 2015;24(4):371-7.
3. Brierley JB, Corsellis JAN, Hierons R, Nevin S. Subacute encephalitis of later adult life. Mainly affecting the limbic areas. Brain. 1960;83(3):357-68.
4. Corsellis JA, Goldberg GJ, Norton AR. "Limbic encephalitis" and its association with carcinoma. Brain. 1968;91(3):481-96.
5. Dalmau J, Gleichman AJ, Hughes EG, Rossi JE, Peng X, Lai M, et al. Anti-NMDA-receptor encephalitis: case series and analysis of the effects of antibodies. Lancet Neurol. 2008;7(12):1091-8.
6. Graus F, Titulaer MJ, Balu R, Benseler S, Bien CG, Cellucci T, et al. A clinical approach to diagnosis of autoimmune encephalitis. Lancet Neurol. 2016;15(4):391-404.
7. Samanta D, Lui F. Anti-NMDA Receptor Encephalitis. Treasure Island (FL): StatPearls Publishing; 2023.
8. Iizuka T, Sakai F, Ide T, Monzen T, Yoshii S, Iigaya M, et al. Anti-NMDA receptor encephalitis in Japan: long-term outcome without tumor removal. Neurology. 2008;70(7):504-11.
9. Marinova Z, Bausch-Becker N, Savaskan E. Anti-N-methyld-aspartate receptor encephalitis in an older patient presenting with a rapid onset of delusions and amnesia. BMJ Case Rep. 2019;12(4):e22851212.
10. Sansing LH, Tüzün E, Ko MW, Baccon J, Lynch DR, Dalmau J. A patient with encephalitis associated with NMDA receptor antibodies. Nat Clin Pract Neurol. 2007;3(5):291-6.
11. Khadem GM, Heble S, Kumar R, White C. Anti-N-methyl-D-aspartate receptor antibody limbic encephalitis. Intern Med J. 2009;39(1):54-6.
12. Espinola-Nadurille M, Flores-Rivera J, Rivas-Alonso V, Vargas-Cañas S, Fricchione GL, Bayliss L, et al. Catatonia in patients with anti-NMDA receptor encephalitis. Psychiatry Clin Neurosci. 2019;73(9):574-80.
13. Wang W, Zhang L, Chi XS, He L, Zhou D, Li JM. Psychiatric Symptoms of Patients With Anti-NMDA Receptor Encephalitis. Front Neurol. 2020;10:1330.
14. Kayser MS, Titulaer MJ, Gresa-Arribas N, Dalmau J. Frequency and characteristics of isolated psychiatric episodes in anti–N-methyl-d-aspartate receptor encephalitis. JAMA Neurol. 2013;70(9):1133-9.
15. Dalmau J, Tüzün E, Wu HY, Masjuan J, Rossi JE, Voloschin A, et al. Paraneoplastic anti-N-methyl-D-aspartate receptor encephalitis associated with ovarian teratoma. Ann Neurol. 2007;61(1):25-36.
16. Wu C-Y, Wu JD, Chen CC. The Association of Ovarian Teratoma and Anti-N-Methyl-D-Aspartate Receptor Encephalitis: An Updated Integrative Review. Int J Mol Sci. 2021;22(20):10911.
17. Buckley C, Oger J, Clover L, Tüzün E, Carpenter K, Jackson M, et al. Potassium channel antibodies in two patients with reversible limbic encephalitis. Ann Neurol. 2001;50(1):73-8.
18. van Sonderen A, Schreurs MW, Wirtz PW, Sillevis Smitt PA, Titulaer MJ. From VGKC to LGI1 and Caspr2 encephalitis: The evolution of a disease entity over time. Autoimmun Rev. 2016;15(10):970-4.
19. Irani SR, Michell AW, Lang B, Pettingill P, Waters P, Johnson MR, et al. Faciobrachial dystonic seizures precede Lgi1 antibody limbic encephalitis. Ann Neurol. 2011;69(5):892-900.
20. Endres D, Prüss H, Dressing A, Schneider J, Feige B, Schweizer T, et al. Psychiatric Manifestation of Anti-LGI1 Encephalitis. Brain Sci. 2020;10(6):375.
21. Teng Y, Li T, Yang Z, Su M, Ni J, Wei M, et al. Clinical Features and Therapeutic Effects of Anti-leucine-rich Glioma Inactivated 1 Encephalitis: A Systematic Review. Front Neurol. 2022;12:791014.

22. van Sonderen A, Ariño H, Petit-Pedrol M, Leypoldt F, Körtvélyessy P, Wandinger KP, et al. The clinical spectrum of Caspr2 antibody-associated disease. Neurology. 2016;87(5):521-8.
23. Lai M, Hughes EG, Peng X, Zhou L, Gleichman AJ, Shu H, et al. AMPA receptor antibodies in limbic encephalitis alter synaptic receptor location. Ann Neurol. 2009;65(4):424-34.
24. Quaranta G, Maremmani AG, Perugi G. Anti-AMPA-Receptor Encephalitis Presenting as a Rapid-Cycling Bipolar Disorder in a Young Woman with Turner Syndrome. Case Rep Psychiatry. 2015;2015:273192.
25. Spatola M, Petit-Pedrol M, Simabukuro MM, Armangue T, Castro FJ, Barcelo Artigues MI, et al. Investigations in GABAA receptor antibody-associated encephalitis. Neurology. 2017;88(11):1012-20.
26. Zhu F, Shan W, Lv R, Li Z, Wang Q. Clinical Characteristics of Anti-GABA-B Receptor Encephalitis. Front Neurol. 2020;11:403.
27. Samra K, Rogers J, Mahdi-Rogers M, Stanton B. Catatonia with GABAB receptor antibodies. Pract Neurol. 2020;20(2):139-43.
28. Gagnon MM, Savard M. Limbic Encephalitis Associated With GAD65 Antibodies: Brief Review of the Relevant literature. Can J Neurol Sci. 2016;43(4):486-93.
29. Hansen N, Widman G, Witt JA, Wagner J, Becker AJ, Elger CE, et al. Seizure control and cognitive improvement via immunotherapy in late onset epilepsy patients with paraneoplastic versus GAD65 autoantibody-associated limbic encephalitis. Epilepsy Behav. 2016;65:18-24.
30. Jang Y, Kim DW, Yang KI, Byun JI, Seo JG, No YJ, et al. Drug Committee of Korean Epilepsy Society. Clinical Approach to Autoimmune Epilepsy. J Clin Neurol. 2020;16 (4):519-29.
31. Pollak TA, Lennox BR, Müller S, Benros ME, Prüss H, Tebartz van Elst L, et al. Autoimmune psychosis: an international consensus on an approach to the diagnosis and management of psychosis of suspected autoimmune origin. Lancet Psychiatry. 2020;7(1):93-108.
32. Lee WJ, Lee HS, Kim DY, Lee HS, Moon J, Park KI, et al. Seronegative autoimmune encephalitis: clinical characteristics and factors associated with outcomes. Brain. 2022;145(10):3509-21.
33. Orozco E, Valencia-Sanchez C, Britton J, Dubey D, Flanagan EP, Lopez-Chiriboga AS, et al. Autoimmune Encephalitis Criteria in Clinical Practice. Neurol Clin Pract. 2023;13(3):e200151.
34. Herken J, Prüss H. Red Flags: Clinical Signs for Identifying Autoimmune Encephalitis in Psychiatric Patients. Front Psychiatry. 2017;8:25.
35. Flanagan EP, Geschwind MD, Lopez-Chiriboga AS, Blackburn KM, Turaga S, Binks S, et al. Autoimmune Encephalitis Misdiagnosis in Adults. JAMA Neurol. 2023;80(1):30-9.
36. Greenlee JE, Carlson NG, Abbatemarco JR, Herdlevær I, Clardy SL, Vedeler CA. Paraneoplastic and Other Autoimmune Encephalitides: Antineuronal Antibodies, T Lymphocytes, and Questions of Pathogenesis. Front Neurol. 2022;12:744653.
37. Vogrig A, Muñiz-Castrillo S, Desestret V, Joubert B, Honnorat J. Pathophysiology of paraneoplastic and autoimmune encephalitis: genes, infections, and checkpoint inhibitors. Ther Adv Neurol Disord. 2020;13:1756286420932797.
38. Abboud H, Probasco JC, Irani S, Ances B, Benavides DR, Bradshaw M, et al.; Autoimmune Encephalitis Alliance Clinicians Network. Autoimmune encephalitis: proposed best practice recommendations for diagnosis and acute management. J Neurol Neurosurg Psychiatry. 2021;92(7):757-68.

COMMENTARY 16

Autoimmune Encephalitis: Some Current Thoughts

Ambar Chakravarty

INTRODUCTION

Currently, autoimmune encephalitis has become the major differential diagnosis in patients with subacute altered mental status, psychiatric alterations, seizures, or cognitive impairment.[1] Testing for neuronal antibodies, testing for which has significantly increased, as their presence, very significantly confirms the diagnosis and is helpful for identifying different comorbidities, such as the presence of an underlying neoplasia, and can assist to define the prognosis.

SOME CURRENT THOUGHTS

Paraneoplastic neurological syndromes (PNSs) are indeed rare (in <1% of cancer patients); but because of their severity, they have a significant impact on the patient's quality of life. Any type of neoplasia can be associated with PNS, but lung cancer, especially small cell lung cancer (SCLC), is characterized by a high incidence. In a prospective study of 264 patients with SCLC, 24 (9%) developed a PNS, mainly Lambert–Eaton myasthenic syndrome, sensory neuronopathy, and limbic encephalitis.[2] Epidemiological studies to assess the incidence and prevalence of PNSs were unavailable until recent years, when three studies (two Italian and one US) showed the overall prevalence to be around 5 per 100,000 populations.[3-5] Other population-based studies have also observed an increase in the annual incidence of PNSs over the last years.[3,4,6] This increased incidence likely reflects a greater awareness of PNSs by neurologists and a wider accessibility to onconeural antibody testing.

Another likely explanation for this increase may be the increasing use of monoclonal antibodies against immune checkpoint molecules that normally inhibit T-cell activation in the treatment of cancer. These immune checkpoint, inhibitors, particularly those against programmed cell death 1 (PD-1) and its ligand (PDL1), have been associated with an increased risk for developing PNS. The likely mechanism may lie in the effect of the immune checkpoint inhibitors in the activation of the immune system.[7]

A very crucial step in the management of PNSs is the early identification of the underlying neoplasia which, in many instances, is not detectable at the time of PNS diagnosis.[8] Full-body computed tomography (CT) or fluorodeoxyglucose positron emission tomography combined with CT (FDG-PET/CT) are preferred screenings for a vast majority of neoplasia.[9,10] Other imaging procedures may be needed in special situations, like mammography or breast MRI in suspected breast cancer, testicular ultrasound for suspected testicular cancer, and transvaginal ultrasound for ovarian teratoma.[11,12]

The question arises as to how to proceed for patients with suspected PNS when the first search for cancer is negative.[13] In the report of the EFNS task force of 2011, it was recommended repeating screening every 6 months up to 4 years.[14] However, in a more recent communication, this period was reduced to 2 years as the vast majority of neoplasia in patients with PNS can be diagnosed <2 years after PNS onset.[15] Patients with classical PNS should be re-evaluated throughout at least 2 years, unless they present antibodies that do not associate with cancer (e.g., limbic encephalitis and LGI1 antibodies).

Autoimmune brainstem encephalitis can be classified as idiopathic, either primary or secondary to systemic autoimmune diseases, and paraneoplastic.[16] Differential diagnosis in primary brainstem encephalitis would lie between multiple sclerosis (MS), neuromyelitis optica spectrum disorder (NMOSD), and myelin oligodendrocyte glycoprotein antibody-associated disease (MOGAD) and this may sometimes be difficult. In a retrospective observational study, brainstem manifestations occurred in 62/185 (34%) MOGAD patients.

Isolated attacks were less frequent in MOGAD (23%) than MS (73%) and NMOSD (47%). Middle cerebellar peduncle fluid-attenuated inversion recovery (FAIR)/T2-weighted hyperintensity was also more common in MOGAD (46%) over MS (10%) and NMOSD (10%). On the other hand, cerebrospinal fluid (CSF) oligoclonal bands were present in 82% of patients with MS, but much lesser (in <20%) of those with MOGAD or NMOSD.[17]

The standard treatment of autoimmune encephalitis and PNSs consists of intravenous methylprednisolone (1 g/d for 3-5 days) or intravenous immunoglobulins (2 g divided in 5 days) and less frequently oral prednisone (1 mg/kg/day). These regimens are usually not very effective in PNS associated with onconeural antibodies, as they likely cause neuronal death mediated by T-cell cytotoxicity. However, in patients with autoimmune encephalitis triggered by antibodies against synaptic receptors and other surface antigens, a partial improvement or complete recovery may occur in at least 75% of the cases. The role of plasma exchange as an alternative or add-on therapy is debatable.[18] Rössling and Prüss by a systematic review of the literature using the Preferred Reporting Items for Systematic reviews and Meta-Analyses (PRISMA) guidelines and screening the articles independently, addressed the issue, for their respective eligibility.[19]

Although the design of the analyzed studies prevented drawing firm conclusions, two messages are important: First, as expected, apheresis did not work on neurologic syndromes associated with antibodies against intracellular antigens; and second, in autoimmune encephalitis, a better outcome was strongly associated with an early start of the treatment.[19] Indeed better treatment protocols for autoimmune encephalitis and PNSs are urgently needed.

REFERENCES

1. Dalmau J, Graus F. Antibody-Mediated Encephalitis. N Engl J Med. 2018;378:840-51.
2. Gozzard P, Woodhall M, Chapman C, Nibber A, Waters P, Vincent A, et al. Paraneoplastic neurologic disorders in small cell lung carcinoma: A prospective study. Neurology. 2015;85:235-9.
3. Vogrig A, Gigli GL, Segatti S, Corazza E, Marini A, Bernardini A, et al. Epidemiology of paraneoplastic neurological syndromes: A population-based study. J Neurol. 2020;267:26-35.
4. Hébert J, Riche B, Vogrig A, Muñiz-Castrillo S, Joubert B, Picard G, et al. Epidemiology of paraneoplastic neurologic syndromes and autoimmune encephalitides in France. Neurol Neuroimmunol Neuroinflamm. 2020;7:e883.
5. Lorusso L, Precone V, Ferrari D, Ngonga GK, Russo AG, Paolacci S, et al. Paraneoplastic Neurological Syndromes: Study of Prevalence in a Province of the Lombardy Region, Italy. J Clin Med. 2020;9:3105.
6. Shah S, Flanagan EP, Paul P, Smith CY, Bryant SC, Devine MF, et al. Population-Based Epidemiology Study of Paraneoplastic Neurologic Syndromes. Neurol Neuroimmunol Neuroinflamm. 2022;9:e1124.
7. Vogrig A, Fouret M, Joubert B, Picard G, Rogemond V, Pinto A-L, et al. et al. Increased frequency of anti-Ma2 encephalitis associated with immune checkpoint inhibitors. Neurol Neuroimmunol Neuroinflamm. 2019;6:e604.
8. Yshii LM, Gebauer CM, Pignolet B, Mauré E, Quériault C, Pierau M, et al. et al. CTLA4 blockade elicits paraneoplastic neurological disease in a mouse model. Brain. 2016;139:2923-34.
9. Opalińska M, Sowa-Staszczak A, Wężyk K, Jagiełła J, Słowik A, Hubalewska-Dydejczyk A. Additional Value of [18F]FDG PET/CT in Detection of Suspected Malignancy in Patients with Paraneoplastic Neurological Syndromes Having Negative Results of Conventional Radiological Imaging. J Clin Med. 2022;11:1537.
10. Sheikhbahaei S, Marcus CV, Fragomeni RS, Rowe SP, Javadi MS, Solnes LB. Whole-Body (18)F-FDG PET and (18)F-FDG PET/CT in Patients with Suspected Paraneoplastic Syndrome: A Systematic Review and Meta-Analysis of Diagnostic Accuracy. J Nucl Med. 2017;58:1031-6.
11. García Vicente AM, Delgado-Bolton RC, Amo-Salas M, López-Fidalgo J, Caresia Aróztegui AP, García Garzón JR, et al. (18)F-fluorodeoxyglucose positron emission tomography in the diagnosis of malignancy in patients with paraneoplastic neurological syndrome: A systematic review and meta-analysis. Eur J Nucl Med Mol Imaging. 2017;44:1575-87.
12. Ruiz-García R, Martínez-Hernández E, Saiz A, Dalmau J, Graus F. The Diagnostic Value of Onconeural Antibodies Depends on How They Are Tested. Front Immunol. 2020;11:1482.
13. McKeon A, Apiwattanakul M, Lachance DH, Lennon VA, Mandrekar JN, Boeve BF, et al. Positron emission tomography-computed tomography in paraneoplastic neurologic disorders: Systematic analysis and review. Arch Neurol. 2010;67:322-9.
14. Titulaer MJ, Soffietti R, Dalmau J, Gilhus NE, Giometto B, Graus F, et al. Screening for tumours in paraneoplastic syndromes: Report of an EFNS Task Force. Eur J Neurol. 2011;18:19-e3.
15. Graus F, Vogrig A, Muñiz-Castrillo S, Antoine JG, Desestret V, Dubey D, et al. Updated Diagnostic Criteria for Paraneoplastic Neurologic Syndromes. Neurol Neuroimmunol Neuroinflamm. 2021;8:e1014.
16. Zoghaib R, Sreij A, Maalouf N, Freiha J, Kikano R, Riachi N, et al. Autoimmune Brainstem Encephalitis: An Illustrative Case and a Review of the Literature. J Clin Med. 2021;10:2970.
17. Banks SA, Morris PP, Chen JJ, Pittock SJ, Sechi E, Kunchok A, et al. Brainstem and cerebellar involvement in MOG-IgG-associated disorder versus aquaporin-4-IgG and MS. J Neurol Neurosurg Psychiatry. 2021;92:384-90.
18. Dubey D, Kryzer T, Guo Y, Clarkson B, Cheville JC, Costello BA, et al. Leucine Zipper 4 Autoantibody: A Novel Germ Cell Tumor and Paraneoplastic Biomarker. Ann Neurol. 2021;89:1001-10.
19. Rössling R, Prüss H. Apheresis in Autoimmune Encephalitis and Autoimmune Dementia. J Clin Med. 2020;9:2683.

CHAPTER 22

Neuropsychiatric Aspects of Central Nervous System Infections

Madhu Nagappa, Sanjib Sinha

INTRODUCTION

Meningitis and encephalitis refer to infection of the meninges and the brain parenchyma respectively. Meningitis is characterized by the triad of fever, headache, and neck rigidity. Signs of meningeal irritation such as the Kernig's sign and the Brudzinski's sign are often elicited at the bedside. Seizures, depressed sensorium, and raised intracranial tension may also be present. Encephalitis, on the other hand is characterized predominantly by alteration in sensorium, which ranges from mild lethargy, drowsiness, and confusion to coma. Features of focal or diffuse cerebral dysfunction such as weakness, aphasia, ataxia, movement disorders, cranial nerve palsies, and hypothalamopituitary dysfunction may be present depending upon the regions of the brain that are affected.[1] Psychiatric symptoms such as altered behavior or personality, delusions, hallucinations, agitation, and frank psychosis may also be present. Infection of the meninges, subarachnoid space, and brain parenchyma often coexist giving rise to the syndrome of meningoencephalitis. The clinical course ranges from (1) acute fulminant, evolving over hours to a few days, (2) subacute, with symptoms evolving over days to weeks and, (3) chronic, wherein the disease progresses over >4 weeks.[2] The etiologies include (1) infective, (2) neoplastic, (3) noninfective inflammatory disorders, (4) chemical or drug-induced, and (5) parameningeal infections. This chapter focusses on the infective causes of meningitis, encephalitis, and meningoencephalitis with an emphasis on those that cause predominant neuropsychiatric manifestations.

BACTERIAL INFECTIONS

Whipple's Disease

Whipple's disease is a rare, chronic or relapsing, and multisystem disease caused by the gram-positive bacillus, *Tropheryma whipplei*, which affects the gastrointestinal tract, joints, eyes, heart, lungs, lymph nodes, skin, kidneys, thyroid gland as well as the testes and epididymis. The infection is most likely acquired by fecal–oral transmission, and the clinical course is marked by a "prodromal" phase followed by a "steady state" phased separated by an interval of approximately 6 years.[3] The central nervous system (CNS) involvement occurs in majority of the infected patients (90%) and based on the clinical course, it is classified as "classical", relapse in a patient with "classical" Whipple's disease or isolated nervous system involvement. The clinical manifestations of CNS involvement are complex and protean. Altered sensorium, ranging from confusion to coma, delirium, seizures, status epilepticus, ataxia, and headache occur. Cognition is impaired in the form of reduced attention and memory or frontal lobe syndrome. Hypothalamic involvement manifested as hyperphagia, weight gain, polydipsia, hypersomnia, and altered libido. Evidence for pyramidal and extrapyramidal dysfunction including myoclonus, chorea, and oculomasticatory or oculofacial-skeletal myorhythmia occur, of which the latter is considered to be the clinical hallmark of Whipple's disease. Psychiatric manifestations in the form of depression and altered personality are seen in nearly 50% of the affected subjects. Brain MRI may be normal, or it may show the presence of focal or multifocal tumor-like lesions in the medial temporal lobes, thalamus, hypothalamus and brainstem, periventricular hyperintensities, ventricular dilation, diffuse atrophy, or pachymeningitis. Ischemic lesions from cardiac emboli may also be seen. Rarely the spinal cord is also abnormal. The diagnosis is established by demonstrating the presence of periodic acid–Schiff (PAS) positive macrophages and *Tropheryma whipplei* deoxyribonucleic acid (DNA) by polymerase chain reaction (PCR) in the cerebrospinal fluid (CSF) or other body fluids/tissue.[3,4]

Clinical Clue

The history of systemic involvement, particularly gastrointestinal symptoms, together with oculomasticatory myorhythmia, in a patient with a complex encephalopathy should raise the suspicion of Whipple's disease.

Brucellosis

This is the most common bacterial zoonoses and is caused by the gram negative, nonmotile coccobacillus, *Brucella melitensis*. Infection is acquired by direct contact with infected animals or their tissues/secretions, consumption of uncooked meat or unpasteurized dairy products, blood transfusion, bone marrow transplantation, and sexual intercourse. The organism disseminates hematogenously and any organ system can be affected including the gastrointestinal tract, heart, lungs, skin, eyes, skeletal and hemotopoietic systems, in addition to the nervous system. The incubation period ranges from 1 to 3 weeks and the course is acute, subacute, or chronic. The organism is intracellular and it remains dormant for a variable latent period before reactivation and relapse of infection. Clinical features include nonspecific systemic features such as fever, malaise, night sweats, headache, and weight loss.[5] Severe infection is characterized by involvement of the heart and nervous system. Neurobrucellosis occurs in up to 25%, and can occur at any stage of the infection, either in isolation or as a part of the multisystem involvement. Seizures, meningismus, and cranial nerve palsies occur. Altered sleep, agitation, depression, anxiety, disorientation, abnormal behavior, psychosis, dementia, euphoria, and episodic crying are some of the psychiatric manifestations. Neurobrucellosis was identified by serological tests in 7.6% of patients with various psychoses such as schizophrenia and bipolar disorder and these patients did not have any systemic features to suggest brucellosis.[6] Depression is common among patients with brucellosis including those without CNS involvement. Depression and anxiety predominate in the chronic stages and contribute to 15% of emotional disorders.[7,8]

Clinical Clue

History of exposure to infected animals or their tissues such as placenta and uncooked milk should be enquired in all patients who present with neuropsychiatric syndrome, with MRI showing acquired white matter changes, meningeal involvement, and CSF pleocytosis and it gives a clue for possible neurobrucellosis.

Neurosyphilis

Syphilis is caused by *Treponema pallidum*, a highly motile spirochete. Infection is transmitted from human-to-human through microabrasions in skin and mucosa, blood transfusion, transplant recipients as well as by vertical transmission. The organism disseminates quickly to virtually all organs. The clinical course progresses through the (1) primary syphilis, characterized by spontaneously healing chancre and regional lymphadenopathy, (2) secondary syphilis, characterized by multisystem involvement with fever, skin rash, lymphadenopathy, hepatitis, nephritis, periostitis, etc., (3) latent infection, characterized by an asymptomatic phase, and (4) tertiary syphilis, characterized by end-arteritis, with involvement of the cardiovascular and nervous systems and gummas. The nervous system is involved early in the disease course, but the infection is cleared by the immune system in majority of the cases. A minority develop neurosyphilis, which can be classified as early and late.[9,10]

During early neurosyphilis, asymptomatic or symptomatic meningitis occurs defined by abnormal CSF, which takes the form of pleocytosis, increased protein, and positive venereal disease research laboratory (VDRL) test. Symptoms of meningitis include headache, nausea, vomiting, and impaired vision. Meningovascular syphilis results in stroke, usually in the territory of the middle cerebral artery, and manifests as acute onset of hemiparesis and aphasia. During late neurosyphilis, the classical neurological syndromes are general paresis of insane (GPI) and tabes dorsalis. The symptoms of GPI include impaired memory and judgement, disorientation, dysarthria, tremor, and parkinsonism. Psychiatric manifestations predominate and they include depression, psychosis, labile affect, grandiose delusion, megalomania, and catatonia. Tabes dorsalis, on the other hand, manifests with shooting or lightening pains, abdominal crisis, abnormal stamping gait, ataxia, areflexia, and bowel, bladder, and sexual dysfunction. Argyll Robertson pupil is a classical clinical sign that aids in the diagnosis. Seizures occur as a part of meningovascular syphilis, gumma, and GPI. Simultaneous presence of ocular and/or ontological involvement in the form of uveitis, impaired hearing, and vestibular dysfunction also aid in the clinical diagnosis.[11]

An MRI shows hyperintensities in the brain parenchyma, such as the mesial temporal region, atrophy, infarcts, meningeal enhancement, and gummas **(Figs. 1A and B)**. Spinal cord may show dorsal column involvement and meningeal enhancement. Treponemal and nontreponemal serological tests are used for making the diagnosis.[12]

Clinical Clue

Neurosyphilis has protean manifestations and is a differential diagnosis for nearly all encephalitic, stroke, dementing, and psychiatric syndromes. MRI brain might show medial temporal, infarcts, and posterior column

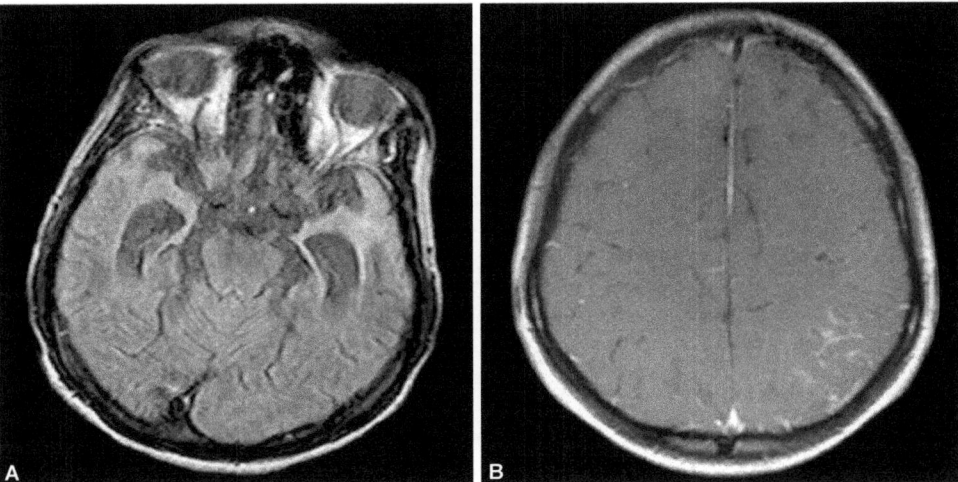

FIGS. 1A AND B: (A) MRI of brain shows hyperintensities in bilateral temporal region and atrophy as evidenced by dilation of the temporal horns in the axial fluid-attenuated inversion recovery (FLAIR) section of a patient with general paresis of insane; (B) Axial postcontrast T1-weighted image shows enhancement of the leptomeninges in the left parietal region in a patient with meningovascular syphilis.

spinal cord changes. Appropriate serological tests should be carried out in all these case scenarios since the history of chancre and other systemic symptoms may not be present or remembered by the patient.

Lyme's Disease

The causative organism is *Borrelia burgdorferi*, a spirochete. Humans acquire the infection by the bite of the *Ixodes* tick. The infection occurs in three stages. Stage 1 is characterized by erythema migrans, an annular lesion, at the site of the tick bite. During stage 2, hematogenous dissemination of the organism to the joints, heart, and nervous system occurs.[13] Clinical features include fatigue, fever, chills, malaise, and sometimes, conjunctivitis, hepatomegaly, splenomegaly and cough, in addition to cardiac conduction block, myocarditis, and cardiomegaly. Headache and meningeal signs may occur and most improve spontaneously. A small proportion (approximately 15%) develops neurological manifestations in the form of meningoencephalitis, ataxia, cranial nerve palsies, myelopathy, radiculopathy, and neuropathy. Symptoms of meningitis may fluctuate. During stage 3 or the late/persistent infection stage, which occurs months after the initial inoculation, recurrent oligoarticular arthritis occurs. Rarely, the nervous system is affected leading to neuropathy, encephalopathy, or encephalomyelitis and clinical manifestations include impaired memory, low mood, and reduced sleep. Post-Lyme syndrome is seen in 10% after the resolution of infection and is characterized by pain and fatigue; this resembles chronic fatigue syndrome and lasts for months to years.[14] The diagnosis is established by the history of erythema multiforme. Culture of *Borrelia burgdorferi* requires a special media and is useful when performed early in the disease course; culture from the skin lesion has higher yield as compared to plasma or CSF. Serological diagnosis requires combination of enzyme-linked immunosorbent assay (ELISA) and Western blot for optimal yield, but it does not distinguish asymptomatic versus active infection versus post-treatment status. These tests need to be interpreted in the context of the clinical status.[15]

Clinical Clue

Tick bite and erythema multiforme are the most important history which aid in the clinical diagnosis with MRI showing acquired white matter (MS-like) changes and sometimes CSF pleocytosis.

Rickettsia

Rickettsiae are a group of gram-negative coccobacilli that include *Rickettsia typhi*, *Rickettsia prowazekii*, *Rickettsia rickettsii*, and *Coxiella burnetii* among others. They are transmitted by the bite of ticks, mites, fleas, or lice. Common clinical features include fever, headache, myalgia, and anorexia. A macular skin rash that evolves to become maculopapular with nonblanching hemorrhages in the center of the lesions is characteristic. An eschar at the site of bite may be present. Encephalitis in Rocky Mountain spotted fever (RMSF) due to *Rickettsia rickettsii*, manifests with delirium, insomnia, and restlessness, particularly at the peak of fever. Epidemic typhus caused by *Rickettsia prowazekii* causes delirium, coma, and sometimes dysphoria. Brain MRI may show patchy hyperintensities in the white matter that have restricted diffusion due to infarcts in the perivascular distribution ("starry sky" appearance), diffuse cerebral edema, and meningeal enhancement. Sequelae in the form of deafness and other cranial nerve palsies, dysarthria, and confusion may occur.[16]

Clinical Clue

The triad of fever, skin rash/eschar, and tick bite should raise the suspicion of rickettsiosis. Empirical treatment with doxycycline is justified since the encephalitis is rapidly progressive and fatal unless timely treatment is administered.

VIRAL INFECTIONS OF THE CENTRAL NERVOUS SYSTEM

Human Immunodeficiency Virus Infection

Central nervous system involvement occurs in nearly all patients with human immunodeficiency virus (HIV) infection and contributes significantly to the morbidity of the condition. Evidence for CNS involvement in the form of abnormal CSF is seen in majority of the patients. This includes CSF pleocytosis, increased protein as well as the presence of HIV-ribonucleic acid (RNA) and anti-HIV antibodies. Clinical manifestations arise from direct infection of the nervous system or secondary to opportunistic infections, neoplasms, and/or medications used for the treatment of HIV. Aseptic meningitis develops at any time during the course of HIV infection, except during the advanced stages. This resembles other viral meningitis clinically, with headache, photophobia, meningismus, and sometimes cranial nerve palsies, which subside spontaneously within 2-4 weeks. Seizures and focal neurological deficits may occur as a result of opportunistic infections or neoplasms. HIV encephalopathy per se causes seizures, and concomitant electrolyte disturbances also contribute to reduction in the seizure threshold. Recurrence of seizures is common necessitating the use of antiseizure medications; these need to be administered with careful monitoring because of their potential interactions with the antiretroviral drugs. A sudden onset of focal neurological deficits signifies stroke and HIV itself is a risk factor for stroke. The presence of other traditional vascular risk factors such as diabetes mellitus and smoking as well as syphilis, varicella zoster, or septic emboli also predispose patients with HIV to stroke. Delirium in a patient with HIV is usually multifactorial with infections, stroke, seizures, trauma, metabolic and endocrine disturbances, substance abuse, and withdrawal contributing to varying extent.[17]

The HIV-associated neurocognitive disorder (HAND) encompasses a spectrum of conditions ranging in clinical severity from asymptomatic or mild-to-severe. In asymptomatic neurocognitive impairment (ANI), patients have mild cognitive deficits and mild impairments in formal neuropsychological testing in two domains which are one standard deviation (SD) less than the normative data derived from the population. These patients do not have impaired function and thus do not fulfil the diagnostic criteria for dementia (**Box 1**).[18] Mild neurocognitive disorder (MND) is similar to ANI, but causes some impairment in the activities of daily living. In HIV-associated dementia (HAD), there occurs moderate to severe cognitive decline by at least two SD as compared to the normative data, which significantly interferes with the activities of daily living (**Box 2**).[18] Insidiously progressive decline in cognitive functions such as reduced attention, executive dysfunction, impaired episodic and working memory, and difficulty in new learning are some of the cognitive symptoms. The dementia is "subcortical" and apraxia and agnosia are uncommon. The dementia is accompanied by signs of motor dysfunction in the form of impaired balance, unsteady gait, and difficulty in performing rapid alternating movements.[19] Psychiatric

---

BOX 1: The American Academy of Neurology AIDS Task Force diagnostic criteria for HIV-associated minor cognitive and motor disorder.[18]

I. Acquired cognitive, motor or behavioral abnormalities (must have both A and B)
   A. At least two of the following symptoms present for at least 1 month, verified by a reliable history:
      – Impaired attention or concentration
      – Mental slowing
      – Impaired memory
      – Slowed movements
      – Incoordination
      – Personality change, irritability or emotional lability
   B. Acquired cognitive or motor abnormality, verified by clinical neurologic examination or neuropsychological testing

II. Cognitive, motor or behavioral abnormalities causing mild impairment of work or activities of daily living (objectively verifiable or by report of key informant)

III. Does not meet criteria for HIV-associated dementia

IV. Absence of another cause of the above cognitive, motor or behavioral abnormalities (e.g., active CNS opportunistic infection or malignancy, psychiatric disorders, and substance abuse)

(AIDS: acquired immunodeficiency syndrome; CNS: central nervous system; HIV: human immunodeficiency virus)

> **BOX 2: The American Academy of Neurology AIDS Task Force diagnostic criteria for HIV-associated dementia.[18]**
>
> I. Acquired abnormality in at least two of the following cognitive abilities, present for at least 1 month and causing impairment in work or activities of daily living:
>   - Attention or concentration
>   - Speed of information processing
>   - Abstraction or reasoning
>   - Visuospatial skills
>   - Memory or learning
>   - Speech or language
>
> II. At least one of the following:
>   - Acquired abnormality in motor functioning
>   - Decline in motivation or emotional control or change in social behavior
>
> III. Absence of clouding of consciousness during a period long enough to establish presence of I, above
>
> IV. Absence of another cause of the above cognitive, motor or behavioral symptoms or signs (active CNS opportunistic infection or malignancy, psychiatric disorders, and substance abuse)
>
> (AIDS: acquired immunodeficiency syndrome; CNS: central nervous system; HIV: human immunodeficiency virus)

symptoms in HAD include psychomotor slowing, apathy, inertia, emotional lability, and irritability. Incontinence occurs in late stages. A number of nosological terms have been used to describe the spectrum of neurocognitive deficits in the setting of HIV infection. While HAD usually occurs as a late complication of HIV infection, this term is preferred to acquired immunodeficiency syndrome (AIDS) dementia complex (ADC) since it can occur without the development of AIDS.[20]

Patients with HIV also suffer from a number of psychiatric symptoms that include depression, anxiety, mania, psychosis, post-traumatic stress disorder, and personality disorders. Patients with HIV are at increased risk of developing depression, anxiety, and apathy as compared to the general population. Symptoms of subjective fatigue, pain, anorexia, and insomnia are reported by patients with HIV even in the absence of syndromic depression. Depressive symptoms may also be a part of HAD or a result of chronic stress related to the diagnosis of HIV. Depression, social isolation, and sense of demoralization contribute to poor compliance to antiretroviral therapy. Mania is characterized by increased impulsivity, impaired judgement, and risk-taking behavior. On the other hand, "AIDS mania" is seen in late stages of HIV infection, wherein manic symptoms are accompanied by impaired cognition, and there is less euphoria and more irritability as compared to mania. Besides, AIDS mania is more chronic and does not remit unless treated. Schizophrenia, post-traumatic stress disorder, and antisocial personality probably contribute to the high-risk behavior associated with HIV.[21]

Some of the antiretroviral drugs also cause psychiatric side effects. The most widely recognized is efavirenz, which causes mood disorders, anxiety, psychosis, aggression, hallucinations, reduced sleep, vivid dreams, and catatonia. Suicidal ideation is higher with efavirenz. These psychiatric manifestations occur within few weeks of intake of efavirenz, and continued intake may lead to habituation. Abacavir and zidovudine have also been reported to cause psychosis and depression.[21]

Clinical Clue

All patients who have been detected to have HIV infection should undergo cognitive and psychiatric assessment at the time of diagnosis for documentation of higher mental functions at the baseline as well as during follow-up, as and when the symptoms appear. An active search for alternative etiologies such as opportunistic CNS infections, neoplasms such as lymphoma, in addition to metabolic encephalopathy such as dyselectrolytemia, and drug-induced encephalopathy should be made.

Herpes Virus Infections

The herpes simplex virus-1 (HSV-1) is the most common cause of sporadic encephalitis. The clinical features are characterized by fever and headache, followed by the development of neuropsychiatric manifestations in the form of changes in personality, altered sensorium, disorientation, cognitive deficits, seizures, and aphasia. Brain MRI shows hyperintensities in the limbic structures, i.e., medial temporal lobes, insular cortex, inferior and lateral frontal lobes, and cingulate gyri **(Figs. 2A and B)**.[22] It is interesting to note that about a third of these patients develop antibodies to the N-methyl-D-aspartate (NMDA) receptor and these patients experience "relapse" of the neuropsychiatric symptoms which may be accompanied by choreoathetosis and other movement disorders.[23]

Any part of the neuraxis can be infected by varicella zoster virus (VZV). Para- or postinfectious cerebellitis and encephalomyelitis accompanying VZV infection is seen in children. On the other hand, in older subjects, VZV reactivation leads to vasculopathy and encephalitis. In immunocompetent individuals, the large vessels in the anterior cerebral circulation are affected leading to strokes. In immunocompromised patients, multifocal vasculopathy of small- and medium-sized arteries results in hemorrhagic infarcts. Patients manifest with altered sensorium and focal neurological deficits. Other

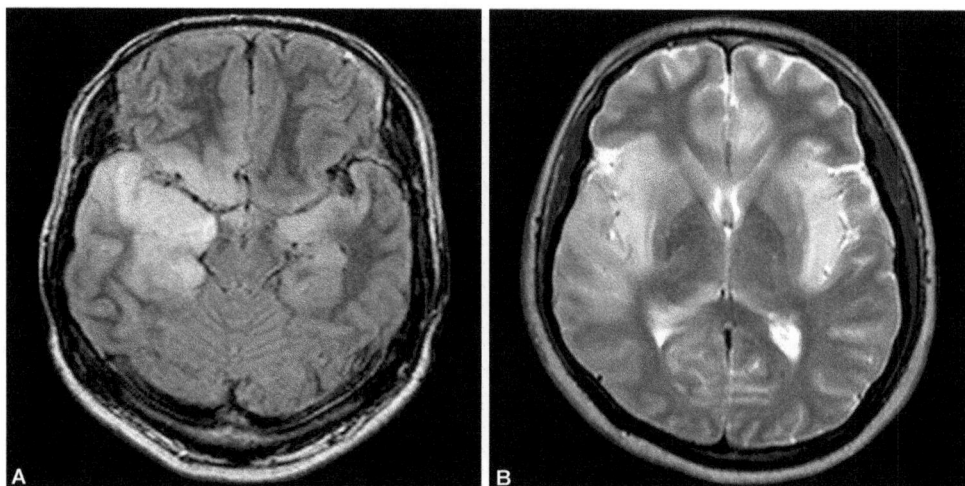

FIGS. 2A AND B: Axial fluid-attenuated inversion recovery (FLAIR) (A) and T2-weighted (B) images of brain show hyperintensities in bilateral temporal, basifrontal, insula, and cingulate regions, associated with edema and mass effect on the ventricles in a patient with herpes simplex encephalitis.

neurological manifestations include aseptic meningitis, giant cell arteritis, myelitis, and segmental zoster.[24,25]

Infection with cytomegalovirus (CMV) is usually asymptomatic, but can rarely result in aseptic meningitis. Severe clinical manifestations occur in the setting of congenital infection or in immunocompromised subjects such as AIDS. The latter develop encephalitis, myeloradiculitis or Guillain–Barré syndrome.[21] Epstein–Barr virus (EBV) only rarely causes neurological complications and they include meningitis, encephalitis, cerebellitis, and cranial nerve palsies in addition to myelitis and peripheral neuropathies. A peculiar symptom complex called as the "Alice in wonderland" syndrome may occur, wherein an individual perceives his/her own body or parts of the body or environmental objects as being abnormally large or small. This may be accompanied by visual hallucinations, mistaken perception of certain events, and misconception regarding the pace of time (either too slow or too fast). An acute limbic encephalitis can arise from infection with human herpes virus-6 (HHV6) in transplant recipients. The diagnosis of herpes virus infections is usually established by demonstrating the presence of the DNA of these viruses in the CSF by PCR. EBV infection may also show atypical lymphocytes in CSF (Tselis, 2014).[26]

Clinical Clue

Among the herpes group of viruses, herpes simplex encephalitis can be recognized by the characteristic involvement of limbic structures in brain MRI in a patient presenting with acute encephalitic syndrome. A high index of suspicion is required for other herpes virus infections; the presence of immunocompromised state and previous history of segmental zoster, etc., may give a clue for initiating further laboratory workup.

Rabies

Rabies is a rapidly progressive fatal disorder caused by the rabies virus that belongs to the Rhabdoviridae family (genus: *Lyssavirus*). The incubation period is variable, and ranges from weeks to several years. Patients develop a prodrome of fever, headache, and pain/paresthesias at the site of bite. Rabies causes encephalopathy that rapidly progresses to coma. Hyperactive delirium occurs in "furious" rabies with agitation, hallucination, dysautonomia, and seizures. A variety of stimuli, such as touch, sound, smell, and induce spasms of the pharyngeal and nuchal muscles, which manifest as aerophobia and hydrophobia. In "paralytic" rabies, the clinical course comprises of paresthesias and flaccid paralysis of the bitten limb, followed by quadriplegia and thereafter the development of encephalopathy. Pleocytosis in CSF is common. Brain MRI shows hyperintensities in the gray matter of the medial temporal lobes, basal ganglia, thalami, and brainstem **(Figs. 3A to C)**. The diagnosis can be established antemortem by demonstrating the rabies virus antigen in the nuchal skin biopsy by immunofluorescence and rabies antibodies in the serum, CSF, and saliva by reverse transcription-PCR (RT-PCR). The Australian bat *Lyssavirus* also causes a clinical syndrome that resembles rabies.[27]

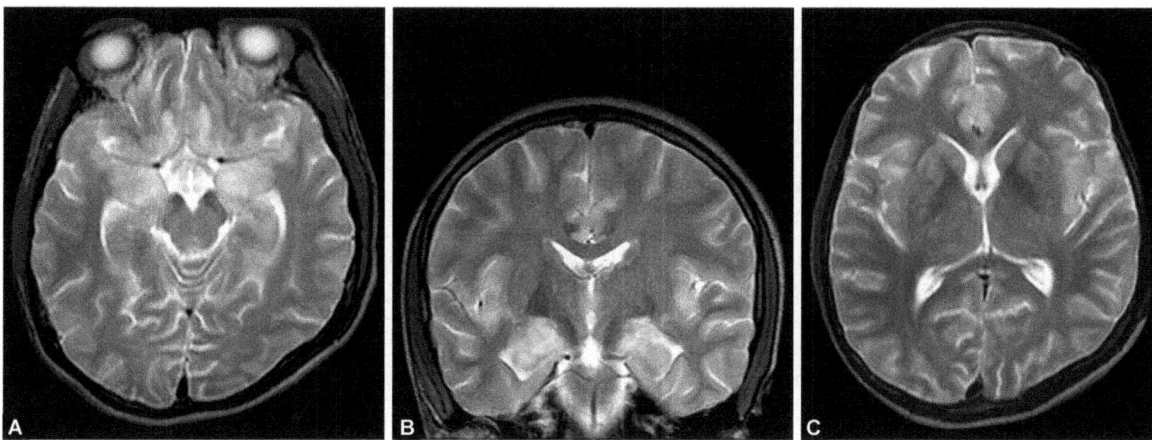

FIGS. 3A TO C: Axial (A and C) and coronal (B) T2-weighted images of brain show hyperintensities in bilateral temporal, basifrontal, insula, caudate, and putamen in a patient with rabies.

Clinical Clue

Aerophobia and hydrophobia are important features that warrant workup for rabies, even if the history of bite from an infected animal is not forthcoming.

Influenza Including Severe Acute Respiratory Syndrome Coronavirus 2

An important cause for seasonal epidemics, influenza causes neurological complications in the form of seizures, encephalopathy, encephalitis, meningitis, and posterior reversible encephalopathy syndrome (PRES), in addition to peripheral nervous system involvement (Guillain–Barré syndrome and myositis). Recognized named syndromes include: (1) acute infantile encephalopathy that affects frontal lobes predominantly, (2) acute necrotizing encephalopathy that affects the basal ganglia, thalami, and brainstem, (3) encephalopathy with hemorrhagic shock, and (4) acute hemorrhagic leukoencephalopathy.[28] During the recent pandemic, the causative organism, the novel coronavirus, severe acute respiratory syndrome coronavirus 2 (SARS-CoV-2), and involvement of the CNS occurs as a part of the systemic infection or direct invasion of the brain. Clinical manifestations include altered sensorium, agitation, seizures, and executive dysfunction, which occur in the setting of multiorgan dysfunction. Reduced or altered smell and taste sensations is common. Interestingly, strokes occur about 1–3 weeks following the acute infection. Brain MRI may show diffuse white matter hyperintensity with petechial hemorrhages in the corpus callosum and juxtacortical white matter.[29]

Arboviral Infections

These are arthropod-borne viral infections, with the vectors being mosquitoes or ticks. There are over 100 arboviruses that infect humans and as a group these constitute the leading cause of encephalitis. Arboviruses comprise of four families, which are the Togaviridae (alphaviruses), Flaviviridae (flaviviruses), reoviruses, and bunyaviruses.[30]

The Japanese encephalitis (JE) virus is the most common mosquito-borne encephalitis and is transmitted by the bite of the *Culex*, *Aedes*, or *Anopheles* mosquitoes. Aseptic meningitis or encephalitis can occur. The prodromal symptoms consist of fever, headache, nausea, vomiting, and dizziness. The clinical features of encephalitis include hyperactive delirium, seizures, parkinsonism, oculomotor disturbances, and ataxia. A significant proportion is left with sequelae in the form of depressed cognition, parkinsonism, and other psychiatric disorders. Investigations show CSF pleocytosis, hyperintensities in the basal ganglia and thalami in brain MRI and JE virus antibodies in the serum and CSF by ELISA or plaque reduction neutralization test (PRNT). The virus can also be detected in the blood or CSF by RT-PCR.[31]

Flaviviruses such as dengue and yellow fever are transmitted by the bite of the *Aedes aegypti* mosquito. Dengue causes a plethora of neurological complications that range from meningitis, meningoencephalitis, rhombencephalitis, hemorrhagic encephalitis, acute disseminated encephalomyelitis (ADEM), strokes, cranial nerve palsies, opsoclonus-myoclonus, and cerebellitis, to myelitis, Guillain–Barré syndrome, brachial plexitis, hypokalemic palsy, and myositis. On the other hand, the *Zika virus*, which is a related *Flavivirus*, predominantly causes peripheral nervous system involvement in the form of Guillain–Barré syndrome, with meningitis, encephalitis, seizures, and ADEM being less common manifestations.[32] Chikungunya virus (CHIKV) is also transmitted by the bite of the *Aedes* mosquito. While chronic debilitating arthritis is the predominant complication of CHIKV infection, a proportion of patients (approximately 1 in 1,000) develop neurological manifestations in the form of encephalitis or encephalopathy, ADEM, and myelitis. These are common in the elderly, while younger individuals are more predisposed to developing the peripheral nervous system complications.[33] Combined flaviviral infections are also recognized.

Filoviruses such as Ebola and Marburg viruses cause severe or fatal hemorrhagic fever. Marburg virus causes psychosis, amnesia, depression, and fatigue, in addition to neuropathy and restless leg syndrome.[28] Neurological manifestations of Ebola virus include acute encephalitis, delirium, myoclonus, and oculomotor disorders.[34] Chronic neuropsychiatric sequelae can occur.

The West Nile Virus (WNV) and St. Louis encephalitis (SLE) virus are transmitted by the bite of the *Culex* mosquito. Infection with WNV is asymptomatic in 80%, but in the rest, there occurs a nonspecific febrile illness following an incubation period of 3–14 days. A fraction of these patients develops encephalitis, meningitis, or lower motor neuron type of paralysis. Tremor, myoclonus, and parkinsonism are the salient neurological manifestations of WNV infection. The elderly are more vulnerable to developing encephalitis, while the neurological complications are uncommon in children. CSF nearly always shows pleocytosis, with neutrophilic predominance in up to one-half of the patients. Brain MRI shows involvement of the basal ganglia, thalami, brainstem, and cerebellum. WNV antibodies can be demonstrated in the serum or CSF. SLE also causes fever with/without meningitis and encephalitis, with increased frequency of neurological involvement in the elderly.[35]

Clinical Clue

Many of these viral encephalitic syndromes do not have specific features that aid at clinical diagnosis at the bedside. The laboratory diagnosis is influenced to a large extent by the epidemiological scenario including travel to regions where these infections are prevalent.

Progressive Multifocal Leukoencephalopathy

This is caused by infection with the John Cunningham (JC) virus, which leads to single or multiple lesions in the white matter and neuropsychiatric manifestations. The clinical manifestations reflect the site of involvement. Patients develop cognitive decline, aphasia, agnosia, apraxia, akinetic mutism, dysarthria, and catatonia in varying combinations. Visual field defects, cortical blindness, oculomotor palsies, impaired sensation, and cerebellar dysfunction may also occur. MRI of brain shows T2/fluid-attenuated inversion recovery (FLAIR) hyperintense lesions in the white matter which are hypointense on T1 and do not enhance with contrast **(Figs. 2A and B)**. The subcortical "U" fibers are spared. CSF analysis shows normal or mildly increased cell count, increased protein, and normal glucose. PCR for JC virus is used to establish the diagnosis, but it has a sensitivity of only 58%.[21]

Clinical Clue

Progressive multifocal leukoencephalopathy (PML) should be suspected in any patient with immunocompromised state who presents with progressive focal or diffuse neurological dysfunction.

Other Viruses

Measles, mumps, and rubella viruses cause exanthematous fever and CNS involvement in the form of acute meningoencephalitis and postinfectious encephalomyelitis. The latter occurs about 1–2 weeks after the acute infection and mimics ADEM. Clues for clinical diagnosis include Koplik spots, keratitis and corneal ulcerations in measles, vestibular labyrinthitis, and enlarged salivary glands in mumps. In addition, acute encephalopathy associated with mumps virus can occur, which is characterized by rapidly progressive coma, raised intracranial tension, and seizures. The CSF is acellular, in contrast to mumps meningoencephalitis where CSF pleocytosis of up to 3,000 cells can occur. Besides this, the measles inclusion body encephalitis (MIBE), which occurs 1–9 months postmeasles infection in individuals with reduced cellular immunity, is characterized by rapidly progressive encephalopathy with abnormal behavior, altered sensorium, delirium, seizures, and myoclonus. The CSF is normal and the diagnosis is established by demonstrating the presence of measles virus by PCR in the CSF or brain (in case of autopsy diagnosis).[36]

A peculiar and delayed syndrome complicating measles infection is subacute sclerosing panencephalitis (SSPE). This arises from defective maturation of the measles virus in the neural cells leading to persistent infection of the neurons and glia in immunocompetent subjects. SSPE occurs 2–12 years after acute measles infection (median = 8 years). The initial manifestations include alterations in behavior and personality and decline in scholastic performance. Subsequently, slow myoclonus, seizures, movement disorder (chorea, athetosis, and ballism), spasticity and ataxia develop. In the late stages, optic atrophy, akinetic mutism, and signs of autonomic dysfunction occur, and the child becomes vegetative. The diagnosis is established by the presence of periodic complexes in electroencephalogram (EEG) and increased measles antibody titers in the CSF.[37]

The arena viruses are rodent borne viruses and they include the lymphocytic choriomeningitis virus (LCMV), argentine hemorrhagic fever, and West African viral hemorrhagic fever (Lassa fever), which cause meningitis and severe encephalomyelitis. LCMV also causes sensorineural hearing loss, bulbar dysfunction and parkinsonism. Argentine hemorrhagic fever causes ataxia as well as oculomotor and other cranial nerve dysfunction. Lassa fever causes sensorineural hearing loss, dystonia, tremor, ataxia, and other neuropsychiatric sequelae.[38]

FUNGAL INFECTIONS

Cryptococcal Meningitis

The causative organism is *Cryptococcus neoformans*. In patients infected with HIV, it usually occurs in the setting of low CD4 count (<100 cells/mm^3). Clinically, the patients develop headache, photophobia, fever and signs of raised intracranial tension. Abnormal behavior and psychosis can also occur. The neuropsychiatric manifestations may persist even after successful treatment of cryptococcal meningitis. CSF analysis shows increased opening pressure, increased protein, and reduced glucose. The yeast forms can be demonstrated in the CSF by India Ink Preparation; detection of cryptococcal antigen and culture of the organism in the CSF also aid in the diagnosis.[39]

Clinical Clue

Raised intracranial tension, particularly in a patient with immunocompromised state, should prompt the workup for cryptococcal meningitis.

PROTOZOAL/PARASITIC INFECTIONS

Cerebral Malaria

Cerebral malaria is common in the low- and middle-income countries and is caused by the *Plasmodium* species and transmitted by the bite of the *Anopheles* mosquito. The most severe manifestations are caused by *Plasmodium falciparum*. Patients develop fever and chills and signs of CNS involvement in the form of delirium, obtundation of consciousness, coma, seizures, and death. Systemic features include anemia, thrombocytopenia, increased bilirubin, renal failure, hypoglycemia, acute respiratory distress syndrome (ARDS) and disseminated intravascular coagulation (DIC). The diagnosis is established by the conventional peripheral blood smear. Rapid diagnostic kits are also available.[40]

Clinical Clue

A rapidly progressive encephalitis/encephalopathy, in combination with hypoglycemia, hepatic, and renal dysfunction gives the clue for cerebral malaria. Patient may be treated empirically in case of delay or lack of facilities for appropriate testing.

Neurocysticercosis

Neurocysticercosis (NCC) is the most common parasitic infestation of the brain and is caused by the ingestion of the eggs of *Taenia solium* from contaminated food or fecal-oral route. On reaching the brain, the NCC pass through the vesicular, colloidal, granular, and calcified stages. The neurological manifestations are related to the number and location of the NCC within the brain (parenchymal, subarachnoid, and intraventricular), as well as the host immune response. NCC is an important cause of epilepsy. Seizures are the most common clinical manifestation of NCC, being present in 50–80%. Focal deficits, seen in about 20%, include subacute or chronically progressive pyramidal weakness, aphasia, impaired sensation, movement disorders, parkinsonism, ataxia, and brainstem dysfunction. Stroke-like presentations also occur. Syndrome of raised intracranial tension, with reduced sensorium, impaired vision, headache, vomiting, and papilledema, is seen with cysticercal arachnoiditis, ependymitis, ventricular cysts, or massive infection leading to cysticercal encephalitis. Cognitive decline leading to impaired memory and recall can occur, and the severity ranges from mild to severe, fulfilling the diagnostic criteria for dementia. Psychiatric manifestations include delirium, confusion, depression, anxiety, and personality disorders. Frank psychosis with delusions, hallucinations, psychomotor agitation, and aggression may occur. Preexisting psychiatric illnesses may predispose to the acquisition of infection because of poor hygienic practices.[41,42]

Imaging of the brain, CT, and MRI, plays a key role in the diagnosis, and also reveals the number, size, and location of the cysticercal lesions. NCC is seen as rounded cystic lesion with an eccentric scolex **(Figs. 4A to C)**. Additional perilesional edema, peripheral enhancement, and calcification depend upon the stage of NCC. Other findings include hydrocephalus and leptomeningeal enhancement. Serological tests have poor sensitivity and specificity.[43] The diagnostic criteria are provided in **Box 3**.[44]

Clinical Clue

Since, imaging of the brain is indicated in all patients presenting with neuropsychiatric manifestations in order to exclude infections such as NCC. The differential diagnosis includes other.

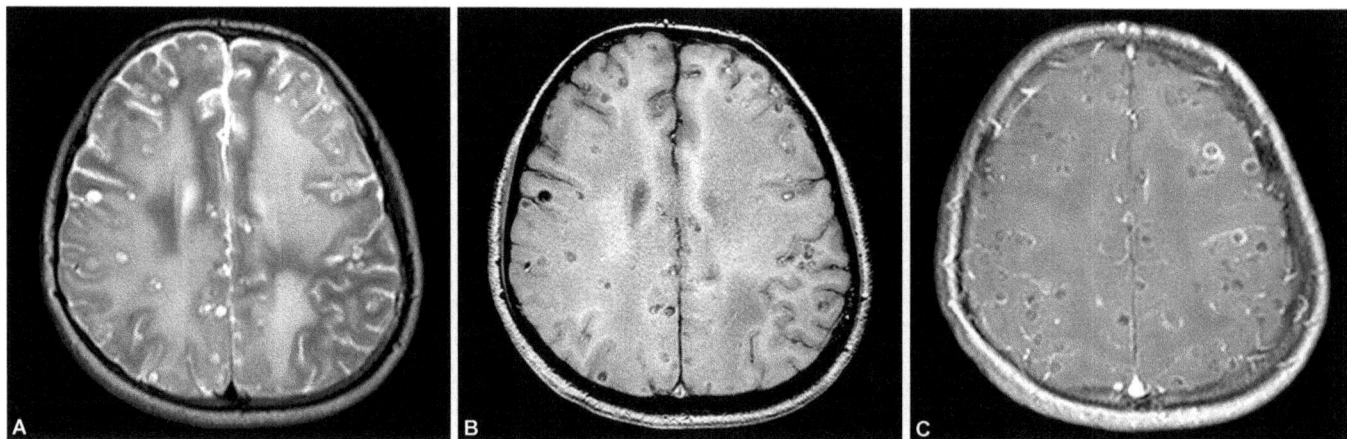

FIGS. 4A TO C: Axial T2-weighted (A) and fluid-attenuated inversion recovery (FLAIR) (B) images of the brain show numerous cystic lesions in bilateral cerebral hemispheres with an eccentric scolex and varying degrees of perilesional edema in a patient with neurocysticercosis. Some of the cysts show peripheral rim enhances in post-contrast T1-weighted images (C).

BOX 3: Criteria for the diagnosis of neurocysticercosis.[44]

Diagnostic criteria

Absolute criteria:
- Histologic demonstration of the parasite from biopsy of a brain or spinal cord lesion
- Evidence of cystic lesions showing the scolex on neuroimaging studies
- Direct visualization of subretinal parasites by fundoscopic examination
- Spontaneous resolution of small single enhancing lesions

Major criteria:
- Evidence of lesions highly suggestive of neurocysticercosis on neuroimaging studies
- Positive serum immunoblot for the detection of anticysticercal antibodies
- Resolution of intracranial cystic lesions after therapy with albendazole or praziquantel

Minor criteria:
- Evidence of lesions suggestive of neurocysticercosis on neuroimaging studies
- Presence of clinical manifestations suggestive of neurocysticercosis
- Positive CSF ELISA for detection of anticysticercal antibodies or cysticercal antigens
- Evidence of cysticercosis outside the central nervous system

Epidemiological criteria:
- Individuals coming from or living in an area where cysticercosis is endemic
- History of frequent travel to disease-endemic areas
- Evidence of household a contact with Taenia solium infection

Diagnostic categories

Definite NCC:
- One absolute criterion
- Two major plus one minor or one epidemiological criterion

Probable NCC:
- One major plus two minor criteria
- One major plus one minor and one epidemiological criterion
- Three minor plus one epidemiological criteria

(CSF: cerebrospinal fluid; ELISA: enzyme-linked immunosorbent assay; NCC: neurocysticercosis)

Central Nervous System Toxoplasmosis

Primary infection with *Toxoplasma gondii* is acquired by ingestion of raw or undercooked meat or food that is contaminated by fecal matter of infected animals. While the primary infection is asymptomatic in vast majority, cerebral toxoplasmosis is caused by reactivation of the cysts of *Toxoplasma gondii* within the brain during conditions of immunosuppression such as HIV infection and low CD4 count (<100 cells/mm^3). Patients develop fever, headache, lymphadenopathy, splenomegaly, and features of encephalitis such as seizures, altered sensorium, and localizing deficits such as hemiparesis, aphasia, and hemianopia. Extrapyramidal features in the form of parkinsonism, hemiballismus, and involuntary movements may occur. Delirium, psychosis, and mania are the other manifestations.

An MRI shows ring-enhancing, hemorrhagic and necrotic lesions in the cerebral cortex, basal ganglia, brainstem, and cerebellum. The diagnosis is established

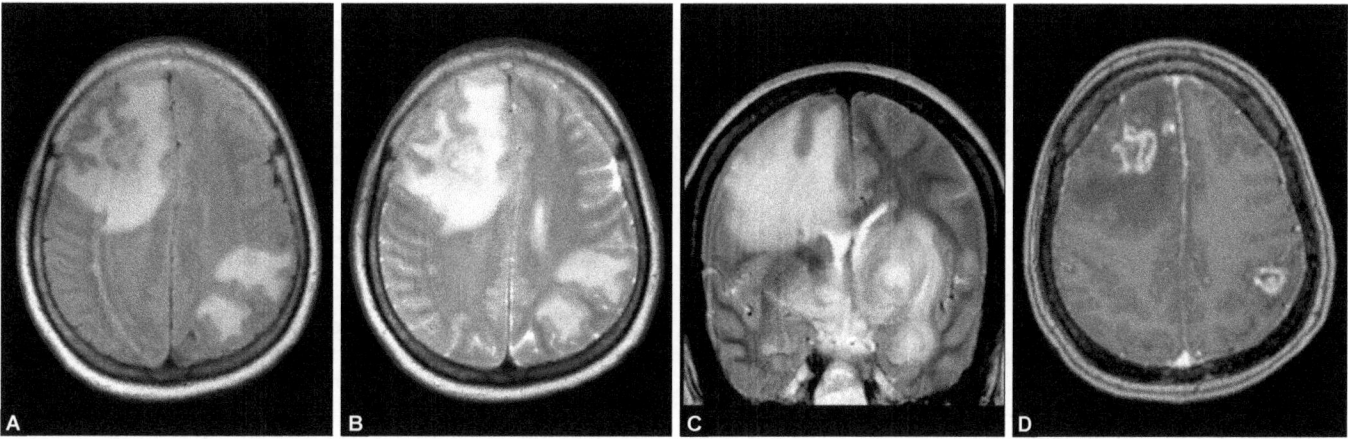

FIGS. 5A TO D: Axial fluid-attenuated inversion recovery (FLAIR) (A) and T2-weighted (B) images and coronal T2-weighted (C) images show multiple variable-sized heterogeneous signal intensity lesions in bilateral cerebral hemispheres, in the basal ganglia and corticomedullary junction, with perilesional edema in a patient with human immunodeficiency virus (HIV) positive status and central nervous system (CNS) toxoplasmosis. Post-contrast T1-weighted (D) images show peripheral enhancement of the lesions with eccentric nodule.

by PCR, which carries a sensitivity of 50% and a sensitivity of 96–100%. Alternately, empirical treatment with pyrimethamine and sulfadiazine or clindamycin supports the diagnosis of toxoplasma encephalitis.[45]

Clinical Clue

Toxoplasmosis should be considered as a differential diagnosis in a patient with acute/subacute encephalopathy who develops movement disorder, particularly hemiballismus and the MRI of brain shows ring-enhancing lesions with hemorrhage within the lesions **(Figs. 5A to D)**.

CONCLUDING REMARKS

Infections of the CNS can be caused by a number of organisms, including bacteria, viruses, protozoans, and parasites. While some present acutely/subacutely, others present as a delayed manifestation due to reactivation of latent infection. Some of these cause meningitis or encephalitis or meningoencephalitis exclusively or predominantly, while in others, the CNS manifestations occur as a part of the systemic illness. A number of psychiatric symptoms such as delirium, depression, mania, anxiety, and psychotic behavior occur and overshadow the systemic or neurological features, potentially delaying the diagnosis. Physicians, psychiatrists, and neurologists should be aware of these pitfalls and actively investigate these patients with the necessary imaging and microbiological and serological tests in order to establish or exclude the diagnosis.

LEARNING POINTS

- A number of infections of the nervous system have prominent psychiatric manifestations.
- An acute/subacute onset and concurrent neurological features such as raised intracranial tension, altered sensorium, and movement disorders necessitates the workup for an underlying organic etiology, before making the diagnosis of a primary psychiatric disorder.
- Presence of non-neurological features such as gastrointestinal, cardiac, and other organ system involvement is useful pointers for diagnosis, e.g., gastrointestinal symptoms in Whipple's disease, hypoglycemia in cerebral malaria, and chancre in neurosyphilis.
- Occupational and epidemiological history should not be neglected at the bedside, e.g., exposure to animal products in brucellosis and epidemics of viral encephalitis.
- Imaging of brain shows characteristic features, which may be diagnostic, e.g., involvement of the limbic structures in herpes simplex encephalitis.

REFERENCES

1. Richie MB, Josephson SA. A Practical Approach to Meningitis and Encephalitis. Semin Neurol. 201535(6):611-20.
2. Bystritsky RJ, Chow FC. Infectious Meningitis and Encephalitis. Neurol Clin. 2022;40(1):77-91.
3. Fenollar F, Puéchal X, Raoult D. Whipple's disease. N Engl J Med. 2007;356(1):55-66.
4. Boumaza A, Ben Azzouz E, Arrindell J, Lepidi H, Mezouar S, Desnues B. Whipple's disease and Tropheryma whipplei

4. infections: from bench to bedside. Lancet Infect Dis. 2022;22(10):e280-91.
5. Franco MP, Mulder M, Gilman RH, Smits HL. Human brucellosis. Lancet Infect Dis. 2007;7(12):775-86.
6. Moogahi S, Rostami H, Salmanzadeh S, Cheraghi M, Tadibeni F. Undiagnosed Brucellosis in Psychiatric Patients: A Cross-Sectional Study. Arch Clin Infect Dis. 2023;18(2):e136729.
7. Shehata GA, Abdel-Baky L, Rashed H, Elamin H. Neuropsychiatric evaluation of patients with brucellosis. J Neurovirol. 2010;16(1):48-55.
8. Kechagia M, Mitka S, Papadogiannakis E, Kontos V, Koutis C. Molecular Detection of Brucella spp. DNA in Patients with Manifestations Compatible with Emotional Disorders. Open Infect Dis J. 2011;5:8-12.
9. Ghanem KG, Ram S, Rice PA. The Modern Epidemic of Syphilis. N Engl J Med. 2020;382(9):845-54.
10. Peeling RW, Mabey D, Kamb ML, Chen XS, Radolf JD, Benzaken AS. Syphilis. Nat Rev Dis Primers. 2017;3:17073.
11. Ropper AH. Neurosyphilis. N Engl J Med. 2019;381(14):1358-63.
12. Corrêa DG, de Souza SR, Freddi TAL, Fonseca APA, Dos Santos RQ, Hygino da Cruz LC Jr. Imaging features of neurosyphilis. J Neuroradiol. 2023;50(2):241-52.
13. Ross Russell AL, Dryden MS, Pinto AA, Lovett JK. Lyme disease: diagnosis and management. Pract Neurol. 2018;18(6):455-64.
14. Garcia-Monco JC, Benach JL. Lyme Neuroborreliosis: Clinical Outcomes, Controversy, Pathogenesis, and Polymicrobial Infections. Ann Neurol. 2019;85(1):21-31.
15. Bransfield RC. Neuropsychiatric Lyme Borreliosis: An Overview with a Focus on a Specialty Psychiatrist's Clinical Practice. Healthcare (Basel). 2018;6(3):104.
16. Sekeyová Z, Danchenko M, Filipčík P, Fournier PE. Rickettsial infections of the central nervous system. PLoS Negl Trop Dis. 2019;13(8):e0007469.
17. Paruk HF, Bhigjee AI. Review of the neurological aspects of HIV infection. J Neurol Sci. 2021;425:117453.
18. Dubé B, Benton T, Cruess DG, Evans DL. Neuropsychiatric manifestations of HIV infection and AIDS. J Psychiatry Neurosci. 2005;30(4):237-46.
19. Sacktor N, Robertson K. Evolving clinical phenotypes in HIV-associated neurocognitive disorders. Curr Opin HIV AIDS. 2014;9(6):517-20.
20. Clifford DB, Ances BM. HIV-associated neurocognitive disorder. Lancet Infect Dis. 2013;13(11):976-86.
21. Singer EJ, Thames AD. Neurobehavioral Manifestations of Human Immunodeficiency Virus/AIDS: Diagnosis and Treatment. Neurol Clin. 2016;34(1):33-53.
22. Bradshaw MJ, Venkatesan A. Herpes Simplex Virus-1 Encephalitis in Adults: Pathophysiology, Diagnosis, and Management. Neurotherapeutics. 2016;13(3):493-508.
23. Armangue T, Spatola M, Vlagea A, Mattozzi S, Cárceles-Cordon M, Martinez-Heras E, et al.; Spanish Herpes Simplex Encephalitis Study Group. Frequency, symptoms, risk factors, and outcomes of autoimmune encephalitis after herpes simplex encephalitis: a prospective observational study and retrospective analysis. Lancet Neurol. 2018;17(9):760-72.
24. Kennedy PGE, Gershon AA. Clinical Features of Varicella-Zoster Virus Infection. Viruses. 2018;10(11):609.
25. Nagel MA, Gilden D. Neurological complications of varicella zoster virus reactivation. Curr Opin Neurol. 2014;27(3):356-60.
26. Tselis AC. Epstein-Barr virus infections of the nervous system. Handb Clin Neurol. 2014;123:285-305.
27. Fooks AR, Cliquet F, Finke S, Freuling C, Hemachudha T, Mani RS, et al. Rabies. Nat Rev Dis Primers. 2017;3:17091.
28. McEntire CRS, Song KW, McInnis RP, Rhee JY, Young M, Williams E, et al. Neurologic Manifestations of the World Health Organization's List of Pandemic and Epidemic Diseases. Front Neurol. 2021;12:634827.
29. Román GC, Spencer PS, Reis J, Buguet A, Faris MEA, Katrak SM, et al; WFN Environmental Neurology Specialty Group. The neurology of COVID-19 revisited: A proposal from the Environmental Neurology Specialty Group of the World Federation of Neurology to implement international neurological registries. J Neurol Sci. 2020;414:116884.
30. Young PR. Arboviruses: A Family on the Move. Adv Exp Med Biol. 2018;1062:1-10.
31. Griffiths MJ, Turtle L, Solomon T. Japanese encephalitis virus infection. Handb Clin Neurol. 2014;123:561-76.
32. Trivedi S, Chakravarty A. Neurological Complications of Dengue Fever. Curr Neurol Neurosci Rep. 2022;22(8):515-29.
33. Arpino C, Curatolo P, Rezza G. Chikungunya and the nervous system: what we do and do not know. Rev Med Virol. 2009;19(3):121-9.
34. Jacob ST, Crozier I, Fischer WA 2nd, Hewlett A, Kraft CS, Vega MA, et al. Ebola virus disease. Nat Rev Dis Primers. 2020;6(1):13.
35. McCarthy M. St. Louis Encephalitis and West Nile Virus Encephalitis. Curr Treat Options Neurol. 2001;3(5):433-8.
36. Fisher DL, Defres S, Solomon T. Measles-induced encephalitis. QJM. 2015;108(3):177-82.
37. Garg RK, Mahadevan A, Malhotra HS, Rizvi I, Kumar N, Uniyal R. Subacute sclerosing panencephalitis. Rev Med Virol. 2019;29(5):e2058.
38. Wilson MR, Peters CJ. Diseases of the central nervous system caused by lymphocytic choriomeningitis virus and other arenaviruses. Handb Clin Neurol. 2014;123:671-81.
39. Kumar A, Gopinath S, Dinesh KR, Karim S. Infectious psychosis: cryptococcal meningitis presenting as a neuropsychiatry disorder. Neurol India. 2011;59(6):909-11.
40. Albrecht-Schgoer K, Lackner P, Schmutzhard E, Baier G. Cerebral Malaria: Current Clinical and Immunological Aspects. Front Immunol. 2022;13:863568.
41. El-Kady AM, Allemailem KS, Almatroudi A, Abler B, Elsayed M. Psychiatric Disorders of Neurocysticercosis: Narrative Review. Neuropsychiatr Dis Treat. 2021;17:1599-610.
42. Garcia HH, Nash TE, Del Brutto OH. Clinical symptoms, diagnosis, and treatment of neurocysticercosis. Lancet Neurol. 2014;13(12):1202-15.
43. Del Brutto OH. Neurocysticercosis. Handb Clin Neurol. 2014;121:1445-59.
44. Del Brutto OH. Neurocysticercosis. Continuum (Minneap Minn). 2012;18(6 Infectious Disease):1392-416.
45. Graham AK, Fong C, Naqvi A, Lu JQ. Toxoplasmosis of the central nervous system: Manifestations vary with immune responses. J Neurol Sci. 2021;420:117223.

CHAPTER 23

Essentials of Sleep Medicine for the Psychiatrist

Joy D Desai

■ INTRODUCTION

Sleep is conserved across most mammals and vertebrates as an evolutionary necessity for survival. This made the pursuit of its science and physiology a tantalizing research prospect for the last century. For some sleep researchers, it paradoxically resulted in sleepless night of toil as the drive to fathom its functions became their "raison d'être". Since humans sleep for approximately a third of their lives, the biology of sleep and its neurophysiological correlates is of relevance to all physicians who treat patients, irrespective of their specialty leanings. This chapter is an introduction to sleep essentials that may be particularly relevant to psychiatrists. It is not meant to be a holistic treatise on sleep disorders and its clinical evaluation.

■ THE BIOLOGY AND NEUROANATOMY OF SLEEP

Sleep is characterized by a gradual process of disengagement of vigilance, awareness, and responsiveness to environmental change leading to a dominant cessation of mobility while breathing and vital functions are preserved albeit languorously. Polysomnography (PSG) is a tool that objectively measures the sequential physiological changes that accompany sleep. Humans are physiologically ordained to sleep for approximately 8 hours throughout adulthood, in synchrony with the day-light cycle (circadian rhythm), with an ideal sleep onset 4 hours from sunset and awakening with the sunrise. Biological feedback loops maintain a sensing of preparatory activities and initiate reciprocal neuronal and biochemical alterations that maintain sleep. Understandably, habitual consistency of sleep timings and investment in sleep hygiene measures preserve the physiological efficiency of sleep.[1]

Adult 8 hours of sleep is characterized by five or six repetitive cycles of physiological changes that represent a hypnogram on the PSG. Each hypnogram lasting from 90 to 100 minutes is identifiable by a three-stage graded transition of physiologies called nonrapid eye movement (NREM), followed by a rapid eye movement phase called REM. NREM constitutes 75–85% of sleep and is divided into N1, N2, and N3 stages. REM sleep is also known as paradoxical sleep because the eyes move rapidly and breathing is deep and stertorous, while the rest of the somatic muscles are completely atonic. During the first two hypnograms REM phases are shorter, with subsequent incremental increases in REM duration with the longest REM just prior to awakening. Each phase of NREM from 1 to 3, and REM has a characteristic electroencephalographic (EEG) signature.[1] The awake EEG is typified by a low amplitude, high-frequency rhythm that progressively slows down on transiting to NREM sleep. In N2 sleep spindles and K complexes dominate, while delta waves are the hallmark of N3 sleep. These are also known as synchronized slow-wave oscillations and are deemed vital for memory consolidation and other sleep-related restorative functions. During REM sleep (again paradoxically) the EEG becomes a desynchronized, low amplitude, high-frequency spiky rhythm akin to that observed in wakefulness.[1,2] During NREM sleep, the EEG progressively slows down, and the heart rate, breathing, spinal reflexes, and cerebral blood flow decreases. The body temperature drops, and growth hormone levels increase. During REM sleep, cerebral blood flow and body temperature increase while spinal reflexes are absent, and dreaming dominates sleep physiology in this phase.[3]

Sleep and wakefulness are maintained by a discrete network of cerebral neurons within the rhombencephalon extending into the diencephalon. Within this region caudorostrally aligned clusters of neurons produce wake promoting neurotransmitters, e.g., dopamine, serotonin, norepinephrine, histamine, and acetylcholine. A parallel system of cell clusters produce a wake promoting peptide called orexin. Galanin, melanocortin, and gamma-aminobutyric acid (GABA) produced by a cell cluster in the ventrolateral preoptic (VLPO) area, have sleep promoting actions. The release of these two sets of neurotransmitters is regulated akin to a flip-flop switch with the wake promoting ones being inhibited during sleep onset and activated during wakefulness. The sleep promoting (inhibitory for wakefulness) neurotransmitters are inhibited during wakefulness and activated during sleep initiation and maintenance.[1,3] The ebb and flow of these polarized chemicals' effect on differing neurotransmitter systems (promoting either wakefulness or sleep) exhibit a finely nuanced process of regulation that merits consideration. The pedunculopontine and laterodorsal tegmental nuclei in the pons and midbrain respectively, are key regulators of the network that precipitates a physiological transition from NREM to REM sleep.[4,5] Cholinergic and glutamatergic neurotransmitter systems are thought to be pivotal for this process. Recent work also implicates a hitherto unrecognized role for dopaminergic regulation in the REM sleep dovetailing with NREM in a normal hypnogram.[4] This is driven by dopaminergic amygdala inputs in the basolateral diencephalon.

The pressure to sleep is orchestrated by a circadian drive known as *process C* and a chemically mediated drive due to accumulation of adenosine (from cerebral neural exhaustion during wakeful work), known as *process S*. The circadian drive is mediated by the induction of melatonin release from the pineal gland triggered by the loss of ambient light at dusk. Dopaminergic amacrine cells in the retia relay this information to the pineal gland via a special network and the gradual increase in melatonin creates a biochemical sequence ultimately inducing the pressure to sleep via this process C. It is implied that lifestyle habits and voluntary abeyance from sleep by wakefulness replete activities can overcome this feedback loop, derailing the harmonious balance ordained by physiology.[6]

Successful sleep via the induction of slowing of the EEG in stage 1 of NREM sleep followed by sleep spindle and K-complex formation in stage 2 NREM, ultimately leading to slow-wave (delta waves) oscillations of stage 3 NREM sleep, require epinephrine, norepinephrine, and cortisol levels to be at the lowest.[7] Physiological stress response is characterized by an increase in these hormones. Therefore, it is not surprising that interpersonal or financial upheavals leading to mental stress can lead to impairment of the sleep induction process resulting in sleep initiation or maintenance failure.[7]

These sleep/wake changes occur bihemispherically as a norm in humans. However, sleep occurs physiologically as a unihemispheric phenomenon in some species, e.g., sea lions, manatees, and porpoises. A similar phenomenon occurs in migratory birds like frigates and the arctic tern. One-half of the brain is asleep while the opposite half is awake and vice versa in a cyclical fashion during the sleep period. It appears that this phenomenon is an adaptation amongst these species to avoid predation both in the oceans and in the skies.[8] In humans, "the first night effect" represents this phenomenon. When sleeping in a novel environment many humans exhibit a noteworthy physiology wherein the dominant cerebral hemisphere maintains a night watch of wakeful rhythms while the nondominant hemisphere sleeps with a signature sleep-associated slow delta rhythm.[9] Physiological interhemispheric sleep associated EEG rhythm asymmetry of this kind reflects the modulable and adaptive nature of sleep biorhythms, perhaps an evolutionary necessity.

The functions of sleep have intrigued researchers since the early part of the last century. The last 70 odd years of untiring research efforts have yielded some thought-provoking insights into the lesser-known functions of sleep. Sleep is vital for memory consolidation. During NREM sleep, the signature EEG rhythms of the brain have nuanced patterns. (Transient events of highly synchronous neuronal activity that typically occur during "offline" brain states; 8–12 Hz) are yoked by sleep spindles (12–16 Hz) to synchronize with slow-wave oscillations (<1.25 Hz) of deep sleep. This results in memory transfer from temporary storage in the human hippocampus to the cerebral cortices for permanent availability for retrieval. This process is called memory consolidation and hence deep sleep is chief the nourisher of human memories.[10,11] If sleep is hampered in duration, timing, consistency, or quality, then this process is impaired. The efficiency of this process is dependent on the anatomical robustness of the prefrontal cortices. In the elderly, prefrontal atrophy leads to uncoupling of these rhythms precipitating forgetfulness and poor hippocampal-dependent memory.[12] Matthew Walker showed that REM sleep is associated with an intense amygdala to prefrontal cortex neural exchange that depotentiates the emotional burden of traumatizing memories.[13] In other words, REM sleep is vital for emotional stability. It has been postulated that insomniacs are haunted by their pasts as distressing memories remain salient in them compared to individuals who sleep well. The maintenance and integrity of REM sleep quantity and quality during a lifetime are directly linked to longevity and mortality.[14] This is mediated by the emerging understanding of the contributory role of REM sleep in neuronal autophagy maintenance.[15] Other studies have correlated polysomnographic suboptimal REM duration and sleep percentages with an enhanced risk of incident dementia.[16]

The NREM sleep contributes to maintenance of blood pressure via a complex interaction exchange between neural networks that connect the amygdala to the prefrontal cortex and insula. Sleep deprivation (SD) can increase daytime blood pressure in normotensive young healthy adults which thankfully reverses on sleep replenishment.[17] Thus, chronic SD from suboptimal duration, timing, quality, and consistency of sleep may contribute to essential hypertension. Not surprisingly, sleep disorders such as obstructive sleep apnea (OSA) perpetuate and worsen existing hypertension. Similarly, sleep is a physiological regulator and modulatory of glucose and adipose tissue storage homeostasis.[18] Sleep contributes to maintenance of body morphology. Sustained SD produces a maladaptive weight gain driven by a hypothalamic imbalance in the activity of leptin and ghrelin.[19] Sleep health is vital for telomere preservation and hence intimately linked to longevity. SD is associated with upregulation of oncogene transcriptases and is implicated in the precipitation of some malignancies, e.g., breast, colorectal, and lung cancer.[20]

In 2013, Nedergaard discovered a unique excretory system solely functional during sleep and called it the "glymphatic system". Herein, the cerebrospinal fluid (CSF) is driven gently in a unidirectional manner from the arterial to the venous system across an expanded interstitium of the brain by the rhythmic arterial pulsations, respiratory effort, and slow-wave oscillations of sleep.[21] The polarization of aquaporin-4 molecules on the foot processes of the astrocytes in the brain impart this directionality to CSF flow. Sleeping in the prone position reduces glymphatic efficiency by 40%, while supine and lateral positions during sleep are optimal for its efficiency. Voluntary exercise, low-dose alcohol consumption, and intermittent fasting can improve glymphatic efficiency by enhancing polarization of aquaporin-4 on the astrocytes.[22] Sleep apnea and lacunar strokes are associated with reduced glymphatic function. The glymphatic system contributes to the clearance of tau and amyloid proteins from the cerebral interstitium. Impairment of this glymphatic system due to sleep apnea contributes to an enhanced risk of cognitive impairment and Alzheimer's disease. Two independent studies have derived a causal association between shorten sleeping hours in midlife with a significantly enhanced risk of developing dementia in late life after the seventh decade.[23] A recent study implies that genetic variations in aquaporin-4 determine its polarization sustenance through life and via glymphatic/sleep efficiency secondarily affect amyloid burden in the brain.[24]

Sleep supports all aspects of the human immune function repertoire and promotes host defense mechanisms against infection and inflammatory insults. SD is associated with alterations of innate and adaptive immune parameters, leading to a chronic inflammatory state, and an increased risk for many infectious/inflammatory pathologies, including autoimmune, neoplastic, cardiometabolic, and neurodegenerative diseases.[25] Some studies have correlated sleep disruption to an enhanced risk of colorectal cancer.[26] Others have proposed that sleep disruption results in increased risk-taking behavior and an enhanced vulnerability to somatic pain of any organ origin.[27] Human creativity has been linked to sleep physiology in numerous studies and sleep onset is perceived to be a creativity sweet spot.[28] Salvador Dali and Edison have been famously linked to have utilized this knowledge to enhance their creative prowess by ingeniously triggering additional sleep-onset transitions in their sleeping times. *"Hypnagogia"* is the term used to describe such sleep–wake transitions. Hypnagogia is observed to be associated with dissociative states, hypnagogic or hypnopompic hallucinations, and sometimes limb jerking. Charles Dickens is believed to have suffered from insomnia and fractured sleep–wake transitions akin to hypnagogia, reflected in his writings when describing experiences of his literary characters Oliver Twist and Ebenezer Scrooge.[29]

In a rare physiological aberration, a stuporous state mimicking sleepiness is accompanied by a near complete disruption of slow-wave sleep on PSG due to dysautonomic sympathetic activation and marked clinical signs of agitation despite visible altered consciousness. This condition is known as *"agrypnia excitata"* and encompasses three distinct conditions—(1) delirium tremens, (2) Morvan's chorea, and (3) familial fatal insomnia.[30] A near complete disruption of normal sleep physiology is a unifying feature of these conditions of variable etiology—alcohol withdrawal, autoimmune dysfunction, and a gene ordained abnormality, respectively.

INSOMNIA

The definitions and classification of insomnia have undergone a remarkable change in recent times leading to a shedding of terminologies such as primary/secondary insomnia, and idiopathic or paradoxic insomnia. The essential understanding is that insomnia can be considered as a working diagnosis in any individual who has difficulty initiating and sustaining sleep despite having an adequate opportunity and/or appropriate circumstance to do so, resulting in a negative daytime consequence on his/her quality of life. A diagnosis of chronic insomnia is considered when these symptoms persist for at least 3 day a week for at least 3 months. Those who suffer from an established psychiatric disorder, sleep disordered breathing, restless legs syndrome, bladder dysfunction, and chronic pain afflictions are understandably excluded from this diagnosis. The symptoms mandatory for this diagnosis to be entertained are:

- Resistance in going to bed at the desired time (4 hours from sunset according to circadian synchrony)
- Difficulty in initiating or maintaining sleep
- Earlier and/or frequent awakening from sleep
- Difficulty in sleeping without parent/caregiver attention

The daytime symptoms wedded to insomnia include fatigue, troublesome mood changes, memory disturbances, impaired social, vocational, or academic performance, lethargy, impaired attention, or concentration leading to performance errors/accidents. These could be reported either to the patient or a caregiver. In a physiologically normal individual, the pressure to sleep arises about four hours from sunset and the signal to awaken is usually sunrise. Habitual over-riding of this urge to sleep by indulgent participation in recreational activities (late night partying and dancing, or television binge watching) or consumption of stimulants that impede sleep initiation (coffee, cocaine, and recreational drugs) are common contributors to the development of a phase shift in sleep onset. A tendency for rumination or being chronically anxious from any interpersonal conflict (perceived or real) can also impede the harmony of sleep onset and maintenance. The scientific analysis of these factors has led to the proposal of a model of chronic "hyperarousal" as the key contributor to the development of chronic insomnia.[31]

The following measures of sleep hygiene are to be promoted in the community to harmonize sleep physiology and decrease the risk of insomnia due to habitual lifestyle investment errors.

- Exercise in the morning hours and avoid heavy exercises within 3 hours of bedtime.
- Remove laptops, cell phones, and TVs from the bedroom.
- Restrict screen time after 9:30 PM.
- Listen to relaxing music.
- Avoid caffeinated drinks after 3 PM and alcohol within 2 hours of bedtime.
- Ensure a comfortable ambient temperature, low/floor level night lighting, and a fragrant aroma in the bedroom.
- Avoid daytime naps.
- If vulnerable to anxiety, invest in meditation and mindfulness as a sleep enhancing activity.

A unique pattern of sleep behavior has emerged in urban settings driven by the pressure to perform target driven work-related projects. City dwellers now predominantly work late into the night on weekdays (usually beyond midnight) and wake early by 6 in the morning to go to work as a result of public transport necessity. Thus, they are sleep deprived on weekdays to about 6 hours only. On weekends, they sleep in late and wake after ten in the morning in the notion that they need to catch up on sleep. The disruption of circadian rhythms and an absence of a sleep pattern consistency results in misaligned biological clock systems in all tissue. The individual clinically behaves as if jetlagged.[32] This pattern has been called *"social jetlag"*. Persistent social jetlag is now implicated in a host of medical disorders that include hypertension, diabetes, metabolic syndrome, cyclothymic mood disorders, polycystic ovarian syndrome, and some autoimmune conditions. This illustrates the important contribution of consistency of circadian synchrony for brain and somatic health maintenance.

Virtually all life forms demonstrate biological circadian rhythms. Human studies show that rhythmic yoking of biological processes to the day-night cycle is driven by different physiological timekeepers or *"zeitgebers"*. These timekeepers are light or its abeyance, timing of meals and physical activity to enumerate a few. At dusk the waning ambient light triggers a signal from the retinal ganglionic cells to the suprachiasmatic nucleus (SCN) resulting in the initiation of melatonin secretion from the pineal gland. The onset is between 9 and 11 PM and it peaks around 1 AM to dissipate completely by 7 AM in the morning. The SCN is the master biological clock and acts as the symphony organizer for all tissue clocks. Its chemical mediator is suspected to be melatonin. Circadian tissue clocks are formed through transcription–translation feedback loops (TTFLs) that are gene driven.[6] The following genes have been recognized as relevant in human circadian biology.

- *Circadian locomotor output cycles kaput (CLOCK)*: A gene encoding protein that affects the length and persistence of a circadian cycle.
- *Brain and muscle aryl hydrocarbon receptor nuclear translocator-like protein 1 (BMAL1)*: A basic helix-loop helix transcription factor

- *PER1, PER2, and PER3 (period):* A negative element in the circadian transcription loop by interacting with other circadian regulatory proteins and transporting them to the nucleus.
- *CRY1 and CRY2 (cryptochrome):* A negative element inhibiting CLOCK-mediated transcription in maintaining period length and circadian rhythmicity.
- *Rev-ErbA (orphan nuclear receptor):* An alpha thyroid receptor splice variant that regulates CLOCK and BMAL1 expression.

Humans are biologically ordained to sleep 4 hours from sunset and to waken with the sunrise. The behavioral expression of the setpoint of an individual's circadian rhythm is known as the *chronotype*. The "morningness" or "lark" chronotype is characterized by early morning awakening, sleeping early, and peak physical performance in the first half of the day. The "eveningness" or "owl" chronotype is characterized by waking up late, taking time to kickstart peak daytime prowess, and working late into the night. The eveningness chronotype is associated with a higher risk of weight gain, metabolic syndrome, sarcopenia, and depressive ideation.[33] Circadian asynchrony is now independently implicated in the genesis of an increased risk for degenerative dementia. This perhaps gives an added credo to the adage "early to bed and early to rise......."

In a world driven by a pressure to deliver relentlessly and in increased appetite for media consumption on devices, maintenance of circadian synchrony is going to be a serious health challenge.

EXCESSIVE DAYTIME SOMNOLENCE

Excessive daytime somnolence (EDS) is one of the most common complaints with which patients may seek medical assistance across any specialty. In a nutshell, EDS may be a symptom worthy of medical analysis and evaluation when a patient (seemingly inexplicably) feels sleepy when he/she ought to be awake. Lethargy and absence of a feeling of energy or zest are usual accompaniments. Like other medical ailments, the analysis is critically clinical. The approach to EDS ideally should address the following questions:
- *Is the patient's sleep hygiene optimal*: Duration, quality, timing of sleep, and consistency of this schedule across a broad timeframe?
- Once duration, timing, and consistency are out of the reckoning, attempts have to be made to assess potential impediments to sleep quality: what can be understood about the frequency of awakenings during sleep time, snoring during sleep, perceived episodes of choking during sleep, perceived sense of excessive of limb movements in sleep, vocalization, or bedpartner reported physical movements in sleep suggestive of dream enactment?
- Is the EDS related to an adverse effect of any medication administered for other systemic medical ailments?

The commonly taught primary disorder of impaired daytime wakefulness maintenance, known as narcolepsy, is actually rare. Patients with narcolepsy cannot stay wake due to a failure of orexin generation. In some patients, excessive daytime episodic somnolence is accompanied by other features of sleep architectural disarray—cataplexy (a reflection of episodic daytime REM sleep associated atonic intrusions), hypnogogic or hypnopompic hallucinations, sleep paralysis, and occasionally sleep myoclonus.[34] The precipitation is often perceived to be autoimmune after a viral infection on a background of genetic susceptibility. Low CSF levels of orexin, the demonstration of two or more REM periods within 15 minutes of sleep onset on a PSG or multiple sleep latency test are diagnostic hallmarks. Most patients are treated with modafinil or solriamfetol.

In the clinic, the most common cause of daytime somnolence is either poor sleep hygiene or sleep disordered breathing. In normal individuals, suboptimal breath excursions (hypopnea) or skipped breaths (apnea) may occur up to five times in an hour of sleep. The calculated apnea-hypopnea index (AHI) on PSG reflects this number. An AHI of between 6 and 15/hours is considered mild sleep apnea that between 16 and 30/hours is considered moderate, and an AHI above 30/hours is deemed severe. Obesity, a short neck, a neck circumference above 17 cm, smoking, and frequent alcohol consumption, late night meals, and even sleeping late frequently are considered predisposing risk factors OSA.[35] Central sleep apnea may occur as an accompaniment of OSA, as a manifestation of obesity hypoventilation syndrome, due to ascent to high altitudes without adequate acclimatization, and as a result of congestive cardiac failure associated Cheyne-Stokes breathing.[36] Rarely, it may accompany neuromuscular conditions like myotonic dystrophy. Sleep disordered breathing if left untreated can pose numerous health-related hazards—perpetuation of hypertension, diabetes, obesity, an enhanced risk of vascular catastrophes such as myocardial infarction, stroke, and cardiac arrhythmias. In the elderly it is associated with an acceleration of neurodegenerative processes. The assessment of sleep disordered breathing and its correction by lifestyle modification and continuous positive airway pressure (CPAP) therapy requires training and experience.

SLEEP PHYSIOLOGY AND SYMPTOMS ASCRIBED TO PSYCHIATRIC DYSFUNCTION

Sleep disturbance is a recognized symptom across the entire spectrum of anxiety disorders—generalized anxiety disorder, panic disorder, post-traumatic stress disorder, and social anxiety disorder. That restorative sleep has anxiolytic biological/physiological properties, was first theorized by the elegant experimental data backed research by Ben Simon and Matthew Walker.[37] Through their experimental demonstration, it was clarified that the anxiogenic outcome of sleep loss was mediated by the suboptimal downregulation of amygdala activity by the medial prefrontal cortices during slow-wave NREM sleep. Replenishment of sleep as a biological investment resulted in sustained improvement in anxiety scores in susceptible individuals.

Their data implies that in normal individuals during NREM sleep a selective network-based functional interplay between the medial prefrontal cortex and amygdala, serves to allay daytime anxiety. Ergo NREM sleep replenishment keeps us physiologically calmer.[37] The same group in a different study convincingly demonstrated that REM sleep depotentiates amygdala activity linked to traumatizing daytime emotional experiences, ultimately resulting in a persistent memory of the event but without its emotional baggage.[13] Thus, they illustrated that sleep has multifaceted emotional salience enhancing biological properties. Harrington and Cairney propose a framework in which top-down inhibitory control networks are impaired by SD leading to intrusive thoughts and emotional dysregulation. This process leads to a vicious cycle of sleeplessness, persistent unwanted thoughts, and heightened anxiety ultimately leading to an increased risk of mental illness.[38] Shakespeare in Macbeth wrote of this in a moment of epiphany much before the era of sleep research based on functional neurobiology—"Sleep that knits up the ravelled sleeve of care, The death of each day's life, sore labor's bath, *balm of hurt minds*, great nature's second course, Chief nourisher in life's feast".

Flavie Waters adopted a systematic review approach to identify experimental and observational studies of SD in healthy adults, identifying the spectrum of psychopathological changes that occur due to it.[39] Finally, 21 of 476 articles were eligible for inclusion in their assessment. The key finding that emerged was the precipitation of anomalies of multimodal perception and reality integration with progressive SD. Visual distortions, metamorphosis, illusions, somatosensory misperceptions, and sometimes frank hallucinations were observed. The visual modality was the most consistently affected (in 90% of the studies), followed by the somatosensory (52%) and auditory (33%) modalities. A full night of SD was enough to set into motion an almost unidirectional progression of these changes. Irritability, anxiety, perceptual distortions, temporal disorientation, and depersonalization started within 24–48 hours of sleep loss. This was followed by complex hallucinations and disordered thinking after 48–90 hours, and delusions after 72 hours of SD. Beyond this the clinical picture resembled that of toxic delirium or acute psychosis.[39] 3 consecutive days without sleep resulted in hallucinations within all three sensory modalities. A period of normal sleep served to resolve psychotic symptoms in most cases. Thus, sleep neurobiology on a daily basis seems to recalibrate the sense of self, reality perception, and integration of all sensory modalities. Loss of sleep results in a disarrayed churning of aberrant perceptual signaling mimicking the clinical umbrella of acute psychosis related symptoms. Thankfully this seems to be reversible with sleep replenishment.

CASE VIGNETTE

A 70-year-old man presented to the neurology OPD with a history of indolent onset slowing of movements, change in handwriting with micrographia, and difficulty in arising out of low chairs. He had a lean habitus, suffered from diabetes and hypertension that was well controlled on medications. He swam regularly for exercise and his dietary habits were disciplined. Clinical examination revealed congenital retrognathia, an apathetic affect, symmetrical akinetic rigid syndrome with predominant axial rigidity, retropulsion on the pull test, and no overt signs of pyramidal or cerebellar dysfunction. A clinical diagnosis of probable progressive supranuclear palsy (PSP) was entertained, and low-dose levodopa therapy was initiated. MRI of the brain was compatible with early PSP.

A few days later, he was brought to the emergency medical service with escalating disorientation, hallucinations, delusions, and verbal diarrhea. He believed his wife was having sex with his neighbor on a table in the corner of the room, he was convinced his liver and spleen were melting and emanating from his anus in a pool of flesh and blood; he reiterated that his demise was impending and repeatedly asked his son to organize his funeral arrangements. He was convinced that the nurses were poisoning his intravenous drip. He hallucinated that bearded men in dark garments were brandishing scimitars and attempting to decapitate him. He fondled one of treating nurses while she set up his intravenous access much to her distress and chagrin. His family was shattered at the dramatic change in his behavior and personality, the nursing staff were angry, and the treating neurologist was vexed. His hemogram, erythrocyte sedimentation rate (ESR), routine biochemistry, abdominal ultrasonography, and CSF examination were all normal. A serum and CSF assessment for known autoantibodies producing autoimmune encephalitis was fruitless. ^{18}F-fluorodeoxyglucose positron emission tomography (FDG-PET) scan of the brain revealed a mild bilateral frontal hypometabolism for glucose. The flurodopa brain scan revealed an asymmetric caudate and putaminal uptake, compatible with the original clinical diagnosis of PSP.

While he was being examined, he fell asleep and started to snore loudly. Very quickly episodes of hypopnea and apnea were discernible at the bedside. When the family was informed that he required a sleep study, the wife promptly fished out a 2-year-old sleep study wherein his AHI was 64/hour with a REM AHI of 76/hour, and frequent desaturations below 80%. The family sheepishly confessed that he had been advised to implement CPAP usage but had balked at the idea of having an intrusive mask over the face each night. The wife narrated: *"Doctor, he has always snored and in the last few years has slept poorly, waking up often despite sleeping medications. In fact, for three nights prior to this admission he has not slept at all'.*

The patient was initiated on CPAP therapy and prescribed melatonin too. Within 6 days his cognitive symptoms reversed to preexistent normal, and he was able to converse coherently with his family and medical team. He profusely and sheepishly apologized to the nursing team for his misdemeanors. He has now been followed up for 3 years and is cognitively intact, with compliance to CPAP. His PSP features have progressed modestly and require a higher dose of levodopa.

This unusual clinical vignette illustrates the important contributions of sleep hygiene and health to neuropsychiatric equipoise. His untreated OSA may have gradually eroded his cognitive reserve and the preadmission three nights of insomnia probably precipitated the vivid frankly psychotic behavior that reversed after implementation of restorative sleep measures.

CONCLUDING REMARKS

The neuroscience of sleep and its biological and physiological implications has leapfrogged into a gigantic separate subspecialty. While its practice and pursuit may be the professional purview of some specialists, its fundamental tenets, and the awareness of its various deviations from the normal should be known to all medical practitioners. This review has attempted to impart key nuances of sleep neurobiology, physiology, and its practical implications with the perspective of being most relevant to psychiatrists. It is meant to be a bridge between subspecialty teaching and rapidly advancing neuroscience perspectives. Like most such attempts it may not be exhaustively complete but is enough to whet the academic appetite of the reader.

LEARNING POINTS

- Human sleep has evolved as a biological super-pill.
- A complex network of pontomesencephalic neuronal clusters drives this intricate phenomenon through a rich, widespread cerebral network.
- Sleep maintains blood pressure, glucose homeostasis, fat storage balance, and physical looks.
- Sleep serves an essential restorative and recalibrative function spanning almost physiologies vital for organ optimization. This includes the brain.
- Sleep is mandatory for memory consolidation, emotional salience, longevity maintenance, creativity, and brain chemical wet cleaning via the glymphatic system.
- SD has cognitive and seemingly psychiatric ill effects the symptoms of which are immediately visible upon 24 hours of SD. These can escalate if deprivation is sustained.
- It is mandatory for all healthcare workers to be empowered with this understanding of sleep physiology and its health maintenance prowess.

REFERENCES

1. Scammell TE, Arrigoni E, Lipton JO. Neural Circuitry of Wakefulness and Sleep. Neuron. 2017;93(4):747-65.
2. Lambert I, Peter-Derex L. Spotlight on sleep stage classification based on EEG. Nat Sci Sleep. 2023;15:479-90.
3. Carley DW, Farabi SS. Physiology of Sleep. Diabetes Spectr. 2016;29(1):5-9.
4. Hasegawa E, Miyasaka A, Sakurai K, Cherasse Y, Li Y, Sakurai T. Rapid eye movement sleep is initiated by basolateral amygdala dopamine signaling in mice. Science. 2022;375(6584):994-1000.
5. Park SH, Weber F. Neural and Homeostatic Regulation of REM Sleep. Front Psychol. 2020;11:1662.
6. Schwartz WJ, Klerman EB. Circadian Neurobiology and the Physiologic Regulation of Sleep and Wakefulness. Neurol Clin. 2019;37(3):475-86.
7. Hirotsu C, Tufik S, Andersen ML. Interactions between sleep, stress, and metabolism: From physiological to pathological conditions. Sleep Sci. 2015;8(3):143-52.
8. Mascetti GG. Unihemispheric sleep and asymmetrical sleep: behavioral, neurophysiological, and functional perspectives. Nat Sci Sleep. 2016;8:221-38.
9. Tamaki M, Bang JW, Watanabe T, Sasaki Y. Night Watch in One Brain Hemisphere during Sleep Associated with the First-Night Effect in Humans. Curr Biol. 2016;26(9):1190-4.

10. Siapas AG, Wilson MA. Coordinated interactions between hippocampal ripples and cortical spindles during slow-wave sleep. Neuron. 1998;21(5):1123-8.
11. Boutin A, Doyon J. A sleep spindle framework for motor memory consolidation. Philos Trans R Soc Lond B Biol Sci. 2020;375(1799):20190232.
12. Mander BA, Rao V, Lu B, Saletin JM, Lindquist JR, Ancoli-Israel S, et al. Prefrontal atrophy disrupted NREM slow waves and impaired hippocampal-dependent memory in aging. Nat Neurosci. 2013;16(3):357-64.
13. Van der Helm E, Yao J, Dutt S, Rao V, Saletin JM, Walker MP. REM sleep depotentiates amygdala activity to previous emotional experiences. Curr Biol. 2011;21(23):2029-32.
14. Leary EB, Watson KT, Ancoli-Israel S, Redline S, Yaffe K, Ravelo LA, et al. Association of Rapid Eye Movement Sleep With Mortality in Middle-aged and Older Adults. JAMA Neurol. 2020;77(10):1241-51.
15. Chauhan AK, Mallick BN. Association between autophagy and rapid eye movement sleep loss-associated neurodegenerative and patho-physio-behavioral changes. Sleep Med. 2019;63:29-37.
16. Pase MP, Himali JJ, Grima NA, Beiser AS, Satizabal CL, Aparicio HJ, et al. Sleep architecture and the risk of incident dementia in the community. Neurology. 2017;89(12):1244-50.
17. Robillard R, Lanfranchi PA, Prince F, Filipini D, Carrier J. Sleep deprivation increases blood pressure in healthy normotensive elderly and attenuates the blood pressure response to orthostatic challenge. Sleep. 2011;34(3):335-9.
18. Morselli L, Leproult R, Balbo M, Spiegel K. Role of sleep duration in the regulation of glucose metabolism and appetite. Best Pract Res Clin Endocrinol Metab. 2010;24(5):687-702.
19. Cooper CB, Neufeld EV, Dolezal BA, Martin JL. Sleep deprivation and obesity in adults: A brief narrative review. BMJ Open Sport Exerc Med. 2018;4(1):e000392.
20. Chen Y, Tan F, Wei L, Li X, Lyu Z, Feng X, et al. Sleep duration and the risk of cancer: a systematic review and meta-analysis including dose-response relationship. BMC Cancer. 2018;18(1):1149.
21. Hablitz LM, Nedergaard M. The glymphatic system: A novel component of fundamental neurobiology. J Neurosci. 2021;41(37):7698-711.
22. Zhang J, Zhan Z, Li X, Xing A, Jiang C, Chen Y, et al. Intermittent Fasting Protects against Alzheimer's Disease Possible through Restoring Aquaporin-4 Polarity. Front Mol Neurosci. 2017;10:395.
23. Sabia S, Fayosse A, Dumurgier J, van Hees VT, Paquet C, Sommerlad A, et al. Association of sleep duration in middle and old age with incidence of dementia. Nat Commun. 2021;12(1):2289.
24. Rainey-Smith SR, Mazzucchelli GN, Villemagne VL, Brown BM, Porter T, Weinborn M, et al. Genetic variation in Aquaporin-4 moderates the relationship between sleep and brain Aβ-amyloid burden. Transl Psychiatry. 2018;8:47.
25. Garbarino S, Lanteri P, Bragazzi NL, Magnavita N, Scoditti E, et al. Role of sleep deprivation in immune-related disease risk and outcomes. Commun Biol. 2021;4:1304.
26. Lin CL, Liu TC, Wang YN, Chung CH, Chien WC. The Association Between Sleep Disorders and the Risk of Colorectal Cancer in Patients: A Population-based Nested Case-Control Study. In Vivo. 2019;33(2):573-9.
27. Krause AJ, Prather AA, Wager TD, Lindquist MA, Walker MP. The Pain of Sleep Loss: A Brain Characterization in Humans. J Neurosci. 2019 Mar 20;39(12):2291-300.
28. Lacaux C, Andrillon T, Bastoul C, Idir Y, Fonteix-Galet A, Arnulf I, et al. Sleep onset is a creative sweet spot. Sci Adv. 2021;7:eabj5866.
29. da Mota Gomes M, Nardi AE. Charles Dickens' Hypnagogia, Dreams, and Creativity. Front Psychol. 2021;12:700882.
30. Provini, F. Agrypnia Excitata. Curr Neurol Neurosci Rep. 2013;13:341.
31. Kalmbach DA, Cuamatzi-Castelan AS, Tonnu CV, Tran KM, Anderson JR, Roth T, et al. Hyperarousal and sleep reactivity in insomnia: current insights. Nat Sci Sleep. 2018;10:193-201.
32. Wittmann M, Dinich J, Merrow M, Roenneberg T. Social jetlag: Misalignment of biological and social time. Chronobiol Int. 2006;23(1-2):497-509.
33. Partonen T. Chronotype and Health Outcomes. Curr Sleep Medicine Rep. 2015;1:205-11
34. Akintomide GS, Rickards H. Narcolepsy: A review. Neuropsychiatr Dis Treat. 2011;7:507-18.
35. Abbasi A, Gupta SS, Sabharwal N, Meghrajani V, Sharma S, Kamholz S, et al. A comprehensive review of obstructive sleep apnea. Sleep Sci. 2021;14(2):142-54.
36. Muza RT. Central sleep apnoea-a clinical review. J Thorac Dis. 2015;7(5):930-7.
37. Ben Simon E, Rossi A, Harvey AG, Walker MP. Overanxious and underslept. Nat Hum Behav. 2020;4:100-10.
38. Harrington MO, Cairney SO. Sleep Loss Gives Rise to Intrusive Thoughts. Trends Cogn Sci. 2021;25(6):434-6.
39. Waters F, Chiu V, Atkinson A, Blom JD. Severe Sleep Deprivation Causes Hallucinations and a Gradual Progression Toward Psychosis With Increasing Time Awake. Front Psychiatry. 2018;9:303.

CHAPTER 24

Clinical and Radiological Pitfalls in the Diagnosis of Dementias

Gautam Das, Atanu Biswas

INTRODUCTION

Diagnosis of dementia requires good clinical assessment supplemented with laboratory and radiologic investigations. A good history, careful neuropsychological assessment (NPA), and neurological examination are necessary for the diagnosis. Traditionally, investigations are performed to exclude probable treatable causes. However, in recent time, as we are moving toward biomarker-based diagnosis, investigations become part of diagnostic workup. This is to aid in determining specific diseases responsible for dementia.

Degenerative diseases such as Alzheimer's disease (AD), dementia with Lewy bodies (DLB), Parkinson disease dementia (PDD), and frontotemporal lobar degeneration (FTLD) are common causes of dementia in the community. Dementia arising from cerebrovascular disease is also a leading cause of dementia in India and in other Asian countries. Till now, definite diagnosis of a disease requires pathological confirmation and without that a probable diagnosis is made with the help of criteria for these diseases. However, the diagnostic accuracy of these criteria is not very high and there are enough reasons for misdiagnosis. This has been proven in numerous autopsy studies.

To improve the diagnostic accuracy, biomarkers are available in some of these degenerative diseases including AD. These are biological, that is, from body fluid and radiological markers that help in establishing pathological diagnosis even without biopsy. As biomarkers are not universally available and they still require refinement to make them useful in routine clinical practice, clinical exercise is still considered as gold standard in making the diagnosis.

Clinical diagnosis is often challenging due to overlapping features of different dementing illnesses and coexistence of vascular risk factors and vascular changes in imaging. In this chapter, we tried to explore various challenges clinicians face in dealing with patients of dementia.

NORMAL AGING VERSUS PRECLINICAL STAGE OF DEMENTIA

Subjective memory complaints (SMCs) are common in old people. Although they are not serious and often ignored by clinicians, studies have shown that presence of SMC increases the risk of dementia in future.

Vignette: BCC, a 68-year-old male, veteran homeopathic practitioner came with complaints of forgetfulness of immediate and recent things with preserved remote memories for 3 years. Recently, for last 1 year, he became irritable and lost his temper with slightest provocation. His NPA revealed impaired learning and recall in word list recall test, with 27/30 score in Mini Mental State Examination (MMSE) and 86/100 in Addenbrooke's Cognitive Examination (ACE)-III, CDR (Clinical Dementia Rating) score 0.5. All other cognitive domains such as visuospatial, executive function, and language were normal. His instrumental activity of daily living (IADL) was unaffected.

This gentleman had SMC and there was some objective evidence of recent memory impairment without disturbing his ADL. This is termed as mild cognitive impairment (MCI). MCI is considered as preclinical stage of dementia, although all MCI subjects do not convert to dementia. The distinction between normal aging and MCI requires detailed NPA. Cognitive performance deteriorates as we grow older. Performance of a 70-year-old person cannot be same with that of a 20-year-old one. But an elderly person performs equally with his/her age-, gender-, and education-matched peers in the community, and this is normal senescence. When the performance deteriorates in respect to what is normal for the age-, gender-, and education-matched individuals in the community, and the person remains functionally independent, it is called MCI or mild neurocognitive dysfunction. If the subject fails to perform his normal activities with this level of cognitive impairment, an early dementia or major neurocognitive dysfunction is considered. The thin line between MCI and early dementia is the preservation or disturbance of IADL. Thus, a CDR score of 0.5 makes a person MCI, if his/her IADL is preserved, and dementia if IADL is affected.

Mild cognitive impairment is further subdivided as amnestic, nonamnestic, and single- and multi-domain categories. With the help of biomarkers, especially amyloid and tau in cerebrospinal fluid (CSF) and ligand-based positron emission tomography (PET) scan, it is now possible to make a diagnosis of AD in this preclinical stage. This helps in prognostication and use of new antiamyloid agent as disease-modifying treatment.

ALZHEIMER'S DISEASE OR MIXED DEMENTIA: THE DILEMMA

Cerebrovascular diseases are common in old age, so also degenerative dementia such as AD. In the community, these two diseases often coexist and make diagnostic labeling difficult. While AD is a progressive disease, vascular dementia (VaD) has relatively better prognosis as the progression can be halted with effective management.

Vignette: A 72-year-old hypertensive businessman presented with gradually progressive cognitive impairment for last 2 years with walking difficulties and urge incontinence. He has had an episode of stroke with left-sided hemiparesis 7 years back from which there was complete recovery. He scored 76 in ACE and 22 in MMSE. His CDR was 2, and he was detected to have disturbances in IADL.

He was having defect in attention (low scores in forward and backward digit span), with preserved language function and gnosis, with poor learning and recall in verbal as well as visual memory tests; and defect in visuoconstructional (unable to copy cube), visuoperceptual (identifying fragmented letters), and visuospatial ability (unable to properly draw a face of a clock, disturbance in praxis with slow in processing speed; time taken to complete Trail A and B) and executive function. Neurological examination revealed slow ataxic gait with positive Babinski on left side.

The clinical profile suggests probable VaD due to history of stroke in the past, presence of vascular risk factors, e.g., hypertension and walking difficulty and urinary symptoms. The cognitive profile of impairment of attention, slow processing speed, and executive dysfunction corroborates with clinical impression of subcortical dementia commonly seen in patients with cerebral small vessel disease. However, cognitive assessment also shows prominent memory impairment not improving with cues that is more likely due to involvement of bilateral entorhinal cortex and hippocampus. Additionally, disturbance in visuospatial, perceptual, and praxis function suggests bilateral parietal lobe dysfunction. These domains are generally not affected in small vessel disease, and suggest coexistence of other pathology such as AD. As both VaD and AD occur in old age, they often coexist and make the clinical diagnosis difficult. The magnetic resonance imaging [(MRI); **Figs. 1 and 2**] shows presence of white matter hyperintensities (Fazekas 2) with multiple microbleeds in basal ganglia areas suggesting small vessel disease. There is also prominent atrophy of brain especially in temporoparietal areas.

Mixed dementia is not uncommon in India and other low- and middle-income countries (LMICs) due to increased burden of vascular risk factors in the community. It is essential to make a proper diagnosis for (1) deciding treatment strategies as well as for (2) prognostication. While VaD has a relatively better prognosis and the progression can be halted by effective management, degenerative aspect will progress despite best medical management available.

Decision of using newer disease-modifying therapies such as aducanumab in such complex situation is much difficult. This requires documentation of amyloid pathology in brain by CSF analysis or amyloid scan. Moreover, presence of vascular pathology makes the subject susceptible to hemorrhagic amyloid-related imaging abnormalities (ARIA-H).

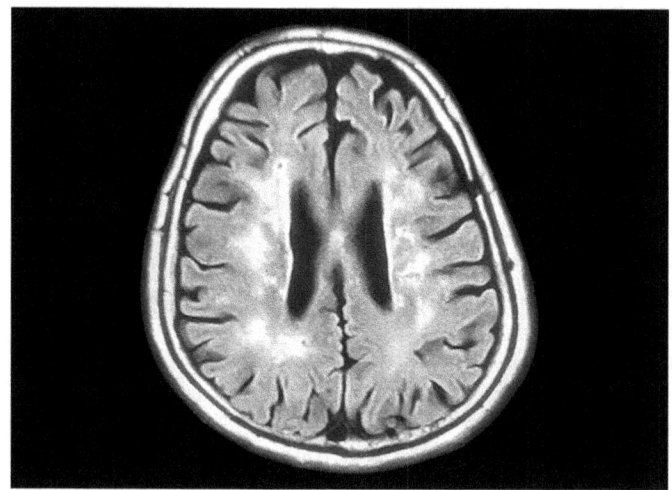

FIG. 1: Axial fluid-attenuated inversion recovery image with periventricular hyperintensities.

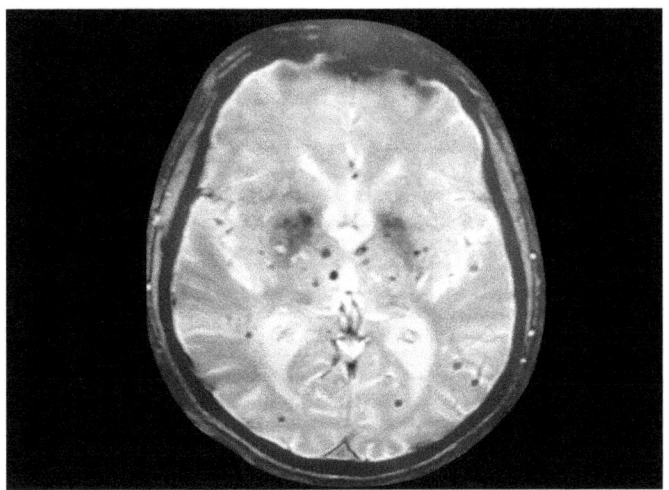

FIG. 2: Axial gradient echo image showing multiple microhemorrhages in basal ganglia area.

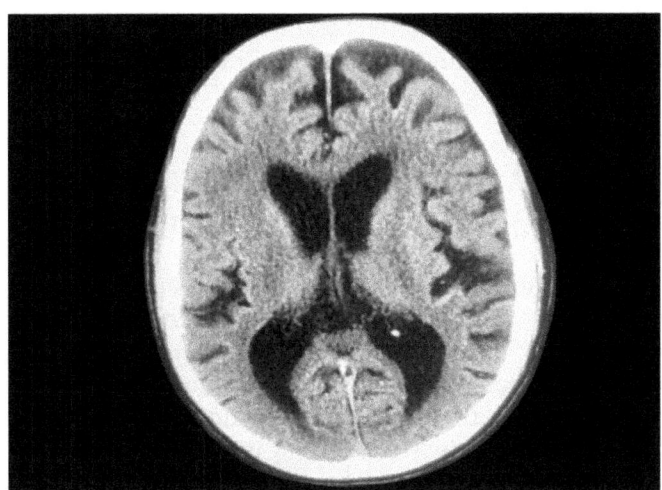

FIG. 3: Axial computed tomography image shows bilateral frontal atrophy.

FRONTAL LOBE SYNDROME: WHAT MAKES THE DIAGNOSIS?

Prefrontal cortex is responsible for social cognition, besides its control over eye movement, planning, execution, and goal-directed behavior. This has extensive subcortical connections with basal ganglia and thalamus and diseases affecting these structures often present with frontal lobe dysfunction. Executive dysfunction is one of the core features of many dementias including AD, frontotemporal dementia (FTD) as well as subcortical diseases such as PD, Huntington disease (HD), and small vessel VaD. Clinical distinction is challenging.[1]

Vignette: A 55-year-old bank manager presented with history of suspiciousness for 6 years. He suspected his wife of cheating, without evidence. One year ago, he suspected his coworker of stealing his mobile phone and confronted with him aggressively. He was suspended from service for his disruptive behavior. His wife complained that he was having multitasking difficulties. There was, however, no disinhibition, no loss of sympathy or empathy, change in dietary pattern, or compulsive behavior.

He scored 26/30 in MMSE with difficulty in serial subtraction and recalling and 78/100 in ACE with poor score in attention and reduced fluency. In Trail-making test, he made two mistakes and was too slow and distracted to finish the test. In neuropsychiatric inventory (NPI), he was found to have delusions, agitation/aggression, anxiety, and irritability/lability. MRI scan was not available as he had claustrophobia. His CT scan (Fig. 3) showed atrophy of bilateral frontal lobes.

The foregoing story of a middle-aged man suggests frontal behavioral abnormalities and dysexecutive syndrome. Numerous possibilities could be considered, such as primary psychiatric illnesses such as severe depression, bipolar disorder, or schizophrenia; behavioral variant of FTD (bvFTD); and frontal variant of AD. Primary psychiatric disorders usually have prominent psychiatric symptoms such as delusions and hallucination, which is lacking in this gentleman. Moreover, presence of executive dysfunction, disturbance in attention, and reduced fluency and reduced psychomotor speed suggest frontal lobar dysfunction. The atrophy of prefrontal lobes corroborated the findings. Differentiating frontal AD from bvFTD is very difficult by clinical and by radiological means. While bvFTD presents with early and prominent behavioral abnormality, behavioral abnormalities are less conspicuous in frontal variant of AD, which is usually diagnosed with presence of marked executive dysfunction. As focal AD is relatively uncommon and often have an early age of onset, they are often misdiagnosed as bvFTD. Even fluorodeoxyglucose (FDG)-PET would not help in differentiating these two conditions and CSF or ligand-based imaging biomarkers will be needed in differentiating them.

Another difficulty arises in patients when they present with dysexecutive syndrome and parkinsonism. The frontal subcortical connections with basal ganglia and thalamus make the clinical presentation similar in both cortical dementias due to frontal lobe degeneration such as bvFTD as well as in subcortical dementias such as PDD, HD, progressive supranuclear palsy (PSP), and even in small vessels VaD. The common thread of all these conditions is the executive dysfunction as cognitive disturbance. The behavioral symptoms, although common, help making the distinction. Prominent and early loss of social cognition, loss of basic emotion, disinhibition, lack of hygiene, loss of embarrassment, altered feeding behavior, impulsivity, compulsive behavior, hoarding, utilization behavior, and loss of insight suggest a diagnosis of bvFTD.[1]

WHEN LANGUAGE DISTURBANCE IS THE PRIMARY COGNITIVE DISTURBANCE

Acquired language disorder or aphasia is an important component of many dementias. The pattern of language dysfunction often indicates a type of pathology. But differentiating aphasia based on clinical examination is challenging.[2] A thorough and meticulous assessment of language function is essential along with careful analysis of neuroimaging in differentiating these aphasia syndromes.

Vignette: A 58-year-old right-handed retired architect is seen in the clinic. Three years ago, he started to complain about isolated hesitant speech and word-finding difficulties, without any other neurologic symptoms. His neurologic examination reveals only anomia, and he scored 29/30 on the MMSE because of poor repetition of the sentence. His reading and writing ability were preserved. There was no other cognitive disturbance.

When language dysfunction is the only cognitive disturbance and this persists for initial 2 years, developing from degenerative disorder, this is termed as primary progressive aphasia (PPA).[3] The agrammatic variant (PPA-G) presents with effortful and marked word finding hesitation in their speech with marked reduced fluency. Comprehension of complex sentences may be difficult, but otherwise normal. The speech is devoid of preposition appears as "telegraphic speech." There is often associated apraxia of speech. The atrophy is dominant inferior frontal lobe anterior to sylvian fissure. The tau protein dysfunction is the primary cause of PPA-G.

The semantic variant (PPA-S) is characterized by fluent speech with lack of content. Due to loss of word meaning, subject often uses "this" and "that" in place of object and object naming is difficult for these patients. Single word comprehension becomes difficult for them. Grammar and comprehension are preserved. Speech is vague and often contains circumlocutions. Imaging usually shows prominent atrophy in left anterior temporal lobe. The pathology in this case is the TDP-43 protein dysfunction.

The logopenic (PPA-L) variant presents with reduced fluency but with preserved grammar and impaired sentence repetition. There is atrophy of posterior temporal lobe, that is, posterior of sylvian fissure in dominant hemisphere. The foregoing case is an example of logopenic PPA. It always suggests Alzheimer pathology in the brain.

Making clinical distinction of various PPA is often difficult, but a systematic language function assessment helps differentiating them **(Table 1)**. Additional clue comes from the pattern of cortical atrophy in structural **(Figs. 4 and 5)** and functional neuroimaging.[4]

TABLE 1: Clinical radiological and pathological features of different types of PPA.

Type of PPA	Clinical criteria	Radiological features	Common pathology

Nonfluent/ Agrammatic variant (PPA-G)[2]	A. One of the following core features must be present:
	  1. Agrammatism in language production
	  2. Effortful, halting speech with inconsistent speech sound errors and distortions (apraxia of speech)
	B. Two of the following three ancillary features must be present:
	  1. Impaired comprehension of syntactically complex (noncanonical) sentences
	  2. Spared single-word comprehension
	  3. Spared object knowledge
		Left inferior frontal gyrus is atrophied (anterior to sylvian fissure) with prominence of sylvian fissure	The most common pathology is FTLD with taupathy

Semantic variant (PPA-S)[2]	A. Both of the following core features must be present:
	  1. Impaired object naming
	  2. Impaired single-word comprehension
	B. Three of the following ancillary features must be present:
	  1. Impaired object knowledge, particularly for low-frequency or low-familiarity items
	  2. Surface dyslexia or dysgraphia
	  3. Spared repetition
	  4. Spared grammaticality and motor aspects of speech
		Left anterior temporal lobe is atrophied	The pathology is usually FTLD-TDP of type C

Continued

Continued

Type of PPA	Clinical criteria	Radiological features	Common pathology

Logopenic variant (PPA-L)[2]	A. Both of the following core features must be present:
	  1. Impaired single-word retrieval in spontaneous speech and naming
	  2. Impaired repetition of phrases and sentences
	B. Three of the following ancillary features must be present:
	  1. Phonological errors (phonemic paraphasias) in spontaneous speech or naming
	  2. Spared single-word comprehension and object knowledge
	  3. Spared motor speech
	  4. Absence of frank agrammatism
		Left (posterior language area) temporoparietal area is atrophied	Alzheimer pathology is the most common

Mixed variant (PPA-M)[3]	Both of the following features must be present: 1. Agrammatism in language production 2. Word comprehension impairments	Both inferior frontal gyrus and anterior temporal lobe are atrophied	Unknown

(FTLD: frontotemporal lobar degeneration; PPA: primary progressive aphasia)

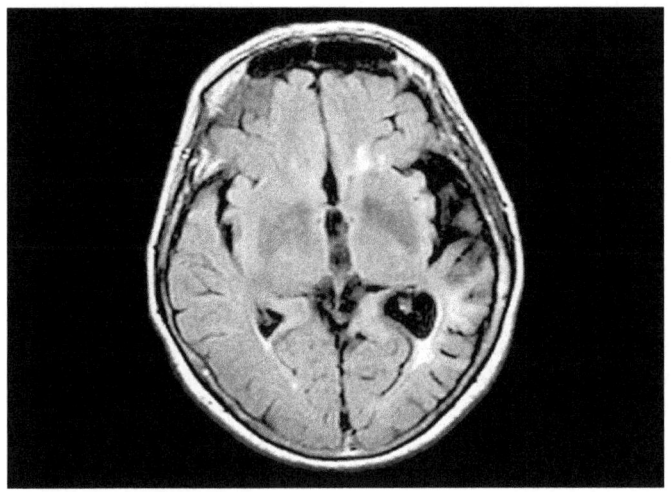

FIG. 4: Axial T2 image showing atrophy of left anterior temporal lobe in primary progressive aphasia-semantic variant.

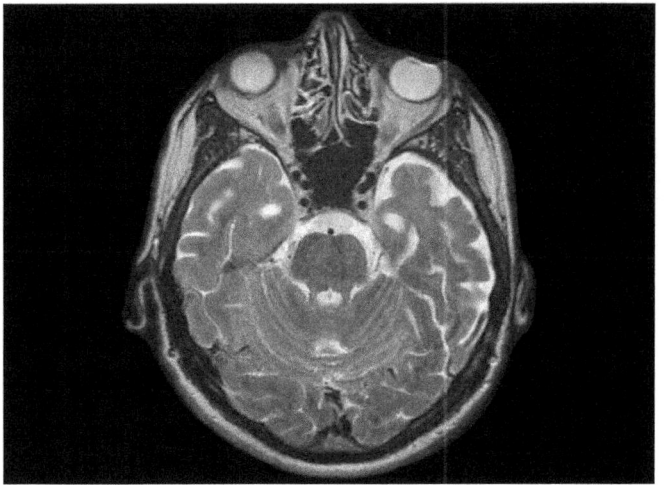

FIG. 5: Axial fluid-attenuated inversion recovery image showing atrophy of left posterior perisylvian (temporal) lobe in primary progressive aphasia-logopenic variant.

PARKINSONISM WITH DEMENTIA: EGG AND THE HEN STORY

Presence of parkinsonism in a demented subject makes the clinical diagnosis difficult. All parkinsonian syndromes are known to produce cognitive abnormalities, the pattern, severity and time of onset vary. On the contrary, patients of FTLD spectrum and even AD may develop parkinsonism. Things get complicated when drugs such as antipsychotic and anticholinergics are implicated.

Vignette: A 72-year-old peasant with 12 years education came with history of slowness of activities, with rest tremor for 3 years with good response to levodopa with history of rapid eye movement (REM) sleep behavioral disorder (RBD), forgetfulness for 1 year, fearfulness, lack of attention, and difficulties in performing multitasking. There were few episodes of formed visual hallucination (VH), but no history of fall or fluctuation. Examination revealed slowness of reflex saccadic eye movement without vertical gaze restriction, features of asymmetrical parkinsonism, without ataxia, pyramidal sign, gait apraxia, and myoclonus. The NPA revealed reduced digit span and problem with serial subtraction, poor learning, and recall that improved with cues in verbal learning test, executive dysfunction, and visuoconstructional deficit with preserved praxis and object naming task. The MRI brain was unremarkable.

The aforementioned patient has asymmetrical parkinsonism, good response to levodopa, prior history of RBD, and subsequent cognitive impairment with inattention, executive dysfunction, and subcortical memory dysfunction—features consistent with cognitive dysfunction of PDD.

Asymmetric parkinsonism is also seen in corticobasal degeneration (CBD) where features of asymmetric dystonia, cortical sensory loss, and cortical myoclonus and apraxia help in making the diagnosis.

Symmetrical parkinsonism may be PSP, multiple system atrophy (MSA), and DLB. The core features of DLB are RBD, fluctuation, autonomic dysfunction with syncope, and formed VH with visuospatial dysfunction with or without other higher order visual dysfunction. Although there are many subtypes of PSP, the classic Richardson variant comes with typical eye movement abnormality and subcortical cognitive impairment. The cognitive variants are (1) PSP-FTD, which comes with typical features with bvFTD with additional features of PSP and (2) PSP-CBD comes with features of CBD mixed with PSP. PSP may also come with language dysfunction with features of PPA-G.

All secondary parkinsonism, for example, drug-induced, normal pressure hydrocephalus, and vascular parkinsonism come with symmetrical parkinsonism. Here, cognitive impairment usually appears simultaneously or after onset of parkinsonism.

Dementia symptoms sometimes come early and parkinsonism becomes prominent subsequently in DLB, FTD-PSP, CBD, and Creutzfeldt–Jakob disease (CJD). The early and late appearance of parkinsonism in a patient of dementia helps in clinical diagnosis of PDD versus DLB.

COMPLEX VISUAL SYMPTOMS: RECOGNIZING THEM AS COGNITIVE DISORDER

Human visual cortex and its upstream connections perform very sophisticated functions. Diseases affecting this area present with myriad of complex visual symptoms. These are often not recognized or misdiagnosed by family physicians, ophthalmologists, and even by neurologists.

*Vignette: A 56-year-old engineer came with the complaint of difficulties in reading billboards and while driving. His complaint was brushed aside by his ophthalmologist. Soon afterward, he found difficulties in reading newspaper headlines, and his wife reported that he had difficulties in finding items in front of him, particularly in more cluttered environments. His vison was tested to be normal and was referred to us. He scored 26/30 in MMSE, with problem in serial subtraction and copying intersecting pentagon. His ACE score was 87/100 with reduced scores in attention and visuospatial function with preserved memory, language, and executive functions. He was found to have alexia with agraphia, color anomia, simultanagnosia, optic ataxia, and oculomotor apraxia. He was also found to have visuospatial deficit and ideomotor apraxia. His MRI showed atrophy of occipitoparietal cortex of both sides (**Fig. 6**).*

This gentleman presented with higher order visual dysfunction with affection of dorsal as well as ventral stream of visual cortex sparing other cognitive domains with radiologic feature of posterior cortical atrophy (PCA). While AD is the most common pathology, DLB, CBD, and CJD are other diseases, which may also present with PCA.

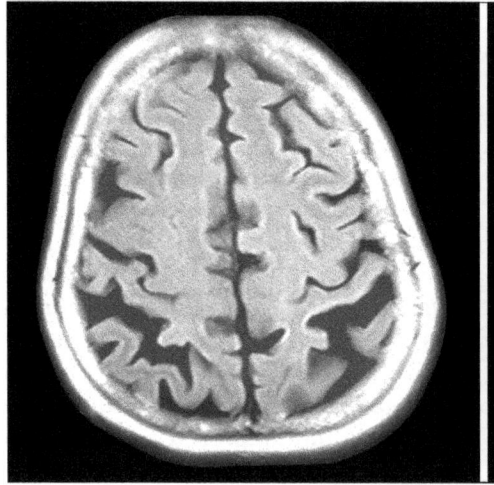 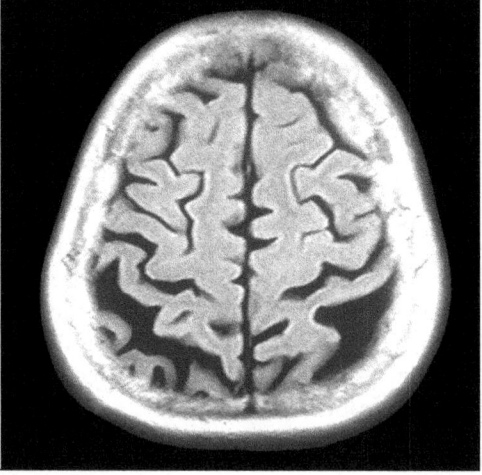

FIG. 6: Axial T1 image showing bilateral parieto-occipital atrophy in posterior cortical atrophy.

Follow-up and looking for appearances of parkinsonian features, VH, myoclonus, etc., help in differentiating these diseases.

STRUCTURAL IMAGING

Neuroimaging report of "diffuse brain atrophy" is common, but it does not make any sense and creates more confusion. Although expertise is essential for better interpretation, there is enough chance of bias and over- or under-reporting of brain images. Neuroimaging is diagnostic in certain conditions, e.g., VaD, normal pressure hydrocephalus, and in some rapidly progressive dementia cases due to infections, autoimmune encephalitis, and CJD. It is also diagnostic for Wilson disease, leukodystrophies, and some metabolic conditions such as Wernicke encephalopathy. However, routine neuroimaging does not provide much information in degenerative diseases. MCI and early dementia from neurodegenerative diseases is often missed in imaging. Atrophy of specific brain areas need to be carefully searched for and correlated with clinical findings. HD, PSP, and some focal atrophies can often be diagnosed with structural MRI. Volumetric study provides good idea about focal and lobar atrophy. Similarly, diffusion tensor imaging (DTI) and vascular imaging provide valuable information in VaD. Functional imaging such as FDG-PET gives better idea and often helps in differentiating degenerative dementias. Ligand-based PET scan, such as amyloid or tau PET, is now not available for routine clinical use.

DEPRESSION AND DEMENTIA

Depression is a common accompaniment of patients with dementia. It is often difficult to make out whether depression is the cause or a manifestation of the disease. Depression is a common neuropsychiatric symptom of dementia, seen in almost all dementing illnesses and shares a common pathobiology with dementia. A careful elicitation of history and recognizing the pattern of deficit in NPA sometimes help in differentiating depression with pseudodementia from true dementia. However, if doubt exists, it is better to treat depression and plan for reassessment after 3 months. In the era of biomarker, it may be possible to differentiate them more easily.

CONCLUDING REMARKS

A good history and clinical assessment are essential for making a diagnosis even when the sophisticated laboratory and imaging facilities are available. Clinician should pay attention to the onset and disease course as well as family history and drug history. Degenerative diseases evolve over time and at a given point of time, a definite diagnosis may not be possible. Follow-up and subsequent assessment often help resolving the issue. Despite these, diagnostic dilemma still exists in clinical practice. These will force more research and refinement of clinical criteria.

In the era of biomarker-based diagnosis, clinical assessment becomes more challenging. The availability of disease-modifying therapies demands an early and accurate diagnosis for their use. While each elderly subject with SMCs needs to be subjected to screening, clinical and NPA must be performed to decide whom to subject for sophisticated biomarker studies. Thus, clinicians need to be prepared to differentiate between normalcy and disease state and to categorize the diseases.

In coming days, artificial intelligence and machine learning processes will also help future clinicians to overcome the challenges faced by present day clinicians. However, scope of clinical differentiation will always remain, and one needs to use clinical acumen judiciously to get benefit from these technological advancements.

LEARNING POINTS

- Dementia diagnosis becomes challenging in early stage of the disease. Careful history and NPA help to differentiate normal aging from MCI and dementia.
- Degenerative disease and cerebrovascular disease occur in same age group and they often coexist. Clinical diagnosis and differentiation is possible if clinical and radiological findings are carefully analyzed. When doubt exists, it is better to consider a mixed pathology for the dementia.
- Depression often makes the diagnosis difficult. Differentiating dementia from depression with consequent pseudodementia is also challenging.
- Making a diagnosis of subjects presenting with frontal dysfunction is also difficult. While many subcortical dementias may have dysexecutive syndrome, pattern of behavioral abnormality usually helps to differentiate.
- Presence of parkinsonism in a subject of dementia poses another diagnostic challenge. The chronology, nature of parkinsonism, pattern of cognitive impairment, and associated other features help determine the diagnosis.
- As things are moving toward biomarker-based diagnosis, it would be possible to make distinction of diseases easier with the use of disease-specific biomarker in near future.

REFERENCES

1. Saini D, Mukherjee A, Roy A, Biswas A. A comparative study of the behavioral profile of the behavioral variant of frontotemporal dementia and Parkinson's disease dementia. Dement Geriatr Cogn Disord Extra. 2020;10(3):182-94.
2. Gorno-Tempini ML, Hillis A, Weintraub S, Kertesz A, Mendez MF, Cappa SF, et al. Classification of primary progressive aphasia and its variants. Neurology. 2011;76(11):1006-14.
3. Mesulam M, Wieneke C, Rogalski E, Cobia D, Thompson C, Weintraub S. Quantitative template for subtyping primary progressive aphasia. Arch Neurol. 2009;66(12):1545-51.
4. Das G, Dubey S, Sinharoy U, Mukherjee A, Banerjee S, Lahiri D, et al. Clinical and radiological pro le of posterior cortical atrophy and comparison with a group of typical Alzheimer disease and amnestic mild cognitive impairment. Acta Neurologica Belgica. 2021;121(4):1009-18.

COMMENTARY 17

Pseudodementia and Pseudodepression: Two Sides of the Coin

Ambar Chakravarty

INTRODUCTION

While evaluating a patient who displays evidence of cognitive dysfunction, a host of reversible causes should be excluded before one can diagnose a neurodegenerative pathology. One well-recognized cause that needs exclusion is depression, which can have significant deleterious effects on cognition, especially in the elderly. If the depression is severe, it may be confused with a number of neurodegenerative disorders causing cognitive decline including Alzheimer's disease. Early identification of such treatable causes of dementia, including severe depression, would go a long way in providing the most appropriate treatment early in the course of the disease process and thus reduce the social and financial burden to the family and society at large. Such disorders should not be labeled as pseudodementia or secondary dementia or reactive depression but simply as dementia or cognitive dysfunction related to a treatable cause. Such conditions may be related to infections [neurosyphilis, human immunodeficiency virus (HIV) acquired immunodeficiency syndrome (AIDS)], autoimmune processes (encephalitic or paraneoplastic), strokes, metabolic (liver disease), or endocrinopathies (hypothyroidism and other thyroid autoantibody-related disorders). The author would argue, in particular, that pseudodementia and other related terms should be used strictly in connection with cognitive dysfunctions solely associated with some underlying primarily psychiatric disorder (depression or otherwise). Such conditions, while not supplanting modern diagnostic criteria, serve an important need by identifying unique groups of patients with atypical presentations of their disorders and highlighting potential pitfalls in clinical decision-making.

PSEUDODEMENTIA: DEFINITION AND EVOLUTION OF CONCEPT

The concept of pseudodementia (Pseudodemenz) was conceived in a specific period of German industrial history, namely the formulation of laws settling claims following railway (1871) and industrial accidents (1884), but also the law of compensation relating to traumatic neurosis (1889).[1,2] The nosological specificity of the lastly mentioned was not clearly defined. This was followed by a near unanimous recognition of traumatic hysteria and the psychogenic hypothesis of its causation. The introduction of the term "pseudodementia" (Pseudodemenz) is usually credited to Carl Wernicke (1848-1905: of Wernicke encephalopathy and Wernicke aphasia fame—German physician, psychiatrist, and neuropathologist). However, this aspect of neurological history remains unclear and the references available are not all accurate.[1,2] "Pseudodemenz" was never mentioned in Wernicke's written works. It is likely that the term originated in relation to Wernicke's discussion of Ganser syndrome. Ganser syndrome[3] is a rare dissociative disorder with features like giving wrong or approximate answers to simple questions and other dissociative symptoms such as fugue, amnesia or conversion disorder, at times with visual hallucinations and unresponsiveness. The syndrome has also been named as *nonsense syndrome, balderdash syndrome, syndrome of approximate answers, hysterical pseudodementia,* or *prison psychosis*. Sigbert Josef Maria Ganser (1853-1931) first described this clinical syndrome in 1898 among prisoners awaiting trial in a penal institution in Halle, Germany. *The characteristic feature had been the production of very approximate answers (or close misses) to simple questions.*[3] *For example, when asked how many legs a dog has, such patients would reply "5," and answers to simple arithmetic* questions would similarly be wrong, but only slightly off the correct answer (e.g., 3 + 3 = 5). Originally labeled as "Vorbeigehen" ("to pass by"), the term "Vorbeireden" ("to talk beside the point") was also often used. Other reported symptoms included "clouding of consciousness," and other suggestive symptoms of conversion disorder, hallucinations, sudden and spontaneous recovery, subsequent amnesia for the episode, premorbid traumatic psychosocial experience (e.g., sexual abuse), and/or history of mild head trauma.[3] Although Ganser viewed it as a form of "twilight hysteria," Wernicke presented it as determined by a "restriction of the field of consciousness," inspired by Janet's view of hysteria (École de la Salpêtrière). Janet[4] proposed a certain limited number of symptoms by which hysteria must be identified and these he called the "*stigmata.*" These included typical symptoms of altered neurological function, namely paralysis, anesthesia, memory loss, unconsciousness, and loss of special senses functions, but not symptoms such as pain, tremor, dystonia, or ataxia. They are "*precipitated,*" as he wrote, by many provocative agents such as "*physical and moral shocks*" and were increased by stress.[4,5] Conversion reactions, Janet felt, were not directly or indirectly symbolic of psychic trauma, but these were "*repressed below the horizon of consciousness.*"[4]

Wernicke rejected the twilight hypothesis of Ganser, and this differential point seems to have initiated the introduction of the concept of pseudodementia.[1,2]

Depressive cognitive decline or pseudodementia is defined as the cognitive and functional impairment mimicking neurodegenerative disorders caused secondary to neuropsychiatric symptoms of depression. Two components need to be present:[6] First, the cognitive dysfunction component (mimicking dementia) and second, the true lack of neurodegenerative dementia accounting for the cognitive impairment—that is the "pseudo" component.

Leslie Gordon Kiloh (1917–1997), a Foundation Professor of Psychiatry, University of New South Wales, Sydney, Australia, argued in 1961 that the concept of pseudodementia does not belong to any well-defined nosological category, is purely descriptive, and does not imply an accurate diagnosis.[7] Depression with cognitive impairment was not well-recognized in the past. Though currently great attention had been given to these disorders. It has been noted that the cognitive symptoms associated with depression often persist after improvement in the mood disorder, as residual symptoms, and in some cases may transform into true organic (neurodegenerative) dementia. Such cognitive impairments affect normal functioning of the individual considerably and increase the risk of recurrence of the depressive disorder. McIntyre et al.[8] more recently opined that cognitive deficits may be considered as important functional predictors of MDD as cognitive deficits accounted for the most common variance factor with respect to the link between psychosocial dysfunction and major depression.

In the 1980s, depressive cognitive disorders were considered as one of the major causes of reversible and treatable forms of dementia, and by the next decade, it had been noted that depression with cognitive dysfunction could be the prodromal phase of irreversible neurodegenerative dementia, at least in some specific individuals, who fail to respond fully to appropriate management of their depression either with antidepressant drugs or electroconvulsive therapy.[6,7] Hence, such subjects would need relevant diagnostic workup. It follows therefore that the term pseudodementia can be considered inappropriate and misleading. In contrast, early features of Parkinson disease such as bradykinesia and bradyphrenia (slowness of movements and thoughts) may be misinterpreted as due to depression. True depression and true cognitive dysfunctions are not uncommon in patients with Parkinson disease. The neuropathology of Parkinson disease-related dementia (PDD) and those of diffuse Lewy body disease are the same and a rather crude way of distinction between the two is based on which features appear first—cognitive dysfunction or motor disabilities.

DEPRESSION AND DEMENTIA: CURRENT STATUS

To summarize, results of a number of studies suggest that several cognitive domains especially those related to memory functions are improved with treatment with antidepressant medications; however, not in all subjects where some of these deficits in mnemonic and executive function tend to persist. Such subjects specifically need to be investigated further because partly reversible cognitive impairment in late life moderate-to-severe depression appears to be a strong predictor of dementia. More studies are needed to exactly understand the relationship of cognitive deficits in depression to crucial epidemiological variables such as age, treatment, duration, and chronicity of illness and number of episodes.[9]

According to the Diagnostic and Statistical Manual of Mental Disorders, Fifth Edition (DSM-5),[10] cognitive impairment such as difficulty in thinking, concentrating, and decision-making are considered as core symptoms of depression. Reversible dementia secondary to neuropsychiatric disorders (such as depression) has not yet been considered as a formal diagnosis in this classification system. In older adults, two distinct forms of mixed mood and cognitive dysfunctions can be recognized. One group may present with an initial mood disorder (such as depression) later developing cognitive dysfunction, and another group of patients may present with initial cognitive decline, which gets associated with depression in course of time. The distinction at times becomes difficult—the inter-relationship between dementia and depression is complex.

Despite the fact that the term pseudodementia (or depressive pseudodementia) is inappropriate and misleading, over the years it had helped clinicians to think about treatable and reversible causes of dementia. It is best to consider it as a descriptive term that should not be used as a diagnostic category. "Depression with cognitive impairment" would be a better diagnostic category than pseudodementia, although the criteria have not yet been defined.

PSEUDO-PSEUDODEMENTIA AND PSEUDODEPRESSION[7]

Back in 1961, Kiloh also noted that a neurodegenerative disorder may, on occasions, be misdiagnosed as a psychiatric disease. This can perhaps be considered as the reverse of pseudodementia—that is an organic dementia masquerading as a purely psychiatric condition. The term "pseudo-pseudodementia" has been used to designate this clinical situation. This term would point to a clinical situation wherein psychiatric symptoms that are typical of a primary psychiatric disorder can be misleading and may mask the actual underlying diagnosis of a neurodegenerative disease. Depression in the older adults can be associated with cerebrovascular disease, detectable as white matter hyperintensities on magnetic resonance imaging (MRI); fluid-attenuated inversion recovery (FLAIR) and T2 sequences]. This has led some to propose a causal relationship, whereby damage to white matter microvasculature in subcortical regions disrupts neural connectivity and produces clinical symptoms. Behavioral changes such as disinhibition and apathy, not very uncommon in the age group under discussion, can be associated with dysfunction of a number of specific brain regions, such as the prefrontal and temporal cortices. These observations, coupled with the existence of pseudo-pseudodementia (as indicated above), suggest greater complexity than the simple dichotomy of dementia and pseudodementia. It also points to the challenges in distinguishing pseudodementia from pseudo-pseudo-dementia and determining whether psychiatric symptoms are a mimic or consequence of neurodegeneration. Apathy, a common symptom of dementia, may be misdiagnosed as depression, thus making the distinction more complex. This has been referred to as "pseudodepression"—meaning disorders, particularly organic dementia, outwardly masquerading as depression. Clearly, there is a need for developing biomarkers or specific functional imaging features to clearly distinguish between these clinically overlapping conditions, namely dementia, depression, pseudodementia, pseudo-pseudodementia, and pseudodepression.[11-13]

CONCLUDING REMARKS

The relationship between depression and neurodegenerative dementias seems to be multifactorial or multipronged; severe depression may be mistaken as a case of dementia (depression with cognitive impairment and not depressive pseudodementia); depression may be an early and overwhelming symptom of a true neurodegenerative dementia and wrongly treated (pseudo-pseudo-dementia), and lastly some subjects with early cognitive dysfunction and apathy may be mistaken as cases of depression (pseudodepression).

REFERENCES

1. Vinet-Couchevellou M, Sauvagnat F. Pseudodémence, de quoi parle-t-on? Partie I: à la recherche de la pseudodémence de Wernicke [Pseudodementia, what are we talking about? Part I: In search of Wernicke's pseudodementia]. Encephale. 2015; 41(2):130-6.
2. Vinet-Couchevellou M, Sauvagnat F. Pseudodémence, de quoi parle-t-on? Partie II: de Stertz à Alzheimer: une maladie psychogène après traumatisme [Pseudodementia, what are we talking about? Part II: From Stertz to Alzheimer: A psychogenic disease after trauma]. Encephale. 2015;41(Suppl 1):S37-43.
3. Dieguez S. Ganser's syndrome. Front Neurol Neurosci. 2018;42: 1-22.
4. Janet P. Major symptoms of hysteria, fifteen lectures given in the medical school of Harvard University. New York: MacMillan; 1920.
5. Carota A, P Calabrese. Hysteria around the World. In: Bogousslavsky J (Ed). Hysteria: The Rise of an Enigma, volume 35. Front Neurol Neurosci. Basel: Karger; 2014. pp. 169-80.
6. Kang H, Zhao F, You L, Giorgetta C, D V, Sarkhel S, et al. Pseudo-dementia: A neuropsychological review. Ann Indian Acad Neurol. 2014;17(2):147-54.
7. Brodaty H, Connors MH. Pseudodementia, pseudo-pseudodementia, and pseudodepression. Alzheimers Dement (Amst). 2020;12(1):e12027.
8. McIntyre RS, Cha DS, Soczynska JK, Woldeyohannes HO, Gallaugher LA, Kudlow P, et al. Cognitive deficits and functional outcomes in major depressive disorder: Determinants, substrates, and treatment interventions. Depress Anxiety. 2013;30(6):515-27.

9. Kessing LV. Cognitive impairment in the euthymic phase of affective disorder. Psychol Med. 1998;28(5):1027-38.
10. American Psychiatric Association: Diagnostic and Statistical Manual of Mental Disorders, Fifth Edition. Arlington, VA, American Psychiatric Association; 2013.
11. Gilles C. Dementia-depression: how are they related? From depressive pseudodementia to pseudodepression in dementia]. Rev Med Brux. 1994;15(5):296-9.
12. Morstyn R, Hochanadel G, Kaplan E, Gutheil TG. Depression vs. pseudodepression in dementia. J Clin Psychiatry. 1982;43(5):197-9.
13. Foerstl H. "Pseudodementia" and "pseudodepression": a short review on the coexistence of cognitive and affective impairment in the elderly. Cesk Neurol Neurochir. 1990;53(5):294-304.

CHAPTER 25

Young-onset Rapidly Progressive Dementias: Recognition and Red Flags

Ambar Chakravarty

INTRODUCTION

Young-onset dementia (YOD), defined as dementia having onset before the age of 65 years, is also often referred to as early-onset dementia. In older literature, it was commonly known as presenile dementia.[1] This age threshold has proved useful for adopting practice strategies and for research. Young-onset dementias differ from the more common late-life occurrences in etiology, phenotypes, handicaps, psychosocial difficulties, and, ultimately, extent of clinical care. Whereas late life dementias are generally neurodegenerative (except the vascular ones), the YOD are more heterogeneous arising from genetic, infectious, autoimmune, vascular, nutritional, and metabolic factors.

Young-onset dementia frequently manifests psychiatric phenomena alongside impairments of cognitive functions, often presenting with disorders of affect, temperament, judgment, dispositions and self-control, perception, ideation, and behavioral problems (feeding, elimination, sexual expression, and sleep). The social problems arising from these conditions are several and include family conflict, financial stress, emotional stress on spouses who provide care, work, and parenting, and suffer social distraction and isolation.[2-4] Owing to the low awareness, and physicians' lack of familiarity with the various conditions from which YOD arises, the diagnosis is frequently missed or are being late.

The etiology in prevalence studies of YOD is broad, including Alzheimer disease (AD), frontotemporal dementia (FTD), vascular dementia (VaD), Huntington disease (HD), Parkinson disease dementia (PDD), and dementia with Lewy bodies (DLB), alcohol-related dementia (ARD), and traumatic brain injury (TBI).[5-20] AD and FTD are the most frequent neurodegenerative causes of YOD.

Hereditary transmission at times occur. Hereditary forms of AD and FTD are well known and arise from autosomal dominant mutations in several genes. Mutations in specific genetic loci are often characterized by phenotypic variants. For example, the mutation in the *C9ORF72* gene gives rise to a variety of FTDs with amyotrophic lateral sclerosis (FTD-ALS), which is often also complicated by psychosis.

Repeated head traumas, typically sustained in sports (typically boxing), are now known to cause chronic traumatic encephalopathy, a neurodegenerative dementia featured by widespread cortical and subcortical tauopathy.[21] No wonder, low cognition, alcohol abuse, high blood pressure, stroke, depression, and neuroleptic use in youth, as also cardiovascular disease—stroke, transient ischemic attack (TIA), chronic kidney disease, and hypertension have been correlated with midlife cognitive decline.[22,23]

Young-onset dementias often demonstrate a predominance of nonmemory and neuropsychiatric features over cognitive deficits in many and (relative to late-onset dementia) a high frequency of syndromes that are defined by motor dysfunctions such as parkinsonism, apraxia, and ataxia. This leads to delayed diagnosis in many.

Three distinct syndromic types may be recognized:
1. *Syndromes that are primarily cognitive (i.e., cognitive > behavioral)*: Examples include AD, the most common form. Young-onset AD is generally alike the classic late-onset phenotype in its presenting features and clinical evolution. However, nonamnesic phenotypes are well known in YOD, that is, syndromes in which visuoperceptual impairments, aphasia, or ideomotor apraxias predominate,[24] and those in which the syndrome is defined by abnormal conduct, affective disturbance, and psychosis, or by motor dysfunctions such as parkinsonism, ataxia, apraxia, or paresis. In posterior cortical atrophy, the highlight is on progressive visual or visuospatial impairment in absence of ophthalmological impairment. Three subforms may occur—a biparietal syndrome (with limb and oculomotor apraxia, visuospatial disturbance, simultagnosia, optic ataxia, and agraphia), an occipital

syndrome (with alexia, apperceptive agnosia, and prosopagnosia), and a visual variant (with primary visual failure and impairment of basic perceptual abilities). Logopenic progressive aphasia (PLA), an aphasia variant (conduction speech disturbance) of AD, is more common in younger patients. There is impaired word retrieval (in spontaneous speech and confrontation naming), severe sentence repetition deficits, and phonological errors in spontaneous speech. In contrast, semantic dementia (SD) is a variant of FTD.[25] SD is characterized by progressive loss of word and object knowledge starts with dysnomia and forgetfulness of words and objects, associated with errors in reading and writing. In later stages, the patient's speech becomes markedly "empty" even though articulation, syntax, and grammar are retained. Speech production, whether spontaneous or in repetition tasks, is also retained in SD. Progressive nonfluent aphasia, PNFA, is a recognized aphasia syndrome of FTD. There is a progressive loss of speech fluency and articulation. There is hesitant, effortful, halting speech, with errors of grammar. Additionally, some are accompanied by speech apraxia. A small number of nonamnesic young-onset AD cases manifest a progressive ideomotor and limb apraxia.

2. *Syndromes that are primarily neuropsychiatric (i.e., behavioral > cognitive)*: Abnormalities of conduct characterize the behavioral variant of FTD (bvFTD) This bvFTD syndrome and the language syndromes discussed earlier are the typical FTD clinical states.[26] Presenting features include a progressive deterioration of temperament, judgment, conduct, and social skills and disordered volition. It is not uncommon for bvFTD to be accompanied by features suggestive of ALS, when the condition is known as FTD-ALS. Parkinsonian features may develop but behavioral features dominate.

3. *Syndromes defined by motor dysfunction (i.e., motor disorder > cognitive/behavioral)*: These syndromes predominantly exhibit motor dysfunction—parkinsonism, motor apraxia, dyscontrol, spastic paresis, abnormalities of posture and gait, chorea, and/or ataxia. DLB and PDD overlap in their clinical and pathological features, differing primarily in the order of emergence of parkinsonism and dementing features and in the symmetry of the motor[27] features—lateral asymmetry being typical of PDD **(Fig. 1)**. In DLB, dementia precedes development of parkinsonism, or both states manifest more or less simultaneously, Generally in PDD, dementia develops after the first decade of the illness, although formal neuropsychological assessment may detect subclinical executive dysfunction in the early stages in some. Parkinsonism is a core feature of either syndrome

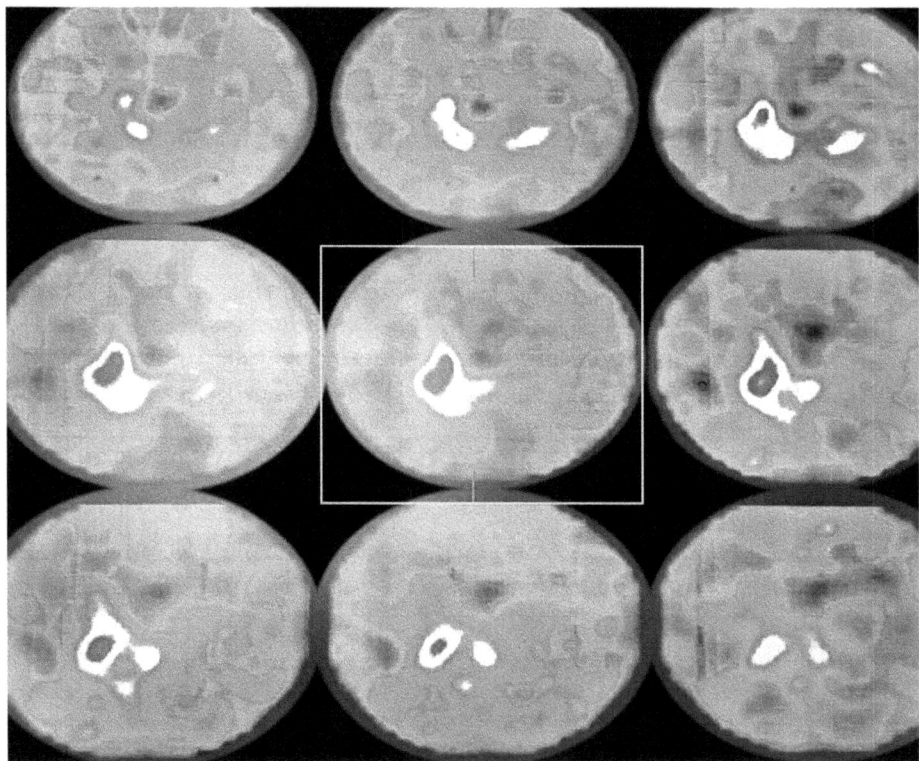

FIG. 1: Dopamine transporter (DaT) scan of 36-year-old left dominant Parkinson disease with early cognitive dysfunction showing very significant low uptake of the tracer in the presynaptic dopamine terminals in the left Putamen.

when fully manifested. The notion that dementia arising within versus 1 year after parkinsonism is the dictum for separating DLB from PDD may not always be true. DLB and PDD both show fluctuations of alertness, attention and mentation, and recurrent formed visual hallucinations. Paranoia and delusions may also be encountered. Chorea and dyskinesias are typical of adult-onset HD. Chorea is present early in the disease course. Impaired involuntary movements such as incoordination, bradykinesia, and rigidity are mainly seen in earlier onset HD (Westphal variant). Executive dysfunction, behavioral rigidity, irritability, and heightened emotions are also early features,[28,29] but are often masked by the dramatic motor phenomena.

Corticobasal degeneration (CBD) and progressive supranuclear palsy (PSP) often exhibit similar features. CBD features asymmetric limb apraxia, akinesia, rigidity, dystonia, along with oral buccal apraxia, dysarticulation of speech (speech apraxia), and dysarthria. Executive dysfunction, which develops early, is overshadowed by the motor phenomena. Some develop behavioral and language dysfunctions like FTD patients.[30] PSP features oculomotor gaze palsy, postural instability with retropulsion, executive dysfunction, behavioral dyscontrol, and symmetric parkinsonian features with the classical restrictions of vertical gaze.

Creutzfeldt–Jakob disease (CJD) mostly occurs in sporadic forms (i.e., sCJD). This is a rapidly progressive dementia manifesting some combination of ataxia, myoclonus, cortical blindness, disordered motor control, spasticity, incoordination, parkinsonism, and akinetic mutism. Several atypical forms occur: An ataxic CJD in which loss of coordination predominates (Oppenheimer type); a visuoperceptual variant that leads to cortical blindness (Heidenhain type); an amyotrophic variant with progressive spastic paresis and muscle atrophy; an encephalopathic type and rapidly progressive dementia with myoclonus and akinetic mutism.[31] CJD is dealt separately later in this chapter.

Spinocerebellar ataxias are a family of hereditary cerebellar degenerations manifesting progressive ataxia, incoordination, dysarthria, and dysphagia. They can be distinguished from ataxic CJD states by their very gradual evolution. Executive dysfunction, cognitive dysfunction, and affective lability can be observed.[32] Dementia is not universal but the gross motor disturbances, especially speech disturbance, may mimic early dementia.

Flowchart 1 may prove to be helpful in ascertaining the cause or underlying neurodegenerative disorder in patients with YOD.[33]

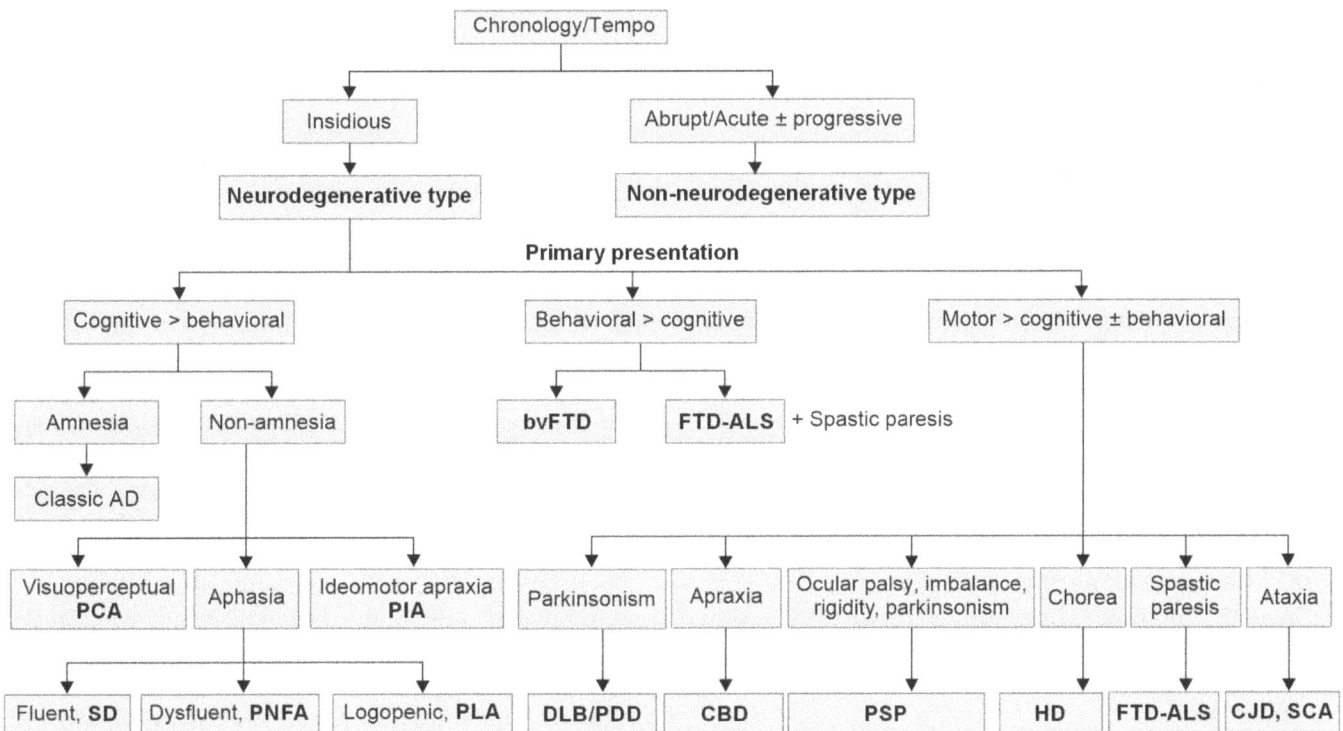

FLOWCHART 1: Causes of neurodegenerative disorder in patients with young-onset dementia.
(AD: Alzheimer disease; ALS: amyotrophic lateral sclerosis; bvFTD: behavioral variant of frontotemporal dementia; CBD: corticobasal degeneration; CJD: Creutzfeldt–Jakob disease; DLB: dementia with Lewy bodies; FTD: frontotemporal dementia; HD: Huntington disease; PCA: posterior cortical atrophy; PDD: Parkinson disease dementia; PIA: progressive ideomotor apraxia; PLA: progressive logopenic aphasia; PNFA: progressive nonfluent aphasia; SCA: spinocerebellar ataxia; SD: semantic dementia)

SOME SPECIFIC YOUNG-ONSET DEMENTIAS

Vascular Dementia

Vascular dementia is not a neurodegenerative disorder and at times arises following an overt stroke, when the diagnosis is straightforward. The clinical picture depends on the mechanism and distribution of the cerebrovascular disease underlying its development and hence may be variable. Though VaD is common after stroke (termed post-stroke dementia), it may follow relatively small infarcts in strategic locations (in thalamus particularly), or arise from chronic cerebrovascular insufficiency with lacunes and white matter leukoaraiosis (through possibly diaschisis on cortical functions). Thus, VaD may arise as a sudden and catastrophic decline in cognitive, mental, and motor functions following a hemorrhagic or large vessel ischemic stroke; as the classical stepwise decline in cognition accompanied by behavioral and motor phenomena with multiple infarcts; or as a hemisyndromic state with focal cognitive deficits (most commonly a nonfluent aphasia). Some may reveal an insidious progression that is difficult to distinguish from AD, FTD, or DLB. The classical features include executive dysfunction, emotional incontinence (pseudobulbar feature), psychomotor slowing, motor dyscontrol, parkinsonism, imbalance, and a gait impairment (small-steppage, apraxic, or parkinsonian gait). An important genetic cause is the cerebral autosomal dominant arteriopathy with subcortical infarcts and leukoencephalopathy (CADASIL).

Cerebral autosomal dominant arteriopathy[34-38] with subcortical infarcts and leukoencephalopathy is an inherited disease with almost exclusively neurological manifestations, primarily migraines with aura and premature onset of small vessel ischemic disease. It has a relatively characteristic appearance on magnetic resonance imaging (MRI) and diagnosis is made via genetic testing or skin biopsy. No disease-modifying therapies are yet available and treatment is targeted mainly at cardiovascular risk reduction.

Earlier, CADASIL was recognized as a heritable early-onset microvascular disease of unknown etiology. The genetic cause of CADASIL was identified in 1996 as multiple mutations involving genes encoding for the Notch3 protein on chromosome 19. CADASIL is the most common small vessel disease caused by mutations involving a single gene with inheritance in an autosomal dominant fashion.

The prevalence of CADASIL has been estimated at approximately 5:100,000. Actual prevalence may be higher due to underdiagnosis. There is no gender predilection, though men tend to be slightly more severely affected than women. No definite ethnic predilection has been identified.

Skin biopsy is the gold standard for diagnosing CADASIL in cases where no genetic studies are possible. Accumulation of granular osmiophilic material (GOM) around smooth muscle in small arteries is the diagnostic appearance. These findings are most seen in the brain but can also be seen in skin and muscle samples throughout the body, thus the diagnosis via skin biopsy is possible. On histopathology, the appearance is typical of any small vessel disease, with degeneration of vascular smooth muscle cells (VSMCs), endothelium, and basal lamina. Notably, atherosclerosis is absent. Again, changes are most prominent in small cerebral vessels as opposed to elsewhere in the body.

Age of onset and disease course are widely variable, with case reports describing onset in children to older adults. On the whole, the average age of onset is around 30 years. A migraine with aura is the most common initial symptom, present in over half of people diagnosed with CADASIL and slightly more common in women. Less commonly, CADASIL may present as an acute encephalopathy. After roughly a decade, TIAs and subcortical/lacunar infarcts manifest with typical clinical syndromes such as a pure motor or sensory deficits or brainstem infarcts. Later still, patients manifest with VaD and often with psychiatric manifestations such as depression and apathy.

The CADASIL should be suspected in patients with a strong family history of early strokes and dementia, keeping in mind that CADASIL is likely underdiagnosed. Though definitive diagnosis is via genetic testing or skin biopsy, a CADASIL scale has been proposed as a less expensive initial clinical screening measure. This scale includes typical symptoms of the disease such as migraines and TIA, typical imaging features, and family history, all with various weightings. In patients where CADASIL is strongly suspected, definitive diagnosis begins with serum genetic testing for a NOTCH3 mutation. Approximately 4% of patients with CADASIL will have a negative genetic test, likely related to unidentified genetic mutations. Thus, for those patients with typical clinical features, the next step is a skin biopsy with histopathologic examination for GOM accumulation.

Alternatively, CADASIL has a somewhat characteristic appearance on MRI and a radiologist may suggest the diagnosis. Abnormal T2/fluid-attenuated inversion recovery (FLAIR) white matter hyperintensities, similar in appearance to those seen with the chronic microvascular disease, are present in CADASIL in the anterior temporal, external capsule, and paramedian superior frontal subcortical white matter with sparing of U fibers. Importantly, these findings are present in younger patients (younger than ~60 years). Though this distribution is reported to be specific for CADASIL, older patients with the severe microvascular disease may have lesions in these locations because they have the diffuse disease. Lacunar or subcortical infarcts can also be seen with CADASIL, which manifest as foci of restricted diffusion on diffusion-weighted imaging (DWI)/apparent diffusion coefficient (ADC) sequences (bright on diffusion, dark on ADC) typically measuring <1.5 cm. Finally, microbleeds are seen with a greater prevalence in CADASIL patients. These are best seen on a T2*-weighted gradient recalled echo (GRE) MRI sequence as multiple punctate foci of susceptibility/hypointensity. These findings of lacunar infarcts and microbleeds in younger patients are less specific but suggestive MRI findings. Retinal abnormalities are encountered with disease progression.

There are numerous differential considerations to keep in mind. Age-related microvascular disease (leukoaraiosis) in the setting of diabetes and/or hypertension should be the first consideration. Besides the expected clinical findings, the traditional microvascular disease would not be expected to have the same MRI distribution of lesions. Multiple sclerosis is another consideration with a different MRI appearance with involvement of the optic nerves and spinal cord that would not be expected with CADASIL. Fabry disease is another heritable cause of early-onset microvascular disease and strokes that also features basal ganglia calcifications and is X-linked. Cerebral autosomal recessive arteriopathy with subcortical infarcts and leukoencephalopathy (CARASIL) is a similar entity to CADASIL that presents with early-onset spinal degenerative disease and hair loss, but typically does not feature migraines. More broadly, other causes of strokes and hemorrhage in younger individuals such as primary central nervous system (CNS) vasculitis, reversible cerebral vasoconstriction syndrome (RCVS), inflammatory amyloid angiopathy, venous thrombosis, septic emboli, metastatic disease, and toxic/metabolic exposures need exclusion. These entities may demonstrate subtly different findings on computed tomography (CT) or MRI. Finally, other heritable conditions such as leukoencephalopathies and mitochondrial encephalomyopathy, lactic acidosis and stroke-like episodes (MELAS) should be considered. *One important practical point needs stressing here and that is to avoid catheter angiography in suspected cases of CADASIL, as this may lead to catastrophic consequences.*

No disease-modifying treatment is available. Recent studies have shown that smoking is a modifiable risk factor for progression of CADASIL. Therapy is very similar to that of traditional chronic microvascular ischemic disease, targeting cardiovascular risk reduction with blood pressure control, smoking cessation, statins, and antiplatelet therapy. However, given that CADASIL is nonatherosclerotic, the role of thrombosis in causing strokes with CADASIL is in question. Thus, antiplatelet therapy may fall out of favor. As CADASIL patients have a higher incidence of microhemorrhages, any anticoagulation therapy must be considered with caution. In addition, therapy for other disease manifestations such as migraines and depression are similar to the general population. Clinical symptoms progress from migraines to infarcts to VaD over decades. Life expectancy is reported to be reduced by 5 years for men and 1-2 years in women. As an additional note, genetic counseling should be offered to patients diagnosed with CADASIL.

The CADASIL coma: This is a medical emergency arising in a patient harboring the NOTCH3 mutation. A high index of suspicion is needed for diagnosis based on the MRI brain appearance and exclusion of other more common causes *including stroke, infections and encephalitis (infective or autoimmune), and amyloid spells*, A reversible acute encephalopathy was the principal presentation in 6 of 70 patients in a British prevalence study. The episodes lasted 7-14 days, presenting with fever, acute confusion, coma, and fits; there was full recovery but in two cases identical episodes recurred some years later. All patients had a previous history of migraine with aura and were originally misdiagnosed as viral encephalitis. CADASIL should be considered in acute unexplained encephalopathies. MRI white matter changes, previous migraine with aura, and a family history of stroke and dementia may be useful pointers to the diagnosis.

Prion Diseases

Prion diseases (PrDs) are diverse disorders caused by misfolded proteins.[39-51] These disorders are also known as transmissible spongiform encephalopathies and are uniformly fatal neurodegenerative diseases. Pathologically, these disorders are characterized by neuronal loss and vacuolation. PrDs that occur in humans are mostly sporadic and rarely acquired. Inherited and familial forms may also occur. Acquired PrDs from infected tissue (transplanted/grafted human tissue or consumed infected animal meat) can have a variable incubation period (usually spanning years) and genetic mutations have variable penetrance and phenotypic expression. Rapidly progressive dementia (RPD) is one of the prototypical phenotypes of PrDs, especially in CJD. Initial symptoms are nonspecific (headache, malaise, cough, dizziness, and change in personality, mood or memory, visual disturbances, giddiness, etc.) and may go unrecognized. In the early stages, possibilities that may be considered are delirium, metabolic encephalopathy, autoimmune neurological disorders, etc. However, clinical evolution into a distinct syndrome characterized by myoclonus and dementia will strongly suggest the possibility of CJD. The proportion of RPD patients eventually diagnosed as PrD may be up to 60% and varies from center to center. The various phenotypes of CJD are described in **Figure 2**.

Atypical presentations of CJD such as pure *cognitive presentations* (~15%) might be mistaken for rapid forms of AD or FTD. *Ataxic presentations* are rare (~10%) and might be misdiagnosed initially for vascular, neoplastic, paraneoplastic, or inflammatory conditions. The *visual presentation* or Heidenhain variant (~5%) are often seen initially by ophthalmologists or optometrists as patients have visual disturbances that are difficult to explain. Very rarely, CJD may mimic a *stroke* (~2%) or a *corticobasal syndrome* (~2%). The *thalamic presentation* (~2%) includes sleep disturbance and distal pain and may include abnormalities of the autonomic nervous system: palpitations, temperature dysregulation, hypertension, or postural hypotension. This presentation is well known as fatal familial insomnia A missense mutation (D178N) in *PRNP*, usually linked to a methionine allele at polymorphic codon 129, is associated with this phenotype. The World Health Organization (WHO) diagnostic criteria have been depicted in **Box 1**.

These symptoms are nonspecific to CJD and can be seen in several other degenerative and acquired neurological and systemic conditions. According to the available criteria to diagnose CJD, one can only make a diagnosis of probable CJD in the absence of a brain biopsy. Considering this "uncertainty," reasonable exclusion of other differentials is strongly recommended.

Prion diseases are uniformly fatal disorders with scope for transmissibility, and hence this diagnosis can have serious implications for the patient's caregivers and family members. Reasonable exclusion of treatable/reversible neurological disorders is necessary. Commonly, degenerative dementias with a relatively rapid course can mimic CJD. Imaging and serial electroencephalograms (EEGs) in this setting may be useful to differentiate between the two. Other mimics such as metabolic disorders (hepatic encephalopathy, hyperammonemia, and Wernicke encephalopathy), immune-mediated conditions (autoimmune and paraneoplastic encephalitis, vasculitis, neurosarcoidosis, etc.), and CNS infections

---

BOX 1: The World Health Organization (WHO) diagnostic criteria for CJD.

I. Rapidly progressive dementia
II. a. Myoclonus
 b. Pyramidal/extrapyramidal signs
 c. Visual disturbances/cerebellar involvement
 d. Akinetic mutism
III. a. Typical electroencephalogram (EEG)
 b. 14-3-3 positive in cerebrospinal fluid (CSF)

Probable: I + II (two out of a-d) + III (a or b)
Possible: I + II (two out of a-d)
Definite: Neuropathologically proven

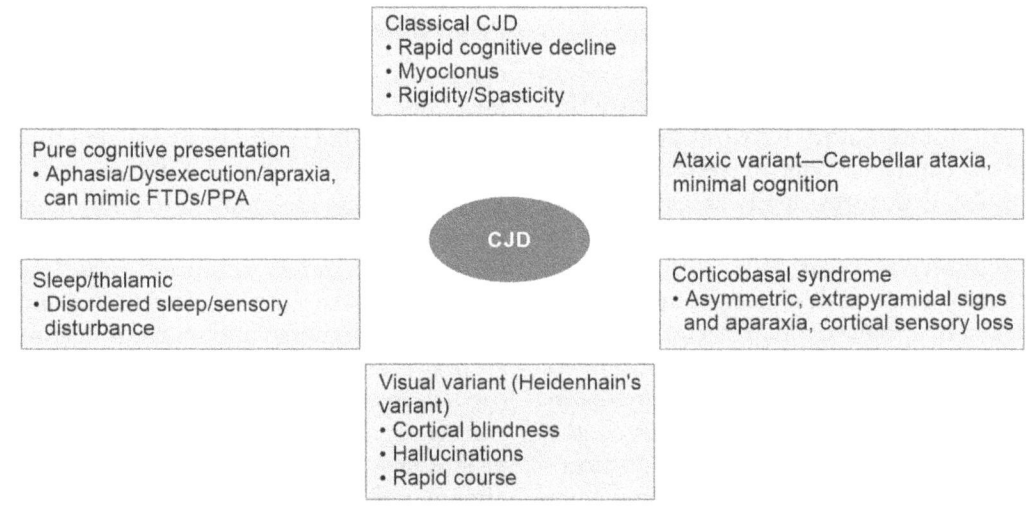

FIG. 2: Clinical features of CJD.
(CJD: Creutzfeldt-Jakob disease; FTD: frontotemporal dementia; PPA: primary progressive aphasia)
Source: Reproduced with permission from Viswanathan LG and Sinha S. Tips for early diagnosis of prion diseases. In: Chakravarty A (Ed). Pitfalls in the Diagnosis of Neurological Disorders. New Delhi: Jaypee Brothers Medical Publishers; 2022.

TABLE 1: Red flags for the diagnosis of CJD.

Red flags	Diseases
Fever/headache/meningeal signs	Infections, immune-mediated disorders, lymphoma
Facial dyskinesias/abnormal facial and/or ocular movements	NMDAR encephalitis, Whipple disease
Hyponatremia	LGI-1 encephalitis
Contrast enhancement of MRI lesions	Lymphoma, vasculitis, infective etiologies
CSF pleocytosis	Infections, immune mediated conditions, carcinomatous meningitis

(CJD: Creutzfeldt–Jakob disease; CSF: cerebrospinal fluid; LGI: leucine-rich glioma inactivated protein 1; MRI: magnetic resonance imaging; NMDAR: N-methyl-D-aspartate receptor)

[human immunodeficiency virus (HIV) dementia, Whipple disease, Syphilis, etc.] are potentially treatable conditions. Some of the red flags that may point to an alternate diagnosis are mentioned in **Table 1**.

Immune-mediated Encephalitis

Immune-mediated encephalitis accounts for a substantial proportion of encephalitis cases in current time.[52-58] This is one of the important differential diagnoses for RPD. This group of conditions includes CNS manifestations of systemic autoimmune disorders and antibody-mediated paraneoplastic and nonparaneoplastic encephalitis.

The "classic" paraneoplastic encephalopathies include those caused by antibodies that target intracellular onconeuronal antigens such as Hu, Yo, and Ri mostly associated with small cell lung cancer and gynecological malignancies. Clinical syndromes include cerebellar syndromes and stiff person syndrome. Nonparaneoplastic immune-mediated encephalitides associated with antibodies against neuronal cell surface proteins, ion channels or receptors, include the N-methyl-D-aspartate receptor (NMDAR) or leucine-rich glioma inactivated protein 1 (LGI1). These may or may not be related to neoplasia in varying degrees (frequently in the case of anti-NMDAR antibodies but rarely in the case of anti-LGI1 antibodies). Limbic system structures are often affected, resulting in prominent memory loss. These syndromes classically present with acute or subacute onset and early occurrence of altered consciousness and seizures. Some may mimic CJD or other neurodegenerative disorders (e.g., anti-IgLON5 disease). The diagnosis of immune-mediated encephalitis in psychiatric practice can be challenging when presenting with acute psychosis.

One immune-mediated encephalitis with good treatment options is steroid-responsive encephalopathy associated with autoimmune thyroiditis (SREAT), previously called Hashimoto encephalopathy. The related thyroid antibodies being not disease-specific and having a high prevalence in the general population pose diagnostic challenges for the clinicians.

Infectious and Parainfectious Encephalitides[59-64]

Subacute sclerosing panencephalitis is an important cause of RPD in some countries, such as India, with low current or past rates of vaccination for the measles virus.

In patients with severe RPD with an accelerated disease course, the possibility of Herpes simplex and Zoster virus infection needs exclusion. Although RPD seems to be a rare presenting clinical finding among acquired immunodeficiency syndrome (AIDS) patients, it is recommended that an HIV test should be part of the basic diagnostic workup for dementia. Clinicians should also pay attention to less frequent CNS infections with good treatment options (e.g., Whipple disease), regionally highly frequent CNS infections (e.g., Japanese encephalitis in Asia), and emerging pathogens (e.g., Borna virus). Progressive multifocal leukoencephalopathy is a demyelinating disease that is associated with reactivation of the JC virus and typically affects patients with immunodeficiency. This condition can cause various progressive neurological symptoms, affecting cognition or behavior in nearly half of the patients.

The coronavirus disease 2019 (COVID-19) pandemic has brought new challenges for the differential diagnosis of RPD. It is possible that severe acute respiratory syndrome coronavirus 2 (SARS-CoV-2) infection can cause encephalopathy with cognitive disturbance, either directly or delayed through immune-mediated mechanisms. The long-term effects of these on the CNS would only be known over the next few years.

Metabolic and Toxic Encephalopathies

Metabolic and toxic encephalopathies are frequent causes of RPD and a large number of these are potentially treatable and reversible. Hence, their early recognition. Alcohol abuse and related cognitive decline is probably the most important of these encephalopathies.[65,66] Alcohol-related dementia is common, accounting for up to 10% of cases of early-onset dementia. Alcoholism is often associated with malnutrition and organ injuries, potentially leading to Wernicke encephalopathy, other vitamin deficiency-related encephalopathies or hepatic encephalopathy. In addition, alcohol abuse may be related to the occurrence of seizures, and this is a major precipitant of status epilepticus.

Other potentially treatable metabolic causes of RPD include recurrent hypoglycemia, severe hypothyroidism, hyponatremia, and osmotic extrapontine myelinolysis, thus stressing the importance of screening for basic metabolic markers in the initial diagnostic evaluation. Clinical history would direct attention toward acute or chronic intoxications with drugs, other toxic agents, and a good drug screening may be needed.

CONCLUDING REMARKS

In recent years, tremendous advances in knowledge in the pathogenesis of various forms of dementias have been made, which has helped potentially treatable pathologies to be identified early. The chances of treatment success are better the earlier the diagnosis is made. Significant improvement of imaging techniques, the development of biomarkers—including blood-based biomarkers—for the diagnosis of brain pathologies, and the recognition of the expanding spectrum of immune-mediated disorders provide valuable tools to enable clinicians to achieve an early differential diagnosis. Such new knowledge would pave the way to study RPDs systematically to build a basis for rational diagnostic workup and treatment decisions.

LEARNING POINTS

- A full assessment, clinical and laboratory, of patients with YOD is essential as some of the causative conditions are indeed treatable.
- Elicitation of family history is of utmost importance.
- History of addictions
- Three syndromic groups may be identified:
  - Syndromes that are primarily cognitive (i.e., cognitive > behavioral)—AD
  - Syndromes that are primarily neuropsychiatric (i.e., behavioral > cognitive)—FTD
  - Syndromes defined by motor dysfunction (i.e., motor disorder > cognitive/behavioral)—VaDs, parkinsonian syndromes, and CJD
- Laboratory investigations must include complete hemogram, full biochemical profile including liver functions tests, thyroid profile, B12 assay, renal functions, and electrolytes.
- Immunological assays to include are as follows: Autoantibody screening including those against systemic connective tissue diseases, onconeuronal and cell surface antibodies, thyroid antibody profile, HIV serology, and serological tests for neurosyphilis.
- CSF study for viral antibodies and prion protein where a PrD is suspected.
- Structural and if possible molecular/nuclear brain imaging

REFERENCES

1. Van Vliet D, De Vugt ME, Bakker C, Pijnenburg YA, Vernooij-Dassen MJ, Koopmans RT, et al. Time to diagnosis in young-onset dementia as compared with late-onset dementia. Psychol Med. 2013;43(2):423-32.
2. Van Vliet D, De Vugt ME, Bakker C, Koopmans RTCM, Verhey FRJ. Impact of early onset dementia on caregivers: A review. Int J Geriatr Psychiatry. 2010;25:1091-100.
3. Gelman CR, Greer C. Young children in early-onset Alzheimer's disease families: Research gaps and emerging service needs. Am J Alzheimers Dis Other Demen. 2011;26: 29-35.
4. Millenaar JK, van Vliet D, Bakker C, Vernooij-Dassen MJ, Koopmans RT, Verhey FR, et al. The experiences and needs of children living with a parent with young onset dementia: results from the NeedYD study. Int Psychogeriatr. 2014;26(12):2001-10.
5. Yokota O, Sasaki K, Fujisawa Y, Takahashi J, Terada S, Ishihara T, et al. Frequency of early and late-onset dementias in a Japanese memory disorders clinic. Eur J Neurol. 2005;12:782-90.
6. McMurtray A, Clark D, Christine D, Mendez M. Early-onset dementia: frequency and causes compared to late-onset dementia. Dement Geriatr Cogn Disord. 2006;21:59-64.
7. Shinagawa S, Ikeda M, Toyota Y, Matsumoto T, Matsumoto N, Mori T, et al. Frequency and clinical characteristics of early-onset dementia in consecutive patients in a memory clinic. Dement Geriatr Cogn Disord. 2007;24:42-7.
8. Nandi SP, Biswas A, Pal S, Basu S, Senapati AK, Das SK. Clinical profile of young-onset dementia. A study from Eastern India. Neurol Asia. 2008;13:103-8.
9. Papageorgiou SG, Kontaxis T, Bonakis A, Kalfakis N, Vassilopoulos D. Frequency and causes of early-onset dementia in a tertiary referral center in Athens. Alzheimer Dis Assoc Disord. 2009;23:347-51.
10. Picard C, Pasquier F, Martinaud O, Hannequin D, Godefroy O. Early onset dementia: characteristics in a large cohort from academic memory clinics. Alzheimer Dis Assoc Disord. 2011;25:203-5.
11. Croisile B, Tedesco A, Bernard E, Gavant S, Minssieux-Catrix G, Mollion H. Diagnostic profile of young-onset dementia before 65 years. Experience of a French Memory Referral Center. Rev Neurol (Paris). 2011;168(2):161-9.
12. Harvey R, Skelton-Robinson M, Rossor M. The prevalence and causes of dementia in people under the age of 65 years. J Neurol Neurosurg Psychiatry. 2003;74:1206-9.
13. Ikejima C, Yasuno F, Mizukami K, Sasaki M, Tanimukai S, Asada T. Prevalence and causes of early-onset dementia in Japan: a population-based study. Stroke. 2009;40:2709-14.
14. Borroni B, Alberici A, Grassi M, Rozzini L, Turla M, Zanetti O, et al. Prevalence and demographic features of early-onset neurodegenerative dementia in Brescia county, Italy. Alzheimer Dis Assoc Disord. 2011;25(4):341-4.

15. Renvoize E, Hanson M, Dale M. Prevalence and causes of young onset dementia in an English health district. Int J Geriatr Psychiatry. 2011;26:106-7.
16. Withall A, Draper B, Seeher K, Brodaty H. The prevalence and causes of younger onset dementia in Eastern Sydney, Australia. Int Psychogeriatr. 2014;26:1955-65.
17. Mercy L, Hodges JR, Dawson K, Barker RA, Brayne C. Incidence of early-onset dementias in Cambridgeshire, United Kingdom. Neurology. 2008;71:1496-9.
18. Garre-Olmo J, Genís Batlle D, del Mar Fernández M, Marquez Daniel F, de Eugenio Huélamo R, Casadevall T, et al. Incidence and subtypes of early-onset dementia in a geographically defined general population. Neurology. 2010;75:1249-55.
19. Abraham MS, Scharovsky D, Romano LM, Ayala M, Aleman A, Sottano E, et al. Incidence of early-onset dementia in Mar del Plata. Neurologia. 2015;30(2):77-82.
20. Ferran J, Wilson KE, Doran M, Ghadiali E, Johnson F, Cooper P, et al. The early onset dementias: A study of clinical characteristics and service use. Int J Geriatr Psychiatry. 1996;11:863-9.
21. Baugh CM, Stamm JM, Riley DO, Gavett BE, Shenton ME, Lin A, et al. Chronic traumatic encephalopathy: Neurodegeneration following repetitive concussive and subconcussive brain trauma. Brain Imaging Behav. 2012;6:244-54.
22. Nordström P, Nordström A, Eriksson M, Wahlund LO, Gustafson Y. Risk factors in late adolescence for young-onset dementia in men: a nationwide cohort study. JAMA Intern Med. 2013;173:1612-8.
23. Heath CA, Mercer SW, Guthrie B. Vascular comorbidities in younger people with dementia: A cross-sectional population-based study of 616 245 middle-aged people in Scotland. J Neurol Neurosurg Psychiatry. 2015;86(9):959-64.
24. Mendez MF. Early-onset Alzheimer's disease: Nonamnestic subtypes and type 2 AD. Arch Med Res. 2012;43:677-85.
25. Neary D, Snowden JS, Gustafson L, Passant U, Stuss D, Black SA. Frontotemporal lobar degeneration: a consensus on clinical diagnostic criteria. Neurology. 1998;51:1546-54.
26. Rascovsky K, Hodges JR, Knopman D, Mendez MF, Kramer JH, Neuhaus J, et al. Sensitivity of revised diagnostic criteria for the behavioural variant of frontotemporal dementia. Brain. 2011;134:2456-77.
27. McKeith IG, Dickson DW, Lowe J, Emre M, O'brien JT, Feldman H, et al. Diagnosis and management of dementia with Lewy bodies: Third report of the DLB Consortium. Neurology. 2005;65:1863-72.
28. Rosenblatt A, Leroi I. Neuropsychiatry of Huntington's disease and other basal ganglia disorders. Psychosomatics. 2000;41:24-30.
29. Rosenblatt A. Understanding the psychiatric prodrome of Huntington disease. J Neurol Neurosurg Psychiatry. 2007;78:913.
30. DeJesus-Hernandez M, Mackenzie IR, Boeve BF, Boxer AL, Baker M, Rutherford NJ, et al. Expanded GGGGCC hexanucleotide repeat in noncoding region of C9ORF72 causes chromosome 9p-linked FTD and ALS. Neuron. 2011;72:245-56.
31. Appleby BS, Appleby KK, Crain BJ, Onyike CU, Wallin MT, Rabins PV. Characteristics of established and proposed sporadic Creutzfeldt-Jakob disease variants. Arch Neurol. 2009;66:208-15.
32. Schmahmann JD. Disorders of the cerebellum: Ataxia, dysmetria of thought, and the cerebellar cognitive affective syndrome. J Neuropsychiatry Clin Neurosci. 2004;16:367-78.
33. Ridha B, Josephs K. Young-onset dementia: A practical approach to diagnosis. Neurologist. 2006;12:2-13.
34. Eswaradass VP, Ramasamy B, Kalidoss R, Gnanagurusamy G. Cadasil coma: Unusual cause for acute encephalopathy. Ann Indian Acad Neurol. 2015;18(4):483-4.
35. Federico A, Di Donato I, Bianchi S, Di Palma C, Taglia I, Dotti MT. Hereditary cerebral small vessel diseases: A review. J Neurol Sci. 2012;322(1-2):25-30.
36. Schon F, Martin RJ, Prevett M, Clough C, Enevoldson TP, Markus HS. CADASIL coma: An underdiagnosed acute encephalopathy. J Neurol Neurosurg Psychiatry. 2003;74(2):249-52.
37. Tan RY, Markus HS. Monogenic causes of stroke: Now and the future. J Neurol. 2015;262(12):2601-16.
38. Tikka S, Baumann M, Siitonen M, Pasanen P, Pöyhönen M, Myllykangas L, et al. Cadasil and Carasil. Brain Pathol. 2014;24(5):525-44.
39. Uttley L, Carroll C, Wong R, Hilton DA, Stevenson M. Creutzfeldt-Jakob disease: A systematic review of global incidence, prevalence, infectivity, and incubation. Lancet Infect Dis. 2020;20(1):e2-10.
40. Satishchandra P, Shankar SK. Creutzfeldt-Jakob disease in India (1971-1990). Neuroepidemiology. 1991;10(1):27-32.
41. Prusiner SB. Prions. Proc Natl Acad Sci U S A. 1998;95(23):13363-83.
42. Mead S. Prion disease genetics. Eur J Hum Genet. 2006;14(3):273-81.
43. Manix M, Kalakoti P, Henry M, Thakur J, Menger R, Guthikonda B, et al. Creutzfeldt-Jakob disease: Updated diagnostic criteria, treatment algorithm, and the utility of brain biopsy. Neurosurg Focus. 2015;39(5):E2.
44. Will RG, Ironside JW, Zeidler M, Estibeiro K, Cousens SN, Smith PG, et al. A new variant of Creutzfeldt-Jakob disease in the UK. Lancet. 1996;347(9006):921-5.
45. Goldgaber D, Goldfarb LG, Brown P, Asher DM, Brown WT, Lin S, et al. Mutations in familial Creutzfeldt-Jakob disease and Gerstmann-Sträussler-Scheinker's syndrome. Exp Neurol. 1989;106(2):204-6.
46. Medori R, Tritschler HJ, LeBlanc A, Villare F, Manetto V, Chen HY, et al. Fatal familial insomnia, a prion disease with a mutation at codon 178 of the prion protein gene. N Engl J Med. 1992;326(7):444-9.
47. Pietrini V, Puoti G, Limido L, Rossi G, Di Fede G, Giaccone G, et al. Creutzfeldt-Jakob disease with a novel extra-repeat insertional mutation in the PRNP gene. Neurology. 2003;61(9):1288-91.
48. Geschwind MD. Rapidly Progressive Dementia. Continuum (Minneap Minn). 2016;22(2 Dementia):510-37.
49. Mead S, Rudge P. CJD mimics and chameleons. Pract Neurol. 2017;17(2):113-21.
50. Vitali P, Maccagnano E, Caverzasi E, Henry RG, Haman A, Torres-Chae C, et al. Diffusion-weighted MRI hyperintensity patterns differentiate CJD from other rapid dementias. Neurology. 2011;76(20):1711-9.
51. Steinhoff BJ, Räcker S, Herrendorf G, Poser S, Grosche S, Zerr I, et al. Accuracy and reliability of periodic sharp wave complexes in Creutzfeldt-Jakob disease. Arch Neurol. 1996;53(2):162-6.
52. Dalmau J, Graus F. Antibody-mediated encephalitis. N Engl J Med. 2018;378:840-51.
53. Lancaster E, Dalmau J. Neuronal autoantigens-pathogenesis, associated disorders and antibody testing. Nat Rev Neurol. 2012;8:380-90.
54. Hansen N, Lipp M, Vogelgsang J, Vukovich R, Zindler T, Luedecke D, et al. Autoantibody-associated psychiatric symptoms and syndromes in adults: A narrative review and proposed diagnostic approach. Brain Behav Immun Health. 2020;9:100154.

55. Geschwind MD, Tan KM, Lennon VA, Barajas RF, Haman A, Klein CJ, et al. Voltage-gated potassium channel autoimmunity mimicking Creutzfeldt-Jakob disease. Arch Neurol. 2008;65:1341-6.
56. Sabater L, Gaig C, Gelpi E, Bataller L, Lewerenz J, Torres-Vega E, et al. A novel non-rapid-eye movement and rapid-eye-movement parasomnia with sleep breathing disorder associated with antibodies to IgLON5: A case series, characterisation of the antigen, and post-mortem study. Lancet Neurol. 2014;13:575-86.
57. Do LD, Chanson E, Desestret V, Joubert B, Ducray F, Brugière S, et al. Characteristics in limbic encephalitis with anti-adenylate kinase 5 autoantibodies. Neurology. 2017;88:514-24.
58. Ricken G, Zrzavy T, Macher S, Altmann P, Troger J, Falk KK, et al. Autoimmune global amnesia as manifestation of AMPAR encephalitis and neuropathologic findings. Neurol Neuroimmunol Neuroinflamm. 2021;8:e1019.
59. Granerod J, Ambrose HE, Davies NW, Clewley JP, Walsh AL, Morgan D, et al. Causes of encephalitis and differences in their clinical presentations in England: a multicentre, population-based prospective study. Lancet Infect Dis. 2010;10:835-44.
60. Boucher A, Herrmann JL, Morand P, Buzelé R, Crabol Y, Stahl JP, et al. Epidemiology of infectious encephalitis causes in 2016. Med Mal Infect. 2017;47:221-35.
61. Wang Y, Liu M, Lu Q, Farrell M, Lappin JM, Shi J, et al. Global prevalence and burden of HIV-associated neurocognitive disorder: a meta-analysis. Neurology. 2020;95:e2610-21.
62. Compain C, Sacre K, Puéchal X, Klein I, Vital-Durand D, Houeto JL, et al. Central nervous system involvement in Whipple disease: Clinical study of 18 patients and long-term follow-up. Medicine (Baltimore). 2013;92:324-30.
63. Turtle L, Solomon T. Japanese encephalitis–the prospects for new treatments. Nat Rev Neurol. 2018;14:298-313.
64. Niller HH, Angstwurm K, Rubbenstroth D, Schlottau K, Ebinger A, Giese S, et al. Zoonotic spillover infections with Borna disease virus 1 leading to fatal human encephalitis, 1999-2019: An epidemiological investigation. Lancet Infect Dis. 2020;20:467-77.
65. Picard C, Pasquier F, Martinaud O, Hannequin D, Godefroy O. Early onset dementia: Characteristics in a large cohort from academic memory clinics. Alzheimer Dis Assoc Disord. 2021;25:203-5.
66. Hillbom M, Pieninkeroinen I, Leone M. Seizures in alcohol-dependent patients: Epidemiology, pathophysiology and management. CNS Drugs. 2003;17:1013-30.

CHAPTER 26

Neuroimaging in the Diagnosis of Dementias

Sukalyan Purakayastha, Soumik Das

■ INTRODUCTION

The diagnostic criteria for major neurocognitive disorders (or dementia) as defined in the Diagnostic and Statistical Manual of Mental Disorders, Fifth Edition published by the American Psychiatric Association in 2013[1] are as follows:
A. Evidence of significant cognitive decline from a previous level of performance in ≥1 cognitive domains (complex attention, executive function, learning and memory, language, perceptual–motor, or social cognition) based on:
  1. Concern of the individual, a knowledgeable informant, or the clinician that there has been a significant decline in cognitive function; and
  2. A substantial impairment in cognitive performance, preferably documented by standardized neuropsychological testing or, in its absence, another quantified clinical assessment.
B. The cognitive deficits interfere with independence in everyday activities (i.e., at a minimum, requiring assistance with complex instrumental activities of daily living such as paying bills or managing medications).
C. The cognitive deficits do not occur exclusively in the context of a delirium.
D. The cognitive deficits are not better explained by another mental disorder. Specify:
  1. Without behavioral disturbance: If the cognitive disturbance is not accompanied by any clinically significant behavioral disturbance
  2. With behavioral disturbance (specify disturbance): If the cognitive disturbance is accompanied by a clinically significant behavioral disturbance (e.g., psychotic symptoms, mood disturbance, agitation, apathy, or other behavioral symptoms), for example, major depressive disorder or schizophrenia.

Diagnosis depends on clinical findings, which are usually nonspecific. Also, patients are mostly diagnosed late in the course of the disease.[2] Definitive diagnosis can only be done by brain biopsy analysis. Advanced neuroimaging coupled with nuclear medicine studies allows accurate diagnosis in doubtful cases. The nuclear medicine and radiologic modalities are complementary and along with the clinical presentation aid rapid diagnosis and facilitates management.[3]

■ IMAGING THE NORMAL AGING BRAIN

Computed Tomography Findings

The normal aging brain shows somewhat enlarged ventricles and mildly widened sulci. Punctate calcifications in the basal ganglia are physiological. Curvilinear calcification in cavernous segment of internal carotid arteries and vertebrobasilar axis are common.[4]

Magnetic Resonance Findings

T1-weighted Images

T1-weighted image (T1WI) reveals mild symmetric ventricular prominence and proportionate enlargement of subarachnoid space.[5] The corpus callosum appears mildly thinned in sagittal T1-weighted scans.

T2/Fluid-attenuated Inversion Recovery

White matter hyperintensities (WMHs) and focal infarcts on T2/fluid-attenuated inversion recovery (FLAIR) images are common in elderly age group.

Perivascular spaces (PVSs) increase in size with aging and appear on T2-weighted image (T2WI) as round or ovoid cerebrospinal fluid (CSF)-like areas in the basal ganglia, midbrain, subcortical WM, etc. PVSs usually suppress completely in FLAIR sequence. However, a thin hyperintense rim may be seen in 25–30% cases. Lacunar infarcts demonstrate a hyperintense irregular rim surrounding the lesions.

T2* (Gradient Recalled Echo, Susceptibility Weighted Imaging)

T2* hypointensity in medial globus pallidus (GP) is considered normal. Hypointensity in the putamen is less prominent till the eighth decade.

Basal ganglia microbleeds are indicative of chronic hypertensive encephalopathy. Cortical and lobar microbleeds are suggestive of amyloid angiopathy.

DISORDERS PRIMARILY INVOLVING GRAY MATTER

Alzheimer Disease

Computed Tomography Findings

Noncontrast enhanced computed tomography (NECT) may be adopted as a screening procedure to exclude potentially treatable causes of dementia, such as normal pressure hydrocephalus and subdural hematoma **(Figs. 1A to D)**.

Magnetic Resonance Findings

The common changes on magnetic resonance imaging (MRI) include thinning of gyri, widening of sulci, and enlargement of lateral ventricles.[6] The disproportionately affected sites include the medial temporal lobe, especially the entorhinal cortex and hippocampus and the posterior cingulate gyri. The most consistent feature is CA1 volume reduction.

T2* [gradient recalled echo (GRE), susceptibility weighted imaging (SWI)] sequences may reveal cortical microhemorrhages—this suggests associated amyloid angiopathy.

Magnetic resonance spectroscopy (MRS) shows increased myoinositol and decreased N-acetyl aspartate (NAA) in Alzheimer disease (AD), even in the early stages. The NAA:myoinositol ratio is highly specific in differentiating patients of AD from the normal subjects.

Diffusion-tensor imaging (DTI) in patients with AD reveals decreased fractional anisotropy (FA) in corpus callosum splenium and superior longitudinal fasciculus.

Functional neuroimaging: Task-based fMR shows decreased extent of activation and/or intensity in the temporal and frontal regions.

Nuclear Medicine Findings

A positron emission tomography (PET) scan using amyloid-binding radiotracers such as 11[C] PiB (Pittsburgh compound B) is one of the techniques for early diagnosis of AD. Aβ deposition occurs well before symptom onset and likely represents preclinical AD in asymptomatic individuals and prodromal AD in patients with mild cognitive impairment (MCI).[7]

Frontotemporal Lobar Degeneration

Computed Tomography Findings

Severe symmetric volume loss of the frontal lobes with comparatively lesser involvement of the temporal lobes is found in late-stage frontotemporal lobar degeneration (FTLD).

Magnetic Resonance Findings

Voxel-based morphometry can discriminate between various pathologic subtypes of FTLD.[8] The SD subtype reveals bilateral temporal atrophy but little or no frontal volume loss. Behavioral variant of frontotemporal

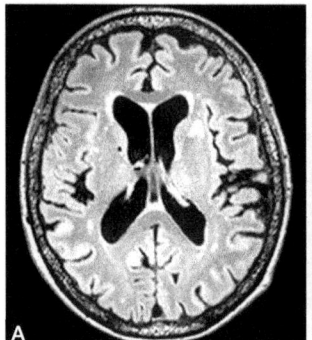
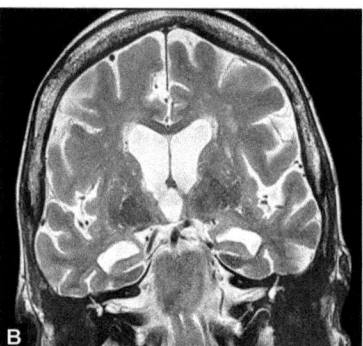
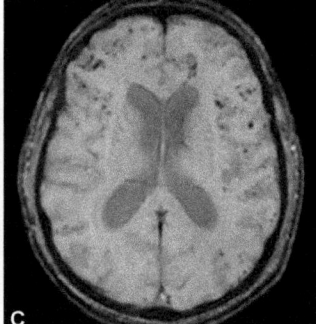
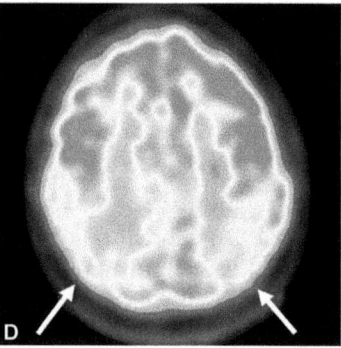

FIGS. 1A TO D: Axial fluid-attenuated inversion recovery (FLAIR) sequence in case of Alzheimer disease reveals moderate supratentorial ventriculomegaly with multiple small FLAIR hyperintense foci in bilateral cerebral white matter and periventricular FLAIR hyperintense rim—suggestive of small vessel ischemic changes. Coronal T2 sequence of the brain reveals prominent temporal atrophy with widening of temporal horns of both lateral ventricles. Axial susceptibility weighted imaging (SWI) sequence reveals multiple tiny blooming foci predominantly in cortical-subcortical region—suggestive of associated amyloid angiopathy. A fluorodeoxyglucose (FDG)-positron emission tomography (PET) scan reveals decreased metabolism of the parietal lobes as demarcated by white arrows.

dementia (bvFTD) and progressive nonfluent aphasia (PNFA) both show bilateral temporal and frontal atrophy, but the left hemisphere is affected in PNFA whereas right-sided atrophy is seen in bvFTD. Diffusion-weighted image (DWI) shows increased mean diffusivity in the orbitofrontal gyri, superior frontal gyri, and the anterior temporal lobes.[9]

Diffusion-tensor imaging shows reduced FA involving the superior longitudinal fasciculus in bvFTD and the inferior longitudinal fasciculus in the SD variant.

Nuclear Medicine Findings

A fluorodeoxyglucose (FDG)-PET scan shows hypometabolism and hypoperfusion in the temporal and frontal lobes **(Figs. 2A to C)**.

Lewy Body Dementias

Lewy body dementias (LBDs) include Parkinson disease dementia (PDD), dementia with Lewy bodies (DLB), and the Lewy body variant (LBV) of Alzheimer disease (LBAD).

General Features

The best neuroimaging technique for specific diagnosis of LBD is dopaminergic imaging of the basal ganglia to differentiate between LBD and other causes of dementia such as PDD.[10]

Magnetic Resonance Findings

Mild generalized atrophy is noted without obvious lobar predominance. Volume reduction in advanced cases is noted in the basal forebrain, hypothalamus, and midbrain. Putaminal atrophy is relatively more compared to medial temporal lobar atrophy in DLB patients.

Diffusion tensor imaging demonstrates elevated mean diffusivity involving the amygdala and reduced FA in inferior occipitofrontal and inferior longitudinal fasciculi.

Nuclear Medicine Findings

An FDG-PET scan reveals occipital hypometabolism. Decreased cerebral blood flow (CBF) on pMR or single-photon emission computed tomography (SPECT)- HMPAO (hexamethylpropyleneamine oxime), especially affecting the primary visual cortex, is highly suggestive of DLB. Presynaptic dopamine transporter (DaT) imaging using the FP-CIT (18F-FP-CIT positron emission tomography for correlating motor and cognitive symptoms of parkinson's disease) ligand reveals almost absent putaminal uptake and significantly decreased uptake in the caudate.[11]

Parkinson Disease

Computed Tomography Findings

A CT scan is primarily used to evaluate electrode position following DBS (deep brain stimulation) placement and to rule out surgical complications.

Magnetic Resonance Findings

Conventional MR imaging studies alone are not sufficient for diagnosing different parkinsonian syndromes. Mild midbrain atrophy may be seen in late stage of PD.[12]

In PD, dopaminergic cell loss occurs in the substantia nigra (SN) mainly in the nigrosomes, maximally in nigrosome 1. At the level of the inferior third of the red nucleus, nigrosome 1 appears as a pocket-like hyperintense indentation at the medial aspect of the hypointense area

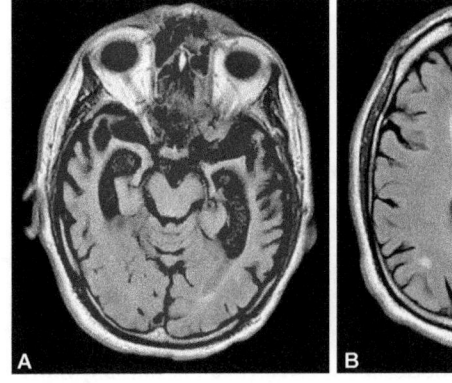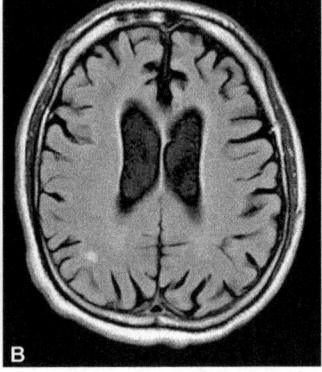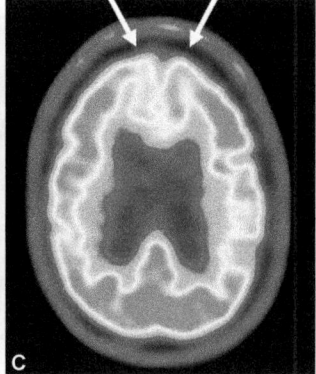

FIGS. 2A TO C: Axial fluid-attenuated inversion recovery (FLAIR) sequence in case of behavior variant of frontotemporal dementia reveals prominent frontotemporal atrophy with widening of temporal horns of both lateral ventricles ("knife blade atrophy") and increased signal intensity in the temporal lobes probably due to gliosis. A fluorodeoxyglucose (FDG)-positron emission tomography (PET) scan reveals frontal hypometabolism as demarcated by white arrows.

attributed to iron deposition in the SN. On 3-T MRI scans, PD patients reveal nigral hyperintensity loss. Also, the asymmetric nigrosomal involvement correlates with the clinical asymmetry in motor symptoms.

Nuclear Medicine Findings

A DaT-SPECT scan is used to assess integrity of dopaminergic nerve cells in movement disorder patients.[13] Reduced uptake of I-123 FP-CIT is highly suggestive of PD.

Progressive Supranuclear Palsy

CT Findings

Noncontrast enhanced computed tomography scans reveal midbrain atrophy with prominent ambient and interpeduncular cisterns.

Magnetic Resonance Findings

Sagittal images reveal midbrain volume loss with concave upper surface (the "penguin" or "hummingbird" sign). Volumetric calculations reveal that the sagittal midbrain is <70 mm³ and the midbrain:pons ratio is <0.15.[14] Axial scans reveal a widened interpeduncular angle and abnormal concave appearance of the midbrain tegmentum. Cerebellar atrophy is commonly seen, and the superior cerebellar peduncles are frequently found atrophic **(Figs. 3A to C)**.

Nuclear Medicine Findings

An FDG-PET scan reveals glucose hypometabolism along medial frontal regions and in the midbrain.

Multiple System Atrophy

Computed Tomography Findings

Noncontrast enhanced computed tomography scans show cerebellar volume loss in multiple system atrophy (MSA)-C with the hemispheres comparatively more affected than the vermis. MSA-P may show shrunken putamina with flattened lateral margins **(Figs. 4A and B)**.

Magnetic Resonance Findings

MSA-P: MRI in MSA-P patients shows putaminal volume loss with hypointensity on T2WI secondary to iron deposition **(Figs. 5A to C)**.

MSA-C: MSA-C patients show cerebellar atrophy, concave-appearing middle cerebellar peduncles (MCPs), and shrunken pons with a cruciform hyperintensity on T2/FLAIR sequences termed the "hot cross bun" sign. Corticospinal tract involvement inapparent on routine T2WI can be clearly demonstrated with DTI.[15]

Corticobasal Degeneration

Conventional studies reveal asymmetric moderate frontoparietal atrophy. The striatum, dorsal prefrontal and perirolandic cortex, and midbrain tegmentum are affected most severely.[16]

The SPECT and PET studies show asymmetric gangliothalamic and frontoparietal hypometabolism.

Huntington Disease

Standard imaging studies (CT and MR) are normal early in the disease course.[17] NECT scans reveal volume loss of caudate nuclei with enlarged, outwardly convex frontal horns with or without cerebellar atrophy **(Figs. 6A to C)**.

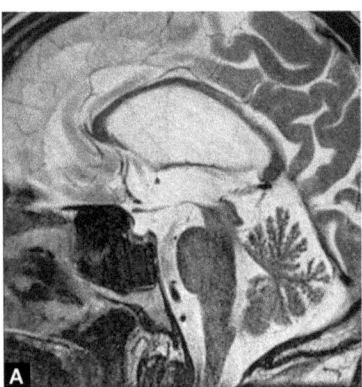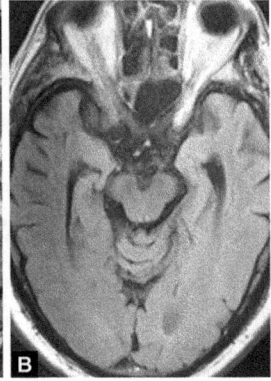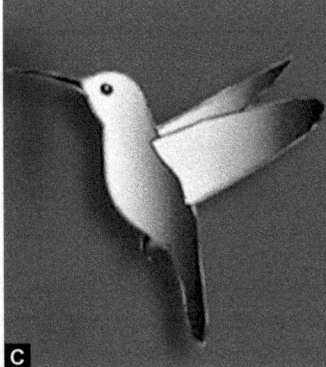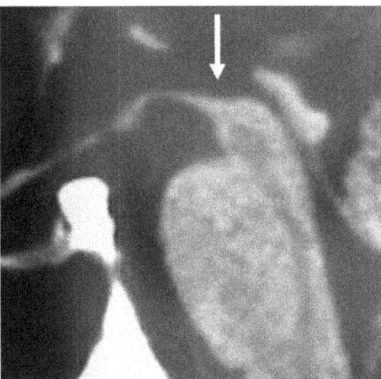

FIGS. 3A TO C: Sagittal T2 sequence of the brain in case of progressive supranuclear palsy reveals midbrain atrophy with loss of concave upper border of the midbrain showing the typical "hummingbird sign." Axial fluid-attenuated inversion recovery (FLAIR) sequence reveals reduction of anteroposterior midline midbrain diameter and loss of the lateral convex margin of the tegmentum of midbrain.

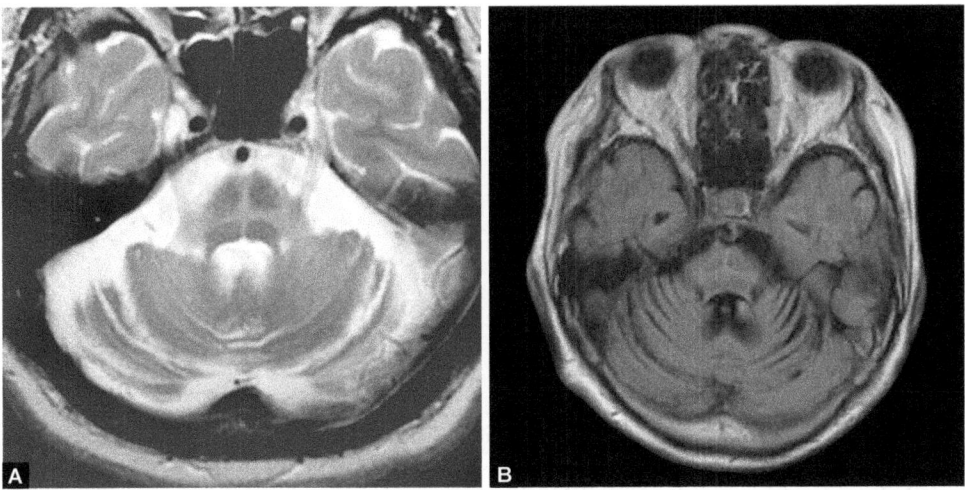

FIGS. 4A AND B: Axial T2 and fluid-attenuated inversion recovery (FLAIR) sequence in case of multisystem atrophy (MSA)-C reveals pronounced cerebellar atrophy and severe atrophy of the pons with characteristic hot cross bun sign.

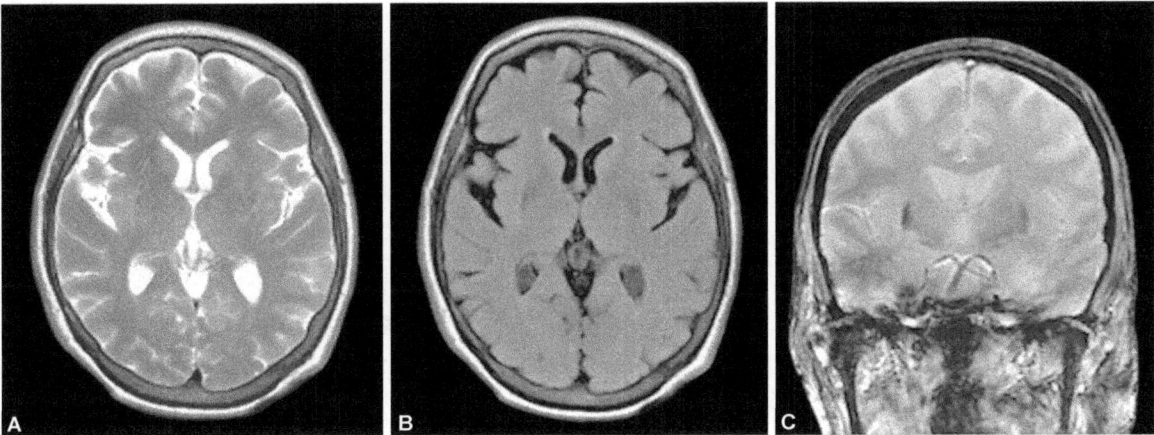

FIGS. 5A TO C: Axial T2 and fluid-attenuated inversion recovery (FLAIR) sequence in case of multisystem atrophy (MSA)—P reveals abnormally high T2 linear rim surrounding the putamen called the putaminal rim sign. Coronal susceptibility weighted imaging (SWI) sequence reveals reduced signal in the putamen relative to the globus pallidus.

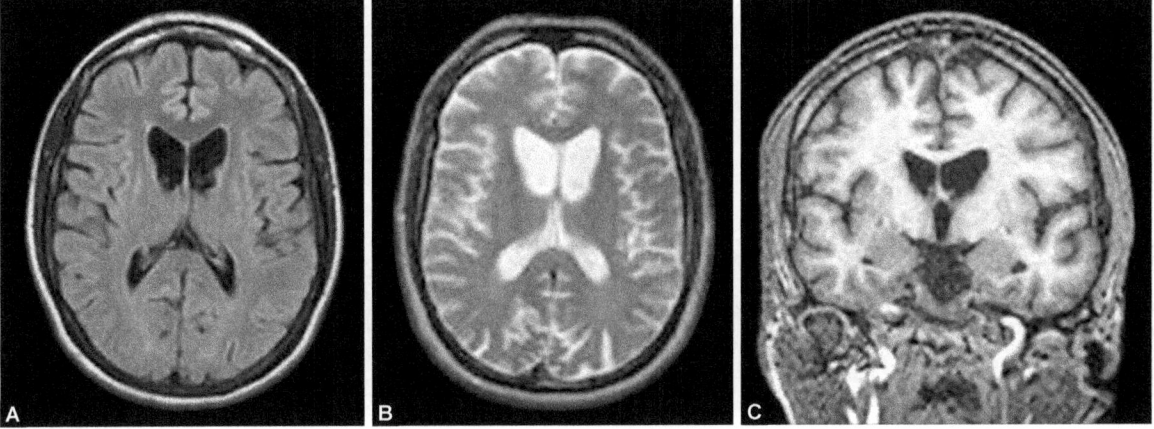

FIGS. 6A TO C: Axial T2 and fluid-attenuated inversion recovery (FLAIR) and coronal T1 sequence in the case of Huntington disease reveals caudate head atrophy and prominent putaminal volume loss with enlargement of the frontal horns showing a "box"-like configuration.

The MR findings reveal generalized cerebral atrophy with T2/FLAIR hyperintensity involving the shrunken caudate heads. Associated putaminal hyperintensity may also be noted.[18]

Wilson Disease

Noncontrast enhanced computed tomography scans may appear normal early in the course of the disease. Generalized brain atrophy with striatal or thalamic hypoattenuation may be seen in advanced cases.

Some cases show subtle T1 hypointensity in the affected regions, whereas others reveal T1 shortening as seen in chronic hepatic encephalopathy.[19]

The common MR imaging findings of WD include bilaterally symmetric T2 hyperintensity in the putamina (70%), caudate nuclei (60%), ventrolateral thalami (55–60%), and midbrain (50%). In 10–12% of cases, diffuse tegmental (midbrain) hyperintensity with sparing of the red nuclei gives an appearance termed the "face of a giant panda."

A PET scan reveals markedly decreased glucose metabolism and reduced dopa-decarboxylase activity suggestive of nigrostriatal dopaminergic pathway dysfunction.

Neurodegeneration with Brain Iron Accumulation

Pantothenate Kinase-associated Neurodegeneration

The T2-weighted images reveal marked hypointensity in GP and substantia nigra. T2 images show pallidal hypointensity along with a focal T2 hyperintensity medially (eye of the tiger) caused by gliosis and tissue vacuolization.[20]

Diffusion-tensor imaging shows markedly elevated FA in GP and substantia nigra. MRS reveals reduced NAA peak—suggestive of neuroaxonal loss (**Figs. 7A and B**).

Prion-linked Dementias

Creutzfeldt–Jakob Disease

The hippocampus, cerebral cortex, thalami, basal ganglia, and cerebellum are frequently affected areas.

The CT scans are usually normal in early stages of the disease although in advanced stages progressive atrophy is evident (**Figs. 8A to C**).

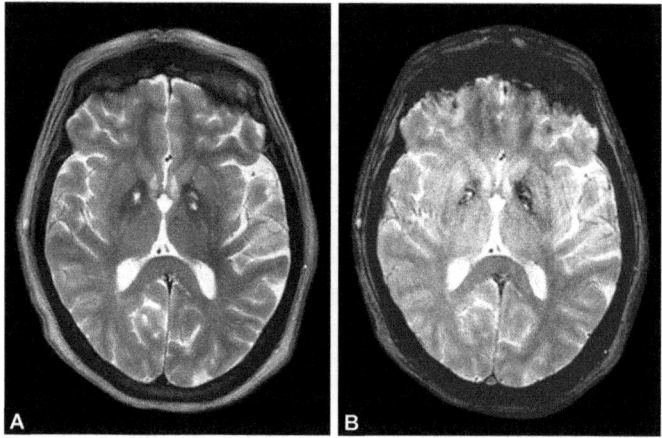

FIGS. 7A AND B: Axial T2 in case of pantothenate kinase-associated neurodegeneration (PKAN) reveals hypointensity in bilateral globus pallidi with internal foci of hyperintensity suggestive of gliosis giving a characteristic "eye of the tiger" appearance. Axial susceptibility weighted imaging (SWI) sequence reveals blooming in bilateral globus pallidi.

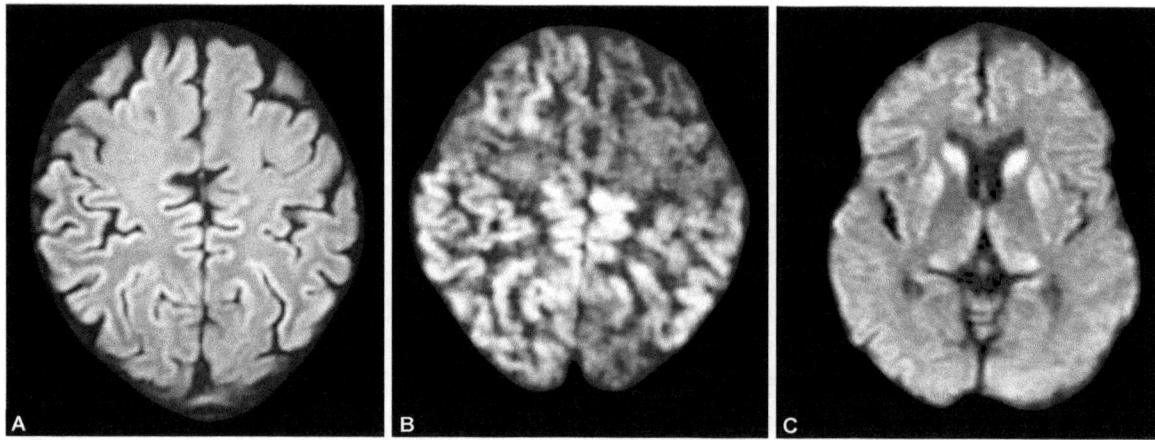

FIGS. 8A TO C: Axial fluid-attenuated inversion recovery (FLAIR) and diffusion-weighted image (DWI) sequence in case of Creutzfeldt–Jakob disease reveals asymmetrical hyperintense signal changes along the cortex bilaterally called the "cortical ribbon sign." Axial DWI sequence in another case reveals hyperintense signal changes in bilateral basal ganglia and thalami.

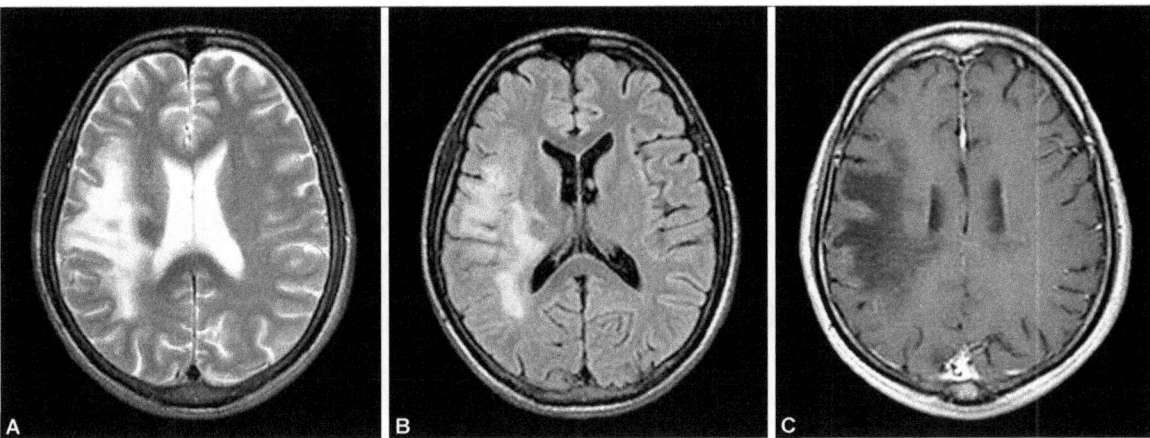

FIGS. 9A TO C: Axial T2 and fluid-attenuated inversion recovery (FLAIR) sequence in case of progressive multifocal leukoencephalopathy (PML) reveals patchy hyperintensity in the right frontoparietotemporal region with involvement of subcortical U fibers. Axial post-contrast T1 sequence reveals no obvious enhancement of the lesion.

Diffusion-weighted imaging is diagnostic in most of the cases. T1 scans may show faint hyperintensity in posterior thalami.[21] Restricted diffusion or FLAIR hyperintensity in putamen and caudate nucleus or at least two cortical regions (temporal-parietal-occipital "cortical ribboning") are highly suggestive of sCJD. Involvement of occipital lobe is seen in Heidenhain variant, whereas cerebellum is the main site of affection in Brownell-Oppenheimer variant. T2/FLAIR hyperintensity in posterior thalamus ("pulvinar" sign) or posteromedial thalamus ("hockey stick" sign) is seen in 90% of vCJD cases **(Figs. 9A to C)**.

Recreational Drugs and Alcohol Abuse

Alcohol-induced Dementia

CT Findings

NECT scans reveal generalized sulcal and ventricular enlargement. Cerebellar atrophy is seen in some cases.

MR Findings

Volume loss involving the prefrontal cortex is common. Focal atrophy involving the superior vermis is seen in many cases.[22]

Chronic hepatic encephalopathy may reveal T1 hyperintensity in the basal ganglia probably due to accumulation of manganese.

Wernicke Encephalopathy

An MRI is more sensitive than CT in evaluating suspected Wernicke encephalopathy (WE) cases. T1WI may reveal hypointensity in the periaqueductal region. In severe cases, T1 hyperintensities in the mammillary bodies and medial thalami are present. T2* SWI sequences may help detecting microhemorrhages in the affected areas.[23] Some cases may show a focus of diffusion restriction on DWI sequence in the splenium of corpus callosum.

Marchiafava–Bignami Disease

Acute Marchiafava-Bignami disease (MBD) reveals hyperintensity in the genu of corpus callosum and frontoparietal cortex followed by splenial lesions. Solid confluent or rim enhancement patterns are noted on postcontrast study.

Chronic MBD with frank callosal necrosis is visualized as corpus callosum thinning with linear hypointensities involving the middle layers.[24]

Cannabis, Ecstasy, and Cocaine

Hippocampal and amygdalar volumes are significantly reduced in chronic cannabis abusers.

Ecstasy (3,4-methylenedioxymethamphetamine or MDMA) is widely used for recreational purposes.[25]

Infections

Herpes Simplex Encephalitis

CT Findings

NECT may reveal hypodensity in the insula and one or both temporal lobes with mild mass effect. Gyriform or patchy enhancement may be seen after 24–48 hours.

MR Findings

T2 scans show predominant cortical/subcortical involvement with relative sparing of adjacent white matter.[26] Asymmetric bilateral temporal lobar and insular involvement is typical of herpes simplex encephalitis (HSE). T2* images may reveal petechial hemorrhages after 24–48 hours.

Autoimmune Limbic Encephalitis

The T2/FLAIR reveals hyperintensity in one or both medial temporal lobes. The main differential diagnosis of limbic encephalitis (LE) is herpes encephalitis.[27]

Autoimmune nonparaneoplastic LE with positive GAD65 antibodies typically shows T2/FLAIR hyperintensity in both hippocampi and amygdalae.

DISORDERS MAINLY INVOLVING WHITE MATTER

Infections

Human Immunodeficiency Virus Encephalitis

CT Findings

NECT scans reveal mild-to-moderate volume loss with patchy white matter hypodensity. No obvious enhancement is noted on contrast-enhanced CT (CECT).

MR Findings

Reduced volume of gray matter involving the superior and medial frontal gyri is a marker of human immunodeficiency virus encephalitis (HIVE).[28] Bilateral symmetric patchy T2/FLAIR hyperintensities in the white matter is characteristic. HIVE usually shows no enhancement on T1 C+ and no diffusion restriction on DWI.

Progressive Multifocal Leukoencephalopathy

CT Findings

Progressive multifocal leukoencephalopathy (PML) cases reveal hypodense areas involving the deep and subcortical white matter on NECT without any enhancement on CECT.

MR Findings

- *Classic PML (cPML)*: Bilateral asymmetric multi-/focal heterogeneously hyperintense lesions on T2/FLAIR sequence extending into the subcortical white matter noted.[29] PML does not show any enhancement on T1 C+ scans.
- *Inflammatory PML (iPML)*: iPML is similar to cPML on imaging except that these lesions show mass effect and/or peripheral enhancement.

Subacute Sclerosing Panencephalitis

An MRI scan shows bilateral asymmetric basal ganglia and subcortical white matter T2/FLAIR hyperintensity. Diffuse volume loss with sulcal and ventricular enlargement occurs in the advanced stages of the disease.

Neuroborreliosis

Imaging features vary according to the nature of central nervous system (CNS) involvement.
- *Cranial neuropathy*: Cranial nerve (CN) VII is the most commonly involved. Uniform enhancement in T1 C+ study is characteristic.
- *Encephalopathy*: The most common MR finding is multiple small periventricular and subcortical white matter hyperintensity in T2/FLAIR.[30]

Neurosyphilis

Two patterns of cerebral gummas are known—dural-based lesions and medial temporal lobe abnormalities mimicking herpes encephalitis. MR reveals the gummata as hypointense on T1 and heterogeneously hyperintense on T2.[31] Marked enhancement in T1 C+ is noted, and a dural tail may also be seen.

Inflammatory Disorders

Multiple Sclerosis

CT findings

NECT may show multiple or solitary ill-defined white matter hypodensities. Acute lesions may reveal varying patterns of enhancement on CECT **(Figs. 10A to D)**.

MR Findings

T1WI—most multiple sclerosis (MS) plaques are hypo- or isointense on T1WI. The hypointensity ("black holes") correlates with axonal destruction.

T2/FLAIR—T2WI shows multiple hyperintense round, linear, or ovoid lesions perpendicular to the margin of the lateral ventricles.[32] One of the earliest findings is alternating areas of linear hyperintensity along the ependyma on sagittal FLAIR, known as the "ependymal dot-dash" sign.

T1 C+—MS plaques reveal varying patterns of transient enhancement during the phase of active demyelination.

Acute Disseminated Encephalomyelitis

CT Findings

CECT may reveal multifocal partial ring-enhancing or punctate lesions.

MR Findings

Multifocal T2/FLAIR hyperintensity varying from small round foci to "cotton ball" lesions with "fuzzy" margins are noted.[33] Asymmetric bilateral involvement is characteristic.

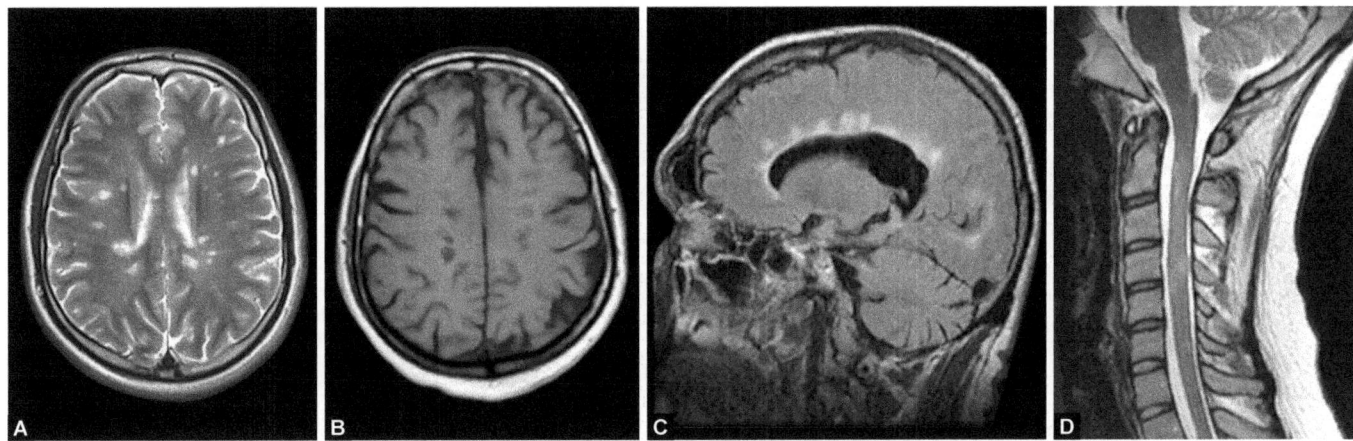

FIGS. 10A TO D: Axial T2 sequence in case of multiple sclerosis reveals multiple T2 hyperintense round or ovoid lesions oriented perpendicular to the margin of lateral ventricles. Some juxtacortical lesions are also noted. Axial T1 sequence reveals hypointensity in some of the lesions called T1 black holes. Sagittal fluid-attenuated inversion recovery (FLAIR) sequence reveals hyperintense lesions arranged perpendicular to the lateral ventricles in a triangular configuration giving a characteristic Dawson fingers appearance. Sagittal T2 image of the cervical spine reveals multiple patchy hyperintense lesions in the cervical cord.

Neurosarcoid

CT Findings

Leptomeningeal disease shows enhancement on CECT. Well-circumscribed punched-out lesions having nonsclerotic margins are seen in bone CT.

MR Findings

Sulci with leptomeningeal infiltrates appear effaced.[34] Infundibular thickening and intense enhancement may be seen.

Celiac Disease

An MRI scan reveals diffuse cerebral atrophy with T2/FLAIR hyperintense lesions.

Inborn Errors of Metabolism

Fragile X-associated Tremor/Ataxia Syndrome

An MRI scan shows symmetric T2 hyperintense lesions in the peridentate region and both middle cerebellar peduncles.

Cerebrotendinous Xanthomatosis

Imaging studies show cerebral and cerebellar atrophy. Hyperintense lesions in the medial GP are seen in most patients,[35] and corticospinal tract involvement is commonly seen.

Neuroaxonal Leukodystrophy

An MRI scan shows frontal subcortical atrophy and confluent T2 hyperintense signal abnormalities involving the frontal lobar white matter.

Adrenomyeloneuropathy

Imaging findings of adrenomyeloneuropathy (AMN) include signal changes in the corpus callosum splenium and posterior limb of internal capsule.

Toxic Leukoencephalopathy and Dementia

Carbon Monoxide Poisoning

Imaging findings in carbon monoxide (CO) poisoning include necrotic lesions involving globus pallidi, subcortical white matter demyelination, and less common involvement of the cerebral and cerebellar cortex with restricted diffusion in acute stage. In the chronic stage, the apparent diffusion coefficient (ADC) values may gradually increase.[36]

Organic Solvent Inhalation

Structural MRI abnormalities can be found in ~20–50% of patients with chronic toluene inhalation and include atrophy and white matter signal changes.[37]

Heroin Vapor Inhalation

Imaging findings in heroin vapor inhalation include confluent white matter changes, involvement of deep gray matter structures, and symmetric involvement of corticospinal tract, medial lemniscus, and tractus solitarius.[38]

Neoplastic Disease and Radiation Necrosis

Gliomatosis Cerebri

In the past, diffuse gliomas with a unique pattern of widespread brain invasion were designated as gliomatosis cerebri (GC). By definition, ≥3 lobes with frequent bihemispheric, basal ganglionic, and/or infratentorial extension were involved.

Intravascular Lymphomatosis

Diffusely infiltrating primary central nervous system lymphomas (PCNSLs), also known as lymphomatosis cerebri, reveal patchy or confluent bi-hemispheric T2/FLAIR hyperintensity involving the deep white matter and basal ganglia. Restricted diffusion may be seen in two-thirds of cases. Enhancement is variable.

Radiation Necrosis

Perfusion MRI and SPECT/PET (thallium/FDG/methionine) may be helpful in differentiating high-grade glioma from necrosis by showing low perfusion/metabolism in the latter.[39] MR spectroscopy will reveal reduced NAA and increased choline concentrations within the tumor, whereas in radiation necrosis lactate may be the only metabolite present.

Trauma

Dementia Pugilistica

Initially called "dementia pugilistica," the term chronic traumatic encephalopathy (CTE) describes a wide spectrum of neurobehavioral abnormalities resulting from multiple blows to the head.[40]

CT Findings

Increased prevalence of a cavum septi pellucidi was present in those boxers with atrophy.

MR Findings

Age-inappropriate volume loss and nonspecific white matter lesions are seen in 15% of cases. Susceptibility-weighted sequences revealed microhemorrhages in some patients with CTE.

Vascular Causes

Vascular Dementia

Operational imaging definitions for the NINDS-AIREN criteria:[41]

Topography Criteria

- *Large vessel stroke*—arterial territorial infarct involving the cortical gray matter
  - Anterior cerebral artery (ACA) infarcts—only bilateral ACA infarcts suffice
  - Posterior cerebral artery (PCA) infarct—involving one of the following regions:
    - Paramedian thalamus (in contact with the third ventricle)
    - Inferior medial temporal lobe
  - Association areas—a middle cerebral artery (MCA) infarct involving:
    - Parietotemporal cortex (e.g., angular gyrus)
    - Temporo-occipital cortex
  - Watershed territories—infarcts between MCA and ACA or between MCA and PCA involving:
    - Superior frontal region
    - Parietal region
- *Small vessel disease*:
  - Ischemic pathology resulting from occlusion of small perforating arteries:
    - Extensive white matter lesions (leukoaraïosis), or
    - Multiple basal ganglia, thalamic and frontal white matter lacunar infarcts:
      - 2 lacunar infarcts in the basal ganglia, thalamus or internal capsule, AND
      - 2 lacunar infarcts in the frontal white matter, or
    - Bilateral thalamic lesions

Severity Criteria

- Large vessel disease of the dominant hemisphere—in the absence of clinical information, the left hemisphere is considered to be the dominant one
- Bilateral large vessel hemispheric strokes—only the infarct located in the nondominant hemisphere should involve an area listed under topography
- Extensive leukoencephalopathy involving at least one-fourth of the total white matter:
  - Confluent lesions—grade 3 on the age-related white matter changes (ARWMC) scale—in at least two regions, AND
  - Beginning confluent—grade 2 on the ARWMC scale—in two other regions

Fulfilment of Radiological Criteria for Probable Vascular Dementia (VaD)

- Large vessel disease—a lesion must be scored in at least one subsection of both topography and severity (both the topography and severity criteria should be met)
- Small vessel disease—for white matter lesions, both the topography and severity criteria should be met; for multiple lacunar infarcts and bilateral thalamic lesions, only the topography criterion is sufficient.

Imaging: The common imaging features include multifocal infarcts and white matter ischemia.

- *CT findings:* NECT scans show diffuse volume loss associated with multiple cortical-subcortical and basal

ganglia infarcts. Patchy hypodensities involving the subcortical and deep white matter are typical.
- **MR findings**: Diffuse volume loss is commonly seen. T2/FLAIR scans reveal multifocal patchy and confluent T2/FLAIR hyperintensities involving the basal ganglia and white matter. T2* sequences may reveal multiple "blooming" foci involving the cortex. DTI may show reduced FA specially involving the inferior fronto-occipital fascicles, superior longitudinal fasciculus, and corpus callosum.

Arteriovenous Malformations

Computed Tomography Findings

The NECT scans usually show numerous hypertrophied serpentine vessels. Calcification within an arteriovenous malformation (AVM) is common. Postcontrast enhancement of feeding arteries, the nidus, and draining veins is intense on a CECT scan **(Figs. 11A to C)**.

Magnetic Resonance Findings

Most AVMs are seen as a tightly packed "honey-comb" of "flow voids" on T1 and T2 scans. Intervening brain parenchyma is gliotic and T2/FLAIR hyperintense.[42] T2* sequences reveal foci of "blooming" within and around the lesion.

Angiography

Digital subtraction angiography (DSA) is considered as "gold standard" in evaluating the angio-architecture of AVMs. All the AVM components, that is, feeding arteries, the nidus, and draining veins must be evaluated in detail. Flow-induced feeding artery aneurysm may be present. Superficially located AVMs may have transdural arterial supply, so complete evaluation of dural vasculature is a must. Intranidal aneurysms may also be present. Draining veins opacify in mid arterial phase—"early draining" veins. Stenosis of the "outlet" draining veins may contribute to hemorrhage.

Dural Arteriovenous Fistula

Computed Tomography Findings

Hemorrhage is unusual except in the presence of cortical venous reflux or venous dilatation. Enlarged transcalvarial channels due to dilated transosseous feeding arteries may be found on bone CT images. Contrast-enhanced scans reveal hypertrophied feeding arteries and draining veins **(Figs. 12A and B)**.

Magnetic Resonance Findings

The most common finding of dural arteriovenous fistula (dAVF) is thrombosed dural venous sinus containing "flow voids."

Angiography

DSA is considered as "gold standard" in evaluating dAVFs. The arterial supply may be derived from both the internal and external carotid systems. Dural branches may also arise from the vertebral arteries.[43] An enlarged tentorial branch of the meningohypophyseal trunk commonly contributes to dAVFs at the transverse/sigmoid sinus junction. The Borden and Cognard classifications are commonly used.

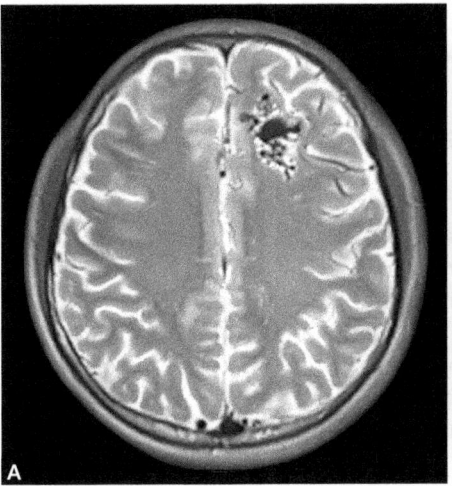 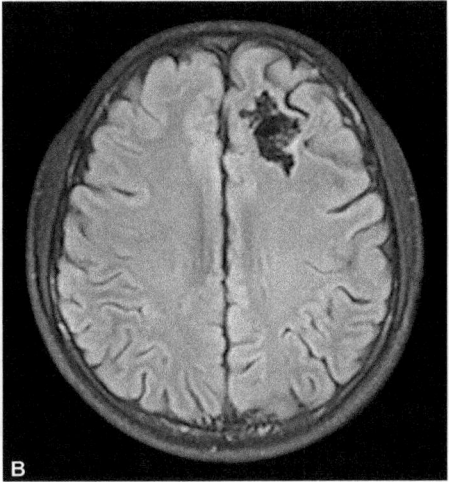 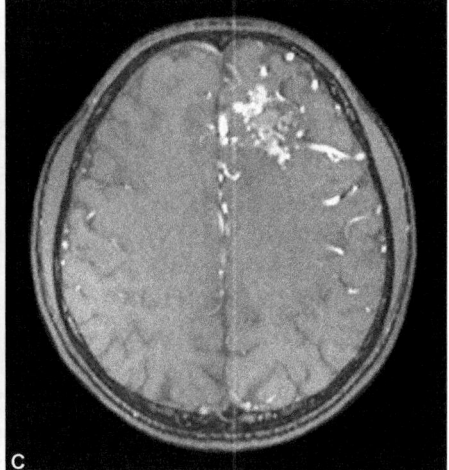

FIGS. 11A TO C: Axial T2 and fluid-attenuated inversion recovery (FLAIR) sequence in case of cerebral arteriovenous malformation reveals a tightly packed "honey-comb" of "flow voids" with gliosis in the adjacent neuroparenchyma. Time-of-flight (TOF) magnetic resonance (MR) angiogram of the brain reveals prominent arterial feeders and early draining veins in relation to the lesion.

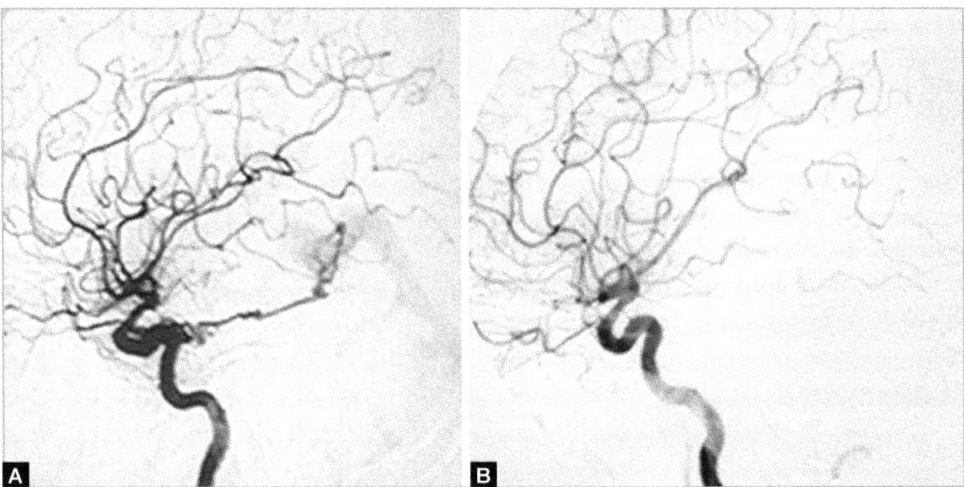

FIGS. 12A AND B: Lateral view digital subtraction angiography in case of cerebral dural arteriovenous fistula reveals a prominent arterial feeder arising from a meningeal branch of internal carotid artery. Postembolization digital subtraction angiography in the same patient reveals complete obliteration of the fistula.

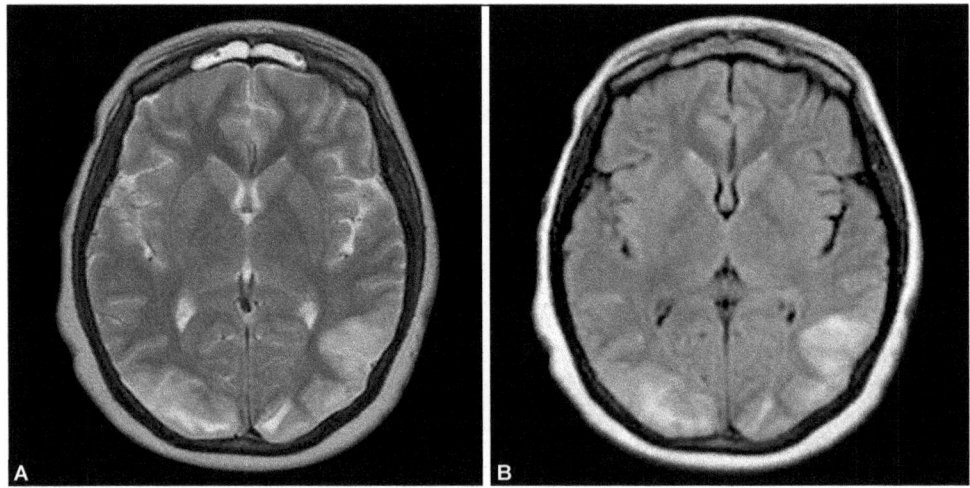

FIGS. 13A AND B: Axial T2 and fluid-attenuated inversion recovery (FLAIR) sequence in case of posterior reversible encephalopathy syndrome (PRES) reveals hyperintensity within bilateral occipital and temporal regions representing vasogenic edema.

Borden Classification of Dural Arteriovenous Fistula

- Type I: Dural arterial supply with antegrade drainage into venous sinus
    - Type Ia: Simple dAVF with single meningeal arterial supply
    - Type Ib: Complex dAVF with multiple meningeal arteries
- Type II: Dural supply + ↑ intrasinus pressure → antegrade sinus, retrograde cortical venous drainage
- Type III: Dural arteries drain into cortical veins

In either classification, presence of cortical venous reflux puts a dAVF into a higher risk category.

Posterior Reversible Encephalopathy Syndrome

Computed Tomography Findings

Subtle cortical/subcortical hypodensities, commonly involving the occipitoparietal lobes, watershed areas, and/or cerebellum may be found on NECT. Three different types of posterior reversible encephalopathy syndrome (PRES)-associated hemorrhage occur: parenchymal hemorrhage, multifocal hemorrhages, and convexal subarachnoid hemorrhage **(Figs. 13A and B)**.

Magnetic Resonance Findings

Posterior reversible encephalopathy syndrome has both classic and atypical MR imaging features.

Classic PRES typically reveals bilateral cortical/subcortical parieto-occipital areas, hypointense on T1 and hyperintense on FLAIR.[44] T2* sequences may show hemorrhagic foci.

Imaging in atypical PRES shows frontal lobar involvement, watershed areas, thalami and/or basal ganglia, cerebellum, brainstem, and spinal cord. DWI is usually negative in PRES due to vasogenic edema.

Angiography

Diffuse vessel constriction or narrowing, focal irregularity, and beaded appearance are typical but nonspecific angiographic findings in PRES.

Normal Pressure Hydrocephalus

General Features

The most common imaging feature of normal pressure hydrocephalus (NPH) is ventriculomegaly (Evans index of at least 0.3) out-of-proportion to the degree of sulcal enlargement ("ventriculo-sulcal disproportion").

Computed Tomography Findings

The NECT scans reveal moderate supratentorial ventriculomegaly. Compared to the extent of ventriculomegaly, sulcal enlargement is mild. Periventricular hypodensity is commonly seen **(Figs. 14A to D)**.

Magnetic Resonance Findings

The T1 scans demonstrate enlarged lateral ventricles. The high frontoparietal convexity sulci appear "tight," whereas sylvian fissures are usually widened. Thinning of corpus callosum is noted. Periventricular T2/FLAIR hyperintensity is noted. Prominent "hyperdynamic" aqueductal "flow-void" may be seen.

Cerebrospinal fluid flow studies are usually undertaken for assessment of shunt responsive normal pressure hydrocephalus.[45] An aqueductal stroke volume >42 μL is associated with shunt responsiveness.

Nuclear Medicine Findings

Prominent ventricular activity after 24 hours on ^{111}In-diethylenetriaminepentaacetic acid (DTPA) cisternography is taken as a sign of NPH.

CONCLUDING REMARKS

Dementing neurodegenerative disorders are a diverse and clinically devastating group of diseases. It is important that practicing radiologists and nuclear medicine physicians work hand in hand with neurologists to arrive at a conclusive diagnosis and prognosticate and counsel patients and their relatives accordingly.

LEARNING POINTS

- Dementias encompass a wide variety of neurodegenerative as well as nonneurodegenerative pathologies, which may be difficult to differentiate on the basis of clinical findings.
- Conventional structural MRI including newer MR imaging sequences such as MR perfusion, MR spectroscopy, DTI, and functional MRI are necessary to narrow down the differential diagnosis in doubtful cases.

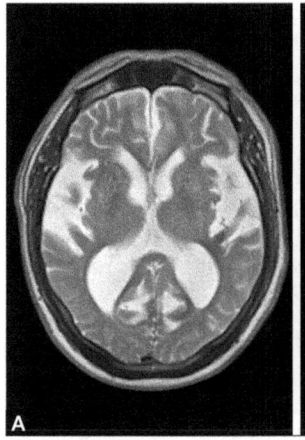 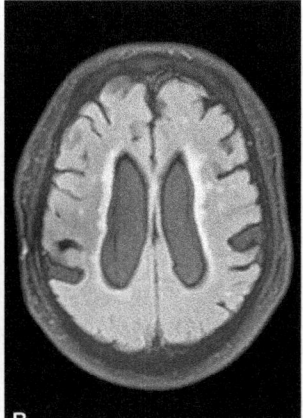 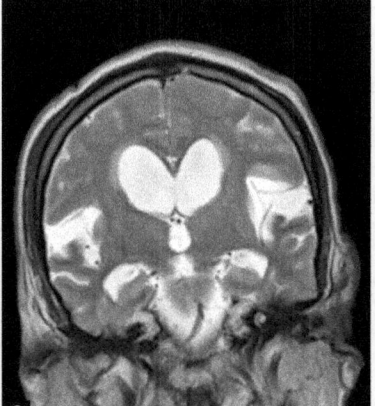 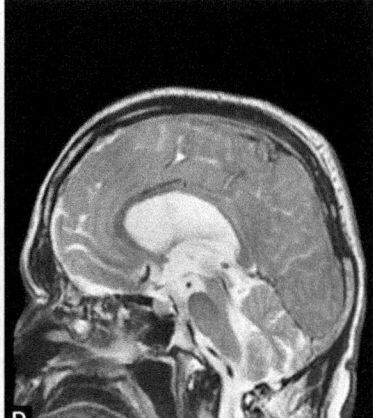

FIGS. 14A TO D: Axial T2 and fluid-attenuated inversion recovery (FLAIR) sequence in case of normal pressure hydrocephalus reveals ventriculosulcal disproportion with periventricular FLAIR hyperintensity. Coronal T2 sequence reveals prominent sylvian fissures and reduced callosal angle. Sagittal T2 sequence reveals prominent flow-void across the cerebral aqueduct.

- Nuclear imaging techniques such as SPECT and PET imaging may be complementary to MR imaging in arriving at a definite diagnosis in certain cases.
- No isolated technique achieves 100% accuracy. So, effective communication among neuroradiologists, neurologists, neurosurgeons, pathologists, and nuclear medicine specialists is essential to avoid the potential diagnostic pitfalls and facilitate early diagnosis.

REFERENCES

1. American Psychiatric Association. Diagnostic and statistical manual of mental disorders: DSM-IV. Washington, DC: American Psychiatric Association; 1994.
2. Bradford A, Kunik ME, Schulz P, Williams SP, Singh H. Missed and delayed diagnosis of dementia in primary care: prevalence and contributing factors. Alzheimer Dis Assoc Disord. 2009;23(4):306-14.
3. Patel KP, Wymer DT, Bhatia VK, Duara R, Rajadhyaksha CD. Multimodality imaging of dementia: clinical importance and role of integrated anatomic and molecular imaging. Radiographics. 2020;40(1):200-22.
4. Osborne AG. Osborne's Brain: Imaging, Pathology and Anatomy. Salt Lake City: Amirsys; 2013.
5. Spiegel AM, Sewal AS, Rapp PR. Epigenetic contributions to cognitive aging: disentangling mindspan and lifespan. Learn Mem. 2014;21(10):569-74.
6. Dallaire-Théroux C, Callahan BL, Potvin O, Saikali S, Duchesne S. Radiological-pathological correlation in Alzheimer's disease: systematic review of antemortem magnetic resonance imaging findings. J Alzheimers Dis. 2017;57(2):575-601.
7. Donohue MC, Sperling RA, Petersen R, Sun CK, Weiner MW, Aisen PS; Alzheimer's Disease Neuroimaging Initiative. Association between elevated brain amyloid and subsequent cognitive decline among cognitively normal persons. JAMA. 2017;317(22):2305-16.
8. Mann DMA, Snowden JS. Frontotemporal lobar degeneration: Pathogenesis, pathology and pathways to phenotype. Brain Pathol. 2017;27(6):723-36.
9. Olney NT, Spina S, Miller BL. Frontotemporal Dementia. Neurol Clin. 2017;35(2):339-74.
10. Gomperts SN. Lewy body dementias: dementia with Lewy bodies and Parkinson disease dementia. Continuum (Minneap Minn). 2116;22(2 Dementia):435-63.
11. Agosta F, Galantucci S, Filippi M. Advanced magnetic resonance imaging of neurodegenerative diseases. Neurol Sci. 2017;38(1):41-51.
12. Braak H, Del Tredici K. Neuropathological staging of brain pathology in sporadic Parkinson's disease: Separating the Wheat from the Chaff. J Parkinsons Dis. 2017;7(s1):S71-S85.
13. Booth TC, Nathan M, Waldman AD, Quigley AM, Schapira AH, Buscombe J. The role of functional dopamine-transporter SPECT imaging in parkinsonian syndromes, part 1. AJNR Am J Neuroradiol. 2015;36(2):229-35.
14. Lee Y, Lee DK, Lee JM, Chung SJ, Lee JJ, Sohn YH, et al. Volumetric analysis of the cerebellum in patients with progressive supranuclear palsy. Eur J Neurol. 2017;24(1):212-8.
15. Chen B, Fan G, Sun W, Shang X, Shi S, Wang S, et al. Usefulness of diffusion-tensor MRI in the diagnosis of Parkinson variant of multiple system atrophy and Parkinson's disease: a valuable tool to differentiate between them? Clin Radiol. 2017;72(7):610.e9-610.e15.
16. Yokoyama JS, Karch CM, Fan CC, Bonham LW, Kouri N, Ross OA, et al. Shared genetic risk between corticobasal degeneration, progressive supranuclear palsy, and frontotemporal dementia. Acta Neuropathol. 2017;133(5):825-37.
17. Ho V, Chuang H, Rovira M, Koo B. Juvenile Huntington disease: CT and MR features. AJNR Am J Neuroradiol. 1995;16(7):1405-12.
18. Negi R, Manchanda K, Sanga S. Imaging of Huntington's Disease. Med J Armed Forces India. 2014;70(4):386-8.
19. King AD, Walshe JM, Kendall BE, Chinn RJ, Paley MN, Wilkinson ID, et al. Cranial MR imaging in Wilson's disease. AJR Am J Roentgenol. 1996;167(6):1579-84.
20. Sener RN. Pantothenate kinase-associated neurodegeneration: MR imaging, proton MR spectroscopy, and diffusion MR imaging findings. AJNR Am J Neuroradiol. 2003;24 (8):1690-3.
21. Kallenberg K, Schulz-Schaeffer WJ, Jastrow U, Poser S, Meissner B, Tschampa HJ, et al. Creutzfeldt-Jakob disease: comparative analysis of MR imaging sequences. AJNR Am J Neuroradiol. 2006;27(7):1459-62.
22. Logan C, Asadi H, Kok HK, Looby ST, Brennan P, O'Hare A, Thornton J. Neuroimaging of chronic alcohol misuse. J Med Imaging Radiat Oncol. 2017;61(4):435-40.
23. Hattingen E, Beyle A, Müller A, Klockgether T, Kornblum C. Wernicke encephalopathy: SWI detects petechial hemorrhages in mammillary bodies in vivo. Neurology. 2016;87(18):1956-7.
24. Gambini A, Falini A, Moiola L, Comi G, Scotti G. Marchiafava-Bignami disease: longitudinal MR imaging and MR spectroscopy study. AJNR Am J Neuroradiol. 2003;24(2):249-53.
25. Mueller F, Lenz C, Steiner M, Dolder PC, Walter M, Lang UE, et al. Neuroimaging in moderate MDMA use: A systematic review. Neurosci Biobehav Rev. 2016;62:21-34.
26. Bulakbasi N, Kocaoglu M. Central nervous system infections of herpesvirus family. Neuroimaging Clin N Am. 2008;18(1):53-84.
27. Oyanguren B, Sánchez V, González FJ, de Felipe A, Esteban L, López-Sendón JL, et al. Limbic encephalitis: a clinical-radiological comparison between herpetic and autoimmune etiologies. Eur J Neurol. 2013;20(12):1566-70.
28. Mahan M, Karl M, Gordon S. Neuroimaging of viral infections of the central nervous system. Handb Clin Neurol. 2014;123:149-73.
29. Smith A, Smirniotopoulos J, Rushing E. From the Archives of the AFIP: Central nervous system infections associated with human immunodeficiency virus infection: Radiologic-pathologic correlation. Radiographics. 2008;28(7):2033-58.
30. Agarwal R, Sze G. Neuro-lyme disease: MR imaging findings. Radiology. 2009;253(1):167-73.
31. Bash S, Hathout GM, Cohen S. Mesiotemporal T2-weighted hyperintensity: neurosyphilis mimicking herpes encephalitis. AJNR Am J Neuroradiol. 2001;22(2):314-6.

32. Filippi M, Rocca MA, Ciccarelli O, De Stefano N, Evangelou N, Kappos L, et al; MAGNIMS Study Group. MRI criteria for the diagnosis of multiple sclerosis: MAGNIMS consensus guidelines. Lancet Neurol. 2016;15(3):292-303.
33. Hynson JL, Kornberg AJ, Coleman LT, Shield L, Harvey AS, Kean MJ. Clinical and neuroradiologic features of acute disseminated encephalomyelitis in children. Neurology. 2001;56 (10):1308-12.
34. Shah R, Roberson GH, Curé JK. Correlation of MR imaging findings and clinical manifestations in neurosarcoidosis. AJNR Am J Neuroradiol. 2009;30(5):953-61.
35. Barkhof F, Verrips A, Wesseling P, van Der Knaap MS, van Engelen BG, Gabreëls FJ, et al. Cerebrotendinous xanthomatosis: the spectrum of imaging findings and the correlation with neuropathologic findings. Radiology. 2000;217(3):869-76.
36. Kim DM, Lee IH, Park JY, Hwang SB, Yoo DS, Song CJ. Acute carbon monoxide poisoning: MR imaging findings with clinical correlation. Diagn Interv Imaging. 2017;98(4):299-306.
37. Jayanth SH, Hugar BS, Praveen S, Girish Chandra YP. Glue sniffing. Med Leg J. 2017;85(1):38-42.
38. Lefaucheur R, Lebas A, Gérardin E, Grangeon L, Ozkul-Wermester O, Aubier-Girard C, et al. Leucoencephalopathy following abuse of sniffed heroin. J Clin Neurosci. 2017;35:70-2.
39. Balentova S, Adamkov M. Molecular, cellular and functional effects of radiation-induced brain injury: A review. Int J Mol Sci. 2015;16(11):27796-815.
40. McKee AC, Stern RA, Nowinski CJ, Stein TD, Alvarez VE, Daneshvar DH, et al. The spectrum of disease in chronic traumatic encephalopathy. Brain. 2013;136 (1):43-64.
41. van Straaten EC, Scheltens P, Knol DL, van Buchem MA, van Dijk EJ, Hofman PA, et al. Operational definitions for the NINDS-AIREN criteria for vascular dementia: an interobserver study. Stroke. 2003;34(8):1907-12.
42. Geibprasert S, Pongpech S, Jiarakongmun P, Shroff MM, Armstrong DC, Krings T. Radiologic assessment of brain arteriovenous malformations: what clinicians need to know. Radiographics. 2010;30(2):483-501.
43. Gandhi D, Chen J, Pearl M. Intracranial dural arteriovenous fistulas: classification, imaging findings, and treatment. AJNR Am J Neuroradiol. 2012;33(6):1007-13.
44. Fugate JE, Claassen DO, Cloft HJ, Kallmes DF, Kozak OS, Rabinstein AA. Posterior reversible encephalopathy syndrome: associated clinical and radiologic findings. Mayo Clin Proc. 2010;85(5):427-32.
45. Bradley W, Scalzo D, Queralt J, Nitz W, Atkinson D, Wong P. Normal-pressure hydrocephalus: Evaluation with cerebrospinal fluid flow measurements at MR imaging. Radiology. 1996;198(2):523-9.

COMMENTARY 18

Utility and Limitations of Neuroimaging and Cerebrospinal Fluid Biomarkers in Diagnosis of Dementia Subtypes

Ambar Chakravarty

INTRODUCTION

Current neuroradiological practice has advanced tremendously with structural neuroimaging being supplemented with functional, metabolic, and receptor imaging. The impact of this is much felt in the field of dementias, especially in differentiating the different subtypes discussed in the preceding chapter. Researchers are focusing attention on human, brain networking, and their imaging features. ^{18}Fluorodeoxyglucose positron emission tomography (^{18}FDG-PET) brain, single-photon emission computed tomography (SPECT) brain, PET Pittsburgh Compound B (PIB), and PET receptor (Dopa) imaging are being included in the routine evaluation of patients with cognitive decline in many centers. ^{18}FDG-PET brain in particular has become an important tool in the early diagnosis of cases with mild cognitive impairment (MCI) as well as in differentiating between different dementia subtypes such as frontotemporal disorders (FTDs) and Alzheimer disease (AD). Newer molecular markers such as beta amyloid, alpha synuclein, TDP-43, tau, and fused in sarcoma (FUS) have been found to be involved at the synaptic and neuronal level at the earliest stages in these diseases. Neuroimaging is being increasingly utilized to decipher these early changes long before the clinical state even emerges or the extensive atrophy seen on structural scans appear. PET scans offer the most accurate diagnostic method for the five main dementia subtypes, namely AD, FTD, vascular dementia (VaD), diffuse Lewy body disease (DLBD), and Parkinson disease associated dementia (PDD).

The frontotemporal hypometabolism seen in FTD and the temporal, parietal, and posterior cingulate hypometabolism noted in AD can be relatively easily identified.[1] Furthermore, it is now possible to differentiate between the posterior cortical atrophy syndrome (Benson syndrome) from slowly progressive AD variant with relatively retained cognition but having complex visual impairments including visual agnosia and Balint syndrome.[2] However, with PDD and DLBD, the differentiating features on PET scanning are less distinct and considerable overlap in the patterns are encountered, resulting in diagnostic confusion. This may not be very surprising as DLDB and AD share features at a clinical, neuroimaging, pathological, and pharmacotherapeutic level. In fact, Parkinson disease (PD), PDD, DLBD, and AD represent a pathological spectrum with loss of both cholinergic and dopaminergic neurons initially. The diagnostic dilemma gets more complicated when in individual cases, there is an overlap of AD and vascular cognitive impairment (VCI)/VaD, or of the frontal variant of AD and the frontal variant of FTD.

Diagnosis and differentiation of evolving dementia subtypes may not be possible by clinical means alone especially in the presymptomatic phase when no cognitive impairment exists particularly in the context of presumed high cognitive reserve. PET brain scan imaging and cerebrospinal fluid (CSF) biomarkers are becoming increasingly important to diagnose early dementia syndromes especially in such situations and in the setting of overlap syndromes.[3-5] AD and FTD have distinct and easily identifiable patterns and VCI/VaD diagnosis is guided primarily by stroke related imaging. The situation with DLBD can be difficult due to the overlap of neuropathologies; but therapy essentially depends upon a correct diagnosis. The increased sensitivity of patients with DLBD to neuroleptics is well recognized, and hence a definitive diagnosis is of extreme importance to avoid such critical drug related situations such as neuroleptic malignant syndrome or malignant catatonia. No doubt the neuroradiological findings of DLDB may be initially confused with those of AD. Hallucinations, a hallmark of DLDB, can occur in AD, as well as in other dementias and can be drug induced. These make diagnostic decision making very difficult at times. There indeed are some recognized metabolic features in PET scanning, which

have been identified in patients with DLBD. These include the following:
- Diffuse glucose hypometabolism in the entire cortex including the occipital region in DLBD and distinctive from AD
- Lateral occipital hypometabolism, which may have the highest sensitivity
- Posterior cingulate preserved metabolism or posterior cingulate island sign (PCIS), which may have the highest specificity.

Hypometabolism is seen very early in the medial portions of the parietal lobes as well as the posterior cingulate region in patients with AD. The difficulty posed by the fluctuating symptomatology in both conditions adds to the diagnostic dilemma. Specific panel of biomarkers such as amyloid β1–42, protein tau, and phosphorylated tau (p-tau 181) have been validated to reflect the pathology in AD. The advent of biomarker-assisted diagnosis has already initiated new diagnostic criteria for AD that enable a premortem diagnosis that is heavily reliant on positive CSF and PET findings.[6] Uptil now, there are no specific CSF biomarkers for DLB and PDD. This is partly related to the occurrence of mixed pathology in DLB and/or PDD. A varying degree of concomitant AD pathology frequently found in DLB is associated with a more rapid disease course and more pronounced cognitive dysfunction compared to "pure" DLB pathology. With the advent of MR perfusion scanning giving similar information to PET brain scanning, this modality may become more desirable in view of its availability and lack of radiation.

The Default Mode Network (DMN) connects selective brain regions that include the posterior cingulate, the precuneus, lateral parietal, lateral temporal, and medial frontal areas. These networks can be visualized by functional MRI (fMRI; resting state without activation procedures) and reflects the basal or default mode activity of the brain. DMN impaired connectivity had been shown in AD, FTD, schizophrenia, epilepsy, autism, and later life depression. The DMN is active during rest and becomes less so during cerebral tasking. DMN is implicated in the pathogenesis of AD as the distribution of the DMN is similar to the fibrillar amyloid deposition in patients with AD, as demonstrable by amyloid PET imaging. The amyloid-beta deposition overlaps considerably with DMN and the tau deposition overlaps with the DMN component that is concerned with episodic memory. It had been hypothesized that overactivity of DMN (posterior cingulate, later parietal, and medial frontal) in younger life may lead to a metabolic impairment predisposing people to amyloid deposition in later life.

Pattern of cortical atrophy in different subtypes of dementia as detectable by standard MR imaging are generally noted at a later stage of the process and perhaps the least sensitive. However, some common observations may be helpful in routine clinical practice and are summarized here.
- *Alzheimer disease*: Temporoparietal, medial hippocampus, precuneus
- *Frontotemporal disorders behavioral variant*: Frontotemporal
- *Parkinson with dementia*: Temporoparietal
- *Diffuse Lewy body disease*: Parietal atrophy but no hippocampal atrophy
- *Huntington disease*: Caudate
- *Vascular cognitive disorder*: Subcortical and periventricular rimming leukoaraiosis are frequent
- *Progressive supranuclear palsy*: Midbrain atrophy (Hummingbird/Penguin signs)
- *Corticobasal ganglionic degeneration*: Pronounced frontoparietal atrophy, often asymmetric; corpus callosum atrophy

The big question remains—how would we image a patient suffering from dementia due to a neurodegenerative disorder in future years with ready availability of all these newer modalities? Perhaps a hierarchical approach as mentioned would be logical: (1) resting state network imaging (DMN) by fMRI; (2) beta amyloid accumulation assessed by PET brain PIB (also CSF assays); (3) the subsequent synaptic dysfunction assessed by FDG-PET brain; (4) finally, neuronal loss follows as assessed by volumetric MRI.

REFERENCES

1. Foster NL, Heidebrink JL, Clark CM, Jagust WJ, Arnold SE, Barbas NR, et al. FDG-PET improves accuracy in distinguishing frontotemporal dementia and Alzheimer's disease. Brain. 2007;130(Pt 10):2616-35.
2. Berti V, Pupi A, Mosconi L. PET/CT in diagnosis of dementia. Ann NY Acad Sci. 2011;1288:81-92.
3. Migliaccio R, Agosta F, Rascovsky K, Karydas A, Bonasera S, Rabinovici GD, et al. Clinical syndromes associated with posterior atrophy: early age at onset AD spectrum. Neurology. 2009;73(19):1571-8.
4. Standley K, Brock C, Hoffmann M. Advances in functional neuroimaging in dementias and potential pitfalls. Neurol Int. 2012;4(1):e7.
5. Gmitterová K, Gawinecka J, Llorens F, Varges D, Valkovič P, Zerr I. Cerebrospinal fluid markers analysis in the differential diagnosis of dementia with Lewy bodies and Parkinson's disease dementia. Eur Arch Psychiatry Clin Neurosci. 2020;270(4):461-70.
6. Dubois B, Feldman HH, Jocava C, Cummings JL, Dekosky ST, Barberger-Gateau P, et al. Revising the definition of Alzheimer's disease: a new lexicon. Lancet Neurology 2010;9(11):1118-27.

Neurological Aspects of Autism Spectrum Disorder

Anaita Udwadia Hegde, Omkar P Hajirnis

INTRODUCTION

Autism spectrum disorder (ASD) is a neurodevelopmental disorder characterized by persistent difficulties in social communication and interaction, as well as restricted and repetitive patterns of behavior, interests, or activities.[1] In Diagnostic and Statistical Manual of Mental Disorders—5th edition (DSM-5), the concept of a "spectrum" ASD diagnosis was introduced, combining the DSM-4's separate pervasive developmental disorder (PDD) diagnoses—autistic disorder, Asperger's disorder, childhood disintegrative disorder, and PDD not otherwise specified (PDD-NOS), into one single spectrum. Rett syndrome is not included under ASD in DSM-5 and is considered a separate neurological disorder. Additional subgroups were established for children with social (pragmatic) communication disorder (SPCD), but lacking repetitive, restricted behaviors. Also, severity level descriptors were included to help categorize the level of support needed by any individual with ASD.[2]

The neurological aspects of ASD are diverse and complex involving various brain regions, with their connectivity patterns and neurotransmitter systems. Delving deep into these neurological aspects is crucial for gaining knowledge about the underlying mechanisms of ASD and developing effective interventions. In this chapter, we will explore some of the key neurological aspects of ASD starting with neuroanatomical and biochemical aspects and then talk about the clinical implications of ruling out neurological conditions mimicking autism and also the investigations required for the same.[3,4]

NEUROANATOMICAL AND PHYSIOLOGICAL ASPECTS

Brain Structure and Function

Neuroimaging studies have shown several differences in brain structure and function in individuals with ASD compared to typically developing individuals. These differences are observed particularly in the prefrontal cortex, amygdala, and corpus callosum. The prefrontal cortex, which is responsible for higher cognitive functions, shows altered connectivity patterns in individuals with ASD. The amygdala, which deals with processing emotions and social information, may also exhibit atypical responses in individuals with ASD. Additionally, the corpus callosum which is responsible for interhemispheric communication has shown to have abnormalities in its size or connectivity in individuals with autism.[5-7]

Neural Connectivity

Several studies have shown that individuals with ASD often show atypical patterns of neural connectivity. Functional connectivity which refers to the synchronized activity between different brain regions may be altered in ASD. There may be both over connectivity and under connectivity between certain brain regions, leading to disruptions in information processing and its integration. These connectivity differences can impact social communication, sensory processing, and the coordination of cognitive processes. Research suggests that this altered connectivity in ASD may arise from impaired development during early brain maturation.[8,9]

Neurotransmitter Systems

Neurotransmitters as we know play a crucial role in transmitting signals between neurons and regulating multiple brain functions. Neurotransmitter systems which have been implicated in ASD include but not limited to serotonin, dopamine, and glutamate regulation. Serotonin excess has been linked to social and repetitive behaviors seen in ASD. Dopamine dysregulation may contribute to attention and reward processing difficulties. Glutamate, an excitatory neurotransmitter, has been associated with sensory hypersensitivity and repetitive behaviors in ASD.

Learning about these neurotransmitter abnormalities provide insights into the chemical underpinnings of ASD and subsequent potential targets for therapeutic interventions.[10,11]

Genetic and Epigenetic Influences

The neurological aspects of ASD are influenced by both genetic and environmental factors. Research has identified numerous genes associated with ASD, many of which are involved in brain development, neuronal connectivity, and synaptic function. However, it is important to note that the genetic landscape of autism is highly complex and more than a single gene, autism is considered a polygenic disorder, meaning that it is influenced by the combined effects of multiple genes. Researchers estimate that hundreds of genes may contribute to autism susceptibility, each exerting a small effect. This complex genetic architecture makes it challenging to pinpoint specific genes or genetic variations responsible for the disorder. Still at present about 30% cases of ASD are estimated to arise due to genetic factors. Along with this, it is increasingly recognized that gene-environment interactions play a role in autism. Certain genetic factors may increase vulnerability to environmental influences, such as prenatal exposure to certain toxins or maternal immune activation during pregnancy. The interplay between genetic susceptibility and environmental factors is an area of active investigation in autism research. Other factors, such as epigenetic modifications such as DNA methylation and histone modifications along with prenatal factors, and interactions with the broader environment, also play a role in the development of autism.

Thus it is important to note that while genetic factors are significant contributors to autism risk, they do not fully explain all cases of the disorder. Further research is needed to better understand the complex interplay between genetic and environmental factors and how they contribute to the genesis of ASD.[12,13]

NEUROLOGICAL DISORDERS ASSOCIATED WITH ASD

As discussed ASD although itself is a distinct diagnostic category but there are several neurological disorders that are commonly associated with or frequently co-occur with ASD.

Here are some examples.

Epilepsy

Epilepsy is frequently observed in individuals with autism and its co-occurrence suggests shared underlying mechanisms and genetic factors. Seizures can further impact cognitive functioning and behavior in individuals with ASD. Several genes have been identified that are associated with both conditions, suggesting a genetic overlap. For example, mutations in genes such as SCN1A, SHANK3, and NRXN1 have been implicated in both epilepsy and autism.

Estimates suggest that approximately 20–30% of individuals with ASD also have epilepsy, making it one of the most common co-occurring conditions. Though epilepsy can occur at any age, but it is more commonly seen in individuals with autism during early childhood. Epilepsy can have a significant impact on cognitive functioning, behavior, and overall development in individuals with autism with impairment in attention, memory, language skills, and social interactions. The presence of epilepsy may itself complicate the assessment and management of ASD symptoms. When treating epilepsy in an autistic child, it is essential to consider potential interactions with other medications and most importantly to take behavioral adverse effects of antiepileptics into consideration. Frequent seizures may limit independence, increase safety concerns, and impact educational and social opportunities. Comprehensive support and interventions are necessary to address the needs of individuals with both conditions. It is also pivotal to note that not all individuals with autism will develop epilepsy, and not all individuals with epilepsy will have autism. Nonetheless, recognizing the association between epilepsy and autism and providing appropriate monitoring, early detection, and intervention can improve outcomes and quality of life for individuals with both conditions.[12-17]

Intellectual Disability

Intellectual disability (ID) is often seen in individuals with autism with the severity of ID ranging from mild-to-severe. ID is seen in approximately 30–70% of individuals with ASD and its wide range is primarily because it is difficult to determine the true intellectual potential of an autistic child. ID which is typically diagnosed based on standardized intelligence tests, such as IQ tests are difficult to be done in individuals with ASD and hence IQ is often underestimated. ID can affect various aspects of a person's functioning, including their cognitive abilities, learning capacity, adaptive skills, and daily living skills. It is important to recognize that individuals with autism and ID display a wide range of abilities and strengths. While some individuals may have significant limitations in intellectual functioning, others may have higher cognitive abilities but are still often unfortunately tagged in the severe ID category.[18]

Attention-deficit/Hyperactivity Disorder

Attention-deficit/hyperactivity disorder (ADHD) is a neurodevelopmental disorder characterized by difficulties with attention, hyperactivity, and impulsivity. Many individuals with autism also exhibit symptoms of ADHD, such as inattention, impulsivity, and restlessness. Managing both ASD and ADHD symptoms may require tailored interventions.[19]

Developmental Coordination Disorder

Developmental coordination disorder (DCD), also known as dyspraxia, is a condition characterized by difficulties with motor coordination and planning. While ASD and DCD are distinct neurodevelopmental conditions, research suggests a higher prevalence of motor coordination difficulties in individuals with ASD compared to the general population. Individuals with autism often display motor coordination challenges, including clumsiness, poor handwriting, and difficulties with fine and gross motor skills.[20]

Sensory Processing Issues

Many individuals with autism have sensory processing issues, where they may be hypersensitive or hyposensitive to certain sensory stimuli. These sensory differences can affect their perception and response to sensory input, including touch, sound, light, and taste. The presence of these disorders can vary among individuals. Occupational therapy (OT) is commonly used to address sensory processing difficulties in individuals with ASD. It focuses on improving sensory modulation, self-regulation, and adaptive responses to sensory stimuli.[21]

Stereotypies and Tics

Stereotypies and tics are more prevalent in individuals with ASD compared to the general population and estimates suggest that up to 80% of individuals with ASD may exhibit stereotypies and about 20% may have tics. The tics in ASD are usually milder and more of simple motor tics, such as eye blinking, facial grimacing, or shoulder shrugging unlike complex motor and vocal tics seen in Tourette's syndrome. There may be an association between the presence of tics and increased severity of autism symptoms, such as repetitive behaviors and social communication difficulties.[22]

Anxiety Disorders

Anxiety disorders, including generalized anxiety disorder, social anxiety disorder, and obsessive-compulsive disorder (OCD), frequently co-occur with autism. Individuals with autism may experience heightened levels of anxiety, which can impact social interactions, daily functioning, and overall well-being. It is important to differentiate anxiety symptoms from ASD-specific behaviors or sensory sensitivities. The physician needs to understand the specific anxiety profiles and individual needs of individuals with ASD for providing appropriate support and intervention.[23]

NEUROLOGICAL DISORDERS MIMICKING AUTISM

While ASD is a distinct neurodevelopmental disorder, there are various other neurological conditions that may present with autistic symptoms as a part of their neurological presentation. These conditions can sometimes be mistaken for autism, leading to misdiagnosis or delayed diagnosis. It is essential to differentiate between these disorders to provide appropriate interventions and support. Here are a few neurological disorders written in the form of case briefings for better understanding.

CASE HISTORY 1

A 5-year-old female child was born as a healthy baby and reached developmental milestones within the expected time frame. She had normal speech development and was able to communicate effectively with her family and peers. However, around the age of 3 years, her parents started noticing changes in her language abilities and behavior. She gradually became less responsive to verbal cues and began showing signs of language regression along with behavioral symptoms of hyperactivity and oppositional defiance. Her parents also observed episodes of staring spells where she appeared to be unresponsive for few seconds.

Medical Evaluation

Her parents sought medical help and she underwent a thorough medical evaluation, including neurological examinations and various diagnostic tests. An awake electroencephalogram (EEG) **(Fig. 1A)** did not show any significant abnormality but a sleep EEG **(Fig. 1B)** performed clinched the diagnosis.

The EEG findings were consistent with Landau–Kleffner syndrome (LKS), a childhood disorder characterized by language regression and seizure activity. The classical EEG findings show presence of continuous bihemispheric spike-and-wave discharges during nonrapid eye movement (NREM) which are often irregular, high-

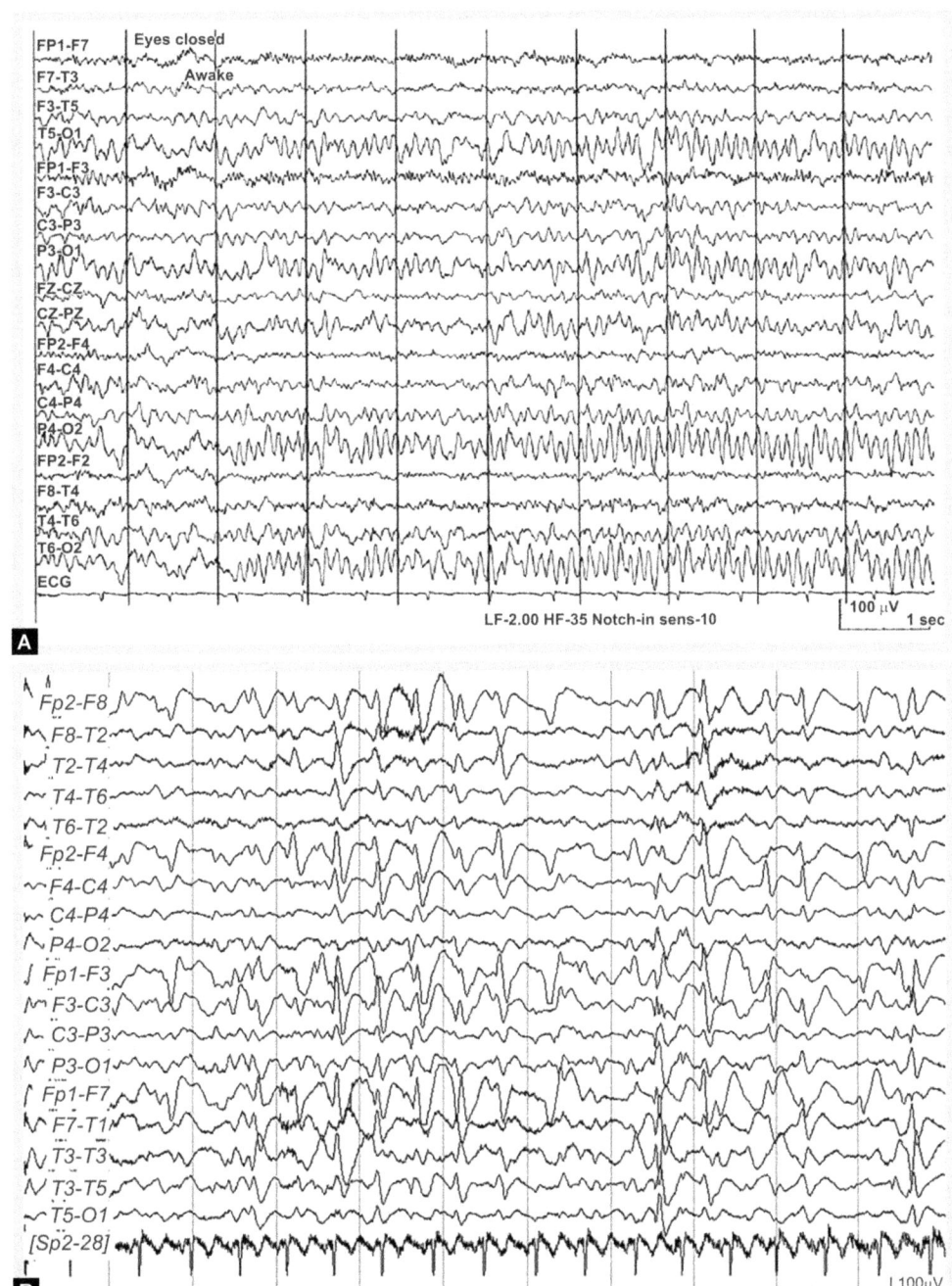

FIGS. 1A AND B: (A) Electroencephalogram (EEG) in awake state; (B) EEG in sleep state.

voltage, and sometimes may be asymmetrical. Hence it is imperative to do a sleep EEG in children suspected with LKS as an EEG done only in awake state may miss the condition. Her treatment plan involved antiepileptic medication along with intensive speech and behavioral therapy. Over time, her seizure activity became better controlled with medication. However, her language progress was slow but remained steady and she started regaining some language abilities and improvement in her communication with others.

Thus here are some ways in which LKS can mimic autism:
- *Language regression*: One of the hallmark features of LKS is the loss or regression of language skills, similar to the speech regression seen in some individuals with ASD. This can easily be mistaken for the language and communication challenges associated with ASD.

- *Social communication difficulties*: Children with LKS may also exhibit social communication difficulties, including challenges in engaging in reciprocal conversations, understanding social cues, and maintaining social relationships which can resemble the social interaction deficits seen in individuals with ASD, making it challenging to differentiate between the two conditions based on this symptom alone.
- *Behavioral abnormalities*: Both LKS and ASD may display behavioral changes such as hyperactivity, inattention, irritability, and difficulties with self-regulation.
- *Sensory issues*: Children with LKS may demonstrate atypical responses to sensory input, such as being overly sensitive to certain sounds or touch. These sensory issues can be mistaken for the sensory processing challenges commonly associated with ASD.

Distinguishing between LKS and ASD requires a comprehensive evaluation by medical professionals, including neurologists, speech-language pathologists, and psychologists. The presence of seizures or abnormal EEG findings is a key differentiating factor for LKS. Additionally, language regression that occurs after previously acquiring language skills is characteristic of LKS but less common in ASD. Accurate diagnosis is crucial for appropriate management and intervention strategies, as LKS requires specific medical treatments, including antiepileptic medications and speech therapy targeted at language recovery.[24]

CASE HISTORY 2

An 8-year-old female child who was previously healthy and active and achieving all developmental milestones on time started having significant changes in his behavior, cognition, and overall functioning. She became increasingly irritable with difficulty concentrating, and started experiencing episodes of confusion and memory lapses. Her parents also observed motor abnormalities, such as tremors and uncoordinated movements. Concerned about these sudden changes, they sought medical help.

Medical Evaluation

She was referred to a pediatric neurologist for a comprehensive evaluation. The medical team conducted a thorough physical examination, neurological assessment, and ordered various diagnostic tests. In the work up certain blood and cerebrospinal fluid (CSF) tests were performed to check for specific autoantibodies associated with autoimmune encephalitis. Additionally, an EEG and magnetic resonance imaging (MRI) were done.

Diagnosis and Treatment

She was thereafter diagnosed with anti-NMDA receptor encephalitis based on his autoimmune markers which came positive for it and treatment involved a combination of immunotherapy and supportive care. An ultrasonography of the abdomen revealed an ovarian mass which on further investigations was an ovarian teratoma which was removed by the surgeon. She additionally needed antiepileptic medications to manage her seizures.

Progress and Follow-up

Following the initiation of treatment, her symptoms gradually started to improve. Her irritability decreased, and her cognition and her memory began to recover. The tremors and motor abnormalities also diminished over time.

Conclusion

- Autoimmune encephalitis can present with symptoms that mimic ASD, which can complicate the diagnostic process. Here are some ways in which autoimmune encephalitis can resemble autism:
- *Social communication and interaction*: Children with autoimmune encephalitis can present with challenges in social communication and interaction in form of poor understanding and limited use of social cues, decreased eye contact, and issues engaging in reciprocal conversations, similar to those seen in individuals with ASD.
- *Behavioral and cognitive changes*: Behavioral changes such as irritability, agitation, mood swings, sleep disturbances, hyperactivity, and difficulties with attention and concentration seen in both can lead to misinterpretation and potentially result in an initial diagnosis of ASD.
- *Language impairments*: Individuals with autoimmune encephalitis may also experience language impairments further complicating the diagnostic process.
- *Sensory processing issues*: Individuals with autoimmune encephalitis may exhibit atypical responses to sensory input, similar to individuals with ASD.
- Distinguishing between autoimmune encephalitis and ASD apart from strong clinical suspicion requires specific diagnostic tests such as serum and CSF autoantibody analysis. The sudden onset of symptoms, rapid progression, and associated neurological findings may suggest autoimmune encephalitis rather than a developmental disorder like ASD.[25]

CASE HISTORY 3

A 7-year-old girl who was a previously healthy and active child and suddenly started experiencing difficulty walking, slurring of speech, and appeared weak on one side of her body. Symptoms were subacute and progressed over few months. Concerned about these changes, they sought medical attention.

Medical Evaluation

Apart from a thorough physical examination and neurological assessment, imaging studies, such as MRI of the brain and spine, were performed to identify any structural abnormalities. Various blood tests were run to check for specific antibodies associated with autoimmune and paraneoplastic syndromes.

Diagnosis and Treatment

She was detected with a neuroblastoma and thereafter treatment involved a multidisciplinary approach. She was referred to an oncologist and an oncosurgeon for subsequent management.

Prognosis and Follow-up

Simultaneously, she received supportive care to manage her paraneoplastic syndrome symptoms. This involved corticosteroids and other immunosuppressive medications. Her weakness and difficulty walking diminished over time, and her speech became clearer over time.

Conclusion

Paraneoplastic syndromes though a group of rare disorders typically manifest with various neurological symptoms, there have been rare cases where these syndromes mimic symptoms of ASD. Here are some common resembling symptoms.
- *Social and behavioral changes*: Paraneoplastic syndromes can sometimes cause social and behavioral changes such as difficulties in social interactions, communication, and behavior regulation, similar to individuals with ASD.
- *Cognitive impairments*: Some paraneoplastic syndromes can lead to cognitive impairments, such as recall/memory issues, concerns with executive function deficits, and inattention. These cognitive impairments can overlap with some of the cognitive challenges seen in individuals with ASD.
- *Language and communication difficulties*: Children with paraneoplastic syndromes can exhibit expressive or receptive language impairments, difficulties with verbal expression, and trouble understanding and using social cues which overlap with those seen in ASD.

It is important to note that while although there have been rare instances where paraneoplastic syndromes mimic symptoms of ASD, the vast majority of individuals with ASD do not have an underlying paraneoplastic syndrome. But it is crucial to consider it as an autism mimic as early detection and treatment of paraneoplastic syndromes is of utmost importance.

CASE HISTORY 4

A 4-year-old boy child was referred for developmental delay particularly for concerns about her speech and motor skills. His birth history was unremarkable along with no significant complications reported during pregnancy. He started walking around 2 years of age but still had poor coordination and balance. He was noted to have significant speech impairments and did not use any meaningful words. He always had a happy sociable demeanor, often smiling and laughing. However, he also showed signs of hyperactivity along with frequent hand flapping and repetitive movements.

Medical History

During the evaluation, it was discovered that he had a history of seizures in form of episodes of brief staring spells and occasional generalized tonic-clonic seizures.

Diagnosis and Treatment

After a detailed physical examination and developmental assessment, an EEG was done in view of history of seizures. The results showed the presence of a characteristic pattern of slow waves and spikes which was suspicious of Angelman syndrome (**Fig. 2**).

Genetic Testing

Based on the clinical presentation and EEG findings, genetic testing was conducted to confirm the diagnosis. A deletion of the *UBE3A* gene on chromosome 15 was identified, confirming the diagnosis of Angelman syndrome.

Follow-up and Progress

A multidisciplinary approach to address his specific needs included speech and OT along with antiepileptic medication to manage his seizures.

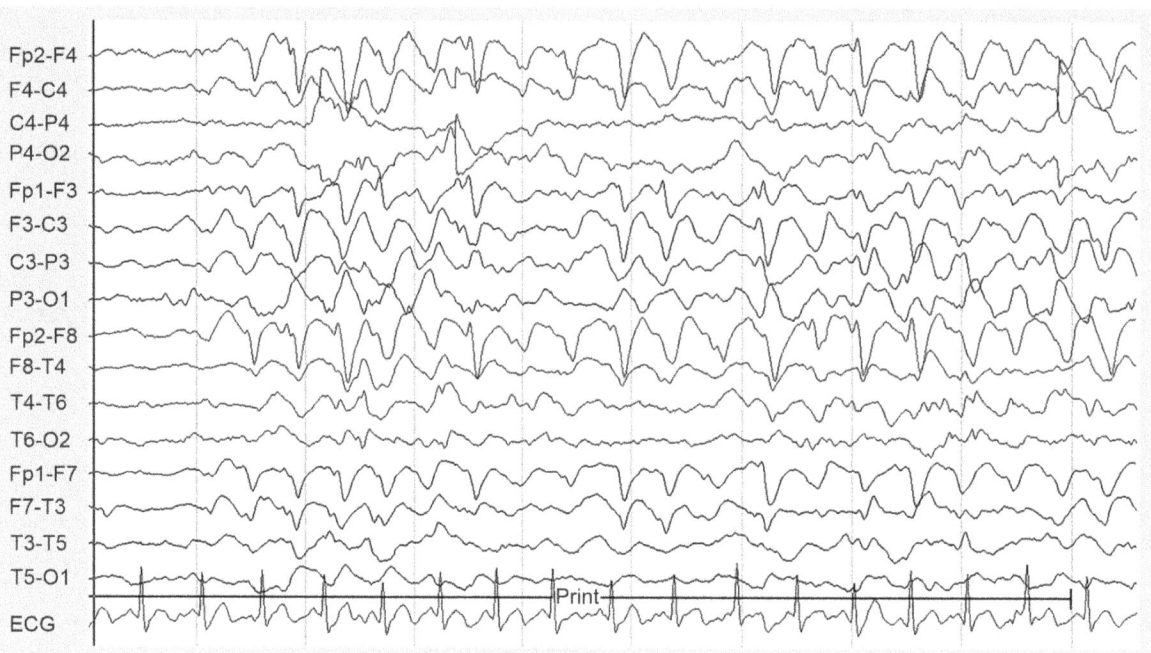

FIG. 2: Electroencephalogram (EEG) in Angelman syndrome.

Conclusion

Both children with Angelman syndrome and those with ASD exhibit repetitive behaviors like hand flapping or body rocking along with restricted interests. Individuals with Angelman syndrome typically have severe speech impairments, with little to no functional speech (usually less than five words) and often rely on nonverbal communication methods unlike children with ASD who though delayed can develop speech gradually over time. Clinical suspicion and recognition of typical syndromic features and timely genetic testing are crucial for early diagnosis and management.[26]

CASE HISTORY 5

A 6-year-old boy child was noted to not meet his developmental milestones at the expected age with symptoms of delayed speech and language development. He also struggled with his fine and gross motor skills, and exhibited difficulties in social interactions. Concerned about his slow progress, his parents sought medical assistance.

Medical Evaluation

After a detailed physical examination and developmental assessment various diagnostic tests in form of neuroimaging, metabolic and genetic tests were performed.

Diagnosis and Treatment

Magnetic resonance imaging findings were unremarkable but magnetic resonance spectroscopy (MRS) revealed an absent to significantly decreased creatine peak in the brain and hence he was suspected with having a cerebral creatine deficiency syndrome (CCDS). Further genetic testing revealed a mutation in the *SLC6A8* gene, which is responsible for the impaired transport of creatine in the brain.

Treatment for him involved creatine supplementation to address the deficiency. He was prescribed a specific dosage of creatine to be taken orally under medical supervision. The creatine supplementation aimed to enhance brain energy metabolism and support cognitive and neurological development.

Progress and Follow-up

Following the initiation of treatment and therapy gradual improvements in his speech and social abilities was noted improved with enhanced coordination and increased independence in daily activities.

Conclusion

Cerebral creatine deficiency syndromes are a group of rare genetic disorders characterized by impaired transport or synthesis of creatine in the brain. These syndromes can lead to neurological symptoms that may mimic ASD. Here

are some ways in which cerebral creatine deficiency can resemble autism:
- *Language and communication difficulties*: Children with CCDS may have delayed speech development or expressive language difficulties like in individuals with ASD.
- *Social interaction and behavioral changes*: The social and behavioral changes which are the core symptoms of ASD can be seen in these children.
- *Cognitive impairments*: Cerebral creatine deficiency can cause cognitive impairments, including ID, deficits in attention and executive functioning, and learning difficulties.
- *Sensory abnormalities*: Sensory processing issues, such as sensory sensitivities or aversions to certain stimuli, may be present in individuals with CCDS, similar to individuals with ASD.

Distinguishing between cerebral creatine deficiency and ASD requires a strong clinical suspicion and awareness of the condition to determine if cerebral creatine deficiency is present along with radiological (especially MRS) and genetic confirmation. Early detection and intervention for CCDS can help improve outcomes and prevent further neurological impairments.

INVESTIGATIONS TO RULE OUT NEUROLOGICAL CONDITIONS PRESENTING AS AUTISM SPECTRUM DISORDER

As seen from the clinical briefings above it is pivotal to evaluate any child with symptoms of autism to rule out other neurological disorders that may present with similar features. The specific investigations can vary depending on the individual's clinical presentation and symptoms. Mentioned below are some common investigations that may be considered to help rule out neurological disorders:

Genetic Testing

Genetic tests such as whole exome sequencing (WES) and chromosomal microarray analysis (CMA) are very commonly done now in view of their availability and decreasing costs which have helped to identify various genetic disorders and also genetic reasons for autism itself. Numerous genetic syndromes may present with autism-like symptoms. Few examples include Fragile X syndrome, Angelman syndrome, Rett syndrome, and Phelan–McDermid syndrome, etc., to name a few.[27]

Metabolic Screening

Blood and urine tests for abnormalities in amino acids, organic acids, lysosomal enzymes, or mitochondrial function can be conducted to evaluate for metabolic disorders that can present with autistic features. A thyroid screening to rule out hypothyroidism is a must in all cases.

Hearing Test

In all children with ASD, a hearing assessment is a must at the first consultation itself as hearing impairment leading to speech delay cannot be missed at any cost.

Serological Testing

Testing for auto antibodies in serum and CSF is necessary to rule out autoimmune encephalitis when suspected in appropriate settings.

Electroencephalogram

Epileptic encephalopathies which can present at various ages usually present with seizures and autistic symptoms and EEG helps in treating the seizures. It should be noted that neither is there any role for performing an EEG in all patients with ASD nor all incidental EEG abnormalities in children with ASD should be treated. The child should be investigated and treated if has clinical seizures or rarely for acute regression after normal development with EEG abnormalities.

Brain Imaging

Structural brain imaging, such as MRI, can help identify any anatomical abnormalities or structural brain lesions that may be causing autistic symptoms along with spectroscopy (MRS) helps in evaluating the metabolite peaks in the brain in conditions such as cerebral creatine deficiencies. Functional imaging techniques, such as functional MRI (fMRI) or positron emission tomography (PET) can provide additional insights into brain function and connectivity in selected cases.

Last but not the least a consultation with a pediatric neurologist or developmental pediatrician experienced in neurodevelopmental disorders can help to guide the evaluation and recommend further investigations based on the individual's specific symptoms and clinical presentation to rule out other neurological disorders.

CONCLUDING REMARKS AND LEARNING POINTS

- Autism is a spectrum and no two patients will have the same combination of features.
- To understand autism, it is important to know how it affects individuals, as the range of symptoms and behaviors can be quite diverse, making it challenging to pinpoint a specific set of characteristics.

- Associations with ASD range from epilepsy, ADHD, movement disorders such as stereotypies and tics, ID, sensory processing issues, anxiety, and other behavioral concerns.
- It is important to know that several disorders may mimic autistic symptoms. It is pivotal to not miss them, especially the treatable ones.
- ASD is ideally diagnosed before 3 years of age. All children who exhibit ASD features after a period of normal development must be thoroughly investigated.
- Any child with ASD features along with dysmorphisms, we must rule out syndromes/genetic etiologies.
- ASD presenting with epilepsy with no perinatal history or MRI abnormality should be evaluated for genetic causes.
- Metabolic causes, though rare, can occasionally be treated and thus should be investigated in appropriate clinical settings.

REFERENCES

1. American Psychiatric Association. Diagnostic and statistical manual of mental disorders, 5th ed. Arlington: American Psychiatric Publishing, 2013.
2. Hodges H, Fealko C, Soares N. Autism spectrum disorder: Definition, epidemiology, causes, and clinical evaluation. Transl Pediatr. 2020;9(Suppl 1):S55-65.
3. Levy SE, Mandell DS, Schultz RT. Autism. The Lancet. 2009;374 (9701):1627-38.
4. Lai MC, Lombardo MV, Baron-Cohen S. Autism. The Lancet. 2014;383(9920):896-910.
5. Amaral DG, Schumann CM, Nordahl CW. Neuroanatomy of autism. Trends Neurosci. 2008;31(3):137-45.
6. Belmonte MK, Allen G, Beckel-Mitchener A, Boulanger LM, Carper RA, Webb SJ. Autism and abnormal development of brain connectivity. J Neurosci. 2004;24(42):9228-31.
7. Courchesne E, Pierce K. Why the frontal cortex in autism might be talking only to itself: Local over-connectivity but long-distance disconnection. Curr Opin Neurobiol. 2005;15(2): 225-30.
8. Müller RA, Fishman I. Brain connectivity and neuroimaging of social networks in autism. Trends in Cognitive Sciences. 2008;12(10):403-12.
9. Zoghbi HY, Bear MF. Synaptic dysfunction in neurodevelopmental disorders associated with autism and intellectual disabilities. Cold Spring Harb Perspect Biol. 2012;4(3):a009886.
10. Muller CL, Anacker AM, Veenstra-VanderWeele J. The serotonin system in autism spectrum disorder: From biomarker to animal models. Neuroscience. 2016;321:24-41.
11. Coghlan S, Horder J, Inkster B, Mendez MA, Murphy DG, et al. GABA system dysfunction in autism and related disorders: From synapse to symptoms. Neurosci Biobehav Rev. 2012;36(9), 2044-55.
12. Ronemus M, Iossifov I, Levy D, Wigler M. The role of de novo mutations in the genetics of autism spectrum disorders. Nat Rev Genet. 2014;15(2):133-41.
13. Geschwind DH, State MW. Gene hunting in autism spectrum disorder: On the path to precision medicine. Lancet Neurol. 2015;14(11):1109-20.
14. Hara, H. Autism and epilepsy: A retrospective follow-up study. Brain Dev. 2017;39(4):318-24.
15. Stefanatos GA, Grover W. An update on autism and childhood epilepsy: What is the relationship? Curr Deve Disord Rep. 2020;7(4):263-9.
16. Ekstein D, Glick B, Weill M, Kay B. Epilepsy and autism spectrum disorder: An epidemiological study. J Child Neurol. 2020;35(14):970-3.
17. Gabis LV, Kesner-Baruch Y, Feldman R, Brezner A. Developmental epilepsy in autism spectrum disorder: Prevalence and risk factors. J Child Neurol. 2021;36(4);296-303.
18. Ghosh A, Lai MC. Understanding the association between autism and intellectual disability: A scoping review. Front Psychiatry. 2020;11:956.
19. Antshel KM, Zhang-James Y, Wagner KE, Ledesma A, Faraone SV. An update on the comorbidity of ADHD and ASD: A focus on clinical management. Exp Rev Neurother. 2016;16(3):279-93.
20. Martini R, Battaglia, MA, Rizzello A. Motor skills assessment in children with autism spectrum disorders: A critical review. Euro J Paediatr Neurol. 2018;22(2):232-41.
21. Nickels KC, Wirrell EC. Electrical status epilepticus in sleep: Mimicry of autism spectrum disorders and other childhood neuropsychiatric disorders. Pediatric Neurol. 2008;39(6):419-23.
22. Chen MH, Lan WH, Hsu JW, Huang KL, Su TP, Li CT, et al. Risk of developing tic disorders in children with autism spectrum disorder: A nationwide population-based cohort study. J Autism Dev Disord. 2019;49(4):1394-402.
23. Leyfer OT, Folstein SE, Bacalman S, Davis NO, Dinh E, Morgan J, et al. Comorbid psychiatric disorders in children with autism: Interview development and rates of disorders. Journal of Autism and Developmental Disorders. 2006;36(7):849-61.
24. Schaaf RC, Lane AE. Toward a best-practice protocol for assessment of sensory features in ASD. J Autism Dev Disord. 2015;45(5):1380-95.
25. Leypoldt F, Armangue T, Dalmau J. Autoimmune encephalopathies. Ann N Y Acad Sci. 2019;1456(1):48-61.
26. Peters SU, Beaudet AL. Autism spectrum disorder in individuals with Angelman syndrome. Am J Med Genet Part C.2019;181(1): 104-14.
27. Bartnik M, Derwińska K. Genetic testing in children with autism spectrum disorder—Current recommendations and challenges. Pharmaceuticals. 2020;13(10):330.

CHAPTER 28

Hyperventilation Syndrome, Panic Disorders, and Related Conditions

Debasish Roy, Ambar Chakravarty

■ HYPERVENTILATION SYNDROME

Hyperventilation (HV) syndrome is defined *"as a syndrome characterized by a variety of somatic symptoms induced by physiologically inappropriate HV and usually reproduced in whole or in part by voluntary HV"*.[1] William Gower in his book Borderland of Epilepsy[2] conceptualized the occurrence of "vagal attacks" which included cases who most likely had HV—*"The symptoms comprehend subjective gastric, respiratory, and cardiac discomfort... often combined with a slight mental change (difficulty in thinking or concentrating) and also disturbance of the vasomotor center, causing constriction of the vessels and coldness, especially of the extremities. Associated with the latter may be some sensory impairment and a form of slight tetanoid spasm... Women suffer more frequently."*

The HV syndrome is characterized by a habit of hyperventilating, breathing in excess of the metabolic needs of the body, eliminating more carbon dioxide causing respiratory alkalosis and elevated blood pH. While this becomes particularly marked in presence of a psychosocial stress or any emotional triggers, certain organic pathologies may also be implicated. This is a very common clinical syndrome, producing myriads of clinical symptoms, while the underlying problem is often missed. On occasions, especially when the alkalosis is severe, motor manifestations might occur and the condition mistaken for epileptic seizure. More commonly; however, HV attacks are mistaken for panic attacks with which it often coexists.[1,3-9]

To further complicate matters, HV can precipitate seizures due to hypocalcemia produced by systemic alkalosis. HV is used as an activating procedure during conduction of an electroencephalogram (EEG).

Clinical Manifestations

The term HV was coined by Kerr, Dalton, and Gliebe in 1937,[10] who described a variety of clinical symptoms caused by a physical phenomenon precipitated by anxiety states and these could be reproduced in the clinic by the HV test. Further observations over the years revealed myriads of physical phenomena which may be summarized as follows:[1,3-11]

- *General*: Fatiguability, exhaustion, weakness, sleep disturbance, nausea, and sweating
- *Cardiovascular*: Chest pain, palpitation, tachycardia, and Raynaud's phenomenon
- *Gastrointestinal*: Aerophagia, dry mouth, pressure in throat, dysphagia, globus hystericus, epigastric fullness or pain, belching, and flatulence
- *Neurologic*: Headache, pressure in head, fullness in head, head warmth, blurred vision, tunnel vision, momentary flashing lights, diplopia, dizziness, faintness, giddiness, unsteadiness, tinnitus, numbness, tingling coldness of face, extremities and trunk, muscle spasms, muscle stiffness, carpopedal spasms, generalized tetany, tremor, ataxia, weakness, syncope, and seizures.
- *Psychologic*: Impairment of concentration and memory, feeling of unreality, disorientation, confusion and dream-like state, déjà vu, hallucinations, anxiety, apprehension, nervousness, tension, fits of crying, agoraphobia, neuroses, phobia, and panic.
- *Respiratory*: Shortness of breath, suffocating feeling, smothering spell, inability to get a good breath or breathe deeply enough "sighing dyspnea", and yawning.

Illustrative Cases

Case 1

A 19-year-old girl with history of idiopathic generalized seizures was referred for re-evaluation because of uncontrolled seizures. The seizure started when she was 19 years old and it did not cause complete loss of consciousness but she had post-ictal sleepiness. It was interpreted as a generalized seizure. An EEG done then showed high voltage sharp and slow waves, especially during HV. She was subsequently treated with varying doses of phenobarbitone, phenytoin, carbamazepine, and sodium valproate because of poor control of seizures. The initial and repeat EEGs on being reviewed was found to be normal, showing only a normal degree of high voltage slow activity induced by HV. In most of the attacks, she fell and became rigid, with wrists and hands flexed and turned outward. She sometimes slept after the spells, but most often her mother noted that she was irritable, sweating, and breathing more deeply. She underwent video-telemetric EEG study, which clearly showed that rapid deep breathing and high voltage slow waves on EEG occurred together during her typical spells. When overbreathing and slow waves were seen on telemetry monitor, she was asked to rebreathe in a paper bag and her symptoms remitted completely.

Case 2

A 40-year-old man presented with near fainting episodes. He had been having such spells almost daily for the past 2 months. The spells lasted about 1-2 minutes during which he would feel lightheaded and sweat and felt that he might pass out and fall from his seat in his office. There had been no history of shortness of breath, heavy breathing, or chest pain. He had been investigated by a physician previously and his electrocardiogram (ECG), chest X-ray, and EEG were all normal. In the clinic, a HV Test was performed and his symptoms were reproduced. Detailed enquiry revealed that his work performance had not been very satisfactory and he had been warned by his boss that he might lose his job. He was very anxious about that and had not been sleeping well.

He was counseled by a professional counselor and was taught to terminate the faint like spells either by holding his breath or breathing into a paper bag.

Case 3

A 20-year-old girl presented with some 3 years history of spells characterized by feeling strange and confused for about 5-6 minutes during which she also felt a tingling sensation in her left side. She never lost consciousness and had no motor phenomena ever. Initial clinical impression had been one of focal seizure likely of temporal lobe origin. EEG studies done on two occasions were essentially normal and HV activation revealed some degree of slowing. She was started on carbamazepine after she had a normal magnetic resonance imaging (MRI) of brain. She continued to have these spells two to three times a week in spite of increasing the dosage of carbamazepine to 900 mg/day. A 24 hours video EEG (VEEG) was done which again was normal. Once she complained of chest tightness which prompted doing a HV test. The symptoms of strange feeling along with left sided paresthesia were reproduced after about 8 minutes of HV. This was terminated by asking her to breathe in a paper bag. She was taught to do the same whenever she would have a spell which worked and the antiepileptic was gradually tailed off. Detailed interview revealed significant degree of anxiety out of her differences of opinion with her parents regarding her marriage. She was asked to see a counselor.

Case 4

A 25-year-old woman was seen when she complained of tightness in her chest and feeling out of breath several times a day for past 5 days. She was initially seen in the emergency room (ER) where her ECG and chest X-ray were normal. She had a resting tachycardia and a fine tremor of hands. HV for 5 minutes reproduced her symptoms but breathing into a paper bag did not terminate her HV fully and she continued to hyperventilate stopping only briefly when the paper bag was applied over her mouth. This continued for about 30 minutes when she developed early carpopedal spasm. A slow intravenous (IV) injection of calcium gluconate was given under ECG monitoring and soon her HV was terminated as well as the carpopedal spasm. It appeared that an altercation with her husband precipitated the episode. Both of them were asked to see a counselor.

The last two cases merit some comments. Case 3 poses a difficult diagnostic problem namely distinguishing between HV spell and a focal seizure. EEG, even done for a prolonged period, can be normal interictally and may even be normal ictally, in cases of focal seizures depending on the location and depth from surface of the seizure focus. Case 3 is really lies in the borderland between epilepsy and paroxysmal nonepileptic events.

In Case 4, the distinction needed to be made between HV spell and panic attack. However, these two conditions may often overlap in the same patient. This probably happened in this particular case as well. The resting tachycardia and fine hand tremor were likely related to an underlying panic disorder. Case 4 also highlights another practical issue in conducting a HV test in a clinic namely the somewhat uncommon possibility of totally terminating a HV attack by using a paper bag for the patient to breathe in and out in the bag to raise the CO_2 level in the inspired air. In the present case, this probably happened due to the co-occurrence of both HV and panic disorder simultaneously.

Interestingly in some subjects, HV may be a "bad habit" of exaggerated thoracic breathing, with spells triggered by emotional disturbances that induce increased ventilation thus producing symptoms causing anxiety about the symptoms and a vicious cycle of sympathetic arousal which causes increased ventilation and increased symptoms.[11]

Case 5

A 45-year-old lady presented with history of having brief spells several times a day for past 3 weeks when she felt dizzy and had tingling sensations over her lips, left half of face, and left upper and lower limbs. There was no alteration of consciousness and she could talk and carry on with whatever she had been doing during such spells. Only she felt a little worried because of these symptoms. She had bipolar disorder and had been on Lithium' Divalproate and a selective serotonin reuptake inhibitor (SSRI). She had no neurological deficit but was found to be hypertensive for which no medication was prescribed. She had been extensively investigated by another neurologist and all test results were normal.

A HV test for 3 minutes reproduced all her symptoms and she was taught the technique of breathing in a paper bag to terminate her spells. The problem was discussed with her family as well as her treating psychiatrist and at 3 months follow-up, she was free of these spells.

This was indeed a difficult problem to start with. The differentials were multiple and included diverse pathologies namely transient ischemic attacks (TIAs), focal seizures, multiple sclerosis, and somatoform disorder. Detailed investigations excluded all the organic brain pathologies mentioned. The HV test clinched the diagnosis.

Apart from the organic pathologies mentioned earlier, the psychiatric differential diagnoses of such spells include agoraphobia, panic attacks, somatization, generalized anxiety, post-traumatic stress disorder, and psychotic disorders. Panic disorder patients may have an increased sensitivity to the vasoconstrictive effect of basilar artery blood flow by the HV-induced hypocapnia (which may cause the sensory symptoms) and some may have hypersensitive CO_2 chemoreceptors which perpetuate the HV syndrome.[12,13]

Etiology and Pathophysiology

Lowry's book *"Hyperventilation and Hysteria"* published in 1967[14] divides the conditions producing HV syndrome into four categories namely organic (neurological), physiological, emotional, and habit.

Neurological Causes[15]

Conditions causing HV syndrome have been described to occur in Rett's syndrome, Joubert's syndrome, Reye's syndrome, pyruvate dehydrogenase deficiency syndrome, biotin-dependent multiple carboxylase deficiency, malignant hyperthermia, brainstem tumors, primary cerebral lymphoma, encephalitis, brainstem strokes, thalamic hemorrhage, syringobulbia, and neurogenic pulmonary edema due to raised intracranial pressure. In all cases of HV syndrome presenting in the ER, it is essential to exclude bronchial asthma and pulmonary embolism (PE). Checking arterial oxygen saturation (SaO_2) with a pulse oximeter is simple but highly useful.

Illustrative Case

Some 10 years back, a 55-year-old professor of Chemistry in USA (cousin brother of the present author) while shaving in the morning had a black out and fell down. Consciousness returned within a few minutes but he had been having breathing difficulty. His wife called the paramedics who arrived shortly. Some of them seeing the gentleman hyperventilating, started laughing and asked him whether he was anxious and tensed up. A young lady paramedic did not join others but quickly brought out a pulse oximeter and shouted that SaO_2 was down to 78% and mentioned that the subject must have got a PE. He was rushed to hospital where ECG and angiography confirmed the diagnosis and he had an emergency pulmonary embolectomy. A mesh umbrella was inserted in the inferior vena cava to prevent further embolization and he was anticoagulated. Later it was found that two days back, he took a flight for over 5 hours, during which he slept continuously in his seat without moving his legs at all.

Physiologic Causes

True physiological HV with lowering of arterial partial pressure of carbon dioxide (pCO_2) occurs during heavy unaccustomed exercise, at high altitude before acclimatization, during high fever and on exposure to heat, in otherwise healthy individuals.

Emotion and Habit

Reports linking HV and anxiety emotions can be traced as far back as the 16th century. During the last several decades, research has been carried out into breathing in psychiatric disorders but truly speaking there had been only few studies in psychiatric literature focusing on the HV syndrome. Though generally believed that HV occurs as a response to anxiety, currently it is felt that HV in reality is due to a bad breathing habit. Whatever the case might be, the distress experienced by patients who hyperventilate may by themselves cause anxiety and exacerbate the HV, and thus sets up a vicious circle. This becomes fully established by the time the patient is seen by a doctor.

The Oxford English Dictionary defines the word *"sigh"* as *"deep audible breath expressing sadness, weariness,..."*

Charles Darwin[16] in connection with body's reaction to fear and anxiety, wrote: *"Men during numberless generations, have endeavoured to escape from their enemies or danger by headlong flight, or by violently struggling with them; and such great exertions will cause the heart to beat rapidly, the breathing to be hurried, the chest to heave, and the nostrils to be dilated."* He later mentioned *"And now, whenever the emotion of fear is strongly felt, though it may not lead to any exertion, the same results tend to reappear, through the force of inheritance and association."*

Canon[17] made similar observations in his book "Bodily Changes in Pain, Hunger, Fear and Rage" as *"And one of the most characteristic reactions of animals in pain and emotional excitement is deep and rapid respiration. Again the reflex response is precisely what would be most serviceable to the organism in the strenuous efforts of fighting or escape that might accompany or follow distress or fear or rage."*

Christie[18] in 1935, on basis of spirometric studies in subjects with respiratory symptoms with no clinical signs, identified two groups:

1. Those with neurosis presenting with chest pain, palpitation, breathlessness, and sweating all being worse with exercise, and
2. Those with "conversion hysteria", complained of being unable to get enough air into their lungs with a sensation of oppression and suffocation. These patients hyperventilated and the spirogram showed deep sighing respiration. Other workers also noted that some emotionally unstable persons tended to over-breathe with lowering of pCO_2.

Further spirometric studies in psychiatric patients by Finesinger and Mazick[19] revealed that sighing respiration occurred in 60% of patients with anxiety neurosis and 54% of patients with hysteria and reactive depression.

Somewhat similar observations[20,21] were made by other workers as well with some commenting that "neurotic women breathed thoracically and wondered if this might be for social reasons so as not to make the stomach protrude" while others reasoned that "respiratory patterns varied with emotional status and that complaints of dysfunction depended not solely on objective respiratory change but also on the attention the subject paid to his body".

In the 1960s, Dudley and his coworkers[22-24] noted that anxiety produces increased respiratory depth and rate with lowering of pCO_2 level whereas depression produced decrease in respiratory rate and depth similar to those that occur in sleep. However, somewhat opposing observations were made by others.

Damas Mora et al.[25] noted that neurotic and nonretarded endogenous depressives breathe faster and have a lower end-tidal pCO_2 than controls, whereas retarded endogenous depressives show an opposite deviation from the controls and schizophrenics, although they breathe faster, tend to have an increased pCO_2.

Few studies have addressed the psychiatric aspects of the HV syndrome. Most studies, quite rightly, had stressed on the development of the vicious cycle produced by anxiety induced HV which tends to increase the anxiety which in its turn perpetuates the HV.

Among military recruits, Lowry[14] found that those who hyperventilate felt themselves to be physically inferior, suffered from fear of heights and closed places and often had family history of cardiac and chest diseases. He felt that HV was not indicative of any one mode of adaptation or personality type.

Rice[26] on the other hand opined that overbreathing is indeed a habit and considered the HV syndrome in this light. Some workers like Lum[12] also subscribed to this view and stated that thoracic breathing, the hallmark of the HV syndrome, had been conditioned *"throughout schools, in physical training classes and in the Army. In men the posture is a symbol of virility and a warning against aggression."* In women, he stated,[12] it serves *"to draw attention to the bosom as a sexual come on"*. He thought the vicious cycle, referred earlier to be of much importance, and hence the habit is primary and the anxiety neurosis secondary. He felt HV syndrome occurs in obsessional people and in those with mild phobic traits but mentioned that <4% of his patients appear to be of primary psychogenic etiology. He did not approve of the diagnosis of anxiety neurosis in subjects with HV syndrome.[12]

The concept of the vicious cycle was well conceived by many and Lazarus and co-authors[27] stated that those who hyperventilate were "typically running scared", their anxiety so severe as to produce thanatophobia (fear of death), nosophobia (fear of having or developing a fatal illness), lyssophobia (fear of losing one's mind), and monophobia (fear of being alone). Some workers added agoraphobia to this list. Many thought that the precipitating factor leading to the initial attack of HV was anxiety about the loss or death of a loved one and that this had to be fully explored during treatment. The present author does not support this notion fully as several other factors might contribute to developing severe anxiety such as stress of education, stress at work place, and marital stress. The present author agrees with Tyrer[28] who felt that the HV syndrome lies at the *"somatic extreme of a somatic-psychic continuum of morbid anxiety."*

Physiological Effects of Hyperventilation[1,29-33]

Acute HV causes lowering of arterial pCO_2 and respiratory alkalosis. The latter produces the Bohr effect, i.e., a leftward shift of the oxygen dissociation curve. This results in increased binding of oxygen to hemoglobin which results in reduced oxygen delivery to tissues. The alkalosis causes hypocalcemia manifested as tetany with carpopedal spasm and even seizures. Hypophosphatemia may also result from altered glucose metabolism. In chronic HV, plasma HCO^- and K^+ levels decrease due increased renal loss. The cause of the vicious cycle discussed earlier is stress-induced hyperadrenergic state which causes β-adrenergic stimulation perpetuating the HV.

These biochemical changes produce alteration in cerebral blood flow (CBF). This accounts for the various neurologic symptoms[1,3-11] mentioned earlier resulting from reduced cerebral hypoperfusion. CBF is reduced in the order of 30–40% due to hypocapnia resulting from HV.

Brief period of HV is often used as an activation procedure during EEG recording. This causes slowing of the background and an increase in the amplitude (build up). This can, on occasions, unmask latent epileptiform activity, especially in cases of absence seizures. Generalized slowing also occurs in habitual hyperventilators. Mostly seen in children and young adults, a brainstem-mediated response to hypocarbia had been suggested but is doubted. The slowing disappears as soon as HV is stopped even when cerebral oxygenation and end-tidal volume CO_2 continue to remain low. Other metabolic factors may be contributory; one such factor is hypoglycemia.

Alkalosis and hypocalcemia cause muscle spasm and tetany. Associated hypophosphatemia may contribute toward such symptoms such as dizziness and paresthesia. This may also account for tiredness, poor concentration, and disorientation in chronic HV syndrome. A hyper-adrenergic state accounts for tachycardia, tremor, and sweating. Hypokalemia is the likely cause for muscle weakness and lethargy again in chronic cases.

Both central and peripheral mechanisms are likely to be involved in production of bilateral and unilateral paresthesia, although the exact mechanism is not certain. Extracellular reduction of Ca^{++} may cause neuronal/axonal hyperexcitability causing spontaneous firing which may manifest as paresthesia. It is difficult to explain the often noted unilateral sensory symptoms; this may be due to anatomic difference in the organization of the autonomic nervous system (ANS) between the two sides. Furthermore the cerebral hypoperfusion, discussed earlier, may be symmetric (bilateral symptom) or asymmetric (unilateral symptom). No definite angiographic proof of this hypothesis is available to date. It is also interesting to note that unilateral symptoms mostly affect the left side of body and/or the face. Why so? One hypothesis may be that the right hemisphere is generally more activated during stress and emotional arousal. However, this theory may not be totally evidence based.

Treatment of Hyperventilation Syndrome[34-36]

It is essential to exclude a secondary cause like neurological disease in all cases of HV syndrome. Secondly, the psychological status needs also to be looked into. Therapeutic approach includes counseling, breathing exercises, physiotherapy, and relaxation exercises. Rebreathing into a paper bag, though universally practiced, ideally should be discouraged (and often so by some neurologists/psychiatrists), because significant hypoxia and even death have been recorded in organic causes of HV syndrome. Furthermore in severely anxious subjects, it may not give adequate benefit due to persistence of the vicious cycle discussed earlier (Case 4). Simple reassurance along with explanation of how HV produces symptoms generally serves the purpose of terminating the spell. Physically compressing the upper chest and asking the patient to exhale maximally reduce the chance of hyperinflation of the lungs. Teaching the patient how to breathe abdominally, using the diaphragm more than the rib cage, often relieves the dyspnea and helps in correcting many of the associated symptoms.

Patients should ideally be in a recumbent position with one hand placed on the chest and the other on the abdomen. Usually the chest excursion is much greater than abdominal excursion. Patients must be gradually taught to decrease the chest excursion and increase the abdominal excursion. If the symptoms do not subside a short-acting benzodiazepine like lorazepam or alprazolam may be effective.

Long-term training with breathing retraining exercises can reduce the frequency of attacks. These exercises must be done twice daily under the supervision of a physiotherapist initially. These exercises can be supplemented with cognitive behavioural therapy (CBT). There is also some role of pharmacotherapy; SSRIs such as sertraline and S-citalopram are effective in chronic cases. Benzodiazepines should not be used long-term for fear of developing dependence. Treatment of the underlying psychiatric disorder, if any, must be given due attention.

Concluding Remarks

The HV syndrome is characterized by a habit of hyperventilating, breathing in excess of the metabolic needs of the body, eliminating more carbon dioxide causing respiratory alkalosis, and elevated blood pH. While this becomes particularly marked in presence of a psychosocial stress or any emotional triggers, certain organic pathologies may also be implicated. This is a very common clinical syndrome, producing myriads of clinical symptoms, while the underlying problem is often missed. On occasions, especially when the alkalosis is severe, motor manifestations might occur and the condition mistaken for epileptic seizure. More commonly; however, HV attacks are mistaken for panic attacks with which it often coexists.

PANIC DISORDERS

There is a lot of overlap between panic disorders and other medical conditions and a typical patient may visit several physicians before a correct diagnosis is made. As some of the symptoms mimic those in different types of epileptic seizures, they are often evaluated by neurologists and epileptologists. Proper differentiation of these types of disorders is necessary for correct treatment. This chapter aims to highlight the different aspects of panic disorders and panic attacks and its overlap with epilepsy and provides tips on how to differentiate one from the other.[37]

Panic attacks are characterized by an intense fear or discomfort which usually reaches its peak very fast, mostly only in a few minutes. There are many somatic accompaniments such as palpitations, chest discomfort, choking, dry mouth, shortness of breath, tingling and numbness of the extremities, and sense of derealization or depersonalization. Four of thirteen recognized symptoms must be present to constitute a panic attack.[38] These include:

1. Palpitations, pounding heart, or accelerated heart rate
2. Sweating
3. Trembling or shaking
4. Sensation of shortness of breath or smothering
5. Feeling of choking
6. Chest pain or discomfort
7. Nausea or abdominal distress
8. Feeling dizzy, unsteady, or faint
9. Derealization or depersonalization
10. Feeling of losing control or going crazy
11. Feeling of dying
12. Paresthesias
13. Chills or hot flushes

All of these symptoms do not occur together in all patients. Symptoms are usually very abrupt in onset usually lasting for about 5-30 minutes but may last longer. There are some patients who live in constant fear of these attacks and develop anticipatory anxiety and avoidance of specific situations to constitute a panic disorder. Agoraphobia is an overlapping disorder but defined separately by the Diagnostic and Statistical Manual of Mental Disorders, Fifth Edition of the American Psychiatric Association. It is defined as anxiety over experiencing a panic attack in a situation where it would be difficult to escape or get help. It leads to avoidance of such situations like driving a car or riding a bus.

Panic attacks are mainly daytime events but can also occur during sleep in a small subset of patients to constitute a nocturnal panic attack. There are a small group of patients who develop only nocturnal attacks. Most panic attacks occur suddenly and spontaneously but others occur as a result of a specific situation or trigger like driving or riding in a crowded bus. Patients develop anticipatory anxiety and avoid these situations. Patients with psychogenic nonepileptic seizure (PNES) report transient loss of consciousness associated panic symptoms more commonly than those with epilepsy or syncope. Although panic symptoms are reported infrequently by most patients with PNES, a composite symptom score, as developed by Rawlings et al.,[39] may contribute to the differentiation between PNES and the other two common causes of transient loss of consciousness.

Panic disorders affect about 2% of the population and are difficult to diagnose. They often visit different physicians before a correct diagnosis is made. They go on to develop physical disorders such as hypertension, migraine, peptic ulcers, irritable bowel syndrome, asthma, and can coexist with epilepsy. Panic disorder patients have a poor quality of life and may have comorbid depression and substance abuse.[40]

There are several theories to explain panic attacks. The behavioural theory suggests that the individual identities certain cues and triggers which precipitates an attack and as a conditioned reflex learns to avoid them.

The cognitive theory suggests that some physical symptoms are identified as life-threatening or dangerous and these precipitate unnecessary anxiety. As, for example, a mild increase in heart rate, may be identified as a potential serious illness which can cause death and can lead to fear of death and severe anxiety.

Some workers opine that panic attacks and panic disorders are due to imbalance and dysregulation of the different neurotransmitters. The norepinephrine and serotonergic systems are linked and connected to different brain nuclei and can play a role in the genesis of these disorders. This is further indirectly supported by the fact that the drugs used to treat these disorders act on the serotonergic and norepinephrine systems. Gamma-aminobutyric acid (GABA) is the main inhibitory neurotransmitter and the benzodiazepines act on these receptors. They also play a role and reduced activity of the GABAergic system may trigger attacks.[41] Glutamate is the main excitatory neurotransmitter and excessive activity of this is believed to trigger panic attacks. Some other substances like caffeine which is an adenosine agonist can trigger attacks in susceptible patients. Cholecystokinin can also be a trigger. Corticotropin-releasing factor can be associated with anxiety and panic disorders. Panic disorder patients are hypersensitive to carbon dioxide and lactate. Most panic disorder patients hyperventilate and have lower carbon dioxide levels and chronic metabolic alkalosis. From the neuroanatomical point, the locus coeruleus has been associated with anxiety, fear, and panic.[42] Recent interest is primarily on the amygdala and the adjacent hippocampus.[43] They have extensive afferent and efferent connections which can explain the multiple somatic symptoms that a patient with panic disorder experiences.

The amygdala and the hippocampus are also thought to play a key role in the genesis of certain types of epilepsies particularly the complex partial seizures (CPSs). The symptoms overlap and are difficult to differentiate.[44] Fear is a key component of both panic attacks and certain types of seizures as the same brain structures are involved in both disorders. There is also a similarity at the neurotransmitter level as both are associated with excessive activity of the excitatory ones like glutamate and the aminergic neurotransmitters and low activity of the inhibitory GABAergic system.

Without astute observation by experienced clinicians and help from EEG, particularly VEEG, the two conditions may resemble each other. However, some symptoms which are observed in seizures are absent in panic attacks such as motor automatisms, transient amnesia, urinary or fecal incontinence, convulsions, and loss of consciousness. Most panic attacks last from 5 to 30 minutes, but most uncomplicated seizures are <2 minutes in duration. Of note, HV in panic attacks can lead to carpal spasms that can be confused with dystonic posturing of seizures of temporal lobe origin.

Final means of differentiating the two conditions would rest on recording a normal ictal VEEG. It is often practiced procedure to reduce or withdraw completely the antiepileptic or sedative drug that the patient might had been on before doing VEEG with the idea that such withdrawal would bring to surface any latent epileptic feature that had not been seen in the interictal record. A note of caution is that abrupt or rapid discontinuation of benzodiazepines (which had been prescribed for treatment of presumed panic attacks) immediately before the VEEG study may precipitate the occurrence of panic attacks or epileptic seizures. Thus, the use of this medication should be slowly tapered before performing the VEEG study or lowered only slightly at the time of admission.

Panic attacks are usually treated by SSRIs or serotonin norepinephrine reuptake inhibitors (SNRIs). These drugs take time to act and adequate duration of therapy is needed before therapeutic response occurs. Benzodiazepines are effective for acute relief but long-term use is not recommended for the risk of drug abuse and dependence.[45] Medical therapy is often combined with CBT.[46] Combination therapy is more useful than either pharmacotherapy or CBT.[47] The role of behavioural therapy becomes very important when benzodiazepines are tailed off.

Panic disorders may be difficult to treat and may be refractory.[48] It causes physical and psychosocial impairment. Medical comorbidities are common and these patients usually have a poor quality of life. It may be difficult to withdraw medications but it must be tried if patients are symptom free for 6 months or longer. Some patients may have recurrence of symptoms on discontinuation of drugs and may need long-term or even lifetime therapy.

Concluding Remarks

Panic attacks are difficult to diagnose as there is considerable overlap with medical conditions where there is overlap of symptoms. Most notable of them is epilepsy where the two conditions may be difficult to differentiate. Proper identification is necessary for optimal therapy in these subsets of patients.

Panic attacks and panic disorders form a very important group of patients who are imitators of epilepsy. Proper history taking and clinical and psychological assessment complemented with appropriate investigations help in proper identification and treatment of these groups of disorders.

POTS AND PANIC: HOW ARE THEY RELATED AND MIMIC EPILEPTIC SEIZURE?

The previous two sections discuss panic attacks and HV syndrome, both being intimately related to each other and both may mimic epileptic seizure. Panic symptoms at times occur in epilepsy and syncope: Partial and complex partial epileptic seizures arising from the limbic system often generate auras with panic symptoms,[49] and such symptoms also commonly occur in syncope.[50] Additionally, often there are overlapping of presyncopal symptoms and autonomic manifestations of panic attacks. In some patients with PNES, increased levels of ictal panic symptoms have been reported. Other workers have postulated that PNES can be looked upon as "panic without panic" meaning absence of overt panic symptoms.[51] Panic symptoms often constitute an integral part of the HV syndrome. A vicious cycle is often generated with panic inducing HV which in turn worsens the panic symptoms. HV is often noted in PNES and may be used to induce a PNES in combination with suggestion. HV may precipitate seizures by lowering arterial pCO_2 with respiratory alkalosis and producing hypocalcemia. The last feature needs differentiation from true epileptic seizure. The inter-relation of the four conditions (panic attack, PNES, syncope, and epilepsy) mentioned earlier is easily understandable.

Postural orthostatic tachycardia syndrome (POTS), a feature of orthostatic intolerance (OI), standing upright from sitting or lying position, can evoke symptoms, such as lightheadedness, headache, nausea, fatigue, cognitive deficits, and exercise intolerance, relieved by lying down. Development of such features constitutes OI. physical signs include marked changes in heart rate, blood pressure (BP), or respiration. POTS is a common form of chronic OI in which significant standing tachycardia is associated with OI symptoms in the absence of postural hypotension. Postural HV can occur in HV syndrome,[52] and is thought to be a psychologically induced event.[53] Their inter-relationship can be like this: HV is present in many but not all patients with panic disorder, and postural stress may trigger onset of panic symptoms, including HV.[54] HV is ventilation out of proportion to metabolic demand, as a result partial pressure of arterial carbon dioxide ($PaCO_2$) falls and a respiratory alkalosis develops.

Dyspnea, HV, and hypocapnia, in the absence of significant heart and/or lung pathology, can occur in POTS in the form of postural hypocapnic hyperpnea.[55] Scientists have observed hypocapnic hyperpnea in POTS in response to a rapid orthostasis on a tilt table resulting in decrease in cardiac output (CO) and CBF[55] during poikilocapnic (uncontrolled CO_2) experiments. Poikilocapnic HV results in sinus tachycardia[56] and hypocapnia reduces CBF. Interestingly scientists have recently demonstrated that postural hypocapnic hyperpnea can cause POTS, rather than resulting from POTS as had been mentioned earlier.[55] It seems that ischemia of the carotid body ("stagnant hypoxia")[55] is the principal mechanism in the genesis of HV and this results primarily from low CO resulting from orthostasis and secondarily from sympathetic vasoconstriction of the artery to the carotid body, also the result of orthostasis.[55,56]

Concluding Remarks

Postural orthostatic tachycardia syndrome, a feature of OI, standing upright from sitting or lying position, can evoke symptoms, such as lightheadedness, headache, nausea, fatigue, cognitive deficits, and exercise intolerance, relieved by lying down. Development of such features constitutes OI.

The inter-relationship of POTS, panic, and HV revolves round orthostasis resulting in lowering of CO and sympathetic hyperactivity. POTS usually does not cause loss of consciousness resulting in drop attacks, unless associated with vasovagal syncope. Superimposition of panic symptoms in such cases would closely resemble features of epileptic seizures with aura of panic attacks. Clinical differentiation of panic attacks and epileptic seizures had been discussed in the previous section.

A NOTE ON ICTAL FEAR (PANIC)

Illustrative Case: A Boy who Felt Panicky at Times!

A 6-year-old boy was brought to the clinic for consultation. Over the last fortnight, he had at least five to six attacks during which he would get up from whatever he had been doing and would run to his mother and clinch to her saying "*I am very scared, I am very scared*". This episode would last for about half a minute after which he would feel well; only on one occasion he was unresponsive for a minute or so but had no motor movements. When asked later, he could not specify exactly for which he felt so scared. He had no neurological deficit. Ictal EEG recording was not possible but the interictal record revealed left anterior temporal spikes. MRI revealed left-sided mesial temporal sclerosis (MTS). He needed combination of oxcarbazepine and lacosamide for total seizure control.

Ictal fear (IF) is a relatively common emotional aura, characterized by "*unprovoked fear without object of dread*" which spontaneously appears associated with epileptic discharges arising from any of the structures included in the limbic system controlling semotions.[57] It may be the singular manifestation of a simple partial seizure (focal aware seizure) or may be the initial expression of a CPS or focal unaware seizure having its origin from the mesial temporal region.[57] It classically manifests as a sudden feeling of extreme fear without any apparent cause or context, having no relation to a preceding causal perception or thought and may or may not proceed to a full blown epileptic seizure. The intensity is variable from feeling just a bit anxious to a feeling of intense panic or terror. The feeling lasts only for a short while, 30–60 seconds usually, but may be followed by other ictal features such as automatisms and impaired consciousness.[57-59] IF had been reported in epilepsies of extratemporal origin, but is commonly associated with seizures arising from mesial temporal lobe. Its overall prevalence is 15–20% in some recent studies.[57,58]

Brain structures included in the limbic system circuitry, especially the amygdala, the hippocampus, and the parahippocampal gyrus, are involved in the mechanism of inducing an aura of fearful perception. Electrical stimulation performed intraoperatively or during presurgical evaluation using intracranial depth electrodes[59] confirm the earlier mentioned notion. MRI have also demonstrated significant reduction in the volume of the amygdala in subjects with intractable temporal lobe seizures with IF compared with those without this feature.[60]

Oehl et al.[61] reported a patient with IF originating from the right occipital lobe that preceded the discharge from the amygdale. However, whether occipital cortex is also involved in emotional processing in humans, remains debatable.[62] Wang et al.,[63] using stereoelectroencephalography (SEEG), reported a rare case of epileptic seizure with lack of activation in amygdala during IF. Seizure onset in the left posterior brain areas was confirmed by simultaneously recording from the amygdala and the occipital cortex.

In view of the association between IF and its mesial temporal lobe origin, Feichtinger et al.,[59] studied a group of patients with refractory temporal lobe epilepsy (TLE) with temporal lobectomy to ascertain whether patients with IF were more likely to become seizure free after temporal lobe resection compared with those without IF. Their results indicated significantly higher seizure freedom rates in subjects who had experienced IF as an aura. Thus the importance of diagnosing auras with IF in selection of cases for surgical treatment can be highlighted for better surgical outcome.

Ictal fear must be distinguished from a panic attack, and correct identification as an epileptic aura is aided by subsequent ictal phenomena and also their much briefer duration compared to panic attacks. However, this distinction may be difficult if the aura of fear occurs in isolation, as the only manifestation of a seizure phenomenon.[64]

As stated earlier, the intensity of IF is variable, but at times, it is out of proportion to, and quite different from the usual apprehension which commonly occurs at the beginning of a seizure. Rarely it might resemble a real-life experience such as suddenly finding a stranger standing close behind, and may also be associated with an unpleasant psychic hallucination of past events. IF may be accompanied by symptoms and signs of autonomic activation (mydriasis, piloerection, tachycardia, and HV).[65] Also it may coexist with other auras such as epigastric aura, *jamais vu* like feeling, and depersonalization.

Ictal panic (like any other epileptic phenomenon) is a stereotypic paroxysmal event, whereas panic attacks may or may not be stereotypic, with variable semiologies. On the whole, patients with IF may remain partially or totally aware of their surroundings though they may report some degree of lack of full concentration during the ictus. With evolution of IF (aura) into a CPS, unawareness of surroundings develops. With such seizures arising from the mesial temporal region of the nondominant hemisphere, responsiveness may at times remain preserved. However, amnesia for all events which happened during that period develops. In contrast, in patients with panic attacks, consciousness and memory remain intact. The only exception is patients with sensation of impending doom or death, when they may feel totally detached from the surroundings.

Panic attacks and IF (panic) should need to be distinguished from several medical conditions, particularly rare disorders associated with paroxysmal cardiac arrhythmias.[66] These conditions include the Romano–Ward syndrome (most common form of congenital long QT syndrome), other forms of long QT syndrome, carcinoid syndrome, hypoglycemia, pheochromocytoma, and Cushing syndrome. Other conditions to consider include alcohol withdrawal or other sedating drug use withdrawal, illicit drug effects (amphetamines, cocaine, and marijuana-induced tachycardia), vertigo-related disorders, and asthma.

Children with IF are often thought to harbor sleep or psychiatric disorders, such as *pavor nocturnus*, panic attacks, and psychogenic reactions.[67-69] Cases reported in the literature suggest that for most patients with IF, their epilepsy was symptomatic and often intractable to medical therapy.

In a Japanese study reported by Akiyama et al.[70] of five children with IF, the ictal symptoms consisted of sudden fright, clinging to someone nearby, and subsequent impairment of awareness, often accompanied by complex visual hallucinations and psychosis-like picture. IF, in four patients, was conceived as a psychogenic disorder, by their parents. Ictal EEG, in three patients showed frontal onset of seizure, while the other two showed centrotemporal or occipital onsets. Two patients had seizure freedom at follow-up, while seizures continued in the other three children. One patient with seizure onset during infancy had a favorable outcome, which was considered to be compatible with a diagnosis of benign partial epilepsy with affective symptoms. In contrast to observations made by other workers mentioned earlier, the Japanese workers noted that IF was not always associated with a symptomatic cause or a poor seizure outcome. The need for early recognition had been stressed for favorable seizure outcome.

Concluding Remarks

Ictal fear/panic (like any other epileptic phenomenon) is a stereotypic paroxysmal event, whereas panic attacks may or may not be stereotypic, with variable semiologies. On the whole, patients with IF may remain partially or totally aware of their surroundings though they may report some degree of lack of full concentration during the ictus. With evolution of IF (aura) into a CPS, unawareness of surroundings develops.

INSULAR EPILEPSY

Insular epilepsy is a less recognized form of epilepsy, which may imitate other types of focal epilepsies. Because of the myriads of functions of the insula and its extensive connections to various areas of the brain, insular epilepsy may present with various types of ictal semiologies ranging from somatosensory, visceral, olfactory, gustatory, or vestibular features.[71] Depending on spread of epileptic discharges, insular seizures may also cause alteration of consciousness, dystonic posturing, complex motor behaviors, and even autonomic features. Such variability in seizure semiology makes recognition of insular epilepsy a challenge to clinicians and confirmation by noninvasive tests is always needed. MRI detection of an insular lesion is of great help to the clinician in confirming the diagnosis of insular epilepsy. Scalp EEG, especially VEEG findings help in lateralization of the seizure focus. Ictal single photon emission computed tomography (SPECT) and positron emission tomography (PET) studies may be helpful in small number of patients. Magnetoencephalography is of great help. Only semiological aspects of insular seizures will be discussed here. As the epileptogenic area often extends into the opercular area, such seizures are often termed as opercular-insular seizures. On the other hand, temporal lobe onset seizures, at times, extend into the insular area as well.

Back in early 1950s, Penfield[72] describing the semiology of insular epilepsy wrote *"the descriptions of the initial phenomenon are remarkably similar from case to case. A sensation begins in the epigastrium and rises to the throat after which consciousness usually disappears. The sensation may be sickening or pressing and may end in a feeling of choking."* He also reported a patient with *"recurring blank spells preceded by a feeling of numbness in hands and lips."*

Diagnosis of insular epilepsy was established in those days with the help of preoperative EEG, operative electrocorticography, direct visual inspection of the cortex at surgery, intraoperative electrical stimulation of the cortex after craniotomy under local anesthesia, and postoperative observation after focal cortical resection. With advent of MRI, more cases can be diagnosed and the seizure semiology can be further ascertained.

Penfield[72] recognized this complexity of seizure semiology and wrote *"it is not surprising that the results of stimulation of the insula are confusingly varied since it is surrounded by such a remarkable variety of functional areas;... it follows, too, that local epileptic discharges often produce a great variety of seizure patterns."* The insula not only can generate visceral sensory symptoms, which may masquerade as temporal lobe seizures, but also may present with somatosensory symptoms, mimicking parietal lobe epilepsy. Lastly, insular seizures may manifest complex motor behavior suggestive of frontal lobe epilepsy.[71,73]

- *Somatosensory auras*: Painful or nonpainful paresthesias involving large areas of limbs (mostly contralateral; may be ipsilateral or bilateral); trunk; face including perioral areas and pharynx; at times feeling of chocking or suffocation. These need differentiation from auras arising from primary somatosensory cortical area—involve large cutaneous nerve territories, rare bilateral distribution, absence of true Jacksonian march, and throat constriction/suffocating feeling.
- *Visceral auras*:
  - Viscerosensory—epigastric rising sensation, abdominal pain/fullness, chest tightness, and throat tightness/chocking.
  - Visceromotor—retching, borborygmi, and vomiting.
  - Both visceromotor and viscerosensory auras are often associated with vegetative and psychic symptoms such as dyspnea, fear, and panic. This association can be mistaken as mesial temporal lobe origin of the seizure. It may be noted that the anterior insula from where these visceral auras originate is intimately connected bidirectionally with the mesial temporal cortex. Hence, the difficulty in differentiation as epileptic discharges may pass rapidly either way. The only clinical clue is early alteration of awareness in TLE than insular onset seizures. Other accompaniments which may help in seizure characterization of insular seizure are co-occurrence of somatosensory, auditory, and vestibular auras like vertigo and autonomic auras such as piloerection and flushing.
- *Hypermotor seizures*: These seizures, characterized by mostly nocturnal occurrence of dystonic posturing of limbs and/or trunk, repetitive leg movements, body rocking, or pelvic thrusting, are generally of frontal lobar origin, especially orbitofrontal cortex. However, these may also arise from the anterior or posterior insular cortex. Even VEEG differentiation may be difficult as the ictal record may not reveal the focal onset of the seizure recorded with scalp electrodes. Again it is the co-occurrence of visceral, gustatory, auditory, or vestibular auras which can raise suspicion of insular origin of the seizure. However, such auras can be reported only rarely by a patient having a hypermotor seizure. Only intracranial EEG recording would help in differentiation. Possibly it is the spread of epileptic discharge from the insula to the frontal lobe that manifests as a hypermotor seizure.

- Two rare manifestations of insular epilepsy are gelastic seizures and ecstatic seizures. The former is classically associated with hypothalamic hamartoma and the latter is generally of temporal lobar in origin. Reflex somatosensory seizures may also occur in insular epilepsy.

Concluding Remarks

Insular epilepsy may present with various types of ictal semiologies ranging from somatosensory, visceral, olfactory, gustatory, or vestibular features. Depending on spread of epileptic discharges, insular seizures may also cause alteration of consciousness, dystonic posturing, complex motor behaviors, and even autonomic features. Such variability in seizure semiology makes recognition of insular epilepsy a challenge to clinicians and confirmation by noninvasive tests is always needed.

LEARNING POINTS

- The HV syndrome is characterized by a habit of hyperventilating, breathing in excess of the metabolic needs of the body, eliminating more carbon dioxide causing respiratory alkalosis and elevated blood pH. While this becomes particularly marked in presence of a psychosocial stress or any emotional triggers, certain organic pathologies may also be implicated.
- This is a very common clinical syndrome, producing myriads of clinical symptoms, while the underlying problem is often missed. On occasions, especially when the alkalosis is severe, motor manifestations might occur and the condition mistaken for epileptic seizure.
- Though most cases of HV attacks result from underlying generalized anxiety or depressive disorders, HV syndrome have been described to occur in Rett's syndrome, Joubert's syndrome, Reye's syndrome, pyruvate dehydrogenase deficiency syndrome, biotin-dependent multiple carboxylase deficiency, malignant hyperthermia, brainstem tumors, Primary cerebral lymphoma, encephalitis, brainstem strokes, thalamic hemorrhage, syringobulbia, and neurogenic pulmonary edema due to raised intracranial pressure. In all cases of HV syndrome presenting in the ER, it is essential to exclude bronchial asthma and PE. Checking SaO_2 with a pulse oximeter is simple but highly useful.
- Panic attacks are difficult to diagnose as there is considerable overlap with medical conditions where there is overlap of symptoms. Most notable of them is epilepsy where the two conditions may be difficult to differentiate. Proper identification is necessary for optimal therapy in these subset of patients.
- POTS, a feature of OI, standing upright from sitting or lying position, can evoke symptoms, such as lightheadedness, headache, nausea, fatigue, cognitive deficits, and exercise intolerance, relieved by lying down. Development of such features constitutes OI wherein while the heart rate increases significantly, postural hypotension does not occur.
- Ictal fear/panic (like any other epileptic phenomenon) is a stereotypic paroxysmal event, whereas panic attacks may or may not be stereotypic, with variable semiologies. On the whole, patients with IF may remain partially or totally aware of their surroundings though they may report some degree of lack of full concentration during the ictus.
- Insular epilepsy may present with various types of ictal semiologies ranging from somatosensory, visceral, olfactory, gustatory, or vestibular features.[71] Depending on spread of epileptic discharges, insular seizures may also cause alteration of consciousness, dystonic posturing, complex motor behaviors, and even autonomic features. Such variability in presentations makes clinical recognition difficult very often, needing ancillary help.

REFERENCES

1. Evans RW. Neurologic aspects of hyperventilation syndrome. Semin Neurol. 1995;15:115-25.
2. Gowers WR. The Borderland of Epilepsy. Edinburgh: Churchill Livingstone; 1907. pp. 18-21.
3. Morgan WP. Hyperventilation syndrome: a review. Am Ind Hyg Assoc J. 1983;44(9):685-9.
4. Radvila A. The hyperventilation syndrome. Schweiz Med Wochenschr. 1984;114(16):562-5.
5. Han JN, Stegen K, Simkens K, Cauberghs M, Schepers R, Van den Bergh O, et al. Unsteadiness of breathing in patients with hyperventilation syndrome and anxiety disorders. Eur Respir J. 1997;10(1):167-76.
6. Cowley DS, Roy-Byrne PP. Hyperventilation and panic disorder. Am J Med. 1987;83(5):929-37.
7. Hanna DE, Hodgens JB, Daniel WA Jr. Hyperventilation syndrome. Pediatr Ann. 1986;15(10):708-12.
8. Joorabchi B. Expression of the hyperventilation syndrome in childhood. Clin Ped. 1977;16:110-5.
9. Pincus JH, Tucker GJ. Behavioral Neurology. Oxford: Oxford University Press; 1985. pp. 287-92.
10. Kerr WJ, Dalton JW, Gliebe PA. Some physical phenomena associated with the anxiety states and their relation to hyperventilation. Ann Int Med. 1937;11:961-91.

11. Lewis BI. The hyperventilation syndrome. Ann Int Med. 1953;38:918-27.
12. Lum LC. Hyperventilation: The tip and the iceberg. J Psychosom Res. 1975;19:325-83.
13. Pfeffer JM. The etiology of hyperventilation syndrome. Psychother Psychosom. 1978;30:47-55.
14. Lowry TP. Hyperventilation and Hysteria: The Physiology and Psychology of Overbreathing and its Relationship to the Mind-body Problem. Springfield, Illinois: Charles C Thomas; 1967.
15. Perkin GD, Joseph R. Neurological manifestations of the hyperventilation syndrome. J Roy Soc Med. 1986;79:448-50.
16. Darwin C. Expression of Emotions in Men and Animals. John Murray: London; 1872.
17. Cannon WB. Bodily changes in pain, hunger, fear and rage, 2nd edition. New York: Appleton; 1920.
18. Christie RV. Some types of respiration in the neuroses. QJM. 1935;4:427.
19. Finesinger JE, Mazick SE. The effects of a painful stimulus and its recall upon respiration. Psychosom Med. 1940;2:333.
20. Clausen J. Respiratory movements in normal, neurotic and psychotic subjects. Acta Psychiatr Neurol Suppl. 1951;68:1-74.
21. Stevenson I, Ripley HS. Variations in respiration and in respiratory symptoms during changes in emotion. Psychosom Med. 1952;14:476-90.
22. Dudley DL, Martin CJ, Holmes TH. Psychophysiologic studies of pulmonary ventilation. Psychosom Med. 1964;26:645-60.
23. Dudley DL, Holmes, TH, Martin CJ, Ripley HS. Changes in respiration associated with hypnotically induced emotion, pain and exercise. Psychosom Med. 1964;26:46-57.
24. Dudley DL, Martin CJ, Holmes TH. Dyspnoea: Psychologic and physiologic observations. J Psychosom Res. 1968;11:325-39.
25. Damas Mora JD, Grant L, Kenyon P, Patel MK. Respiratory ventilation and carbon dioxide levels in syndromes of depression. Br J Psychiatry. 1976;129:457-64.
26. Rice RL. Symptom patterns of the hyperventilation syndrome. Am J Med. 1950;8:691-700.
27. Lazarus HR, Kostan JJ. Psychogenic hyperventilation and death anxiety. Psychosomatics. 1969;10:14-22.
28. Tyrer P. Role of bodily feelings in anxiety. In: Tyrer P (Ed). Maudsley Monograph No. 23. London: Oxford University Press; 1976.
29. Pincus JH. Disorders of conscious awareness: hyperventilation syndrome. Brit J Hosp Med. 1978;19:312-3.
30. Blau JN, Wiles CM, Solomon FS. Unilateral somatic symptoms due to hyperventilation. Br Med J. 1983;286:1108.
31. O'Sullivan G, Harvey I, Bass C, Sheehy M, Toone B, Turner S. Psychophysiological investigations of patients with unilateral symptoms in the hyperventilation syndrome. Br J Psychiatry. 1992;161:722-7.
32. Raichle ME, Posner JB, Plum F. Cerebral blood flow during and after hyperventilation. Arch Neurol. 1970;23:394-403.
33. Kennealy JA, McLennan JE, Loudon RG, McLaurin RL. Hyperventilation induced cerebral hypoxia. Am Rev Respir Dis. 1980;122:407-12.
34. Kraft AR, Hoogduin CA. The hyperventilation syndrome. A pilot study on the effectiveness of treatment. Br J Psychiatry. 1984;145:538-42.
35. Hoes MJ. Pharmacotherapy of the hyperventilation syndrome. Ann Med Psychol (Paris). 1983;141(8):859-74.
36. Willeput R, Dubreuil C, Prosper M, Compere P, Pujet JC. Hyperventilation syndrome: evaluation of voluntary hypoventilation programs in two rehabilitation centers. Rev Mal Respir. 2001;18(4):417-25.
37. Stahl SM, Soefje S. Panic attacks and panic disorder: the great neurological imposters. Semin Neurol. 1995;15:126-32.
38. American Psychiatric Association. Diagnostic and Statistical Manual of Mental Disorders, 4th Edition. Washington, DC: American Psychiatric Association; 1994. pp. 393-444.
39. Rawlings GH, Jamnadas-Khoda J, Broadhurst M, Grünewald RA, Howell SJ, Koepp M, et al. Panic symptoms in transient loss of consciousness: Frequency and diagnostic value in psychogenic nonepileptic seizures, epilepsy and syncope. Seizure. 2017;48:22-7.
40. Simon NM, Otto MW, Korbly NB, Peters PM, Nicoladau DC, Pollack MH. Quality of life in social anxiety disorder compared with panic disorder and the general population. Psychiatr Serv. 2002;53:714-18.
41. Treiman DM. GABAergic mechanisms in epilepsy. Epilepsia. 2001;42 Suppl 3:8-12.
42. Charney DS, Deutsch A. A functional neuroanatomy of anxiety and fear; implications for the pathophysiology and treatment of anxiety disorders. Crit Rev Neurobiol. 1996;10:419-46.
43. Davis M, Whalen PJ. The amygdala: vigilance and emotion. Mol Psychiatry. 2001;6:13-34.
44. Bernik MA, Corregiari FM, Braunl M. Panic attacks in the differential diagnosis and treatment of resistant epilepsy. Depress Anxiety. 2002;15:190-2.
45. Kasper S, Resinger E. Panic disorder: the place of benzodiazepines and selective serotonin reuptake inhibitors. Eur Neuropsychopharmacol. 2001;11:307-21.
46. Goldberg C. Cognitive-behavioural therapy for panic: effectiveness and limitations. Psychiatr Q. 1998;69:23-44.
47. Bridler R, Umbricht D. Treatment of panic disorder with combination of SSRI and cognitive behavioural therapy. Psychiatr Prax. 2001;28:244-5.
48. Slaap BR, den Boer JA. The prediction of no response to pharmacotherapy in panic disorders: a review. Depress Anx. 2001;14:112-22.
49. Low PA, Opfer-Gehrking TL, Textor SC, Benarroch EE, Shen WK, Schondorf R, et al. Postural tachycardia syndrome (POTS). Neurology. 1995;45:Suppl 5:S19-25.
50. Low PA, Opfer-Gehrking TL, Textor SC, Schondorf R, Suarez GA, Fealey RD, et al. Comparison of the postural tachycardia syndrome (POTS) with orthostatic hypotension due to autonomic failure. J Auton Nerv Syst. 1994;50:181-8.
51. Jacob G, Shannon JR, Black B, Biaggioni I, Mosqueda-Garcia R, Robertson RM, et al. Effects of volume loading and pressor agents in idiopathic orthostatic tachycardia. Circulation. 1997;96:575-80.
52. Malmberg LP, Tamminen K, Sovijärvi AR. Orthostatic increase of respiratory gas exchange in hyperventilation syndrome. Thorax. 2000;55:295-301.
53. Gardner WN. The pathophysiology of hyperventilation disorders. Chest. 1996;109:516-34.
54. Hibbert G, Pilsbury D. Hyperventilation in panic attacks. Ambulant monitoring of transcutaneous carbon dioxide. Br J Psychiatry. 1998;153:76-80.
55. Del Pozzi AT, Schwartz CE, Tewari D, Medow MS, Stewart JM. Reduced cerebral blood flow with orthostasis precedes

55. [continued] hypocapnic hyperpnea, sympathetic activation, and postural tachycardia syndrome. Hypertension. 2014;63:1302-8.
56. Ding Y, Li YL, Schultz HD. Role of blood flow in carotid body chemoreflex function in heart failure. J Physiol. 2011;589: 245-58.
57. Kanner AM. Recognition of various expressions of anxiety, psychosis and aggression in epilepsy. Epilepsia. 2004;45:22-7.
58. Beyenburg S, Mitchell AJ, Schmidt D, Elger CE, Reuber M. Anxiety in patients with epilepsy: systematic review and suggestions for clinical management. Epilepsy Behav. 2005;7:161-71.
59. Feichtinger M, Pauli E, Schäfer I, Eberhardt KW, Tomandl B, Huk J, et al. Ictal fear in temporal lobe epilepsy: surgical outcome and focal hippocampal changes revealed by proton magnetic resonance spectroscopy imaging. Arch Neurol. 2001;58: 771-7.
60. Cendes F, Andermann F, Gloor P. Evans A, Carpenter S, Olivier A. Relationship between atrophy of the amygdala and ictal fear in temporal lobe epilepsy. Brain. 1994;117:739-46.
61. Oehl B, Schulze-Bonhage A, Lanz M, Brandt A, Altenmüller DM. Occipital lobe epilepsy with fear as leading ictal symptom. Epilepsy Behav. 2012;23:379-83.
62. Krolak-Salmon P, Hénaff MA, Vighetto A, Bertrand O, Mauguière F. Early amygdala reaction to fear spreading in occipital, temporal, and frontal cortex. Neuron. 2004;42:665-76.
63. Wang J, Wang Q, Wang M, Luan G, Zhou J, Guan Y, et al. Occipital Lobe Epilepsy With Ictal Fear: Evidence From a Stereo-Electroencephalography (sEEG) Case. Front Neurol. 2018;9:644.
64. So NK. Epileptic auras. In: Wyllie E (Ed). The Treatment of Epilepsy: Principles and Practice. Philadelphia, Lippincott Williams & Wilkins; 2006. pp. 229-39.
65. Ring HA, Gene-Cos N. Epilepsy and panic disorder. In: Trimble M, Schmitz B (Eds). The Neuropsychiatry of Epilepsy. Cambridge: Cambridge University Press; 2002. pp. 226-38.
66. Moore D, Jefferson J. Panic Disorder, 2nd edition. St. Louis (MO): Mosby; 2004.
67. Biraben A, Taussig D, Thomas P, Even C, Vignal JP, Scarabin JM, et al. Fear as the main feature of epileptic seizures. J Neurol Neurosurg Psychiatry. 2001;70:186-91.
68. Alemayehu S, Bergey GK, Barry E, Krumholz A, Wolf A, Fleming CP, et al. Panic attacks as ictal manifestations of parietal lobe seizures. Epilepsia. 1995;36:824-30.
69. Paparrigopoulos T, Kyrozis A, Tzavellas E, Karaiskos D, Liappas I. Left parieto-occipital lesion with epilepsy mimicking panic disorder. Prog Neuropsychopharmacol Biol Psychiatry. 2008;32:1606-8.
70. Akiyama M, Kobayashi K, Inoue T, Akiyama T, Yoshinaga H. Five pediatric cases of ictal fear with variable outcomes. Brain Dev. 2014;36(9):758-63.
71. Isnard J, Guenot M, Ostrowsky K, Sindou M, Mauguiere F. The role of the insular cortex in temporal lobe epilepsy. Ann Neurol. 2000;48:614-23.
72. Penfield W, Faulk ME Jr. The insula; further observations on its function. Brain. 1955;78:445-70.
73. Isnard J, Guenot M, Sindou M, Mauguiere F. Clinical manifestations of insular lobe seizures: a stereo-electroencephalographic study. Epilepsia. 2004;45:1079-90.

CHAPTER 29

Psychiatric Emergencies in Critical Care Units: Recognition and Management

Joshua Battley, Bappaditya Ray, Venkatesh Aiyagari

INTRODUCTION

The American Psychiatric Association defines a psychiatric emergency as "an acute disturbance in thought, behavior, mood, or social relationship, which requires immediate intervention as defined by the patient, family, or social unit". Such emergencies require immediate intervention to save the patient and others from imminent danger. If these patients have a premorbid psychiatric diagnosis of mania, acute psychosis, suicidal, or homicidal ideation, management should focus on clinical work-up for acute precipitants, and symptom control.[1] However, an acute de novo psychiatric emergency presenting to the critical care unit can be challenging and requires a detailed history, review of medications, clinical examination, and ancillary laboratory and radiological testing. This discussion is limited to the latter group of patients, namely those without a previously known psychiatric diagnosis. Autoimmune encephalitis can also present as an acute psychiatric emergency, but a detailed discussion on this condition is beyond the scope of this chapter.

ALCOHOL AND ALCOHOL-RELATED DISORDERS

Alcohol Intoxication

Acute alcohol intoxication (AAI) is often associated with road accidents, pedestrian injuries, and acts of violence, including domestic violence, suicide attempts, and head injuries due to falls and crashes. Binge drinking, as defined by the National Institute on Alcohol Abuse and Alcoholism (NIAAA), is "a pattern of drinking that brings blood alcohol concentration (BAC) levels to 80 mg/dL. This typically occurs after four drinks for women and five drinks for men—in about 2 hours". Currently, 90% of teenagers in the US are "binge drinkers".

Clinical manifestations of AAI, although variable, often correlate with BAC. In an infrequent alcohol drinker, ataxia, nystagmus, slurred speech, impaired judgment, and changes in mood and behavior are frequently seen at a BAC above 100 mg/dL (21.7 mmol/L). Signs and symptoms of central nervous system (CNS) depression manifested as amnesia without loss of consciousness can occur at a BAC of 200 mg/dL, with autonomic manifestations of hypothermia, hypotension, nausea, and vomiting at a BAC of 300 mg/dL and above. BAC above 500 mg/dL can produce coma, hyporeflexia, respiratory compromise, and death.[2] However, it should be noted that the degree of tolerance can be significant for people who drink heavily, permitting sobriety at blood concentrations above 120 mg/dL and survival above 700 mg/dL.

Seizures are frequent clinical presentation of AAI. Prolonged seizures resulting in severe rhabdomyolysis could lead to acute kidney injury and hyperkalemia. Thiamine deficiency, decreased synthesis of gamma-aminobutyric acid (GABA), excitotoxic effects of glutamate, acute imbalance of electrolyte levels (dehydration, low potassium, and magnesium), and acute blood–brain barrier damage are pathophysiologically linked to AAI. Acute alcoholic encephalopathy, also called Wernicke's encephalopathy, is a rare hemorrhagic encephalopathy with a subacute course due to altered thiamine metabolism and can be precipitated with inadvertent use of dextrose-containing fluid infusion without replacing thiamine. Clinical manifestations include oculomotor disorders, cerebellar ataxia, memory deficits, hyperkinesis, and autonomic disorders (e.g., arterial hypertension, orthostatic hypotension, hypo- or hyperthermia, and hyperhidrosis). Thus, parenteral thiamine administration is recommended prior to any dextrose solutions. Other acute manifestations associated with alcoholism are central pontine myelinolysis (symmetric demyelination in the region of the pons usually associated with acute fluctuation of sodium levels) manifesting with miosis, tetraplegia, aphonia, and altered horizontal movements of eyes, configuring the so-called locked-in syndrome; Marchiafava-Bignami syndrome (demyelination of the corpus callosum), manifesting with memory impairment, tremors, seizures, muscle rigidity, confusion, evolving into stupor and coma; tobacco-alcohol amblyopia, consisting in a mono/bilateral optic neuritis due to the direct toxic effects of alcohol and tobacco associated with nutritional deficits (vitamin B12 and lipoic acid).

Alcohol Withdrawal Syndrome

Acute alcohol withdrawal (AWS) develops when patients with severe alcohol use disorder (AUD) abruptly discontinue or decrease alcohol consumption. Clinical manifestation of AWS includes autonomic hyperactivity (tremors, anxiety, hyperreflexia, hypertension, tachycardia, and fever), usually developing within 6-24 hours after the abrupt discontinuation or decrease of alcohol consumption in patients with an underlying severe AUD or in patients being treated for AAI using drugs promoting alcohol metabolism and elimination. An admission BAC > 200 mg/dL should be considered a risk factor for the subsequent development of severe AWS.

Treatment

Early treatment for AAI is essential to prevent the risk of developing respiratory depression and cardiac arrest. In the emergency department (ED), particularly in patients with severe forms of AAI (especially those with BAC > 300 mg/dL), the primary aim is stabilizing vital functions. It may involve securing the airway, controlling seizures, assessing for signs of trauma, fluid resuscitation (especially in dehydrated and hypotensive patients), and correcting metabolic abnormalities (especially electrolyte abnormalities and hypoglycemia). A commonly adopted protocol is based on dextrose (i.e., 500 mL of 10% dextrose), electrolytes (i.e., 500 mL of sodium chloride 0.9% with 2 g of magnesium sulfate), thiamine (100 mg), and folate (1 mg). It is advisable to administer thiamine before any glucose load due to the risk of accelerating the onset of Wernicke's encephalopathy. Recent publications suggest a higher dose of thiamine, 500 mg thrice a day for 2 days, then 250 mg daily for an additional 5 days. The lack of thiamine supplementation in deficient patients could precipitate severe cardiovascular (i.e., heart failure and sudden death) and neurological (i.e., Wernicke's encephalopathy and Korsakoff's psychosis) consequences.

Principles of management of AAI in the critical care units include restoring and maintaining body homeostasis through supporting vital organs using a multidisciplinary team approach. Respiratory failure in AAI that could be secondary to CNS depression, aspiration, or infections, needs oxygen supplementation with low-flow or high devices targeting optimal peripheral oxygen saturation provided patients can maintain airway patency and adequately ventilate. In severe cases, especially with acute respiratory and/or metabolic acidosis and acute hypoxemic respiratory failure, invasive mechanical ventilation may be needed. Since AUD patients are often malnourished, dietician consultation and formulating adequate nutrition regimen and vitamin replacement need special attention. Nausea and vomiting may worsen such deficiencies and need appropriate use of antiemetics. Management of agitation requires the use of typical and atypical antipsychotics such as haloperidol, droperidol, olanzapine, and sedatives benzodiazepines (BDZs), ketamine, dexmedetomidine, and propofol (in intubated patients only). Clinicians need to be cognizant of potential side effects of antipsychotics (e.g., prolongation of QTc and precipitation of ventricular arrhythmias) and sedatives (e.g., dexmedetomidine and propofol causing bradycardia and hypotension, ketamine causing paradoxical effect), in the setting of AAI to prevent patient morbidity.

Metadoxine, a pyrrolidone carboxylate of pyridoxine (pyridoxol L-2-pyrrolidone-5-carboxilate), is currently the only drug indicated for treating AAI. It accelerates ethanol clearance and consequently reduces BAC improving symptoms of intoxication. Mechanisms of action include maintaining and restoring adenosine triphosphate (ATP) levels in the brain and liver by enhancing glutathione synthesis, and pyridoxine promotes the ethanol degradation.[3] Ultimately, the administration of metadoxine increases acetaldehyde dehydrogenase activity, promotes ethanol and acetaldehyde plasma clearance, and promotes urinary elimination of ketones. In a double-blind trial, patients receiving the drug showed a steeper decrease in BAC and a faster improvement of symptoms compared to those receiving a placebo.[4] The recommended dose is 900 mg intravenously, given as a single administration. This treatment is strongly recommended in adolescent patients who are more prone to damage from alcohol intoxication in consideration of the immature enzyme activity used for the degradation of alcohol. Of note, metadoxine is currently approved in some EU countries and is not approved in the US.

Alcohol Withdrawal Syndrome and Delirium Tremens Management

The treatment of severe AWS and delirium tremens (DT) should be focused on ameliorating agitation and other symptoms of delirium, recognition, and treatment of underlying medical comorbidities, and adequate and protocol-driven treatment of alcohol withdrawal. Classically, as needed doses of BDZs, based on the

TABLE 1: Treatment of benzodiazepine refractory delirium tremens.[5,6]

"Persistent CIWA-Ar > 25, frank delirium or inability to control symptoms despite medication" and/or requirement of >200 mg in the initial 3 hours or ≥400 mg of diazepam in the first 8 hours or ≥30 mg in the initial 3 hours or ≥60 mg of lorazepam in the initial 8 hours

First line	• Phenobarbital
	• 60 mg IV bolus every 15–30 minutes
	Alternate regimens for moderate to severe DT:
	   ○ Load with 10 mg/kg IBW and repeat 5 mg/kg after 4–6 hours
	   ○ 260 mg and repeat 130 mg every 30 minutes if DT symptoms persist
	• Maximum dose in 24 hours—1,040 mg
	.....BDZ dose to be halved (if patient is not intubated). Intubation is necessary if there are signs of respiratory depression and BDZ therapy is to be continued

Second line (If intubated and refractory to phenobarbital)	• Propofol infusion 0.3–1.25 µg/kg/h • *RASS*: –3 to –4 • *Maximum dose*: 4 µg/kg/hour • *Maximum duration of administration*: 48 hours
Third line (Alternative to propofol if patient is not intubated)	• Dexmedetomidine 0.2–0.7 µg/kg/hour • *Maximum dose*: 1.4 µg/kg/hour
Other options	*Haloperidol*: Uncontrolled agitation or hallucinations (0.5–5.0 mg intravenously or intramuscularly every 30–60 minutes as needed for severe agitation or hallucinosis—not to exceed 20 mg; or 0.5–5.0 mg orally every 4 hours up to 30 mg ....Monitor QTc on ECG—consider using alternate agent if QTc persistently remains >500 ms *Ketamine*: Total infusion rate of 0.20 mg/kg/hour

(BDZ: benzodiazepine; CIWA-Ar: Clinical Institute Withdrawal Assessment of Alcohol Scale-Revised; DT: delirium tremens; ECG: electroencephalogram; IBW: ideal body weight)

Clinical Institute Withdrawal Assessment of Alcohol Scale-Revised (CIWA-Ar), is employed. DT may be refractory to BDZ use, in which case patients should be admitted to the intensive care unit (ICU) and additional agents, enumerated in **Table 1** should be used.

NEUROLOGIC COMPLICATIONS OF PRESCRIPTION AND RECREATIONAL DRUG OVERUSE

Prescription and recreational drug use can cause neurologic manifestations from acute and chronic intoxication. There is a gradual change in the paradigm for drug overuse of illicit substances to that of prescription medications for recreational use. Abusers need not obtain drugs exclusively on the street; physician offices, pharmacies, and medicine cabinets have become familiar sources of these substances. Awareness of the potential for patient abuse when prescribing these substances and the potential for these drugs to fall into the hands of other users, including family members and acquaintances of patients, is needed.

Standard urinary drug screens are inexpensive and utilized in most EDs when acute intoxication is suspected. They test for commonly used recreational drugs or their metabolites, including alcohol, amphetamines, barbiturates, BDZs, cannabis, opioids, and cocaine. Many of the drugs **(Table 2)** may not be detected in typical urinary screens and either cannot be tested for easily or are only detected using serum screens that tend to be expensive and time-consuming. These serum screens remain the gold standard for testing, especially outside emergency settings. Other options for testing include saliva and hair analysis, the latter having the advantage of detecting some drugs of abuse weeks to even months after ingestion.

DELIRIUM

Introduction

Delirium is a disturbance in attention, awareness, and cognition without significantly decreased level of arousal that develops over a short period of time, represents a change from baseline, and tends to fluctuate during the course of the day.[7] Delirium is very common in critical care units, especially in the elderly population. Classically considered a transient condition, delirium can have long-term effects including increased mortality and impaired cognitive function.[8]

TABLE 2: Clinical manifestations and treatment of drug overuse.

Intoxicant	Clinical features	Treatment
Cocaine	• *Mechanism*: Increases monoamine neurotransmitters through inhibition of reuptake • Can be ingested in different ways including by snorting, smoking (often as "crack" cocaine), and intravenous injection • Neuropsychiatric effects—psychosis and paranoia can occur in addition to the expected euphoria and increased energy • Acute elevation of blood pressure can result in intracerebral hemorrhage (ICH), hypertensive encephalopathy with seizures (posterior reversible encephalopathy syndrome, PRES) • Ischemic cardiovascular and cerebrovascular events—myocardial infarction and stroke • Fulminant acute leukoencephalopathy may occur due to adulterants found in cocaine, including the antiparasitic medication levamisole	• Mostly supportive • Avoid nonselective beta blockers • Avoid haloperidol as first-line agent due to its potency to reduce seizure threshold • BDZ is preferred for agitation • Hyperthermia—cooling devices • ICH, PRES, AIS, AMI management as per guidelines
Methamphetamines	• *Mechanism*: Increases norepinephrine, epinephrine, and serotonin transmission at the synapse while also activating dopamine receptors • Euphoria and increased energy predominating along with the risk of paradoxical reactions including agitation and paranoia. As the effects of the drug wear off, dysphoria and increased sleep commonly occur, mimicking some of the effects of sedatives • Neurologic and non-neurologic complications similar to cocaine intoxication	Mostly supportive and similar to cocaine-related toxicity management
MDMA (Ecstasy, "Molly") 3,4-ethylene-dioxymeth-amphetamine	• *Mechanism*: Serotonergic similar to amphetamine • This became popular at dance parties ("raves") and is often taken in combination with other psychotropic drugs • Causes disinhibition and sexual arousal. In some patients, agitation and anxiety can paradoxically occur at the time of intoxication or once the acute effects of the drug have worn off • Acute hyponatremia often develops both due to primary polydipsia and a drug-induced increase in antidiuretic hormone secretion • Neurologic complications include seizures and fatal cerebral edema from severe hyponatremia and potential central pontine myelinolysis from rapid correction of hyponatremia	• Supportive care • Gastric decontamination • BDZ for psychomotor agitation and shivering • Cyproheptadine for associated serotonin syndrome • Surface cooling for hyperthermia
Gamma hydroxybutyrate (GHB)	• *Mechanism*: Precursor to GABA • Causes euphoria and stimulant effects with purported sexual enhancement and disinhibition • The most cited neurologic effect of GHB intoxication is coma, which may occur rapidly after ingestion and necessitate intubation. Other neurologic complications of acute use include ataxia and nystagmus • Patients with GHB intoxication are at risk of seizures, and myoclonus is typically seen especially when patients are in the agitated phase	• Supportive care • No specific antidotes • Severe withdrawal symptoms are life-threatening and can last up to 15 days

Continued

Continued

Intoxicant	Clinical features	Treatment
Opioids	• *Mechanism*: Inhibition of μ and other opioid receptors • Clinical manifestation includes miosis and altered consciousness that can progress to coma at high doses, especially in those without previous exposure to this class of medications. Some specific opiates can lead to seizures, including fentanyl, meperidine (particularly in the setting of renal insufficiency), tramadol, and pentazocine. Individuals taking opiates demonstrate diffuse myoclonus, which can be mistaken for seizures or other movement disorders • Heroin inhalation after vaporization on a piece of aluminum foil ("chasing the dragon") can cause toxic leukoencephalopathy • *Opiate withdrawal*: Causes dysphoria and akathisia. Muscle pain, nausea, vomiting, yawning, and rhinorrhea are some non-neurologic symptoms	• Treatment of life-threatening acute intoxication • Administration of opiate antagonists such as naloxone
Lysergic acid diethylamide (LSD) and other hallucinogens	• *Mechanism*: Effects on the serotonin receptors can cause serotonin syndrome, especially when LSD is combined with other serotonergic drugs including prescription antidepressants • The intent of use of hallucinogens like LSD is to alter neurologic perception and mood • Causes a cholinergic toxidrome manifested by exhaustion, irritability, muscular cramps, salivation, frothing from mouth, sweating, lacrimation, blurring of vision, miosis, ptosis, bronchorrhea, cough, wheeze, tachypnea, rhonchi, bradycardia, hypotension, abdominal cramps, vomiting, and diarrhea • Rare adverse effects include more permanent visual disturbances and vasospasm leading to cerebral ischemia	• Supportive care • BDZ is safe for agitation management • Avoid haloperidol as it can lower seizure threshold • Serotonin syndrome management as described in the text
Phencyclidine (PCP and "angel dust")	• *Mechanism*: Inhibition of NMDA receptors • Clinical manifestation includes tachycardia, hypertension, violent outbursts, and nystagmus, which classically is vertical in direction. Higher doses of PCP may induce an acute psychosis with hallucinations and agitation, whereas a striking akinetic mutism with unresponsiveness and preserved eye opening may accompany overdose	• Supportive care • Gastric decontamination as applicable • BDZ use for agitation
Tetrahydrocannabinol (THC)	• Intoxicated patients demonstrate decreased coordination and gait along with psychomotor slowing that can impair safe driving • AIS is reported as a complication of overdose. Cerebral vasoconstriction is a known complication	No antidote flumazenil, a selective BDZ antagonist, may have some therapeutic effect

(AIS: acute ischemic stroke; AMI: acute myocardial infarction; BDZ: benzodiazepine; PRES: posterior reversible encephalopathy syndrome; MDMA: 3,4-methylenedioxymethamphetamine)

Clinical Characteristics

The Diagnostic and Statistical Manual of Mental Disorders, Fifth Edition (DSM-5) provides a set of five criteria for diagnosing delirium: Disturbance in attention and awareness; disturbance develops over a short period of time and tends to fluctuate throughout the day; an additional disturbance in cognition; disturbances must not be better explained by preexisting cognitive impairment and do not occur solely in the context of reduced level of arousal; evidence the disturbance is a direct consequence of another medical condition.[7,8]

Delirium can be hypoactive to hyperactive or agitated. Hypoactive delirium is often underrecognized due to its less dramatic clinical presentation and is associated with poorer prognosis.[8]

Diagnosis

Delirium is underdiagnosed with studies suggesting that >65% of cases go unrecognized.[8] This percentage increases with routine active screening.[9] Several clinical tools are available in clinical practice.[8-10] The most widely used screening instrument is the Confusion Assessment

TABLE 3: Risk factors for delirium.[8-10]

Predisposing	Precipitating
Increasing age	Acute illness
Cognitive impairment	Impaired sleep wake cycle
Multiple comorbidities	Immobility
Functional impairment	Length of stay
Male sex	*Medications*: Sedatives, opioids, and anticholinergics
Substance use or withdrawal	Surgery
Visual or hearing impairment	Pain
Neurologic injury	*Agitation*: Restraints, thirst, hunger, anxiety, and frustration

Method (CAM) due to its high sensitivity (94–100%), high specificity (90–95%), and ease of use.[9] CAM consists of four features: (1) Acute onset and fluctuating course, (2) inattention, (3) disorganized thinking, and (4) altered level of consciousness. The diagnosis of delirium by CAM requires the presence of features 1 and 2 and either 3 or 4.[11] This tool has also been adapted and validated for nonverbal and mechanically ventilated patients in the CAM for ICU patients (CAM-ICU).[12]

Other conditions may mimic or coincide with delirium including dementia, depression, mania, psychosis, seizure, and structural brain abnormality and must be evaluated and managed accordingly.[9] Risk factors associated with delirium are enumerated in **Table 3**.

Evaluation

Evaluation of delirium begins with detailed history of patient's baseline cognition, functional status, medical comorbidities, and medication/substance use, and nutrition assessment to understand predisposing factors. Evaluation of modifiable precipitating factors then includes physical examination, vital signs, and detailed neurologic assessment. Laboratory and imaging studies should be obtained to evaluate precipitating factors. Routine studies include comprehensive metabolic panel and complete blood count (CBC), urinalysis, and electrocardiogram. Other, more specific studies are needed based on initial history and workup. These may include blood culture, chest radiography, or CSF analysis if infection is suspected; blood gas analysis if acute respiratory insufficiency is suspected; brain imaging with CT or MRI if structural lesion is suspected; electroencephalogram if seizure is suspected; and metabolic screening with urine/serum toxicology, thyroid function, and serum B12 levels as indicated.[8,9]

Management

Prevention and nonpharmacological management are keys to the management of delirium. General principles to the prevention of delirium are discussed in the **Table 4**. Creating as calm and familiar of an environment as possible and maintaining homeostasis for patients at risk of or experiencing delirium is critical during acute illness.

Pharmacologic Therapy

Pharmacologic therapy for agitated delirium should be reserved for individuals at high risk of immediate harm to self or others. Common antipsychotic agents used for agitated delirium are discussed in **Table 5**. Electrocardiography should be assessed at baseline and monitored periodically when using antipsychotic agents due to potential QTc prolongation. Infusion of dexmedetomidine has been used with some evidence of shorter time to extubation, shorter stay in the ICU, and more rapid resolution of delirium when compared to propofol or midazolam.[10] Scheduled melatonin 3–5 mg or ramelteon 8 mg in the evening may be beneficial for facilitating sleep if refractory to nonpharmacologic methods.[9]

NEUROLEPTIC MALIGNANT SYNDROME

Introduction

Neuroleptic malignant syndrome (NMS) is an uncommon, but potentially life-threatening emergency associated with antipsychotic agent use that must be promptly recognized as mortality rates may be as high as 30%.[13] The classic syndrome of recent exposure to dopamine antagonist, hyperthermia, rigidity, mental status change, and dysautonomia may have a variable presentation requiring a high clinical suspicion and immediate treatment.[14,15] NMS is classically associated with antipsychotic medications. Other central-acting dopamine depleters including antiemetics, amphetamines, cocaine, or tetrabenazine are also risk factors. Abrupt cessation of dopamine precursors, COMT inhibitors, or dopamine agonists may have a similar effect.[15]

Epidemiology/Pathophysiology

Incidence of NMS in individuals treated with antipsychotics is fortunately low, around 0.01–0.02%.[14,16] Pathophysiology is complex and multifaceted. Dopamine antagonist use or cessation of dopamine agonist results in central dopamine depletion. Dopamine depletion in

TABLE 4: General principles to prevent delirium.[8-10]

Issue	Description
Orientation	Provide frequent reorientation to time, place, and situation; provide signs, calendars, white board, clock, and visual messages to reiterate orientation; encourage cognitively stimulating activities
Environment	Noise reduction; provide adequate lighting during awake times; encourage family to provide family objects from home
Sleep	Optimize sleep-hygiene, ideally with a nonpharmacologic sleep protocol; avoid excessive daytime sleep; minimize unnecessary nighttime awakenings (vital signs, examinations, phlebotomy, imaging, etc.); reduce noise and excessive light at night; avoid medications that may disturb sleep
Acute symptoms	Accurately assess and manage acute symptoms including pain, anxiety, and agitation
Mobilization	Encourage early mobilization; physical and occupational therapy evaluation to screen for functional needs; minimize physical restraints
Nutrition	Maintain adequate, preferably oral, nutrition; dietitian and speech therapy evaluation as nutrition needs may be altered during acute illness; nutritional supplement as necessary
Impaired sensory input	Optimize vision and hearing with use of corrective lenses and hearing amplifiers or hearing aids as needed
Prevent complications	Screen and treat for complications of prolong hospital stay including: pressure ulcers, skin breakdown, falls; limit urinary or vascular catheter use; implement infection control precautions as appropriate; avoid hypoxia; assess and treat urinary retention and bowel impaction
Medications	Avoid medication that can precipitate or worsen delirium; minimize sedatives; use low dose, high potency antipsychotics only if necessary for safety of patient or caregivers
Socialization	Encourage communication and interaction with family and caregivers
Family support	Involve family to actively participate with interventions to prevent delirium

TABLE 5: Antipsychotic agents for agitated delirium.[8,9]

Agent	Typical dose	Routes
Haloperidol	0.25–0.5 mg	Oral, IM, IV
Quetiapine	12.5–25 mg	Oral
Olanzapine	2.5–5 mg	Oral, sublingual, IM
Risperidone	0.25–1 mg	Oral, IM
Ziprasidone	5–10 mg	Oral, IM

(IM: intramuscular; IV: intravenous)

BOX 1: Medications associated with neuroleptic malignant syndrome.[13-15]

- *Typical antipsychotics*
  - Haloperidol
  - Fluphenazine
  - Chlorpromazine
- *Atypical antipsychotics*
  - Quetiapine
  - Olanzapine
  - Risperidone
  - Ziprasidone
  - Aripiprazole
  - Clozapine
- *Antiemetics*
  - Metoclopramide
  - Prochlorperazine
  - Promethazine
  - Droperidol
- *Altered dopamine reuptake*
  - Amphetamines
  - Cocaine
- *Dopamine depleters*
  - Tetrabenazine
  - Reserpine

the hypothalamus results in hyperthermia and autonomic instability (labile hypertension, tachycardia, tachypnea, and diaphoresis).[16] Dopamine antagonism in the nigrostriatal pathway results in rigidity and movement symptoms which may lead to rhabdomyolysis and other metabolic effects.[15,16]

Etiology/Risk Factors

High potency, typical antipsychotics pose a greater risk than newer, atypical antipsychotics. Higher total medication dosing or rapid uptitration may be associated with increased risk of NMS **(Boxes 1 and 2)**.[13]

> **BOX 2: Medication discontinuation associated with neuroleptic malignant syndrome.**[13,15]
>
> - *Dopamine precursors*
>   - Levodopa
> - *COMT inhibitors*
>   - Entacapone
>   - Tolcapone
> - *Dopamine agonists*
>   - Bromocriptine
>   - Amantadine

Clinical Characteristics

Classic NMS is characterized by hyperthermia, "lead-pipe" muscle rigidity, mental status changes, and autonomic instability.[13-16] Elevation in temperature can be significant, sometimes exceeding 40°C.[15] Neurologic motor manifestations can also include tremor, akinesia/bradykinesia, dystonia, myoclonus, dysarthria, and dysphagia.[14] When rigidity/bradykinesia is prominent, catatonia may predominate. Mental status changes can range from mild confusion to stupor or coma when severe. Autonomic dysfunction results in labile hypertension, tachycardia, tachypnea, cardiac arrhythmias, diaphoresis, and incontinence.[14,15] Clinical symptoms typically evolve over 24-72 hours after starting/discontinuing offending agent. Most cases are self-limited if offending agents is discontinued in a timely fashion. Symptoms and signs typically resolve within 7 days but can last several weeks, particularly if long-acting offending agents are utilized.[14]

Differential Diagnosis

Alternative diagnoses need urgent evaluation when NMS is considered as management should be enacted as soon as possible. Differential diagnoses that need to be excluded include: Serotonin syndrome, malignant catatonia, malignant hyperthermia associated with inhalation anesthesia, infectious meningitis or encephalitis, acute intoxication (amphetamine, cocaine, anticholinergic, and salicylate poisoning), status epilepticus, heat stroke, thyrotoxicosis, and pheochromocytoma.[13-16]

Evaluation

Laboratory abnormalities are common but nonspecific. Laboratory evaluation is important in excluding alternative diagnoses and assessing severity of the syndrome. Creatine kinase (CK) is often elevated and degree of elevation may correlate with disease severity and worse prognosis.[15] Leukocytosis is also often present ranging from 10,000-40,000/μL. Other laboratory abnormalities include elevated lactate dehydrogenase, elevated transaminases, hypercalcemia, acute renal impairment secondary to rhabdomyolysis, low serum iron, hyperosmolality, and metabolic acidosis.[13,15,16] Electroencephalogram is typically suggestive of nonspecific generalized slowing or is normal. Cerebrospinal fluid analysis is nonspecific or normal. Imaging studies and histopathologic findings are typically normal.[13,14] Additional tests may be helpful to narrow the differential diagnosis or assess provoking factors. This may include urinalysis, blood and urine culture, chest radiograph, blood and urine toxicology, and electrocardiogram.

Management

Discontinuation of the offending dopaminergic agent is the most important step in management of NMS. Discontinuation of contributing medications including serotonergic or anticholinergic agents should be considered.[16]

Supportive Therapy

Supportive measures are the mainstay of management after discontinuation of offending agent. Principles of supportive care are enumerated under alcohol-related disorders.

Pharmacologic Therapy

For severe cases, NMS may require additional pharmacologic intervention in addition to antipsychotic cessation and supportive measures. Oral or parenteral BDZs such as lorazepam, diazepam, or midazolam can be utilized for motor and/or catatonic symptoms. Dopaminergic agents such as bromocriptine and amantadine may hasten recovery and improve mortality.[16] Dantrolene, a skeletal muscle relaxant, can be beneficial in severe NMS with extreme hyperthermia, rigidity, and hypermetabolism. Close monitoring of liver function is indicated while using dantrolene due to risk of hepatotoxicity.[15,16] Electroconvulsive therapy (ECT) may be beneficial if symptoms fail to improve with supportive measures and pharmacologic therapy and is considered relatively safe. A typical ECT regimen consists of 6-10 session with bilateral electrode placement.[13,15,16]

Recurrence

Recurrence of NMS is as high as 30% in individuals restarting antipsychotic medications. If continued antipsychotic medication is warranted after complete resolution of NMS symptoms, it is recommended to use low-potency atypical antipsychotics with slow titration while utilizing the lowest effective dose to avoid recurrence.[16]

SEROTONIN SYNDROME

Introduction

Serotonin syndrome is a condition resulting from therapeutic serotonergic medication use, drug-drug interactions, or intentional overdose. Clinical manifestations range from mild to life-threatening.[17] Classical serotonin syndrome is defined clinically by altered mental status, autonomic hyperactivity, and neuromuscular abnormalities.[17,18] Incidence has increased as serotonergic medication use has become more prevalent in clinical practice.[18]

Risk Factors

Many medications or medication combinations increase serotonin formation or decrease serotonin metabolism increasing risk of developing serotonin syndrome. Increasing total dose, rapid titration, and utilization of multiple serotonergic medications increase risk of toxicity **(Table 6)**.[17]

Clinical Characteristics

Serotonin syndrome is a clinical diagnosis. Prompt recognition of characteristic signs and symptoms is paramount to prevent escalation to more severe disease. Cardinal clinical manifestations include mental status changes, autonomic hyperactivity, and neuromuscular abnormalities.[17,18] The spectrum of mental status involvement ranges from mild agitation, hypervigilance, and pressured speech to coma and delusions when severe. Autonomic hyperactivity results in hyperthermia (temperature > 40°C is not uncommon), hypertension, tachycardia, tachypnea, diaphoresis, hyperactive bowel sounds, diarrhea, and mydriasis. Neuromuscular manifestations may include hyperreflexia, spontaneous or inducible clonus, ocular clonus, muscle rigidity, and hypertonicity that predominately involves the lower extremities.[17] Onset of symptoms often occurs rapidly within hours of starting or increasing serotonergic medication. However, individuals with mild symptoms may slowly progress over the course of weeks. It is rare to develop serotonin syndrome >5 weeks from alteration in serotonergic medication in the absence of other provoking factors.[17]

Diagnostic Criteria

The Hunter Serotonin Toxicity Criteria Decision Rules were proposed by Dunkley et al. in 2003 to clinically diagnose serotonin syndrome with 84% sensitivity and 97% specificity.[19] To diagnose serotonin syndrome by Hunter criteria one must have been exposed to one or more serotonergic agents in the past 5 weeks and exhibit at least one of the following clinical signs: Spontaneous clonus; inducible clonus and agitation or diaphoresis; ocular clonus and agitation or diaphoresis; tremor and hyperreflexia; hypertonia and hyperthermia (>38°C), and ocular clonus or inducible clonus.[19]

Differential Diagnosis

Alternative diagnoses warrant prompt evaluation and exclusion to guarantee proper management. The differential diagnosis when serotonin syndrome is suspected includes: NMS, anticholinergic toxicity, malignant catatonia, and malignant hyperthermia.[17] Accurate medication history is vital in distinguishing amongst these conditions due to similar clinical manifestations.

TABLE 6: Medications associated with serotonin syndrome.[17-19]

Selective serotonin-reuptake inhibitors	Citalopram, escitalopram, fluoxetine, fluvoxamine, paroxetine, and sertraline
Antidepressants	Amitriptyline, buspirone, clomipramine, duloxetine, trazodone, and venlafaxine
Monoamine oxidase inhibitors	Clorgiline, phenelzine, rasagiline, and selegiline
Analgesics	Fentanyl, meperidine, and tramadol
Antiemetics	Metoclopramide and ondansetron
Triptans	Eletriptan, frovatriptan, naratriptan, rizatriptan, sumatriptan, and zolmitriptan
Antibiotics	Linezolid and ritonavir
Drugs of abuse	Amphetamines, cocaine, LSD, and MDMA
Dietary supplements	Ginseng, St. John's wort, and tryptophan
Other	Cyclobenzaprine, dextromethorphan, lithium, and valproic acid

(LSD: lysergic acid diethylamide; MDMA: 3,4-methylenedioxymethamphetamine)

Evaluation

There are no laboratory or imaging findings specific to the diagnosis of serotonin syndrome. Detailed medication history is required to elicit offending agents. Laboratory and imaging studies should be obtained as needed to narrow differential diagnoses and assess complications. Urine and serum toxicology should be obtained to screen for illicit substances. CBC, metabolic profile, and liver function studies may be obtained to screen metabolic abnormalities. Severe rigidity may result in elevated CK and rhabdomyolysis which would warrant aggressive volume resuscitation and serial monitoring. There are typically no imaging abnormalities associated with serotonin syndrome and imaging should only be obtained if there is clinical concern for alternative diagnosis.

Management

Prompt recognition of the clinical syndrome, discontinuation of any offending serotonergic agent, and supportive measures are the mainstay of serotonin syndrome management. Additional pharmacologic agents aimed at minimizing complications may be needed based on severity.

Supportive measures follow similar principles as other emergencies mentioned previously. Agitation, autonomic hyperactivity, and severe neuromuscular abnormalities require sedation with BDZs. Parenteral lorazepam and diazepam are often used. BDZs may not be sufficient in managing more severe hypertension or tachycardia. Short-acting antihypertensive agents may be needed while the offending medication is eliminated. Intravenous push or infusion medication such as labetalol, metoprolol, nicardipine, or esmolol can be used for persistent or symptomatic tachycardia and hypertension.[17]

Hyperthermia can be managed with BDZs and external cooling in mild cases. Severe cases may require deeper sedation and induced neuromuscular paralysis to terminate excessive muscle activity which is driving the elevated temperature. Succinylcholine should be avoided due to increased risk of rhabdomyolysis, hyperkalemia, and cardia arrhythmia that is associated with serotonin syndrome. Antipyretic agents such as acetaminophen are often not beneficial as the etiology of elevated temperature is related to muscle rigidity and not hypothalamic abnormality.[17]

If supportive measures and sedation fail to adequately manage the clinical syndrome, administration of the 5-HT2a antagonist cyproheptadine is recommended. An initial dose of 12 mg with 2 mg doses as needed every 2 hours for 24 hours for continued symptoms binds 85–95% of serotonin receptors.[17] Atypical antipsychotics such as olanzapine can also be used for serotonergic antagonism and sedation.[17]

MALIGNANT CATATONIA

Introduction

Malignant catatonia is a severe, potentially life-threatening subtype of catatonia requiring prompt recognition and treatment. Characterized by rigidity, autonomic instability, and fever there is significant overlap with other acute neuropsychiatric emergencies. Fortunately, malignant catatonia is usually highly responsive to treatment. Rapid response to BDZs is diagnostic and therapeutic and ECT is often necessary.[20,21]

Clinical Characteristics

Catatonia is a motor dysregulation syndrome that can be divided into relatively common nonmalignant catatonia and rare, but critical malignant catatonia. General catatonia is defined by three or more of the following symptoms: Stupor (limited psychomotor activity), catalepsy (passive induction of a posture), waxy flexibility, mutism, negativism (resistance to manipulation), posturing (maintenance of a posture against gravity), mannerism (odd caricature of normal actions), stereotypy (repetitive and non-goal-directed movements), agitation, grimacing, echolalia (mimicking speech), and echopraxia (mimicking movements).[22] Malignant catatonia is characterized by general signs and symptoms of catatonia with the addition of hyperthermia and autonomic hyperactivity including labile blood pressure, tachycardia, tachypnea, and diaphoresis.[20]

Differential Diagnosis

Significant overlap exists between malignant catatonia, NMS, serotonin syndrome, and malignant hyperthermia. Catatonia often coexists with other psychiatric disorders including neurodevelopmental, psychotic bipolar, depressive disorders, and autoimmune or paraneoplastic disorders.[22] A detailed medical and pharmacologic history is instrumental in efficiently distinguishing these syndromes. Seizure is also a consideration warranting electroencephalography if suspected.[20]

Evaluation

Malignant catatonia is diagnosed clinically and supported by response to first- and second-line therapies. A BDZ challenge is warranted if catatonia is suspected. Parenteral lorazepam, typically 1–2 mg, is administered and rapid improvement in symptoms is considered diagnostic. Elevated creatinine kinase and low serum iron levels may be present in malignant catatonia but this is shared with NMS.[20]

Management

Management includes supportive measures for associated autonomic instability and maintenance BDZ. Supportive measures include intensive cardiopulmonary monitoring, treatment of hyperthermia and hypertension, and optimizing nutrition. After diagnostic parenteral BDZ, maintenance parenteral or oral lorazepam should be initiated and increased as needed to resolution of symptoms.[20] In cases of malignant catatonia bilateral ECT is also indicated as first line therapy.[20,21] ECT is typically performed daily for 2-5 days. Lorazepam is associated with 80-100% remission while ECT is associated with 82-96% remission.[21]

CONCLUDING REMARKS

Psychiatric emergencies in the emergency and critical care setting require prompt recognition to prevent excess morbidity. These emergencies may occur with or without known history of psychiatric comorbidities so clinicians of all backgrounds need to aware of presenting signs and symptoms to expedite evaluation and management.

LEARNING POINTS

- *Alcohol intoxication*:
  - Clinical manifestations: Ataxia, nystagmus, slurred speech, impaired judgment → amnesia → hypothermia, hypotension, nausea, vomiting → hyporeflexia, respiratory compromise, and coma
  - Administer thiamine prior to glucose when treating suspected thiamine deficiency.
- *Alcohol withdrawal*:
  - Clinical manifestations: Tremor, anxiety, diaphoresis, tachycardia, fever, hyperreflexia, and hypertension
  - Treatment: Assess and treat respiratory depression, stabilize vital functions, correct metabolic abnormalities, fluid resuscitation, and nutritional supplementation. Metadoxine accelerates ethanol clearance.
  - DT management: Scheduled symptom screening with validated tool such as CIWA; pharmacologic management with scheduled and as needed BDZs and/or phenobarbital; additional pharmacologic options for refractory cases with propofol or dexmedetomidine infusion
- *Delirium*:
  - Disturbance in attention, awareness, and cognition without significantly decreased level of arousal that develops over a short period of time, represents a change from baseline, and tends to fluctuate during the course of the day
  - Predisposing and precipitating risk factors include increasing age; underlying cognitive, sensory, or functional impairment; acute illness; impaired sleep cycle; psychotropic medications; and uncontrolled acute symptoms
  - Management: Optimize precipitating factors: Frequent reorientation, familiarize environment, minimize disturbances, sleep hygiene, early mobilization, optimize nutrition, prevent complications; reserve pharmacologic therapy if delirium refractory to nonpharmacologic therapies, consider antipsychotic agents for agitated delirium
- *NMS*:
  - Characteristics: Recent exposure to dopaminergic medication, hyperthermia, rigidity, mental status change, and dysautonomia
  - Management: Discontinue offending agent, supportive measures, volume resuscitation, external cooling and correction of metabolic derangements as needed; BDZs, bromocriptine, dantrolene, and ECT for sere or refractory cases
- *Serotonin syndrome*:
  - Characterized by altered mentation, autonomic hyperactivity (hyperthermia, hypertension, tachycardia, tachypnea, diaphoresis, and diarrhea), and neuromuscular manifestations (hyperreflexia, spontaneous or inducible clonus, ocular clonus, muscle rigidity, and hypertonicity)
  - Management: Discontinue offending agent, supportive measures, fluid resuscitation, BDZs, and cyproheptadine
- *Malignant catatonia*:
  - Characterized by general symptoms of catatonia with hyperthermia and autonomic hyperactivity (labile blood pressure, tachycardia, tachypnea, and diaphoresis)
  - Supportive measures, BDZs, and ECT

REFERENCES

1. Wheat S, Dschida D, Talen MR. Psychiatric Emergencies. Prim Care. 2016;43(2):341-54.
2. Mirijello A, Sestito L, Antonelli M, Gasbarrini A, Addolorato G. Identification and management of acute alcohol intoxication. Eur J Intern Med. 2023;108:1-8.
3. Díaz Martínez MC, Díaz Martínez A, Villamil Salcedo V, Cruz Fuentes C. Efficacy of metadoxine in the management of acute alcohol intoxication. J Int Med Res. 2002;30(1):44-51.
4. Shpilenya LS, Muzychenko AP, Gasbarrini G, Addolorato G. Metadoxine in acute alcohol intoxication: a double-blind,

randomized, placebo-controlled study. Alcohol Clin Exp Res. 2002;26(3):340-6.
5. Grover S, Ghosh A. Delirium Tremens: Assessment and Management. J Clin Exp Hepatol. 2018;8(4):460-70.
6. Schmidt KJ, Doshi MR, Holzhausen JM, Natavio A, Cadiz M, Winegardner JE. Treatment of Severe Alcohol Withdrawal. Annals of Pharmacotherapy. 2016;50(5):389-401.
7. Association AP. Delirium. 5th edition. Arlington, VA: American Psychiatric Publishing; 2013.
8. Marcantonio ER. Delirium in Hospitalized Older Adults. N Engl J Med. 2017;377(15):1456-66.
9. Oh ES, Fong TG, Hshieh TT, Inouye SK. Delirium in Older Persons: Advances in Diagnosis and Treatment. JAMA. 2017;318(12):1161-74.
10. Reade MC, Finfer S. Sedation and Delirium in the Intensive Care Unit. N Engl J Med. 2014;370(5):444-54.
11. Inouye SK, van Dyck CH, Alessi CA, Balkin S, Siegal AP, Horwitz RI. Clarifying confusion: the confusion assessment method. A new method for detection of delirium. Ann Intern Med. 1990;113(12):941-8.
12. Ely EW, Inouye SK, Bernard GR, Gordon S, Francis J, May L, et al. Delirium in Mechanically Ventilated Patients Validity and Reliability of the Confusion Assessment Method for the Intensive Care Unit (CAM-ICU). JAMA. 2001;286(21):2703-10.
13. Guzé BH, Baxter LR. Neuroleptic Malignant Syndrome. N Engl J Med. 1985;313(3):163-6.
14. Association AP. Medication-Induced Movement Disorders and Other Adverse Effects of Medication, 5th edition. Arlington, VA: American Psychiatric Publishing; 2013.
15. Bhanushali MJ, Tuite PJ. The evaluation and management of patients with neuroleptic malignant syndrome. Neurol Clin. 2004;22(2):389-411.
16. Strawn JR, Keck PE Jr, Caroff SN. Neuroleptic malignant syndrome. Am J Psychiatry. 2007;164(6):870-6.
17. Boyer EW, Shannon M. The Serotonin Syndrome. N Engl J Med. 2005;352(11):1112-20.
18. Wijdicks EFM, Rabinstein AA, Hocker SE, Fugate JE. Treatable Toxicity After Chemotherapy, 2nd edition. New York, USA: Oxford University Press; 2016.
19. Dunkley EJC, Isbister GK, Sibbritt D, Dawson AH, Whyte IM. The Hunter Serotonin Toxicity Criteria: simple and accurate diagnostic decision rules for serotonin toxicity. QJM. 2003;96(9):635-42.
20. Fink M, Taylor MA. The Catatonia Syndrome: Forgotten but Not Gone. Arch Gen Psychiatry. 2009;66(11):1173-7.
21. Heckers S, Walther S. Caring for the Patient With Catatonia. JAMA Psychiatry. 2021;78(5):560-1.
22. Association AP. Catatonia Associated With Another Mental Disorder (Catatonia Specifier), 5th edition. Arlington, VA: American Psychiatric Publishing; 2013. pp. 119-21.

Exploring the Neurobiology of Human Sexuality

Joy D Desai

INTRODUCTION

An anthropological perspective views sexual behavior as an evolutionary necessity that ensures the preservation and propagation of the human species. Its biological necessity has resulted in behavioral paradigms that ensure the likelihood of species propagation (its prime purpose). Evolution and sociological determinants influence the adaptation this behavior has undergone amongst ethnic and religious groups within society.

Observant writers have dwelled on its varied nuances, at times triggering heated debates. *"Graze on my lips, and if those hills be dry stray lower, where the pleasant fountains lie."*—wrote William Shakespeare in *Venus and Adonis*. This literary vignette describes a facet of human sexual behavior exemplifying the close relationship between the pursuit of pleasure and execution of an action that drives the subliminal goal of procreation.

RELEVANT TERMINOLOGIES

Libido, derived from the Latin root for lust, refers to the fluctuating state of sexual motivation in all organisms. It is modified by the internal hormonal milieu and/or multimodal erotic sensory cues moderated by learnt behavior/beliefs and situational propriety of the pursuit of its incentives. Cognitive processing provides variability in sexual arousability, and behavior directed at attaining an anticipated sexual reward.

Both central and peripheral neural networks determine the physiological capability of an individual to be aroused and participate in sexually goal directed behavior. The activation and sustainability of these network driven physiologies at a moment in time is modified by cultural norms, learned associations, perceived propriety, mood, and exposure to recreational chemical compounds. This essay is an exploratory attempt at integrating some of these known neurobiological insights into human sexual behavior.

Sexual desire is defined by some, as the presence or initiation of sexual motivations, fantasies, or thoughts with an intent to engage in sexual behavior in response to relevant internal and external cues.[1] It is modified by mood, health, opportunity and/or partner availability, and prevailing attitudes from experience or learning. According to Masters and Johnson, physiological sexual stimulation is characterized by phases of excitement, plateau, orgasm, and resolution.[2] During the excitement phase, an erotic mental or physical stimulation or situation results in arousal as a preparation for coitus.

In males, arousal is characterized by a physical penile tumescence driven by engorgement by blood within the corpora cavernosa, a reflexogenic parasympathetic activity mediated by endothelial release of nitric oxide.

Female arousal is characterized by a similar parasympathetic mechanism driving clitoral engorgement in conjunction with enhanced activity within the Bartholin glands at the vaginal opening producing mucoid secretary lubrication within the vagina to aid coital engagement with a tumescent penis. Vasoactive intestinal peptide acts as an arterial vasodilator while neuropeptide Y produces venous vasoconstriction contributing to this secretory process.[3]

While these peripheral mechanisms are well known, the neural networks that are activated during various phases of sexual activity were elucidated only with the advent of sophisticated imaging such as functional magnetic resonance imaging (MRI) and brain fluorodeoxyglucose (FDG) positron emission tomography (PET) imaging. The challenges lay in designing paradigms within the imaging devices that could replicate closely normal, unobserved, consensual sexual activity with its implied privacy.

The "sexual pleasure cycle" model proposed by Georgiadis[4] implies similarities with other reward seeking behaviors like consuming food or indulging in exposure to recreational drugs. It assumes that the neurobiological reward system is the basis of "appetitive" sexual behavior as in a "wanting system", followed by a "consummatory" or "liking/wanting system", and a feedback "inhibitory" system that modulates the actual execution of sexual activity based on learned beliefs and social propriety. Naturally, the mesolimbic dopaminergic system network plays an integral role in the initiation of such "appetitive" activity.[5] The core elements of the mesolimbic dopaminergic system form the epicenter of reward seeking behavior that results in the pursuit of pleasure in various forms such as food, gambling, recreational drugs, and sexual forays.

An alternative viewpoint positions sexual behavior as optionally reflexive involving autonomic activation, genital reflexes/sensations, and innate copulatory behavior driven by neural networks integrating parasympathetic and sympathetic peripheral nerves with spinal reflexes, followed by brainstem and hypothalamic activation. Dopamine is the neurotransmitter switch that flips in the medial preoptic area (a component of the mesolimbic dopaminergic network). It is deemed necessary for the regulation of parasympathetic and sympathetic flow within the peripheral genital nerves. The incentive to allow this to progress is moderated by Pavlovian associations between sexual stimuli and putative reward or punishment. This involves limbic and cortical structures that interact with the hypothalamus.

The following discussion will focus on the current understanding of the neuroanatomical basis for the distinct components of the sexual response cycle: Sexual incentive identification, sexual desire, sexual arousal, physical and genital stimulation, and sexual pleasure including orgasm. The brain responses to sexual stimuli are very similar between homosexual and heterosexual individuals, once there is an exposure to the preferred sexual incentives.[6,7] Hence, no separate discussion on gender preference deviations will be included.

KEY ELEMENTS

Sexual drive and the threshold for seeking sexual incentives via motivated behavior or exploration has been attributed to activity within the mesolimbic dopaminergic reward-oriented network. This network connects the ventral tegmental area (VTA) to the nucleus accumbens in the ventral striatum and to the amygdala.[8] Dopamine and endocannabinoids are key transmitters that participate in neural transmissions within this network. A functional MRI (fMRI) study demonstrated that the orbitofrontal cortex encodes both the identity and the value of reward within the mesolimbic system, while modulatory activity of the ventromedial prefrontal cortex (PFC) is probably involved in categorizing stimuli across reward categories.[9] A complex modulatory role is played by endocannabinoids within this system as cannabinoid receptor 1 (CB1) receptors abound in VTA, hippocampus, amygdala, and hypothalamus.

When implicit sensory stimuli are considered to be sexually salient, integration with past experiences and learned behavior are orchestrated through limbic forebrain structures such as hypothalamus, amygdala, hippocampus, and nuclei of the septal region, which are employed in motivational states and emotional processing. The sensorimotor cortices are involved in genital sensations and triggering the voluntary movements during sexual intercourse. Higher order associative areas in the parieto-occipital cortices play a pivotal role in erotic mental imagery whereas the prefrontal cortices are instrumental for the inhibition of sexual pulses.

The spinal cord is mainly involved in penile and clitoral tumescence, vaginal and penile gland lubrication, and rhythmic contraction of perineum muscles whereas the nucleus paragigantocellularis (nPGi), locus coeruleus (LC), raphe nuclei, and periaqueductal gray area, located in the brainstem, are integral for erection and ejaculation. Stimulation of the pelvic plexus and the cavernous nerves induces erection, whereas stimulation of the sympathetic trunk causes detumescence. This clearly implies that the sacral parasympathetic input is responsible for tumescence and the thoracolumbar sympathetic pathway is responsible for detumescence. Similarly, the parasympathetic system is responsible for clitoral erection and vaginal lubrication, while the sympathetic one contributes to female orgasm.[3] The similarities between the regulatory mechanisms determining sexual responsiveness of either gender are thus striking. Thus, it is clear that integrated networks contribute to sexual neurobiology in a flowing manner yet segregated for functionality within different components of the pleasure cycle.

The brain areas that play key roles in human sexual function are depicted in **Table 1**.

While the nucleus accumbens is accepted as a pivotal component of the reward system, the role of the thalamus has been independently evaluated in the complex neurobiology of sexual activation. Thalamic deep brain stimulation and isolated thalamic electrical stimulation have been shown to influence penile erection in humans.[10] The fMRI studies have demonstrated thalamic activation on exposure to erotic visual stimulation and independently implicated in sexual preference processing via its complex connectivity to the limbic network. It may thus play an important role in mate choices and complex behavioral alterations through all phases of the sexual pleasure cycle.[11] The notion that the thalamus is a just relay station for simplex and complex sensory stimulatory pathways needs revisiting.

TABLE 1: The brain areas that play key roles in human sexual function.

Mesolimbic reward system	• Triggers sexual motivation • Mate choice
Thalamus	Relays incoming erotic stimuli from spinal cord to sensorimotor cortices
Hypothalamus	• Co-ordinates autonomic events in sexual behavior • Plays a role in mate choice
Amygdala	• Designates emotional value to incoming erotic stimuli • Mate choice • Modulates sexual drive
Septal region	Modulates sexual drive
Prefrontal cortex	• Moderates initiation of sexual behavior • Modulates sexual drive
Cingulate cortex	• Processing sexual stimuli in context of perceived conflict • Modulates sexual drive
Insula	• Awareness of tumescence of erectile organs • Modulates sexual drive

Source: Adapted from Calabrò RS, Cacciola A, Bruschetta D, Milardi D, Quattrini F, Sciarrone F, et al. Neuroanatomy and function of human sexual behavior: A neglected or unknown issue? Brain Behav. 2019;9(12):e 01389.

ROLE OF HYPOTHALAMUS

The hypothalamus is known to participate in and contribute to complex behavior and varied endocrine biologies, e.g., hunger, thirst, circadian timing, sexual drive, and behavioral responses. The medial preoptic area and the anterior hypothalamus receive information from the hippocampus via the lateral septum and from the amygdala via the bed nucleus of the stria terminalis. In rats, lesioning of the medial preoptic area resulted in muted sexual drive despite being in a sexual-incentive rich environment. The hypothalamus contributes to penile erection through two of its several nuclei: The dorsomedial hypothalamic nucleus (DMHN) and ventromedial hypothalamic nucleus (VMHN). The DMHN projects into the mesencephalic reticular formation via the dorsal and central gray matter and LC. Both the DMHN and VMHN network with the lumbosacral autonomic centers involved in penile erection through the dorsolateral funiculus of the spinal cord. The hypothalamic nuclei also receive information directly from the genital regions. The paraventricular nucleus of the hypothalamus has been demonstrated to be intensely activated in fMRI studies evaluating the female orgasm.[12] Interestingly, the interstitial nucleus of the anterior hypothalamus 3 (INAH3) is demonstrated to be dimorphic. In gay men and in women it is smaller suggesting that sexual orientation may have a biological basis.[13] Similar studies have implicated structural variability within the uncinate nucleus of hypothalamus and the bed nucleus of the stria terminalis with sexual orientation and gender identity.[14-16]

AMYGDALA

The human amygdala is a collection of three distinct cell nuclei populations. The basolateral group is the largest, the centromedial group being smaller, with the cortical nucleus being the smallest. The amygdala has a rich neural networked connectivity with the orbitofrontal cortex (OFC), ventromedial PFC, the hypothalamus (the bed nucleus of the stria terminalis), the nucleus accumbens, and many areas of the sensorimotor cortices. Bilateral damage to the amygdala can result in manifest hypersexuality, as graphically elucidated in the Klüver–Bucy syndrome.[17] The most ancient part of the amygdala, the cortical nucleus receives a rich input from the olfactory bulb and the olfactory cortex. In the animal kingdom, the refined assessment of smell and pheromones due to this input contributes to the fundamental macrosmatic sexual behavior of these animals.

The amygdalae are also contributors to the social brain.[18] In humans, when incoming sexually rich stimuli gain an emotional relevance, the amygdala convey them to the PFC and OFC. The associated connections to the hypothalamus and nucleus accumbens result in a complex cognitive regulation of autonomic responses to sexually salient stimuli. Stimulation of the amygdala results in orgasm like pleasurable sensations.[19]

The relationship of the amygdala to sexual orientation was studied innovatively. MRI based volumetric asymmetry and functional connectivity on PET scan assessment of glucose utilization amongst a cohort of heterosexual men and women (*HeM* and *HeW*) and homosexual men and women (*HoM* and *HoW*) revealed intriguing results.[20] In *HeM* and *HoW*, volumetric measurements showed a rightward cerebral asymmetry, whereas the volumes of the cerebral hemispheres were symmetrical in *HoM* and *HeW*. Moreover, homosexual subjects also showed sex atypical amygdala connections. In *HoM*, as in *HeW*, the connections were more widespread from the left amygdala. In *HoW* and *HeM*, on the other hand, they were more widespread from the right amygdala. In *HoM* and *HeW*, the connections were primarily consolidated with the contralateral amygdala and the anterior cingulate gyri; in *HeM* and *HoW*, they were consolidated with the caudate, putamen, and PFC. These findings suggest that sexual orientation is probably driven by distinct set of neural networks that warrant diligent study.

As the apex species within the evolutionary pyramid, human sexual behavior is modulated by past learned experiences, religious beliefs, moral convictions, and social paradigms of propriety. It is not surprising therefore that the cerebral cortices play an important role in human sexual behavioral patterns. The *PFC*, the *OFC*, the cingulate gyrus, and the insula play pivotal roles in this function.

The PFC contributes to planned activity, experience, and moral value-based decision making, gauging accurate cause and effect relationships, socially accepted behavior, and managing conflict resolution. As a result, it suppresses autonomic sexual arousal and incentive motivated urges/behavior when deemed inappropriate for a given context or social setting. This type of inhibition or suppression represents an approach–avoidance conflict, wherein the expectation of a sexual reward flames the desire, but the actual or perceived negative consequences of engaging in sexual activity blunts the initiation of behavior.[21] Sexual activity promoting social stimulants such as alcohol and cocaine act via an inhibition of these regulatory PFC influences. Serotonin, which induce satiety; endocannabinoids, which induce sedation; and opioids, which moderate sexual reward states, seem to be the three cardinal neurochemical systems involved in PFC mediated sexual inhibition.[22] Hypersexuality or disinhibited sexual behavior is often attributed to OFC lesions. The OFC region is also hyperperfused on fMRI and is the preorgasmic phase of sexual escalation, especially in women.[23] The complex connectivity of this region to the mesolimbic reward system contributes to the cognitive filtering of sexual behavior.[24]

CINGULATE GYRUS

The cingulate cortex or the cingulate gyrus is a conspicuous part of the limbic system, and it anatomically envelopes the corpus callosum from the rostrum to its splenium. It is divided into anterior, a middle, and a genual subregion. The anterior cingulate cortex (ACC) is further divided into two functionally segregated areas, i.e., ventral and dorsal (vACC/dACC). Through its rich connectivity to the limbic cortex, it plays a vital role in motivational behavior.[25] During the sexual act, it plays an important role in decision-making, and on fMRI studies, it lights up during the process of analyzing erotic stimuli irrespective of divergent contexts.[26] Increased cingulate activation is observed in females during orgasm and in males during sustained erection.[27] The cingulate cortex in conjunction with the PFC and OFC acts as a moderator and arbitrator for sexual behavior within contextual conflict assessment and resolution.

INSULA

The insula is an integral part of the salience network, analyzing and conveying complex sensory information/stimuli to varied cortical areas facilitating attention and working memory related activity.[28] In conjunction with the cingulate gyrus, the insula conveys incoming stimulatory information to the brainstem for autonomic responsiveness and is noted to be activated in various fMRI studies of sexual arousal. Once sexual activity is initiated, this activation moves to the posterior insula.[29] Functional coupling of the cingulate gyrus, insula, nucleus accumbens, and the mesolimbic network occurs in most phases of the pleasure cycle. Patients suffering from symptomatic epilepsy due to dysplasia in the insular cortex have been shown to exhibit disorders of genital arousal, an indirect indication of its role in this physiology.[30] It has been suggested that body maps are processed in the posterior parts of the insula, explaining some of its contributory roles in the physiology of the sexual cycle. In men, awareness of tumescence and engorgement of the genitals on viewing erotic visual imagery is associated with insular activation on functional imaging.[31]

The current understanding of neural networks implies that these critical neuroanatomical hubs function within densely recruited, constantly flowing regional connections within the cerebral cortices during different phases of the sexual pleasure cycle. Mutual partner stimulation paradigms of fMRI during sexual activity are now refined enough to demonstrate a "sexual wanting pattern" that encompasses the superior parietal lobule, the temporo-occipital areas, nucleus accumbens, OFC, ACC, amygdala, and the hippocampus during sexual arousal. An alternative "sexual liking pattern" involving the inferior parietal lobule, hypothalamus, insula, ventral premotor cortex, and the middle cingulate cortex, has been demonstrated during the physical sexual activity.[4]

Studies examining brain regions activated on fMRI during orgasm in either gender have revealed striking patterns. In women during self-induced and partner stimulated sexual activity in an MRI scanner, brain activity gradually increased leading up to orgasm, peaked at orgasm, and then decreased. There was no evidence of deactivation of brain regions leading up to or during orgasm. The activated brain regions included sensory, motor, reward, frontal cortical, and brainstem regions, e.g., nucleus accumbens, insula, ACC, OFC, operculum, right angular gyrus, paracentral lobule, cerebellum, hippocampus, amygdala, hypothalamus, VTA, and dorsal raphe.[23]

The same author had earlier studied women with complete spinal injury at D10 or higher in a self-stimulated paradigm. Sexual self-stimulation resulted in activation of the nucleus of the solitary tract implying an ascending sensory pathway utilizing the afferents within the vagus nerve. During orgasm, brain regions activated included the hypothalamic paraventricular nucleus, amygdala, accumbens-bed nucleus of the stria terminalis-preoptic area, hippocampus, basal ganglia (especially putamen), cerebellum, and anterior cingulate, insular, parietal, and frontal cortices, and lower brainstem: central gray, mesencephalic reticular formation, and nucleus of the tractus solitarius.[12] The study concluded that the vagus nerve provides a spinal cord bypass pathway for conveyance of cervical and vaginal sexual sensory stimuli.

Orgasmic perceptual experiences have been described in the absence of genital stimulation more often in women than in men. Some have been described in sleep and others as spontaneous on a background of psychiatric illness. In a singular case study, a woman who claimed to induce orgasms by a "tantric" yoga exercise was confirmed to demonstrate a prolactin surge after such an induced event.[32]

ROMANTIC LOVE AND SOCIAL PAIR BONDING

While these studies are a window to the complexities of neural network activation during the sexual act leading up to and ultimately resulting in orgasm, in actuality the neurobiology may be more complex. The neurobiology of romantic love has also been assessed in fMRI studies. The activity in the brains of 17 subjects who were deeply in love was scanned using fMRI, while they viewed pictures of their romantic partners, and compared with the activity produced by viewing pictures of three friends of similar age, sex, and duration of friendship as their partners. The activity was restricted to foci in the medial insula and the ACC, and subcortically in the caudate nucleus and the putamen, all bilaterally. Deactivations were observed in the posterior cingulate gyrus and in the amygdala and were right lateralized in the prefrontal, parietal, and middle temporal cortices.[33] The authors concluded that functional specialization occurs in the neural networks responsible for affective states too.

Pair bonding and social monogamy in marital or committed relationship have been studied in prairie voles and in humans in many unique ways. These have shed light on the complex interplay between dopamine, oxytocin, and arginine vasopressin in experimental mammals and in humans. Oxytocin released maternally during labor, delivery, and subsequent breast feeding has gained fame as the love hormone or bonding hormone. In ewes, an infusion of oxytocin into the brain results in rapid bonding with a foreign lamb. In male prairie voles, vasopressin stimulates pair bonding, aggression toward potential rivals, and paternal instincts, such as grooming offspring in the nest. Variation in a regulatory region of the vasopressin receptor gene "AVPR1A" predicts the likelihood that a male vole will bond with a female.

A study shows that men with a particular *AVPR1A* variant are twice as likely as men without it to remain unmarried, or when married, twice as likely to report a recent crisis in their marriage.[34] The spouses of men with this variation in vasopressin gene also express a greater dissatisfaction in their marital relationship. This is probably indirect evidence of the role of vasopressin in maintaining behavior relevant for cementing social bonds. In a randomized, placebo-controlled trial, the intranasal administration of oxytocin stimulated men in a monogamous relationship (but not single ones) to keep a much greater distance between themselves and an attractive unattached woman in a first encounter.[35] Oxytocin now came to be perceived as biological promoter of socially bonded monogamous behavior irrespective of gender. While pair bonding has been linked to oxytocin biology, the polar opposite of this behavior, i.e., promiscuity and infidelity in monogamous relationships has been linked to variations in the dopamine D4 gene.[36]

"Love cures people—both the ones who give it and the ones who receive it", claimed psychiatrist Karl Menninger. A recent study at the University of South Carolina shows that pair bonding in monogamous mice is protective against tumor growth, likely via changes in serum factors and cancer cell transcription.[37] They demonstrated in vitro that human lung cancer grows larger when exposed to sera from mice with disrupted pair bonds compared to sera from mice with intact pair bonds. Transcriptomic analyses reveal that tumor cells grown with sera from bonded animals, compared to those grown with sera from either virgin or bond-disrupted animals, exhibit differential expression of several cancer-related genes involved in cell migration and tissue morphogenesis.

Postorgasmic prolactin secretion within the diencephalon is perceived to aid postcoital satiety and induction of sleep. There is some evidence that orgasm from intercourse results in greater such cerebral prolactin surges than that from masturbation.[38] Postorgasmic prolactin is also thought to drive the postcoital inhibitory period for sexual arousal in men.

NEUROTRANSMITTER CONTRIBUTIONS TO SEXUAL NEUROBIOLOGY

Human neurons of the raphe nuclei are the principal source of serotonin release in the brain.[39] Axons of neurons in the *caudal* raphe nuclei terminate in deep cerebellar nuclei, cerebellar cortex, and spinal cord. Axons of neurons in the *rostral* raphe nuclei terminate in the thalamus, striatum, hypothalamus, nucleus accumbens, temporal neocortex, cingulate gyrus, cingulum, hippocampus, and amygdalae. Serotonin receptors abound in the peripheral nervous system wherein they play an important contributory role in vascular responsiveness during sexual arousal through complex effects on vasodilatation and vasoconstriction. The central effects of serotoninergic activation impair erection, ejaculation, sexual interest, and coital lubrication. Not surprisingly, consumption of selective serotonin reuptake inhibitors for endogenous depression is associated with this wide array of sexual dysfunctions. Norepinephrine stimulates penile erection via autonomic activation and can reverse the sexual inhibition that follows sexual exhaustion, thus being useful in the treatment of erectile dysfunction and anorgasmia. Acetylcholine is implicated in penile erection, and it has been shown to be useful in reversing antidepressant induced erectile and ejaculation difficulties. Opioids within the hypothalamic physiology exhibit a complex interplay with testosterone and luteinizing hormone. It has a significant inhibitory effect on most neurobiological mechanisms that drive sexual arousal and performance and chronic opioid excess either for recreational or therapeutic purposes can result in loss of libido, erectile dysfunction, and anorgasmia. Androgens play cardinal roles in both stimulating and maintaining sexual function in man, being critical for sexual motivation, penile tissue development, growth, and maintenance of erectile function. Similarly, estradiol via complex regulatory influences can modulate all aspects of female sexual responsiveness. It is evident that the biological repertoire of sexual behavior is an integrated expression of neural networks driven by situational and incentive driven reciprocity, moderated by social and learnt nuances of propriety, and catalyzed by neurotransmitter fluctuations.

CONCLUDING REMARKS

The different phases of the pleasure cycle resulting in sexually directed behavior are perceived as fascinating from numerous points of view. While a sexual response (given an incentive) is thought to be reflexive or autonomically generated, its regulation by complex cognitive processing makes the contribution of the nervous system vividly evident. Numerous elements within the nervous system act as hubs promoting a specific input into sexual physiology governance, while simultaneously participating in a flowing network richly connected to emotional, cognitive, salience, and motivational circuits. Each of these is intimately connected and intertwined with a complex neurotransmitter functionality. A growing body of neuroscience research has cast an inquiring spotlight on these phenomena. As research paradigms improve with increasing sophistication of imaging of the brain, we will be convinced that (like in other physiologies) in the sexual uniqueness of our behavior, we are our brains. Diversity in neurobiology lends individual colors to this alluring palette.

REFERENCES

1. Buss DM, Schmitt DP. Sexual strategies theory: An evolutionary perspective on human mating. Psychol Rev. 1993;100(2):204-32.
2. Masters WH, Johnson VE. Human sexual response, 1st edition. Boston, MA: Little, Brown and Company; 1966.
3. Levin RJ. The ins and outs of vaginal lubrication. Sex Relatsh Ther. 2003;18(4):509-13.
4. Georgiadis JR, Kringelbach ML. The human sexual response cycle: Brain imaging evidence linking sex to other pleasures. Prog Neurobiol. 2012;98(1):49-81.
5. Alcaro A, Huber R, Panksepp J. Behavioral functions of the mesolimbic dopaminergic system: an affective neuroethological perspective. Brain Res Rev. 2007;56(2):283-321.
6. Safron A, Barch B, Bailey JM, Gitelman DR, Parrish TB, Reber PJ. Neural correlates of sexual arousal in homosexual and heterosexual men. Behav Neurosci. 2007;121:237-48.
7. Ponseti J, Granert O, Jansen O, Wolff S, Mehdorn H, Bosinski H, et al. Assessment of sexual orientation using the hemodynamic brain response to visual sexual stimuli. J Sex Med. 2009;6(6):1628-34.
8. Halbout B, Marshall AT, Azimi A, Liljeholm M, Mahler SV, Wassum KM, et al. Mesolimbic dopamine projections mediate cue-motivated reward seeking but not reward retrieval in rats. Elife. 2019;8:e43551.
9. Howard JD, Gottfried JA, Tobler PN, Kahnt T. Identity specific coding of future rewards in the human orbitofrontal cortex. Proc Natl Acad Sci U S A. 2015;112(16):5195-200.
10. Temel Y, van Lankveld JJDM, Boon P, Spincemaille GH, van der Linden C, Visser-Vandewalle V. Deep brain stimulation of the thalamus can influence penile erection. Int J Impot Res. 2004;16(1):91-4.
11. Mutarelli EG, Omuro AMP, Adoni T. Hypersexuality following bilateral thalamic infarction: Case report. Arq Neuropsiquiatr. 2006;64(1):146-8.
12. Komisaruk BR, Whipple B. Functional MRI of the brain during orgasm in women. Annu Rev Sex Res. 2005:16:62-86.
13. LeVay S. A difference in hypothalamic structure between heterosexual and homosexual men. Science. 1991;253(5023): 1034-7.
14. Hammack SE, Braas KM, May V. Chemoarchitecture of the bed nucleus of the stria terminalis: Neurophenotypic diversity and function. Handb Clin Neurol. 2021;179:385-402.
15. Brunetti M, Babiloni C, Ferretti A, Del Gratta C, Merla A, Olivetti Belardinelli M, et al. Hypothalamus, sexual arousal, and psychosexual identity in human males: A functional magnetic resonance imaging study. Eur J Neurosci. 2008;27(11):2922-7.

16. Calabrò RS, Cacciola A, Bruschetta D, Milardi D, Quattrini F, Sciarrone F, et al. Neuroanatomy and function of human sexual behavior: A neglected or unknown issue? Brain Behav. 2019;9(12):e01389.
17. Lanska DJ. The Klüver-Bucy syndrome. Front Neurol Neurosci. 2018;41:77-89.
18. Adolphs R, Tranel D, Damasio AR. The human amygdala in social judgment. Nature. 1998;393(6684):470-4.
19. Baird AD, Wilson SJ, Bladin PF, Saling MM, Reutens DC. The amygdala and sexual drive: Insights from temporal lobe epilepsy surgery. Ann Neurol. 2004;55(1):87-96.
20. Savic I, Lindstrom P. PET and MRI show differences in cerebral asymmetry and functional connectivity between homo- and heterosexual subjects. Proc Natl Acad Sci USA. 2008;105:9403-8.
21. Berkman ET, Lieberman MD. Approaching the bad and avoiding the good: Lateral prefrontal cortical asymmetry distinguishes between action and valence. J Cogn Neurosci. 2010;22(9):1970-9.
22. Pfaus JG. Pathways of sexual desire. J Sex Med. 2009;6(6):1506-33.
23. Wise NJ, Frangos E, Komisaruk BR. Brain Activity Unique to Orgasm in Women: An fMRI Analysis. J Sex Med. 2017;14(11):1380-91.
24. Baird AD, Wilson SJ, Bladin PF, Saling MM, Reutens DC. Neurological control of human sexual behaviour: Insights from lesion studies. J Neurol Neurosurg Psychiatry. 2007;78(10):1042-9.
25. Touroutoglou A, Andreano J, Dickerson BC, Barrett LF. The tenacious brain: How the anterior mid-cingulate contributes to achieving goals. Cortex. 2020;123:12-29.
26. Arnow BA, Desmond JE, Banner LL, Glover GH, Solomon A, Polan ML, et al. Brain activation and sexual arousal in healthy, heterosexual males. Brain. 2002;125:1014-23.
27. Schober JM, Pfaff D. The neurophysiology of sexual arousal. Best Pract Res Clin Endocrinol Metab. 2007;21(3):445-61.
28. Uddin LQ. Salience processing and insular cortical function and dysfunction. Nat Rev Neurosci. 2014;16(1):55-61.
29. Georgiadis JR. Functional neuroanatomy of human cortex cerebri in relation to wanting sex and having it. Clin Anat. 2015;28(3):314-23.
30. Anzellotti F, Franciotti R, Bonanni L, Tamburro G, Perrucci MG, Thomas A, et al. Persistent genital arousal disorder associated with functional hyperconnectivity of an epileptic focus. Neuroscience. 2010;167(1):88-96.
31. Rupp HA, Wallen K. Sex differences in response to visual sexual stimuli: A review. Arch Sex Behav. 2008;37(2):206-18.
32. Pfaus JG, Tsarski K. A Case of Female Orgasm Without Genital Stimulation. Sex Med. 2022;10(2):100496.
33. Bartels A, Zeki S. The neural basis of romantic love. Neuroreport. 2000;11(17):3829-34.
34. Walum H, Westberg L, Henningsson S, Neiderhiser JM, Reiss D, Igl W, et al. Genetic variation in the vasopressin receptor 1a gene (AVPR1A) associates with pair-bonding behavior in humans. Proc Natl Acad Sci U S A. 2008;105(37):14153-6.
35. Scheele D, Striepens N, Güntürkün O, Deutschländer S, Maier W, Kendrick KM, et al. Oxytocin modulates social distance between males and females. J Neurosci. 2012;32(46):16074-9.
36. Garcia JR, MacKillop J, Aller EL, Merriwether AM, Wilson DS, Lum JK. Associations between dopamine D4 receptor gene variation with both infidelity and sexual promiscuity. PLoS One. 2010;5(11):e14162.
37. Naderi A, Soltanmaohammadi E, Kaza V, Barlow S, Chatzistamou L, Kiaris H. Persistent effects of pair bonding in lung cancer cell growth in monogamous Peromyscus californicus. Elife. 2021;10:e64711.
38. Brody S, Krüger THC. The post-orgasmic prolactin increase following intercourse is greater than following masturbation and suggests greater satiety. Biol Psychol. 2006;71(3):312-5.
39. Calabrò RS, Bramanti P. Neuroanatomy and physiology of human Sexuality. In: Calabrò RS (Ed). Male Sexual Dysfunction in Neurological Diseases: From Pathophysiology to Rehabilitation. New York, NY: Nova Science Publisher Inc; 2011. pp. 1-24.

CHAPTER 31

Neuropsychological Aspects of Traumatic Brain Injury

Sandip Chatterjee, Niloy Biswas

INTRODUCTION

Traumatic brain injury (TBI) is known as the silent epidemic which worldwide produces more deaths and disabilities than most other illnesses. It is a major public health problem in India, today exceeding heart attacks and brain strokes in terms of mortality and morbidity resulting in deaths, injuries, and disabilities of young and productive people of our society. The cost in terms of loss to the country's exchequer is phenomenal, though currently unmeasured.

In the National Institute of Mental Health Neuro Sciences (NIMHANS) study[1] looking at the effect of patients with head injury (7,164 patients), the specific health problems faced by surviving injured persons were difficulty in locomotor activities among 87 subjects, post-traumatic headache ($n = 79$), decreased power and strength in limbs ($n = 57$), memory and information processing deficits ($n = 44$), visual difficulties ($n = 31$), speech and communication problems ($n = 25$), generalized pains and aches ($n = 48$), anxiety features ($n = 30$), giddiness and loss of balance ($n = 32$), hearing problems ($n = 14$), and phobias ($n = 22$). A myriad of behavior problems such as anger, depressive features such as worry and sadness, becoming violent, and complete inability to concentrate were noticed among 74 subjects at 1 year follow-up. A number of patients in the study ended up with long-term epilepsy.

The short- and long-term psychological sequelae results in poor quality of life in a large number of patients with moderate-to-severe head injuries. This chapter will look at some of the common problems encountered.

NEUROPSYCHIATRY OF TRAUMATIC BRAIN INJURY

Phineas Gage is probably the most famous person to have survived severe damage to the brain. He is also the first patient from whom we learned something about the relation between personality and the function of the anterior parts of the brain. On September 13th, 1848, an accidental explosion of a charge he had set while involved in a railroad construction, blew a tamping iron through his head. The tamping iron was 3 feet 7 inches long and weighed 13 1/2 pounds. It was 1 1/4 inches in diameter at one end (not *circumference* as in the newspaper report) and tapered over a distance of about 1 foot to a diameter of 1/4 inch at the other. Some months after the accident, probably in about the middle of 1849, Phineas felt he was physically well enough to resume work. He was blind in the left eye and had left facial weakness but no other focal neurological deficits. Unfortunately for him his personality had changed so much, the contractors who had employed him could not feel confident enough to give him his place again. Before the accident, he had been their most capable and efficient foreman, one with a well-balanced mind, who could be completely relied upon, and who was looked on as a shrewd smart businessman. He was now, as observed by his Physician Dr Harlow, fitful, irreverent, and grossly profane, showing little respect or courtesy for his fellows. He was also impatient and obstinate, yet capricious and vacillating, unable to settle on any of the plans he envisaged for his own future. If Dr Harlow were alive today, he would have witnessed an explosion of research into the amazing powers of the frontal cortex. He would know that the cardinal function of the prefrontal cortex is the temporal organization of behavior supported by the subordinate functions of short-term memory, motor attention, and inhibitory control.[2] The change in Gage's personality would clearly be consistent with damage to the orbitofrontal cortex of the ventral aspect of his frontal lobe, affecting affect, and emotion. He could take comfort, however, in the knowledge that 150 years after his original observations, we have made considerable advancement in our understanding of the relation between mind and brain and the reason why, following his injury, Mr Phineas Gage was "no longer Gage".

The frontal-subcortical circuits that are involved in cognition and social behavior are primarily responsible for the psychiatric changes that occur after trauma. Three circuits are predominantly involved—(1) the circuits in the dorsolateral prefrontal cortex which modulate executive functions which include memory, decision making, problem solving, and mental flexibility. (2) The circuits in the orbitofrontal cortex, which play an important part in intuitive reflexive social behavior, the ability to self-monitor, and self-correct in real time. (3) The circuits in the anterior cingulate which regulate motivation.[3]

PATHOPHYSIOLOGY

The most common short-term complications associated with TBIs include cognitive impairment, difficulties with sensory processing and communication, immediate seizures, hydrocephalus, cerebrospinal fluid (CSF) leakage, cranial nerve injuries, vascular injuries, tinnitus, organ failure, and polytrauma. Long-term complications associated with TBIs include Parkinson's disease, Alzheimer's disease, dementia pugilistica, and post-traumatic epilepsy.

Following TBI, there are acute changes in the neurotransmitters which lead to psychiatric manifestations by altering the levels of acetylcholine, norepinephrine, dopamine, and serotonin. Neuropsychiatric symptoms can arise after penetrating or focal trauma as well as nonpenetrating trauma. Penetrating trauma can produce psychiatric symptoms depending on the function served by that particular area (e.g., aggression and behavioral disinhibition in bifrontal contusion). Symptoms of nonpenetrating injuries can be explained by cytotoxic processes such as Ca^{2+} and Mg^{2+} dysregulation, neurotransmitter excitotoxicity, free radical-induced injury, and diffuse axonal injury.[4,5]

Catecholamines

Damage to the ascending monoaminergic projections may cause pathological functioning of the systems dependent on these pathways. Studies show that TBI in these areas leads to decrease in dopamine levels, which have uncertain outcome. Drugs that increase dopaminergic transmission have shown to cause significant improvement in cognitive functions (e.g., arousal, speed of processing, attention, and memory).[6]

Serotonin

Serotonin pathways in the frontal cortex are interrupted by contusions as well as axonal injuries causing dysfunction in this particular neurotransmitter system. These pathways can also be damaged by secondary mechanisms of neuronal damage such as excitotoxins and lipid peroxidation that mediate serotonin. It has been seen that the levels of lumbar CSF 5-hydroxyindoleacetic acid (5-HIAA) are less than normal in conscious patients, it is true that in unconscious patients, levels were found to be normal. 5-HIAA levels in the CSF vary with the size of lesions, for example, patients with frontotemporal contusions have shown a decrease in 5-HIAA level whereas increased levels are seen in cases of diffuse contusions.[7]

Acetylcholine

Both acute and chronic changes are evident in cholinergic cortical transmission after TBI. Acutely, there is an increase in cholinergic transmission after TBI followed by chronic reductions in neurotransmitter function and cholinergic afferents. Chronically following severe TBI, loss of cortical cholinergic afferents with concurrent preservation of postsynaptic muscarinic, and nicotinic receptors are recognized.

The prevalence of psychiatric illness in the first year following moderate-to-severe TBI has been quoted to be as high as 49% in the first year.[8]

Let us look at some of the common problems.

POST-TRAUMATIC STRESS DISORDER

This is an anxiety disorder that some people get after living through a dangerous event in their lives. The normal "fight or flight" response is altered so that they feel scared or stressed even when the danger has passed. War and terrorist attacks have shown there is a complex relationship between psychological and biomechanical trauma. One study[9] in particular showed that there were higher rates of post-traumatic stress disorder (PTSD) in Iraq war veterans who had suffered on the battlefield previous TBI with loss of consciousness compared with veterans that reported no injuries.

The hippocampus and amygdala are brain regions that have networks associated with contextual memory, consolidation, and fear conditioning. Alterations in these circuits have been shown to trigger PTSD symptoms after exposure to trauma. The biomarker S-100B is an astrocyte protein which when measured to be abnormally high in the acute phase of TBI is predictive of PTSD a year later.[10]

COGNITIVE DEFICITS

Cognitive dysfunction occurs in a significant percentage of people with mild TBI, especially in general cognitive ability (26.4%), learning memory (22.6%), and immediate memory (18.9%).[11] Also, compared to a healthy control group, mild-to-moderate TBI patients showed significantly worse cognitive performance on general cognitive ability, naming, incidental memory, immediate memory, learning memory, delayed recall, and executive functioning.[12] A number of studies have reported significant cognitive deficits in the acute phase of post-TBI, mainly associated with episodic memory losses. It is well recognized that compared with healthy controls, patients with mild-to-moderate TBI performed significantly worse in attention, memory, language, and executive functions at acute phase of TBI and at 6-month follow-up.[13] Those patients who had documented neuropsychological changes in the acute phase were found to have changes in white matter integrity in brain regions such as the splenium of corpus callosum and cingulum.[14]

The cognitive functions mainly affected which prevent early return to independent living, social rehabilitation, and family life include the following—frontal executive functions, attention span, short-term memory and learning, speed of information processing, speech, and language functions.

These cognitive domains are affected mainly due to damage to medial temporal regions, dorsolateral prefrontal cortex, and subcortical white mater in between. Professor Fann published in 2018 their work showing an increased risk of dementia in people who had suffered from TBI. He also showed significant problems associated with activities of daily living caused by psychological changes associated with TBI.[15]

Management consists of neuropsychological testing followed by cognitive rehabilitation and use of psychostimulants and dopaminergic agents. Cholinesterase inhibitors have also been recommended.

AFFECTIVE DISORDERS

Disruption of affective-emotional control following moderate-to-severe brain injury may be related to the disruption at the emotion regulation neural networks. This includes several disorders of affect, such as pathological uncontrollable laughing and crying (PLC), and affective lability, triggered by stimuli that commonly do not cause such emotional feeling state, also known as "pseudobulbar affect" or "emotional incontinence" which represent a prototypical form of affective-emotional dissociation. These events must cause subjective distress and/or interfere with everyday life. The pathophysiology is still unknown. However, it seems that PLC is the result of release of cortical inhibition of upper brainstem centers that incorporate the motor activation patterns involved in laughing and crying. Tateno et al.[16] showed that lesions of the lateral aspect of the left frontal lobe were significantly linked to the presence of PLC.

Depressive disorders associated with TBI are categorized into—(1) with major depressive-like episodes, (2) with depressive features, and (3) with mixed features. Prevalence rates for depression vary from 18 to 61%.[17] Rupture of neuronal circuits involving prefrontal cortex, amygdala, hippocampus, basal ganglia, and thalamus may be implicated in the genesis of depression.

Treatment includes psychoeducation, cognitive behavioral therapy (CBT), and medications. Selective serotonin reuptake inhibitors (SSRIs) are the are the first-line recommendations and include sertraline and citalopram as well as fluoxetine and paroxetine.

MANIA

Mania associated with TBI manifests with higher aggression and less euphoria.[18] Injuries to the brain affecting the inhibitory part of the frontal lobes on the subcortical limbic structures is responsible for the development of mania. It is more common in patients having damage to orbitofrontal or temporal cortex.

Valproate is the drug of choice in treatment. Antipsychotic medications like quetiapine and olanzapine are also useful.

PERSONALITY CHANGE

The following personality changes have been described after TBI:[19]
- *Impulsivity* includes verbal utterances, poor decisions, and physical actions.
- Irritability includes verbal outbursts, aggressiveness, and assaultive behavior that are out of proportion to the precipitating stimulus.
- Affective instability includes emotional expression which have a paroxysmal onset, brief duration, and are followed by significant remorse.
- Apathy which in extreme form is akinetic mutism.

Aggression responds to valproate and carbamazepine. Stimulants, dopaminergic agonists, and cholinesterase inhibitors help in apathy.

PSYCHOSIS

The TBI can result in a chronic psychotic illness like schizophrenia developing in patients. Schizophrenia is a mental disorder characterized by continuous or relapsing episodes of psychosis. Major symptoms include hallucinations, delusions, and disorganized thinking. Delusions are the most common symptom, and the content is most often persecutory. EEG abnormalities in the temporal lobe have been found and some have a history of having had seizures in the acute phase. Risperidone is effective, and clozapine in resistant cases.[20]

CONCLUDING REMARKS AND LEARNING POINTS

- Neuropsychological disability produced by traumatic brain injury is significant, and the effects often can last a lifetime.
- Cognitive disorders and sensory processing remain the two most affected faculties after head injury.
- Changes in the levels of both excitatory and inhibitory neurotransmitters cause all the changes.
- Post-traumatic stress disorders and cognitive disorders impact quality of life often in the long term.
- Affective disorders and mania require long-term medications and cognitive behavioral therapy

REFERENCES

1. Gururaj G. Epidemiology of traumatic brain injuries: Indian scenario. Neurol Res. 2002;24(1):24-8.
2. Fuster JM. The prefrontal cortex: anatomy, physiology, and neuropsychology of the frontal lobe, 3rd ed. New York: Lippincott-Raven; 1997.
3. Timonen M, Meittunen J, Hakko H, Zitting P. The association of preceding traumatic brain injury with mental disorders, alcoholism, and criminality: The Northern Finland 1966 Birth Cohort study. Psychiatry Res. 2003;113(3):217-26.
4. Morrison JH, Molliver ME, Grzanna R. Noradrenergic innervation of cerebral cortex: Widespread effects of local cortical lesions. Science. 1979;205:313-6.
5. Donnemiller E, Brenneis C, Wissel J, Scherfler C, Poewe W, Riccabona G, et al. Impaired dopaminergic neurotransmission in patients with traumatic brain injury: A SPECT study using 123I-beta-CIT and 123I-IBZM. Eur J Nucl Med. 2000;27:1410-4.
6. Hamill RW, Woolf PD, McDonald JV, Lee LA, Kelly M. Catecholamines predict outcome in traumatic brain injury. Ann Neurol. 1987;21:438-43.
7. Pasaoglu H, Inci Karakücük E, Kurtsoy A, Pasaoglu A. Endogenous neuropeptides in patients with acute traumatic head injury, I: Cerebrospinal fluid beta-endorphin levels are increased within 24 hours following the trauma. Neuropeptides. 1996;30:47-51.
8. Dewar D, Graham DI. Depletion of choline acetyltransferase activity but preservation of M1 and M2 muscarinic receptor binding sites in temporal cortex following head injury: A preliminary human postmortem study. J Neurotrauma. 1996;13:181-7.
9. Hoge C, McGurk D, Thomas JL, Cox AL, Engel CC, Castro CA. Mild traumatic brain injuries in US returning from Iraq. N Eng J Med. 2008;358(5):453-63.
10. Scwarzbold M, Dias A, Martins ET, Rufino A, Amante LN, Thais ME, et al. Psychiatric disorders and traumatic brain injury. Neuropsychiatr Dis Treat. 2008;4(4):797-816.
11. McCauley RL, Wilde EA, Barnes A, Hanten G, Hunter JV, Levin HS, et al. Patterns of early emotional and neuropsychological sequelae after mild traumatic brain injury. J Neurotrauma. 2014;31:914-25.
12. Leary JB, Kim GY, Bradley CL, Hussain UZ, Sacco M, Bernad M, et al. The association of cognitive reserve in chronic-phase functional and neuropsychological outcomes following traumatic brain injury. J Head Trauma Rehabil. 2018;33:E28-35.
13. Wilson L, Horton L, Kunzmann K, Sahakian BJ, Newcombe VF, Stamatakis EA, et al. Understanding the relationship between cognitive performance and function in daily life after traumatic brain injury. Neurol Neurosurg Psychiatry. 2021;92:407-17.
14. Andelic N, Løvstad M, Norup A, Ponsford J, Røe C. Editorial: impact of traumatic brain injuries on participation in daily life and work: recent research and future directions. Front Neurol. 2019;10:1153.
15. Fann JR, Ribe AR, Pedersen HS, Fenger-Grøn M, Christensen J, Benros ME, et al. Long term risk of dementia among people with traumatic brain injury in Denmark: a population-based observational cohort study. Lancet Psychiatry. 2018;5(5):424-31.
16. Tateno A, Jorge RE, Robinson RG. Clinical correlates of aggressive behavior after traumatic brain injury. J Neuropsychiatry Clin Neurosci. 2003;15:155-60.
17. Cummings J. The Neuropsychiatric Inventory: Development and Applications. J Geriatr Psychiatry Neurol. 2020;33:73-84.
18. Li AD, Bmed B, Samantha M, Walterfang M. Mania following traumatic brain injury: a systemic review. J Neuropsychiatry Clin Neurosc. 2023;35(4):341-51.
19. Svensson V, Much A, Exner C. Personality changes after acquired brain injury and their effects on rehabilitation outcomes. Neuropsych Rehab. 2023;33(2):305-24.
20. Robert S. Traumatic brain injury and mood disorders. Mental Health Clinician. 2020;10(6):335-45.

Chronic Traumatic Encephalopathy

Ambar Chakravarty

INTRODUCTION

The long-term consequences of repetitive head injury (RHI) evoked interests of the scientific community around a century ago. In fact, people interested in sports had long noted that those boxers who sustained many blows to the head were prone to a deterioration popularly known as "Punchdrunk." Way back in 1928, Martland described a spectrum of neurological and psychological decline[1] in such individuals. By mid-20th century, the later-onset symptoms of RHI in professional boxers became well known and terms such as "dementia pugilistica," "traumatic dementia," and "traumatic encephalopathy" appeared in the literature. It was Macdonald Critchley who first introduced in 1957 the currently used term "chronic traumatic encephalopathy" (CTE) as a "suitable scientific alternative to punch-drunkenness".[2] He described the clinical features as well as the classic pathological features of "gliosis, cortical atrophy, and internal hydrocephalus" at autopsy.[3] Essentially a pathological diagnosis, CTE is characterized by the presence of phosphorylated tau protein in nerve cell bodies and their processes around the small blood vessels at the depth of the cortical sulci.[4] Additional features may be present, but a definitive diagnosis of CTE absolutely requires the presence of perivascular nerve cell p-tau.[5,6]

Scientific and public interests on CTE were triggered after the publication of the first autopsy report of CTE in an American football player who had suffered cognitive impairment, mood disorder, and parkinsonian symptoms.[7] This single neuropathology report in 2005 stimulated hundreds of new studies into the association between repetitive head trauma sustained in contact sports and the armed forces.[8,9] and later life neurological deficits and psychiatric symptoms.

Tau aggregates are not only found in CTE alone, but also noted in multiple neurodegenerative conditions, such as Alzheimer disease (AD), frontotemporal lobar degeneration diseases (FTLDs), and aging-related tau astrogliopathy (ARTAG).[10] But the pathology of the different tauopathies are distinct: The classic pathologic lesion of CTE is p-tau aggregates in neurons and neurites ± astrocytes, while ARTAG is characterized by astrocytic p-tau aggregates alone.[11,12] While the tau isoform in aggregates in ARTAG is 4R, in CTE aggregates in the neurons are composed of both 3R and 4R isoforms, simulating then pathology of AD.[13] CTE indeed has common features with other neurodegenerative disorders, but the detailed histology as detailed above, is specific.

Recent studies have shown that head trauma increases the risk of development of various neurodegenerative disorders. Studies done in current time have identified RHI as risk factor for Parkinson's disease, amyotrophic lateral sclerosis as also frontotemporal dementia.

Interestingly while mortality from heart disease and non-neurodegenerative disorders remains low in soccer players that from neurodegenerative disorders is higher.[14-19] More interestingly, goal keepers seem to have a lower risk than the attacking players in the forward positions who need to head the ball more frequently.[19-25]

In 2020, the Lancet Commission included traumatic brain injury as a definitive modifiable risk factor to target for dementia prevention.[25]

There is at present no clear set of diagnostic criteria for CTE in life. Are there any particular clinical features which might suggest development of CTE in susceptible individuals in life?

Stern et al.[26] noted clinical features from 36 individuals with sports-related RHI diagnosed with only CTE and no comorbid neuropathology.[26] A vast majority of them exhibited a host of psychological symptoms like mood disorders such as major depression, impulse control disorders, loss of memory, headache, language disorders, visuospatial disturbances, executive dysfunction, and even an overall cognitive decline. Stern et al.[26] Identified two clinical subgroups associated with CTE: One with younger age at symptom presentation with predominant behavioral symptoms, and another older age-at-onset more likely to present with cognitive impairment leading to dementia. Montenigro et al., categorized CTE as a "traumatic encephalopathy syndrome"[27] (TES), with mood, behavioral, cognitive, and movement subtypes.[28] Further modifications of these criteria have been made subsequently.[28,29] Corsellis et al. wrote "it is not suggested that this is a common sequence of events but that it has occurred occasionally can scarcely be denied".[30] Unfortunately even in the current era, despite the very large body of evidence linking RHI to later life cognitive and motor decline, significant skepticism and confusion remains, particularly around CTE and its relationship to sports-related RHI.[31-36] Individuals who continue to play games with high rates of head trauma deserve to have the most complete available information regarding the long-term risks of RHI.

REFERENCES

1. Martland HS. Punch drunk. J Am Med Assoc. 1928;91:1103-7.
2. Critchley M. Medical aspects of boxing, particularly from a neurological standpoint. Br Med J. 1957;1:357.
3. Brandenburg W, Hallervorden J. Dementia pugilistica with anatomical findings. Virchows Arch Pathol Anat Physiol Klin Med. 1954;325:680-709.
4. Bieniek KF, Cairns NJ, Crary JF, Dickson DW, Folkerth RD, Keene CD, et al. The second ninds/nibib consensus meeting to define neuropathological criteria for the diagnosis of chronic traumatic encephalopathy. J Neuropathol Exp Neurol. 2021;80:210-9.
5. McKee AC. The neuropathology of chronic traumatic encephalopathy: the status of the literature. Semin Neurol. 2020;40:359-69.
6. McKee AC, Stern RA, Nowinski CJ, Stein TD, Alvarez VE, Daneshvar DH, et al. The spectrum of disease in chronic traumatic encephalopathy. Brain. 2013;136:43-64.
7. Omalu BI, DeKosky ST, Minster RL, Kamboh MI, Hamilton RL, Wecht CH. Chronic traumatic encephalopathy in a national football league player. Neurosurgery. 2005;57:128-34.
8. Goldstein LE, Fisher AM, Tagge CA, Zhang XL, Velisek L, Sullivan JA, et al. Chronic traumatic encephalopathy in blast-exposed military veterans and a blast neurotrauma mouse model. Sci Transl Med. 2012;4:134ra60.
9. McKee AC, Daneshvar DH, Alvarez VE, Stein TD. The neuropathology of sport. Acta Neuropathol. 2014;127:29-51.
10. Gotz J, Halliday G, Nisbet RM. Molecular pathogenesis of the tauopathies. Annu Rev Pathol. 2019;14:239-61.
11. McKee AC, Stein TD, Kiernan PT, Alvarez VE. The neuropathology of chronic traumatic encephalopathy. Brain Pathol. 2015;25:350-64.
12. Mortimer J, Van Duijn C, Chandra V, Fratiglioni L, Graves A, Heyman A, et al. Head trauma as a risk factor for Alzheimer's disease: A collaborative. Front Neurol. 2022;13:880905.
13. Mortimer JA, van Duijn CM, Chandra V, Fratiglioni L, Graves AB, Heyman A, et al. Chronic Traumatic Encephalopathy re-analysis of case-control studies. Int J Epidemiol. 1991;20(Suppl. 2):S28-35.
14. Fleminger S, Oliver D, Lovestone S, Rabe-Hesketh S, Giora A. Head injury as a risk factor for Alzheimer's disease: The evidence 10 years on; a partial replication. J Neurol Neurosurg Psychiatry. 2003;74:857-62.
15. Li Y, Li Y, Li X, Zhang S, Zhao J, Zhu X, et al. Head injury as a risk factor for dementia and Alzheimer's disease: a systematic review and meta-analysis of 32 observational studies. PLoS One. 2017;12:e0169650.
16. Jafari S, Etminan M, Aminzadeh F, Samii A. Head injury and risk of Parkinson disease: A systematic review and meta-analysis. Mov Disord. 2013;28:1222-9.
17. Chen H, Richard M, Sandler DP, Umbach DM, Kamel F. Head injury and amyotrophic lateral sclerosis. Am J Epidemiol. (2007) 166:810-6.
18. Watanabe Y, Watanabe T. Meta-analytic evaluation of the association between head injury and risk of amyotrophic lateral sclerosis. Eur J Epidemiol. 2017;32:867-79.
19. Rosso S, Landweer E, Houterman M, Kaat LD, Van Duijn C, Van Swieten J. Medical and environmental risk factors for sporadic frontotemporal dementia: A retrospective case–control study. J Neurol Neurosurg Psychiatry. 2003;74:1574-6.
20. Kalkonde YV, Jawaid A, Qureshi SU, Shirani P, Wheaton M, Pinto-Patarroyo GP, et al. Medical and environmental risk factors associated with frontotemporal dementia: A case-control study in a veteran population. Alzheimers Dement. 2012;8:204-10.
21. Lehman EJ, Hein MJ, Baron SL, Gersic CM. Neurodegenerative causes of death among retired national football league players. Neurology. 2012;79:1970-4.
22. Mackay DF, Russell ER, Stewart K, MacLean JA, Pell JP, Stewart W. Neurodegenerative disease mortality among former professional soccer players. N Engl J Med. 2019;381:1801-8.
23. Russell ER, Mackay DF, Stewart K, MacLean JA, Pell JP, Stewart W. Association of field position and career length with risk of neurodegenerative disease in male former professional soccer players. JAMA Neurol. 2021;78:1057-63.
24. Livingston G, Huntley J, Sommerlad A, Ames D, Ballard C, Banerjee S, et al. Dementia prevention, intervention, and care: 2020 report of the lancet commission. Lancet. 2020;396:413-46.
25. Stern RA, Daneshvar DH, Baugh CM, Seichepine DR, Montenigro PH, Riley DO, et al. Clinical presentation of chronic traumatic encephalopathy. Neurology. 2013;81:1122-9.
26. Stein TD, Alvarez VE, McKee AC. Chronic traumatic encephalopathy: A spectrum of neuropathological changes following repetitive brain trauma in athletes and military personnel. Alzheimers Res Ther. 2014;6(1):4.
27. Montenigro PH, Baugh CM, Daneshvar DH, Mez J, Budson AE, Au R, et al. Clinical subtypes of chronic traumatic encephalopathy: literature review and proposed research diagnostic criteria for traumatic encephalopathy syndrome. Alzheimers Res Ther. 2014;6:68.
28. Katz DI, Bernick C, Dodick DW, Mez J, Mariani ML, Adler CH, et al. National institute of neurological disorders and stroke consensus diagnostic criteria for traumatic encephalopathy syndrome. Neurology. 2021;96:848-63.

29. Mez J, Alosco ML, Daneshvar DH, Saltiel N, Baucom Z, Abdolmohammadi B, et al. Validity of the 2014 traumatic encephalopathy syndrome criteria for CTE pathology. Alzheimers Dement. 2021;7:1709-24.
30. Corsellis JAN, Bruton CJ, Freeman-Browne D. The aftermath of boxing. Psychol Med. 1973;3:270-303.
31. Smith DH, Johnson VE, Trojanowski JQ, Stewart W. Chronic traumatic encephalopathy—confusion and controversies. Nat Rev Neurol. 2019;15:179-83.
32. Stewart W, Allinson K, Al-Sarraj S, Bachmeier C, Barlow K, Belli A, et al. Primum non nocere: a call for balance when reporting on CTE. Lancet Neurol. 2019;18:231-3.
33. Randolph C. Chronic traumatic encephalopathy is not a real disease. Arch Clin Neuropsychol. 2018;33:644-8.
34. Finkel AM, Brand KP, Caplan AL, Evans JS, Wolpe PR. First report the findings: Genuine balance when reporting Cte. Lancet Neurol. 2019;18:521-2.
35. Casper ST, Golden J, Oreskes N, Largent M, Goldberg DS, Gillett G, et al. First report the findings: genuine balance when reporting Cte. Lancet Neurol. 2019;18:522-3.
36. Howick J, Chalmers I, Glasziou P, Greenhalgh T, Heneghan C, Liberati A, et al; Oxford Centre for Evidence-Based Medicine. (2011). The 2011 Oxford CEBM Levels of Evidence (Introductory Document). [Available from https://www.cebm.ox.ac.uk/resources/levels-of-evidence/ocebmlevels-of-evidence [Last accessed May 1, 2022].

CHAPTER 32

Neurological Side Effects of Psychiatric Medications

Shripad Pujari, Amitkumar V Pande, Rahul Kulkarni

INTRODUCTION

"The person who takes medicine must recover twice, once from the disease and once from the medicine."
—**William Osler**

With the turn of century and haplessness caused by coronavirus disease 2019 (COVID-19), the number of psychiatric consults is on the rise. This in turn has led to increased use of psychotropic drugs and longer duration of therapies. The usage of drugs helps treat the sufferer from his mental travesty, but it is not fraught without the side effects. This chapter reviews the side effects of psychotropic therapies in neurology and general wellbeing.

The neurological side effects of psychiatric medicines (PMs) are not only restricted to movement disorders, but also include cognitive impairment, confusion, reduction of seizures threshold, sleep and weight problems, increased risk of stroke and death and acute conditions such as neuroleptic malignant syndrome (NMS) and serotonin syndrome (SS). Additionally, stopping antipsychotics (APs) and antidepressants (ADs) can lead to discontinuation symptoms.[1] The adverse effects of PMs reduce daily physical, social, and occupational function and further reduce the quality of life of the patients who are already compromised due to their psychiatric illness. Understanding and recognizing these side effects is crucial for healthcare professionals, patients, and their families to make informed decisions about treatment options and effectively manage any potential risks.[1,2]

OVERVIEW OF PSYCHIATRIC MEDICATIONS

Psychiatric medications encompass different classes, including APs, ADs, mood stabilizers, anxiolytics, sedatives, and hypnotics. In general, conventional antipsychotic agents such as chlorpromazine and haloperidol have a much higher incidence of extrapyramidal symptoms (EPSs) and NMS than atypical ones due to their strong dopamine receptor blocking ability. Likewise, within ADs, different types of neurological complications are seen with different categories of ADs. The main mood stabilizers are lithium, valproic acid, carbamazepine, oxcarbazepine, and lamotrigine. Tremor is the most common side effect seen with lithium and valproic acid. Valproic acid can also cause parkinsonism whereas acute lithium toxicity has its own typical manifestations. Carbamazepine, oxcarbazepine, and lamotrigine can cause dizziness, vertigo, diplopia, and ataxia. Sleep disturbances are seen with all drugs and the type of sleep abnormality depends upon the mechanism of action of the medicine. Nonbenzodiazepine hypnotics are known to produce parasomnias.[1-6]

NEUROLOGICAL SIDE EFFECTS

Neurological side effects include EPSs, certain special acute syndromes, and nonextrapyramidal side effects. They are enumerated in the **Box 1**.[1-4,7]

Extrapyramidal Symptoms

Extrapyramidal symptoms include dystonic reactions, parkinsonism, tardive dyskinesia, dystonia, akathisia, and tremor. All EPSs are described hereafter in detail **(Box 2)**.

Parkinsonism

Parkinsonism is the most common movement disorder caused by drugs. It is also one of the most common causes of nondegenerative parkinsonism. The drugs causing parkinsonism are mainly APs, but they are also seen with antiemetics, ADs, and various mood stabilizers. It is commonly seen because of blockade of D2 receptors. Parkinsonism due to drugs is not really dose dependent. It is commonly seen in the age group of 60–80 years and patients with long-term therapy.

> **BOX 1: Neurological side effects of psychiatry medicines.**
>
> *Extrapyramidal symptoms (EPSs):*
> - Parkinsonism
> - Tardive dyskinesia
> - Tardive dystonia
> - Tardive akathisia
> - Drug-induced tremor
>
> *Special acute syndromes:*
> - Neuroleptic malignant syndrome (NMS)
> - Serotonin syndrome (SS)
> - Acute lithium toxicity
> - Acute dystonic reaction
> - Acute akathisia
> - Syncope due to postural hypotension
> - Syncope due to cardiac conduction blockade
>
> *Nonextrapyramidal side effects:*
> - Cognitive impairment
> - Delirium
> - Diplopia, dizziness, and ataxia
> - Sleep disturbances
> - Seizures
> - Catatonia
> - Sexual dysfunction
> - Weight gain
> - Increased risk of stroke and death
> - Discontinuation symptoms

> **BOX 2: Strategies to prevent extrapyramidal symptoms (EPSs).**
>
> Strategies to prevent EPSs are as follows:
> - Given the severity and chronicity of EPSs, if possible, avoidance of antipsychotic (AP) medicines is the best strategy
> - If AP medicines are necessary, avoid high potency first generation agents
> - Reduce dose to the minimum
> - Switch to a drug with the least EPS risk, e.g., quetiapine or clozapine

Drugs causing parkinsonism are:
- *Conventional APs*: Many factors such as potency, route, and dose of these agents influence the development of drug induced parkinsonism. Parenteral route of administration has got a higher chance of developing parkinsonism even if the doses are lower.
- *Atypical APs*: Have higher affinity for other targets including the serotonergic, histaminergic, and muscarinic receptors. Among the atypical APs risperidone, olanzapine, ziprasidone, lurasidone, and paliperidone are associated with higher risk of parkinsonism while quetiapine and clozapine have a lower risk. Aripiprazole and brexpiprazole have got a lower chance of parkinsonism. Pimavanserin is an inverse agonist of the HT_{2A} receptors with no affinity for D2 receptors. It is approved by the Food and Drug Administration (FDA) for Parkinson's psychosis.
- *Antiemetic and prokinetic medications*: Derivatives of benzamide and phenothiazine APs cause both central and peripheral blockade of dopamine D2 receptors. Prochlorperazine and metoclopramide are prototype drugs for causing variety of movement disorders. Domperidone is associated with lower risk of Parkinson's disease.
- Valproic acid rarely causes parkinsonism due to gamma-aminobutyric acid (GABA) induced inhibition of dopamine transport in basal ganglia.
- Other drugs such as lithium, serotonin reuptake inhibitors (SSRIs), and calcium channel blockers especially flunarizine, is known to cause parkinsonism.

Signs and Symptoms

The classical symptoms of bradykinesia, rigidity, resting tremor that are clinically indistinguishable from idiopathic Parkinson's disease form a hallmark. Onset of symptoms can be seen within a few weeks to months. However, it is well known that parkinsonism can occur many years after the exposure to medication. Rigidity is the most common finding on examination seen in about 65–100% of the patients. Bradykinesia and tremor have variable associations. The diagnosis of drug induced parkinsonism can be confirmed if the parkinsonism resolves in 6 months after stopping the offending agent. Majority of parkinsonism due to drugs are symmetrical as compared to idiopathic Parkinson's disease which usually starts unilaterally.

The best way to treat drug induced parkinsonism is to avoid using causative agents. If the symptoms are mild and the psychosis is severe then we can continue psychotropic drugs. Levodopa is the reasonable first option for treatment of disabling parkinsonism albeit it may exacerbate psychosis. Psychiatrists have been using anti cholinergic agents preemptively to negate the extrapyramidal side effects drugs of drugs. Amantadine has also been used in case patients report of worsening psychosis with anticholinergics.[1,7]

Tardive Dyskinesia

Tardive dyskinesia (TD) is a neurological disorder characterized by involuntary and repetitive movements of the face, tongue, lips, and other parts of the body. It is typically associated with the long-term use of certain medications, particularly APs, although it can also occur with other psychotropic medications. Here are some important points to know about TD:

- *Symptoms*: TD is characterized by abnormal movements that can vary in severity and presentation. Common symptoms include repetitive and involuntary movements such as facial grimacing, tongue protrusion, lip smacking, rapid blinking, chewing movements, and finger movements. These movements may be constant or intermittent and can be distressing and socially embarrassing.
- *Medications associated with TD*: TD is mostly associated with the use of APs, especially "conventional" APs like haloperidol or chlorpromazine. However, it can also occur with newer "atypical" APs such as risperidone, quetiapine, or olanzapine. Other medications, such as certain ADs or antiemetics, can also rarely cause TD.
- *Risk factors*: The risk of developing TD is influenced by several factors, including the duration of medication use, higher doses of medication, older age, female gender, and a history of movement disorders. Individuals who have taken antipsychotic medications for an extended period, particularly older adults, are at higher risk.
- *Monitoring and prevention*: Regular monitoring for the development of TD is essential for individuals taking APs. In some cases, switching to a different medication with a lower risk of TD may be considered. Additionally, early recognition and treatment can potentially lead to symptom improvement or resolution.
- *Management*: Adjusting the dose of the offending medication, switching to a different medication, or discontinuing the medication altogether may be considered. Medications such as tetrabenazine and valbenazine specifically approved for the treatment of TD may be prescribed in certain cases. In severe or persistent cases, other treatments such as botulinum toxin injections or deep brain stimulation may be explored.[2,8,9]

Tardive Dystonia

Tardive dystonia refers to a condition in which dystonic manifestations predominate. Dystonia is sustained or repetitive muscle contractions that result in twisting and repetitive movements or abnormal fixed postures. Most common dystonias seen are retrocollis (which may be sustained or jerky), torticollis, opisthotonus, shoulder dystonia, hyperextension of the arms or legs, blepharospasm, and jaw dystonia. It is most seen after the age of 40 years, and it has got lower remission rate as compared to TDs.[2,9]

Tardive Akathisia

It is a form of TD. It is characterized by motor restlessness. Patients may have various manifestations in the form of moving around, stopping to and fro from one foot to other, leg crossing, arm folding, or shifting weight. It is often confused for agitation or worsening of psychosis.[10] Its incidence decreases with age and may be seen in only 15% above 65 years. Akathisia that is tardive is not responsive to treatment. It is one of the most common causes of premature termination of antipsychiatry treatment. The drug of choice for akathisia is propranolol in doses of 30–240 mg/day (mediated through serotonergic receptors that are responsible for antiakathisic properties). The other drug that may help is benzodiazepine. Last resort is to change the neuroleptic to a less potent or a novel one.[2,7]

Drug-induced Tremor

The drug-induced tremor (DIT) with APs is usually a parkinsonian tremor whereas the one with lithium, valproic acid, and SSRIs resembles an essential or enhanced sympathetic tremor. Valproic acid can uncommonly also cause parkinsonism when it produces a parkinsonian tremor. APs can also at times cause a dystonic or a position-dependent tremor. Risk factors for tremor include use of multiple drugs, higher doses, male gender, and older age. DIT usually resolves spontaneously after stopping the offending drug, but occasionally, the tremor may persist (a tardive tremor). If persistent, anticholinergic (trihexyphenidyl) or beta blocker (propranolol) and benzodiazepine (clonazepam) are recommended, respectively for parkinsonian tremor and tremor resembling essential tremor.[4,11]

Medicines recommended for each type of EPS with contraindications are listed in **Table 1**.

Special Acute Syndromes

Neuroleptic Malignant Syndrome

The NMS is a rare but potentially life-threatening condition that can occur as a side effect of certain medications, particularly APs **(Box 3)**. NMS is characterized by a combination of symptoms that affect the central nervous system and the autonomic nervous system. It typically occurs as a reaction to the use of APs, although it has also been reported with other psychotropic drugs.

Various mechanisms for pathogenesis have been proposed. Central to this is (1) involvement of the hypothalamus causing dysautonomia and hyperthermia; (2) interference with the nigrostriatal pathway causing

TABLE 1: Types of extrapyramidal symptoms with contraindications and categories of medicine.

Types of extrapyramidal symptoms	Category of medicine	Drug	Contraindications
Acute dystonia and parkinsonism	Anticholinergic	Trihexyphenidyl	Cognitive impairment, confusion
Akathisia	Beta blocker	Propranolol	Depression, asthma, peripheral vascular disease (PVD)
	Benzodiazepine	Clonazepam	Drowsiness, cognitive impairment
Tardive dyskinesia	Vesicular monoamine transporter 2 (VMAT2) inhibitors	Tetrabenazine, Valbenazine	Depression
Tardive dystonia	VMAT2 inhibitors	Tetrabenazine	Depression
	Anticholinergic	Trihexyphenidyl	Cognitive impairment, confusion
	Muscle relaxant	Botulinum toxin	
Drug-induced (chronic) parkinsonism	Anticholinergic, levodopa, dopa agonist	Trihexyphenidyl, levodopa, amantadine	
Drug-induced tremor	• Anticholinergic • Beta blocker Benzodiazepine	• Trihexyphenidyl • Propranolol • Clonazepam	• Confusion • Depression

BOX 3: Management guidelines for neuroleptic malignant syndrome (NMS).

Management guidelines for NMS are as follows:
- Stop all antipsychotics (APs), antidepressants (ADs), and lithium
- Regular monitoring of clinical status and creatine phosphokinase (CPK) levels
- Detail medical evaluation
- Rehydration
- Cooling—with blankets, intravenous (IV) fluids
- Treat rhabdomyolysis (as per protocol), if present
- Treat intercurrent infection
- Medicines—dopamine agonists—bromoergocriptine, amantadine; muscle relaxants—dantrolene, benzodiazepines
- If AP is direly essential to control symptoms, the guidelines are:
  o Wait for 2–4 weeks after NMS has resolved, before reintroducing AP
  o Avoid the same AP
  o Avoid depot AP
  o Use atypical AP if possible
  o Use low potency AP in low dose
  o Monitor for reappearance of symptoms of NMS

muscular rigidity and slowness; and (3) disrupted modulation of the sympathetic pathway causing increased sudomotor activity and sweating, muscle stiffness, rigidity, and ineffective heat dissipation.
- *Hyperthermia (high body temperature)*: A significant increase in body temperature is one of the hallmark symptoms. The body temperature can rise rapidly and reach dangerous levels.
- *Muscle rigidity*: Severe muscle rigidity or stiffness is another characteristic symptom. The muscles may become rigid and difficult to move, leading to a condition known as "lead pipe rigidity".
- *Altered mental status*: NMS can cause changes in mental status, including confusion, disorientation, agitation, and even coma.
- *Autonomic dysfunction*: NMS can affect the autonomic nervous system, leading to symptoms such as irregular blood pressure, rapid heart rate, profuse sweating, and urinary retention.
- *Other symptoms*: Additional symptoms may include tremors, changes in breathing pattern, elevated white blood cell count, and elevated levels of creatine kinase (a marker of muscle damage) in the blood.[1,3]

Serotonin Syndrome

The SS is a potentially life-threatening condition that occurs due to an excess of serotonin in the central nervous system. It is usually caused by certain medications that increase serotonin levels, such as SSRIs, serotonin-norepinephrine reuptake inhibitors (SNRIs), or monoamine oxidase inhibitors (MAOIs) **(Box 4)**. Here are some key points about SS:
- *Symptoms and signs*: They include agitation, restlessness, confusion, rapid heart rate, dilated pupils, elevated blood pressure, excessive sweating, tremors, muscle rigidity, high body temperature, and in severe cases, seizures, or loss of consciousness.
- *Onset*: The symptoms of SS can develop rapidly, often within hours of taking a new medication or increasing the dosage. However, in some cases, symptoms may appear days after starting a medication or changing the dose.

> **BOX 4: Management guidelines for serotonin syndrome.**
>
> Management guidelines for serotonin syndrome are as follows:
> - Stop all serotonergic drugs
> - Immediate medical opinion
> - Treat medical complications—rhabdomyolysis, renal failure, disseminated intravascular coagulation (DIC)
> - Control seizures
> - Reduce fever
> - Control agitation and excessive muscular activity—use benzodiazepines

- *Risk factors*: SS is more likely to occur when multiple medications or substances that increase serotonin levels are combined. It can also be more common in cases of overdose or when certain medications are used at high doses. Some other drugs and supplements that may increase the risk of SS include certain pain medications (e.g., tramadol) and illicit substances like MDMA (ecstasy).
- *Treatment*: If SS is suspected, it is essential to seek immediate medical attention. Treatment typically involves discontinuing the medications that are contributing to the condition and providing supportive care to manage the symptoms. In severe cases, hospitalization and intensive medical monitoring may be required.
- *Prevention*: To reduce the risk of SS, history of all the medications, supplements, and herbal products one is taking must be sought. They can assess potential interactions and adjust your treatment plan accordingly. It is important to follow prescribed dosages and not exceed recommended limits.[1,3]

Acute Lithium Toxicity

Lithium toxicity is common because of the narrow margin between the therapeutic and toxic levels. Mild-to-moderate toxicity produces gastrointestinal distress and a coarse tremor and drowsiness. Severe toxicity can cause confusion, ataxia, seizures, and coma. Urgent dialysis is recommended for severe toxicity.[3]

Acute Dystonic Reaction

Acute dystonic reactions (ADR) can occur within 6 hours of injection and up to the first week after exposure to the offending drug. Commonly seen with APs such as phenothiazines, butyrophenones, and thioxanthenes, and antiemetics such as prochlorperazine and metoclopramide. Children are more susceptible as compared to adults and it occurs twice as common in males. It is by far, always due to absolute/relative dopaminergic deficiency with cholinergic imbalance.[12,13] They may present as:

- *Oculogyric crisis*: It commences as blepharospasm and evolves into a painful upward or lateral deviation of eyes.
- *Buccolingual crisis*: It is bizarre grimacing involving facial muscles and tongue dysarthria and dysphagia.
- *Torticollic crisis*: It is spasm of the neck musculature.
- *Tortipelvic crisis*: It is spasm of the abdominal wall musculature.
- *Opisthotonus*: It is tetanic spasm of spine and extremities that are bent in convexity forward body resting on head and heels.

Acute dystonic reactions can be life threatening and can involve laryngeal musculature causing respiratory compromise. It may also sometimes cause dislocation of mandible.[14] Conventional APs have the highest risk whereas the atypical ones carry lower risk due to faster dissociation of the medicine from the D2 receptor site. ADR is treated with intravenous diphenhydramine, benztropine, and benzodiazepine (lorazepam).[1,3,13,15]

Acute Akathisia

It is a type of extrapyramidal syndrome characterized by uneasiness and is seen in 6 weeks to 3 months of the drug therapy. It is often confused with nonresponse of underlying psychiatric condition. Early identification and reduction or substitution of therapy along with antiakathisic drug therapy controls the disorder.[1,3,7]

Syncope due to Postural Hypotension

It is mostly seen in elderly. Systolic blood pressure/diastolic blood pressure (SBP/DBP) fall by >20/10 mm Hg. It can be seen in low doses of drugs and is not always dose related. It is commonly seen with tricyclic antidepressants (TCAs) and low potency neuroleptics. MAOIs cause dose-related hypotension the effect of which is exacerbated when used with diuretics and other antihypertensives. Treatment consists mainly of leg elevation or if need be, hydration.[3,8,16]

Syncope due to Cardiac Conduction Blockades

Patients with left bundle branch block, bifascicular block, and prolonged QT interval are at risk. This is commonly seen with TCAs and at times, with APs. SA node dysfunction is seen in patients with preexisting cardiac disease who are on lithium therapy.[3,8,16]

Nonextrapyramidal Side Effects

These include effects on cognition, attention, alertness, seizure threshold, behavior, sexual function as well as appetite, and weight. They also have effects on stroke risk and mortality and lastly, discontinuation also may produce different kinds of neurological symptoms. Such effects are elaborated in detail.

Cognitive Impairment

Psychotropic drugs, particularly certain APs, ADs, and benzodiazepines can be associated with an increased risk of cognitive decline and potentially contribute to the development or worsening of dementia in some individuals. This is more common in older adults with preexisting risk factors for dementia. Here are a few important points to consider:

- *Antipsychotic medications*: Studies have linked the long-term use of certain antipsychotic drugs, particularly older "typical" APs like haloperidol or chlorpromazine, and even "atypical" APs with a higher risk of cognitive decline and the development of dementia in older adults. However, it is important to note that the relationship between APs and dementia is complex, and not all individuals who take these medications will develop dementia.
- *Black box warning*: Due to the potential risks, the US FDA has issued a "black box warning" for antipsychotic medications, highlighting the increased risk of death among older adults with dementia-related psychosis who are treated with these drugs. This warning emphasizes the need for careful consideration and monitoring when using APs in this population.
- *ADs and benzodiazepines*: Both show significant cognitive impairment which to a large extent is reversible after stopping the offending medicine.
- *Mechanism*: Impaired learning and memory are linked to anticholinergic effects whereas other cognitive functions get affected due to differential effects on serotonergic, dopaminergic, α_1-adrenergic, muscarinic and histamine receptors.
- *Individual factors*: The risk of developing cognitive decline because of psychotropic drugs can be influenced by individual factors such as age, preexisting cognitive impairment, genetic predisposition, and other medical conditions.
- *Benefits versus risks*: It is essential to assess risk benefit ratio while prescribing psychotropic drugs in elderly. In some cases, the benefits of treatment may outweigh the risks, especially when nonpharmacological interventions are insufficient or when severe symptoms require pharmacological management.

Regular monitoring for cognitive behavioral functions is recommended especially in older individuals on psychotropic drug therapy.[17-20]

Delirium

Any psychotropic medicine can cause delirium but, it is commonly seen with TCAs and benztropine. Lithium alone or in combination with carbamazepine may cause delirious neurotoxicity.[3]

Diplopia, Dizziness, and Ataxia

These adverse effects (AEs) are mainly seen with carbamazepine, oxcarbazepine, and lamotrigine and usually revere with dose reduction.[6]

Sleep Disturbances

Different ADs affect sleep in different ways. In sleep studies, TCAs, SSRIs, and SNRIs cause rapid eye movement (REM) suppression and increased REM latency. Trazodone and mirtazapine reduce sleep latency and increase slow wave sleep (SWS). Bupropion is one of the few ADs which shortens REM latency and increases total REM sleep time. Clinically, tertiary TCAs (e.g., amitriptyline) are sedating whereas secondary TCAs (e.g., nortriptyline) are activating. SSRIs decrease sleep efficiency and increase the number of awakenings. SNRIs cause insomnia, daytime somnolence, and increase in wakefulness after sleep onset (WASO). Trazodone and mirtazapine increase total sleep time and decrease sleep onset latency, thus producing beneficial effects on sleep. There are reports of insomnia on bupropion.

The APs increase total sleep time (TST) and improve sleep efficiency and have shown positive effects up to moderate doses. APs cause sedation but can also cause daytime somnolence. Nonbenzodiazepine hypnotics (zolpidem and zopiclone) are reported to produce parasomnias.[5,16]

Seizures and Convulsions

The APs are known to reduce seizure thresholds in people with epilepsy. The TCAs (imipramine, bupropion) have the maximum potential to do so. Among the APs, clozapine has the highest risk of seizure frequency (1% at 300 mg and 4.4% at 600 mg). The predisposing factors may include large or sudden changes in drug dosage, organic brain syndrome, history of head injury, or preexisting epilepsy. The seizure activity is preceded by myoclonus which should be a warning symptom. It is advisable to avoid any depot formulations of APs in an epileptic patient, not only for their epileptogenic tendency but if seizures do occur, then, withdrawal of the drug becomes difficult. Benzodiazepines themselves have a relatively low risk of causing seizures. However, abrupt discontinuation or rapid dose reduction of benzodiazepines, especially if used for an extended period, can sometimes lead to seizure activity.

Most seizures due to psychiatry medicines are self-limiting. Prolonged or recurrent seizures should be dealt with benzodiazepines and barbiturates. Propofol can be considered if seizures fail to get controlled.[3,21]

Catatonia

Commonly seen in schizophrenia and major depression but psychotropic medications may cause the same. It has a gradual onset and is slow to respond to withdrawal of neuroleptic. Catatonia is treated well with amantadine.[3]

Sexual Dysfunction

All PMs including serotonergic ADs, APs (especially those increasing prolactin levels), mood stabilizers, and anxiolytics can cause sexual dysfunction (SD). Prime symptoms of psychiatric disorders such as low mood, anxiety, thought disturbances, negative symptoms, irritability, and decreased concentration themselves can cause SD. Decreased sleep, appetite, and energy levels also lead to alteration in sexual function. Surprisingly, only around 20% of patients spontaneously report their sexual problems.

There is not much difference in the incidence and severity of SD among SSRIs. Between SNRIs, venlafaxine has the highest rate whereas duloxetine has the least. In addition to their serotonergic effects, TCAs also affect lubrication because of their anticholinergic properties. Mirtazapine has lower SD than SSRIs and bupropion is observed to have beneficial effect on SD. Actually, it has been shown to improve sexual function in some studies. Trazodone has been found to increase sexual desire and there are case reports of priapism.

Valproic acid can increase testosterone levels and thus cause erectile dysfunction (ED) and reduce sexual desire in men and cause decreased libido and anorgasmia in women. Carbamazepine studies in epilepsy patients showed ED and reduce testosterone levels. Lamotrigine has been specifically associated with improvement in sexual functioning. Benzodiazepines are described to cause decreased sex desire and delayed orgasm. Aripiprazole has the lowest incidence of SD when compared with all other APs.

Sexual problems can be solved by using a medicine with least SD in the given category, lowering the dose, taking intermittent drug holidays, psychotherapy, and adding bupropion.[6,16,22]

Weight Gain and Metabolic Effects

Almost all PMs cause weight gain. Weight gain is associated with several comorbidities such as impaired glucose tolerance, diabetes mellitus, hypertension, hyperlipidemia, coronary heart disease, ischemic stroke, premature death, obstructive sleep apnea, and osteoarthritis. Weight gain also leads to psychosocial disturbances such as body image issues, low self-esteem, inferiority complex, and social stigma. TCAs, SSRIs, SNRIs, all mood stabilizers (including lithium and valproic acid), and all APs cause it. Atypical APs have a higher tendency for weight gain than conventional ones, most severe being with clozapine and olanzapine and the least with ziprasidone.[23]

Several mechanisms implicated are central nervous system alteration of energy balance, changing the resting metabolic rate, food craving, dysregulation of neurotransmitters, hormones and cytokines (such as leptin and tumor necrosis factor alpha), and genetic predisposition. Several management choices include switching to a drug which causes least weight gain, strict diet, increase physical exercise, and behavior therapy. The best way is to avoid weight gain by performing detail pretreatment counseling and putting the appropriate measures in place right at the outset of the treatment.[16,23,24]

Increased Risk of Cerebrovascular Events and Death

Meta-analysis was conducted of studies which had used atypical APs which included aripiprazole, olanzapine, quetiapine, and risperidone prescribed in dementia patients. There was a significant increased risk of cerebrovascular events and a small but significantly increased risk in mortality.[25] One out of the three cohort studies which assessed the risk of stroke and death in elderly patients on conventional versus atypical APs showed an increased risk even with conventional APs.[26] So, the risk with conventional APs is at least same as the atypical agents. Therefore, preexisting cerebrovascular risk factors should be taken into account and benefit versus risk of using APs should be measured before prescribing APs in the elderly.[26]

Discontinuation Symptoms

Discontinuation of APs and ADs can cause neuropsychiatric symptoms different from the original psychiatric disorder. AP discontinuation symptoms are restlessness, anxiety, insomnia, delirium, nausea, and vomiting. Cases of withdrawal dystonia, dyskinesia, and tics have also been reported. The recommendation is to taper APs very slowly over months.

Antidepressant discontinuation symptoms are seen with all ADs which include electric shock-like sensations in head, arms and legs, tinnitus, vertigo, imbalance, and unsteadiness. Mild symptoms resolve spontaneously and only need priming and reassurance. Severe symptoms can be addressed by prescribing benzodiazepines or reintroducing the same AD and tapering very gradually or using fluoxetine, which suppresses the symptoms.[1,27]

RISK FACTORS

Understanding the risk factors associated with neurological side effects is crucial for optimizing patient care. Overall, EPSs were more common in females who are middle aged and overweight. Age has a significant correlation with EPSs. Dystonia occurred in younger patients whereas TD was seen in the older ones.[28] Among the APs, conventional agents are much more associated with parkinsonism, tardive syndromes, akathisia, and NMS than the atypical ones. In the present era, atypical agents are mainly used as long-term therapies, and there is a wide variability in the type of side effects each of them produces. Broadly, the risk of development of EPS is proportionate to their dopamine receptor affinity. So, clozapine and quetiapine have the least, olanzapine have intermediate, and risperidone and ziprasidone have the highest risk of EPS among them.[1] Risk factors for AD side effects include age, sex, genetic predisposition (polygenic), and a high body mass index. AD side effects are generally more common in younger patients except confusion. Sexual dysfunction is more common in males whereas weight gain in females.[29] Benzodiazepine induced side effects are seen more in the elderly.[20]

PATIENT EDUCATION AND COUNSELING

Educating patients and their families about potential neurological side effects is essential for fostering informed decision-making and adherence to treatment. The crucial task is providing patients and families with comprehensive information about the potential side effects, strategies for managing them, and the significance of reporting any concerning symptoms to healthcare providers. A patient centered approach is advocated in which doctor is trained to invite patient and family to take active role in choosing and altering psychiatric therapies. This is called shared decision making (SDM).[30]

CONCLUDING REMARKS

Neurological side effects are important considerations when prescribing psychiatric medications. EPSs are the most common AEs of PMs and they can also manifest with other neurological complications such as cognitive impairment, delirium, sleep disorders, seizures, catatonia, sexual dysfunction, weight gain, metabolic effects and increased risk of ischemic stroke, and mortality. Acute AEs include NMS, serotonin toxicity, acute lithium toxicity, and syncope, either due to postural hypotension or cardiac arrhythmias. Discontinuation symptoms also need to be recognized as management strategies are different from adverse effects. Principles to minimize AEs are avoiding high potency agents, conventional APs and polytherapy, using lowest doses, tailoring appropriate agents after studying patient profile and risks, and stringent monitoring of patients. By understanding the potential risks, recognizing the various neurological side effects, adopting shared decision making, and implementing appropriate management strategies, healthcare professionals can optimize treatment outcomes while minimizing the impact of these side effects on patients' daily lives.

LEARNING POINTS

- Psychotropic drug induced neurological syndromes can be acute and tardive.
- Acute neurological effects can be life threatening and may require stopping of drug and intensive care management.
- Neurological side effects of these drugs are not only confined to movement disorders, but also include cognitive impairment, confusion, reduction of seizures threshold, sleep and weight problems, increased risk of stroke, and death.
- Assess with an electrocardiogram (ECG) before prescribing drugs that may cause cardiac conduction abnormalities.
- Lithium, with its narrow therapeutic window, may cause acute toxicity, tremor, parkinsonism, and encephalopathy.
- Increase in symptoms of psychiatry after starting drugs could be because of the drug itself.
- Newer drugs are with lesser side effects, but they also have a narrower therapeutic spectrum. In future, disease specific drugs may lead to reduction in side effects.
- The best measures to avoid or minimize side effects are avoid psychiatry medicines or use them in minimum doses, stop or switch over to drugs with least side effects, regular monitoring for side effects, and involving patient and family in decision making.

REFERENCES

1. Haddad PM, Dursun SM. Neurological complications of psychiatric drugs: clinical features and management. Hum Psychopharmacol. 2008;23 Suppl 1:15-26.
2. Pierre JM. Extrapyramidal symptoms with atypical antipsychotics: incidence, prevention and management. Drug Saf. 2005;28(3):191-208.
3. Tueth MJ. Emergencies caused by side effects of psychiatric medications. Am J Emerg Med. 1994;12(2):212-6.
4. Baizabal-Carvallo JF, Morgan JC. Drug-induced tremor, clinical features, diagnostic approach and management. J Neurol Sci. 2022;435:120192.
5. Doghramji K, Jangro WC. Adverse Effects of Psychotropic Medications on Sleep. Psychiatr Clin North Am. 2016;39(3):487-502.
6. Murru A, Popovic D, Pacchiarotti I, Hidalgo D, León-Caballero J, Vieta E. Management of adverse effects of mood stabilizers. Curr Psychiatry Rep. 2015;17(8):603.
7. Weiden PJ. EPS profiles: the atypical antipsychotics are not all the same. J Psychiatr Pract. 2007;13(1):13-24.
8. Stroup TS, Gray N. Management of common adverse effects of antipsychotic medications. World Psychiatry. 2018;17(3):341-56.
9. Sachdev P. Early extrapyramidal side-effects as risk factors for later tardive dyskinesia: a prospective study. Aust N Z J Psychiatry. 2004;38(6):445-9.
10. Wirshing WC. Movement disorders associated with neuroleptic treatment. J Clin Psychiatry. 2001;62 Suppl 21:15-8.
11. Tarsy D, Baldessarini RJ, Tarazi FI. Effects of newer antipsychotics on extrapyramidal function. CNS Drugs. 2002;16(1):23-45.
12. Campbell D. The management of acute dystonic reactions. Aust Prescr. 2001;24:19-20.
13. Ribot B, Aupy J, Vidailhet M, Mazère J, Pisani A, Bezard E, et al. Dystonia and dopamine: from phenomenology to pathophysiology. Prog Neurobiol. 2019;182:101678.
14. Munhoz RP, Moscovich M, Araujo PD, Teive HA. Movement disorders emergencies: a review. Arq Neuropsiquiatr. 2012;70(6):453-61.
15. Chang V. Motor side effects of atypical antipsychotic drugs. Therapy. 2009;6(2):249-58.
16. Tandon R. Safety and tolerability: how do newer generation "atypical" antipsychotics compare? Psychiatr Q. 2002;73(4):297-311.
17. Baldez DP, Biazus TB, Rabelo-da-Ponte FD, Nogaro GP, Martins DS, Kunz M, et al. The effect of antipsychotics on the cognitive performance of individuals with psychotic disorders: Network meta-analyses of randomized controlled trials. Neurosci Biobehav Rev. 2021;126:265-75.
18. Moraros J, Nwankwo C, Patten SB, Mousseau DD. The association of antidepressant drug usage with cognitive impairment or dementia, including Alzheimer disease: A systematic review and meta-analysis. Depress Anxiety. 2017;34(3):217-26.
19. Crowe SF, Stranks EK. The residual medium and long-term cognitive effects of benzodiazepine use: an updated meta-analysis. Arch Clin Neuropsychol. 2018;33(7):901-11.
20. Picton JD, Marino AB, Nealy KL. Benzodiazepine use and cognitive decline in the elderly. Am J Health Syst Pharm. 2018;75(1):e6-12.
21. Chen HY, Albertson TE, Olson KR. Treatment of drug-induced seizures. Br J Clin Pharmacol. 2016;81(3):412-9.
22. Clayton AH, Alkis AR, Parikh NB, Votta JG. Sexual dysfunction due to psychotropic medications. Psychiatr Clin North Am. 2016;39(3):427-63.
23. Allison DB, Mentore JL, Heo M, Chandler LP, Cappelleri JC, Infante MC, et al. Antipsychotic-induced weight gain: a comprehensive research synthesis. Am J Psychiatry. 1999;156(11):1686-96.
24. Ruetsch O, Viala A, Bardou H, Martin P, Vacheron MN. Psychotropic drugs induced weight gain: a review of the literature concerning epidemiological data, mechanisms and management. Encephale. 2005;31(4 Pt 1):507-16.
25. Schneider LS, Dagerman K, Insel PS. Efficacy and adverse effects of atypical antipsychotics for dementia: meta-analysis of randomized, placebo-controlled trials. Am J Geriatr Psychiatry. 2006;14(3):191-210.
26. Wang PS, Schneeweiss S, Avorn J, Fischer MA, Mogun H, Solomon DH, et al. Risk of death in elderly users of conventional vs. atypical antipsychotic medications. N Engl J Med. 2005;353(22):2335-41.
27. Brandt L, Bschor T, Henssler J, Müller M, Hasan A, Heinz A, et al. Antipsychotic withdrawal symptoms: a systematic review and meta-analysis. Front Psychiatry. 2020;11:569912.
28. Musco S, Ruekert L, Myers J, Anderson D, Welling M, Cunningham EA. Characteristics of patients experiencing extrapyramidal symptoms or other movement disorders related to dopamine receptor blocking agent therapy. J Clin Psychopharmacol. 2019;39(4):336-43.
29. Campos AI, Mulcahy A, Thorp JG, Wray NR, Byrne EM, Lind PA, et al. Understanding genetic risk factors for common side effects of antidepressant medications. Commun Med (Lond). 2021;1:45.
30. Angell B, Bolden GB. Justifying medication decisions in mental health care: Psychiatrists' accounts for treatment recommendations. Soc Sci Med. 2015;138:44-56.

Central Neurological Manifestations of Alcoholism and Substance Abuse

Sweety Tribedi, Ambar Chakravarty

INTRODUCTION

Alcohol use and substance abuse are often widely associated with social and economic impact on society worldwide. Drug abuse[1] refers to the excessive use of drugs that tends to activate the brain reward system that reinforces behaviors and the production of memories. As per the Diagnostic and Statistical Manual of Mental Disorders, Fifth edition (DSM-5), substance abuse includes 10 separate classes of drugs, including alcohol, caffeine, cannabis, hallucinogens, inhalants, opioids, sedatives, hypnotics and anxiolytics, stimulants, tobacco, and other substances.

Neurologic disorders associated with recreational drug use can be divided into those resulting from overdose or withdrawal and those resulting from additional effects on the nervous system. In this chapter, central neurological manifestations of alcohol consumption and substance abuse have been reviewed. Some of the acute neurological emergencies associated with these are dealt with in chapter on psychiatric emergencies in critical care units.

CENTRAL NEUROLOGICAL MANIFESTATIONS OF ALCOHOLISM

Alcohol abuse and alcohol dependence are now under the umbrella term, alcohol use disorder (AUD).

Initially, it was thought that low doses of alcohol might have healthful benefits. However, >3 standard drinks per day enhances the risk for cancer and vascular disease, and AUDs decrease the life span by about 10 years.

As per a recent systematic review,[2] there is an increased risk of all-cause mortality for drinkers who drank 25 g or more and a significantly increased risk when drinking 45 g or more per day. The all-cause mortality had been higher in men than in women drinking the same amount and even when drinking lesser amount per day. However, mortality risk is similar for both sexes for mean consumption of 25 g/day.

ALCOHOL: FEW POINTS ABOUT PHARMACOLOGY

Alcohol represents a wide range of compounds, but the alcohol suitable for drinking is ethanol or ethyl alcohol. It is a small, water-soluble molecule. Major site of absorption is small intestine followed by modest amount from stomach and large bowel and small amounts from mucous membrane of mouth and esophagus. It is freely distributed throughout the body.[3] Ethanol levels can be measured by blood, urine, saliva, or breath tests. Although toxic concentrations are dependent on individual tolerance and usage, levels >300–400 mg/dL can be fatal due to respiratory depression.

Ethanol blood levels are expressed as milligrams or grams of ethanol per deciliter with values of 0.02 g/dL resulting from the ingestion of one typical drink. Rate of absorption of alcohol is influenced by many factors. It is quickest when drunk on an empty stomach and the concentration of alcohol is 20–30%.[3,4]

More than 90% of alcohol is eliminated by the liver;[3,4] 2–5% is excreted unchanged in urine, sweat, or breath. The first step in metabolism is conversion of ethanol to acetaldehyde in the presence of cofactor by alcohol dehydrogenases. There are four isoenzymes of alcohol dehydrogenase. Acetaldehyde is a highly reactive and toxic carcinogenic substance. Next step is conversion of acetaldehyde by aldehyde dehydrogenases to harmless acetate. Alcohol is much more rapidly absorbed in empty stomach. It roughly peaks about 1 hour after consumption and then declines in a more or less linear manner for the next 4 hours. Alcohol is metabolized at a rate of about

TABLE 1: Blood alcohol levels and clinical manifestations.

Blood level (g/dL)	Stage	Clinical manifestations
0.01–0.05	Sobriety	No apparent influence
0.03–0.12	Euphoria	Mild euphoria, talkativeness, decreased inhibitions, loss of efficiency in fine performance test
0.09–0.25	Excitement	• Emotional instability; decreased inhibitions • Loss of critical judgment, impairment of memory and comprehension • Decreased response; increased reaction time • Incoordination of movements
0.18–0.3	Confusion	• Disorientation, mental confusion, dizziness • Exaggerated emotional states • Disturbance of sensation • Impaired balance, movement incoordination, staggering gait, slurred speech
0.27–0.4	Stupor	• Apathy, inertia of responses, approaching paralysis • Marked incoordination movements; inability to stand or walk • Vomiting; incontinence of urine and feces • Impaired consciousness; sleep or stupor • Markedly decreased response to stimuli
0.35–0.5	Coma	Coma abolished reflexes, subnormal temperature, incontinence of urine and feces, embarrassment of circulation and respiration, possible death
0.45	Death	

Source: Adapted from Dubowski K (1977).[11]

3.3 mmol/h (15 mg/100 mL/h), but this is variable with the amount drunk. In the United States,[5] a "standard alcoholic drink" is equivalent to 14 g of ethanol.

The United States Dietary Guidelines recommend two drinks or less in a day for men and one drink or less in a day for women for healthy adults who choose to drink and do not have any contraindications.[6]

Drinking in moderation can also increase the risk for stroke,[7] cancer,[8] and premature death.[9,10]

Common symptoms, levels of impairment, and risks for various blood alcohol concentration (BAC) levels are presented in **Table 1**.[11]

THE WERNICKE–KORSAKOFF SYNDROME

Wernicke–Korsakoff syndrome (WKS) is a complex and debilitating neurological disorder. This condition is actually a combination of two distinct disorders—Wernicke encephalopathy (WE) and Korsakoff psychosis **(Figs. 1 and 2)**. While WE is characterized by acute neurological symptoms, Korsakoff psychosis presents as a chronic amnestic syndrome.

Wernicke encephalopathy[12] is an acute neurological condition resulting from thiamine deficiency (vitamin B1) that can result from chronic alcoholism, poor nutrition, long-term parenteral feeding, hyperemesis gravidarum, or bariatric surgery.[13]

The increased incidence of WE among alcoholics is due to a combination of inadequate nutritional intake, together with alcohol's inhibitory effects on thiamine

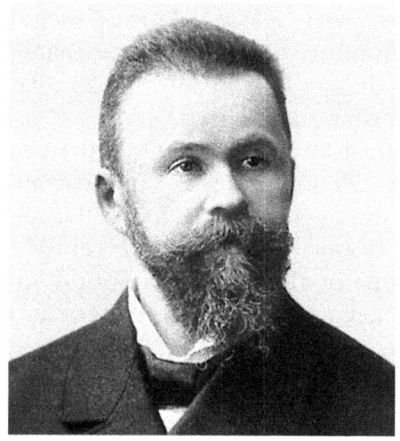

FIG. 1: Carl Wernicke (1848–1905).

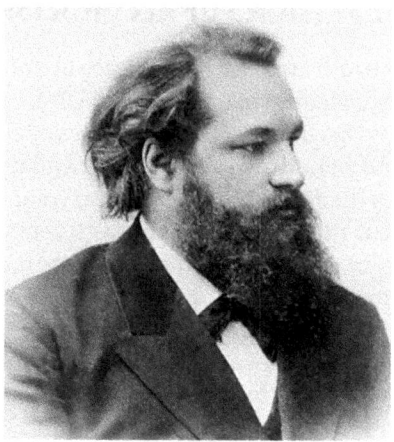

FIG. 2: Sergei Korsakoff (1854–1900).

absorption through the gastrointestinal tract, and on thiamine activation via phosphorylation.[14]

Incidence rates of WE in the general population range from 0.1 to 2.8% but can be as high as 12.5% in patients with alcoholism.[15,16]

Approximately 80% of undiagnosed and untreated WE patients develop KS, a severe, typically permanent neurological disorder characterized by anterograde amnesia.[17,18]

Pathophysiology

The bioactive form of thiamine is thiamine pyrophosphate (TPP), which is required for energy metabolism in all cells and is stored in all cells as thymine diphosphate (TDP).[19] Thiamine is essential to maintain membrane integrity and oncotic pressures across cell membranes. Pathophysiologically, thiamine deficiency causes dysfunction of the Krebs cycle (tricarboxylic acid, TCA cycle) and the pentose phosphate pathway with consequent development of brain cytotoxic edema and vasogenic edema.[20]

Low levels of TPP result in impairment of several biochemical pathways in the brain, including carbohydrate metabolism (for energy production), lipid metabolism (for production and maintenance of myelin), and amino acid metabolism (for production of glucose-derived neurotransmitters; e.g., glutamic acid and gamma-aminobutyric acid).[16]

Thymine diphosphate participates in energy production as an essential cofactor for several enzymes in the TCA cycle and pentose phosphate pathways.[19,21]

Thiamine pyrophosphate acts as a cofactor for transketolase in the pentose phosphate pathway,[22] as a cofactor for pyruvate dehydrogenase in the transition from glycolysis to the TCA cycle and as a cofactor for alpha-ketoglutarate dehydrogenase within the TCA cycle. Thiamine deficiency therefore disrupts cellular metabolism in several ways and limits the availability of adenosine triphosphate (ATP). Thus, due to high metabolic demands, the brain bears the brunt of the disease.

The TCA cycle or Krebs cycle is second part of aerobic respiration pathway that occurs in the mitochondria where acetate derived from carbohydrates, fatty acids, and proteins undergo series of chemical reactions that result in ATP production. The pentose phosphate pathway occurs in cell cytosol in parallel to glycolysis and consists of two parts—first aerobic part resulting in formation of NADPH and second anerobic part resulting in generation of pentoses and ribose-5-phosphate, which is required for nucleotide synthesis. NADPH is necessary for several anabolic processes and also acts as a free radical scavenger during oxidative stress.[19,21]

Brain lesions in WE are often attributed to focal lactic acidosis.[23] In patients with thiamine deficiency, pyruvate accumulates within the cell. The increase in pyruvate causes increase in lactate concentration and there is an accumulation of toxic intermediate metabolic products such as lactate, alanine, and glutamate, resulting in reduced cellular pH and disruption of the homeostasis of cellular electrolytes. The entire cascade results in cytotoxic edema.[24]

Vasogenic edema[20] results when there is blood–brain barrier (BBB) dysfunction. The BBB is composed of capillary endothelial cells (ECs), mesenchymal-like cells pericytes, and astrocytes terminal processes, which form strong tight junctions. When astrocytes are damaged by ATP depletion, oxidative stress, pH reduction, and secondary excitotoxicity by excessive glutamate concentration in the synaptic clefts, these tight junctions are damaged and BBB dysfunction occurs.[25,26]

Another proposed mechanism includes neural cell excitotoxicity. In thiamine deficiency, glutamate transporters in astrocytes are downregulated, which causes extracellular buildup of glutamate leading to sustained depolarization of neurons and subsequent death of the cells. Inflammation is also known to occur in thiamine deficiency, with microglial reactivity and proinflammatory cytokines found throughout the brain.[27,28]

In patients of AUD, there is low thiamine uptake, low absorption rate at mucosal level, and impaired thiamine utilization.[29]

Clinical Presentation

Wernicke encephalopathy was first characterized by Carl Wernicke in 1881, as a triad of altered mental status, ocular signs, and ataxia. Korsakoff syndrome, which is the chronic phase of WKS, was described by Sergei Korsakoff in 1887, as an amnesic disorder with confabulations.[16,30,31]

Although classically described as a triad of ocular motor abnormalities, cerebellar dysfunction, and altered mental state, many patients do not have all the three components. Ocular motor abnormalities occur in approximately 30% of patients with WE. Patients present with nystagmus, which is usually horizontal or ophthalmoplegia. Other presentations are bilateral decreased visual acuity, bilateral abducens palsy, and other ocular muscle or conjugate-gaze palsies. Complete ophthalmoplegia occurs rarely. Anatomically, these clinical manifestations localize to pontine tegmentum including the abducens and oculomotor nuclei.[21]

Cerebellar dysfunction is found in approximately 25% of patients. It manifests as loss of equilibrium, incoordination of gait, trunk ataxia, dysdiadochokinesia, and, occasionally, limb ataxia, or dysarthria.[32] They occur due to involvement of the cerebellar vermis and vestibular dysfunction. Unusual manifestations of WE include hypothermia/hyperthermia due to the involvement of the posterior hypothalamus, deafness, and epileptic seizures.[21]

Most of the patients of WE (approximately 80%) exhibit an altered mental status in the form of mental sluggishness, apathy, impaired awareness, an inability to concentrate, confusion or agitation, hallucinations, behavioral disturbances, which may mimic an acute psychotic disorder and some may also present with coma.[33,34] These symptoms are possibly due to involvement of the reticular system at the level of the midline thalamic nuclei or mammillary bodies.[19]

Retrospective analysis of the clinical signs and symptoms of patients diagnosed at autopsy as having WE revealed that only 20% of patients with this disorder presented with the full triad of clinical features and approximately 30% of such individuals exhibited only cognitive impairment.[34]

If untreated, WE can lead to irreversible brain damage and even death in up to 20% of cases or KS in 85% of survivors.[21]

Patients with untreated WE develop KS, a form of anterograde and retrograde amnesia with confabulation, related to lesions in the dorsal thalamus and mammillary bodies.[19] In discussing confabulation, Korsakoff (1889) himself emphasized the role of real memories, recalled out of temporal sequence, such that they were retrieved inappropriately out of their temporal context. He identified a confusion of "old recollections with present impressions" as the basis of many instances of confabulation.

Korsakoff syndrome affects the patient's working memory. Patients are unable to consolidate short-term memories to long-term memories because of lesions in the diencephalon-hippocampal circuit.[20]

As per a systematic review,[33-35] comparing alcoholic with nonalcoholic WE, the clinical features were unevenly distributed; dietary deficiency and vomiting were more frequent among nonalcoholics, whereas eye and cerebellar signs were more frequent among alcoholics. The classical triad was significantly more frequent in alcoholics than in the nonalcoholics. Magnesium deficiency could also contribute to the poor recovery from WE in alcoholics.[35]

Diagnostic Criteria

As per the European Federation of Neurological Societies (EFNS) recommendation,[35] the clinical diagnosis of WE in both alcoholics and nonalcoholics requires two of the following four signs: (1) Dietary deficiencies, (2) eye signs, (3) cerebellar dysfunction, and (4) either an altered mental state or mild memory impairment.

Caine et al.[36] reported a sensitivity of 94% and specificity of 99% for the diagnosis of WE when these criteria were used. One study showed only 44% of those with postmortem WE diagnosis displayed two or more operational criteria before death.[34]

The erythrocyte transketolase activity assay including TPP effect has been replaced by direct measurement of thiamine and its phosphate esters in human blood by high-performance liquid chromatography (HPLC).[37,38]

Blood sample should be taken before administration of thiamine and should be protected from light. In the presence of thiamine transporter gene mutations, thiamine level may remain normal.[39]

Imaging

Computed tomography (CT) can show areas of reduced attenuation density at the periaqueductal gray matter and the medial portion of thalami but, in most cases, CT findings are normal in the acute phase of WE. Magnetic resonance imaging (MRI) has a low sensitivity of only 53% but high specificity of 93% for the diagnosis of WE **(Fig. 3)**. MRI typically symmetrical increased signal intensity in T2, fluid attenuation inversion recovery (FLAIR), and diffusion-weighted imaging (DWI) of mammillary bodies, dorsomedial thalami, tectal plate, periaqueductal gray matter, and around the third ventricle. This typical pattern of lesions on MRI is observed in only 58% of patients.[21,40]

Sometimes unusual sites of lesions such as putamen, caudate, splenium of the corpus callosum, dorsal medulla, pons, red nucleus, substantia nigra of the midbrain, cranial nerve nucleus (VI, VII, VIII, XII), vermis, dentate nucleus, paravermian region of the cerebellum, fornix and pre- and postcentral gyri may also be involved on MRI. However, they hardly occur in isolation and almost always found in association with the typical imaging findings.[20,21]

Magnetic resonance spectroscopy studies have reported low N-acetylaspartate/creatine ratio (NAA/Cr), suggestive of neuronal metabolic impairment, and an abnormal lactate peak, suggesting anaerobic glycolysis.[41] The low NAA/Cr has been reported to improve in parallel with clinical improvement following thiamine therapy in some cases.[41]

Gadolinium enhancing lesions are more common in alcoholics, whereas cranial nerve nucleus involvement is seen more frequently in nonalcohol WE.[42]

Lesions of the caudate nuclei are frequently observed in patients in a comatose state thus signifying a sign of severity. Cortical involvement indicates irreversible damage and poor prognosis[42] and signal abnormalities of the paramedian thalamic nuclei and contrast enhancement of the mammillary bodies may be a predictor of poor recovery from memory impairment and altered mental state in case of WE.[40]

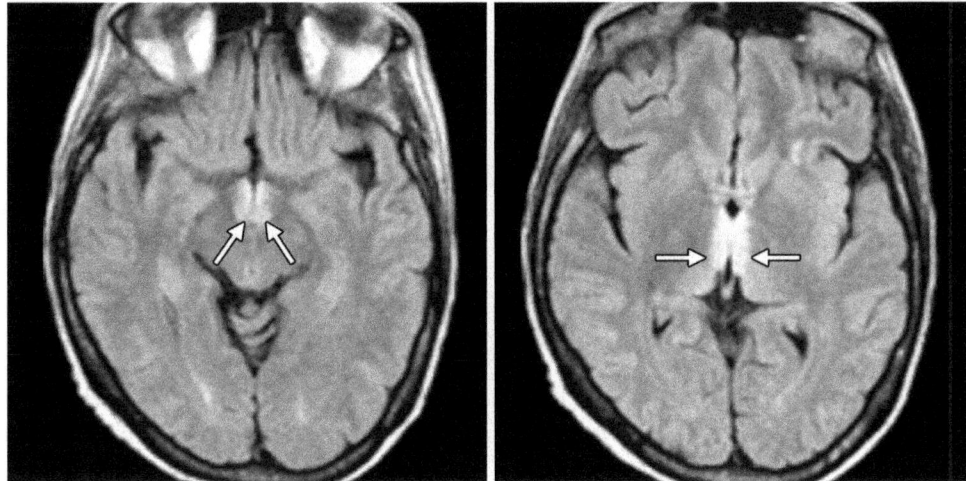

FIG. 3: Magnetic resonance imaging scan of the brain in Wernicke encephalopathy (WE) fluid attenuation inversion recovery sequence showing (on the right) hyperintensity in the mammillary bodies and (on the left) hyperintensity in the medial thalami. Gadolinium enhancing lesions are more common in alcoholics, whereas cranial nerve nucleus involvement is seen more frequently in nonalcohol WE.[42]

Among alcoholics with a clinically verified acute WE, conventional MRI revealed lesions in nearly two-thirds of the subjects, whereas nonalcoholics showed a higher yield of lesions varying from 97% in DWI and 99% in conventional and 100% in FLAIR images.[43] Location of lesions are frequently atypical among nonalcoholic than alcoholic patients whereas contrast enhancement of the thalamus and mamillary bodies are observed to associate more frequently in alcoholics.[42] Reversible cytotoxic edema was considered the most distinctive lesion of WE.[42]

In pediatric patients, abnormal intensity is more often observed in the basal ganglia with a characteristic involvement of the putamen. It is probably due to the high thiamine-dependent metabolism of these areas in children.[40,42]

Treatment

The EFNS recommends intravenous 200 mg thiamine thrice daily until there are no additional improvements in clinical condition, while British authors have recommended 500 mg thrice daily for 2-3 days followed by 250 mg daily until improvements cease.[16,35]

Studies from several countries show a thiamine deficiency in the elderly population.[44] Thiamine has been added to foods in many countries.[12,45] This preventive effort has resulted in a decrease of the occurrence of the disease in some countries. Prophylactic parenteral administration of 200 mg thiamine is recommended before carbohydrates are started in all subjects with a risk condition in emergency and after bariatric surgery.[35]

Prognosis

Approximately 25% of patients with WKS require long-term supervised care or institutionalization.[46] They usually have comorbidity in more than one domain (somatic and psychiatric).[47]

In patients who recover, there is particular sequence of recovery of symptoms. Ocular abnormalities are the earliest to recover, usually occurring within hours of the initial thiamine dose. One should reconsider the diagnosis in case of failure of ocular abnormalities to respond to thiamine.

Vertical nystagmus may persist for months. Fine horizontal nystagmus may persist indefinitely in as many as 60% of patients, but patients completely recover from sixth nerve palsies, ptosis, and vertical-gaze palsies.

Approximately 40% of patients recover completely from their ataxic symptoms. But most patients have incomplete recovery with residual cerebellar signs in the legs. Vestibular dysfunction also shows similar pattern of recovery. The symptoms of global confusional state are the last to resolve and recovery is gradual after treatment is initiated. Amnestic deficits, if present, are unmasked after global confusion resolves. Only 20% of such patients have complete recovery. Many are left with varying degrees of persistent learning and memory impairment. Recovery may take ≥1 years.

The mortality rate is up to 10-15% in severe cases. Prognosis depends on the stage of disease at presentation, severity of the disease, and timing of treatment. Unspecified infections were the cause of death in 77% of one cohort of Wernicke-Korsakoff patients.[33]

MARCHIAFAVA–BIGNAMI DISEASE

Marchiafava–Bignami disease (MBD) is a rare condition characterized by demyelination and necrosis of the entire length and middle layer of corpus callosum with extension into hemispheric white matter.[48,49]

Others such as the optic chiasm and tracts, putamen, cerebellar peduncle, and anterior commissure may also be affected. Cortical gray matter and subcortical U fibers are involved rarely.[50,51] It is seen most often in chronic alcoholism and occasionally occurs in chronically malnourished patients.[52,53]

In 1903, Italian pathologists Marchiafava and Bignami[53] **(Figs. 4 and 5)** described three alcoholic men who died after having seizures and coma. All patients had severely necrotic middle two-thirds of the corpus callosum. Since then, many such cases were reported most frequently in alcoholic men, but some nonalcoholics have also been reported with phenotypic and radiological findings that are typical of MBD.[54-57]

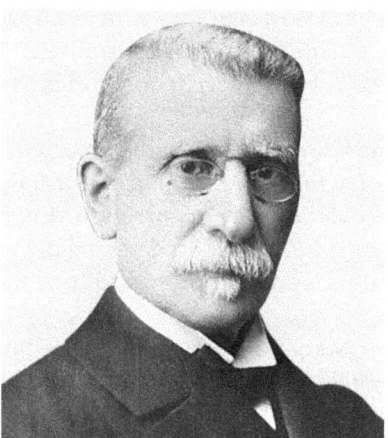

FIG. 4: Ettorre Marchiafava (1848–1935).

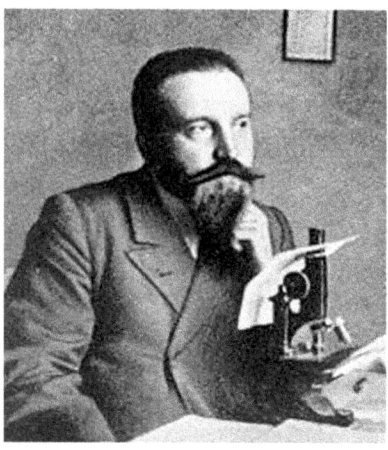

FIG. 5: Amico Bignami (1862–1929).

Heinrich et al.[58] described two clinicoradiological subtypes of MBD:
1. *Type A*: Immediate to subacute development of consciousness disturbance, seizures, pyramidal tract symptoms, hypertonia of limb, and extremely severe swelling of the entire corpus callosum on T2-weighted MR sequences; poor prognosis; and has predominant features of coma and stupor.
2. *Type B*: Hyperintense lesions on T2-weighted MR sequences showing partial or focal corpus callosum lesion, dysarthria, gait disturbance, evidence of disconnection between hemispheres, and normal or mildly compromised level of consciousness. This type has a better prognosis as the underlying lesions more likely are edema than demyelination.

Demography

As per a systematic review,[59] MBD subjects were significantly older than MBD-mimics and most of them were male in both groups. History of alcoholism, malnutrition, and Wernicke disease may be present in MBD subjects. None of the MBD mimics had such history. The nonalcoholic subjects with MBD are usually younger with female predominance.

Clinical Presentation

Marchiafava–Bignami disease might have an acute, subacute, or chronic manifestation:[58]
- *Acute state*:[60] Confusion, dysarthria, limb hypertonicity, ataxia, and delirium/coma, seizures, alterations of consciousness, and death may occur.
- *Subacute state*:[60] Features can be depression, ataxia, apraxia, agraphia, anomia, dysarthria, visual dyslexia. Some of these can be a part of an interhemispheric disconnection syndrome, with a unilateral presentation.
- *Chronic state*:[60,61] Progressive severe global dementia, visual hallucinations, auditory delusions, and behavioral abnormalities. Also, there can be signs of interhemispheric disconnection syndrome. Hemialexia, limb apraxia, unilateral agraphia, and tactile agraphia may be seen. The close differential diagnosis of chronic phase of MBD is Alzheimer's disease, both of which manifest as dementia.

The spectrum of clinical signs and symptoms differ between the MBD patients and the MBD mimics. The MBD patients frequently show an altered mental state, which included confusion, delirium, unconsciousness, impaired memory, and/or disorientation on admission. Impaired walking, dysarthria, mutism, signs of disconnection, pyramidal signs, primitive reflexes, rigidity, incontinence, sensory symptoms, and gaze palsy or diplopia are also more frequently found in the MBD cases than in the MBD mimics. On the other hand, hemi- or quadriparesis, nystagmus, and seizures were more frequent among the mimics.[59]

The cognitive abnormalities in MBD may be related to microhemorrhages. The anatomical sites of microbleeds have been found to correlate with cognitive deficit.[62]

Manifestations of chronic alcohol abuse such as WE, central pontine myelinolysis (CPM), and Morel laminar sclerosis are often associated.

Pathophysiology

Deficiency of all eight forms of vitamin B group results in necrosis and demyelination of the corpus callosum in MBD. Sometimes hemispheric white matter, internal capsule, and middle cerebellar peduncle may also have lesions. Although rare, Morel laminar sclerosis can also be seen.[49]

When hyperintense lesions are observed on DWI in acute phase of the disease, it is due to underlying cytotoxic edema whereas in the later stages necrosis and demyelination predominate.[63]

The pathophysiological mechanism of MBD is currently unclear. Cytotoxic edema, the breakdown of the BBB, demyelination, and necrosis are possible mechanisms. The splenium has more myelin than any other part of the callosum. So, there is a plausible explanation for lesions in callosum. However, the cortical lesions cannot be explained by this hypothesis.[64]

Cortical lesions are considered to indicate Morel laminar sclerosis, which has previously been reported in postmortem examinations.[65]

Cytotoxic edema is proposed as the possible underlying mechanism in the early stage when hyperintense lesions are seen on DWI, while demyelination and necrosis may play a role in later stages.[63] However, neither of these mechanisms could explain why the corpus callosum is vulnerable in MBD.

Diagnosis

Presently, diagnosis of MBD is based on history examination and imaging findings. MRI is the gold standard. A symmetrical lesion encompassing the central region in the body of the corpus callosum leaving out the ventral and dorsal layer also called the sandwich sign is a hallmark of acute MBD. Chronic lesions may develop into well-defined cavitation, except in cases of subacute hemorrhage, in which the lesions can appear as isodense or hyperdense.[60]

Gadolinium-enhancing lesions are frequently reported in MBD patients, but this was not found in the mimics.[59] The MRI features of MBD are symmetric lesions of the corpus callosum, which usually are restricted to the genu, body, or splenium. The impaired area has edematous changes with or without demyelination, which appears as a high signal lesion on T2-weighted imaging (T2WI)/FLAIR and DWI. With resolution of the acute stage, edematous changes gradually subside and the high signal changes are replaced by normal signal. If the impairment progresses to permanent myelin impairment and necrosis, the MRI of the affected region shows atrophy and cystic transformation.[66,67] With early diagnosis and treatment as the patients recover, serial MRI demonstrate gradual disappearance of corpus callosum lesion. Patients with lesions in other regions of the brain, especially cortical lesion portends poor prognosis for recovery.[66,67]

In chronic stage, corpus callosum degenerates and separates into three layers with necrotic cavities mainly in the middle layer. Cortical involvement is extremely rare and when present, it is usually localized in lateral-frontal regions.[49] MR spectroscopy of the lesion shows a higher level of choline and an increased choline to creatine (Cho/Cr) ratio in acute phase along with lactate peak may be present. Single-photon emission computerized tomography (SPECT) scans may reveal bilateral cerebral blood flow decrease.[68]

Treatment

There are no management guidelines or specific proven treatment to date. Most of the case reports of MBD have shown a favorable response to parenteral administration of thiamine, folate, and vitamin B complexes as well as high-dose corticosteroids.[69-72] Some case reports show significant improvement with high-dose intravenous thiamine (500 mg/TID), oral vitamin B complex, amantadine, and folate.[63,70] Early administration of parenteral thiamine particularly within 2 weeks is associated with better outcomes.[59] Trial of corticosteroids to reduce brain edema, suppress demyelination, stabilize the BBB, and reduce inflammation may be given. The dose of thiamine is same as recommended for Wernicke disease, and the therapy is continued as long as recovery is going on.

Prognosis

Heavy alcohol consumption, extracallosal lesions, lobar impairment, and patients with low Glasgow Coma Scale (GCS) may have a poor prognosis.[73] Autopsy reports of alcoholic patients with MBD found that the third layer of the cortex was primarily affected.[74] Some researchers have proposed that the cortex and the corpus callosum are the most vulnerable regions of acute MBD and the cortical lesions might not be caused by heavy alcohol consumption but by deficiency of thiamine.[75] Patients with lesions in other brain regions have poor prognosis and severe residual cognitive impairment. In contrast, patients with circumscribed lesions in the corpus callosum who receive an early diagnosis and appropriate treatment have a favorable prognosis.[76]

Blackouts

These are periods of dense amnesia during and after episodes of heavy alcohol consumption. They are not accompanied by drowsiness, inattentiveness, or impairment of consciousness, and speech and behavior may appear normal. Close differential of such episodes is transient global amnesia. The proposed mechanism for such episodes is ethanol inhibiting the N-methyl-D-aspartate receptor and impairing long-term potentiation. They can arise in social drinkers but are indicative of heavy consumption and risk of developing alcohol dependence.[77]

CENTRAL PONTINE MYELINOLYSIS

Central pontine myelinolysis is a disease affecting alcoholics and the malnourished.[78] In approximately 10% patients, CPM is associated with extrapontine myelinolysis (EPM), which may lead to Parkinson symptoms[79] and psychotic features.[80]

Pathologically, CPM is defined as a symmetric area of myelin disruption in the center of the basis pontis.[81]

It is a condition most frequently related to rapid correction of hyponatremia. Involvement of the corticospinal tracts in the pons and midbrain, resulting in spastic quadriparesis and pseudobulbar palsy, is a characteristic neurological finding.[82]

Risk factors for CPM are dialysis, liver failure and transplantation, advanced lymphoma, carcinoma, cachexia from various causes, severe bacterial infections, dehydration and electrolyte disturbance, acute hemorrhagic pancreatitis, chronic alcoholism, and pellagra.[82-84]

Chronic alcoholics are particularly predisposed for CPM and EPM, and it has been reported that they may be asymptomatic or have relatively few symptoms, with a better outcome of their CPM and EPM than in cases associated with an acute correction of hyponatremia.[85]

The proposed mechanisms include osmotic injury to the vascular ECs and this causes the release of myelinotoxic factors, the production of vasogenic edema and/or brain dehydration. It is possible that chronic alcoholics are unable to maintain protective cerebral mechanisms against osmotic stress compounded by direct toxicity of alcohol.[86]

Extrapontine myelinolysis usually occurs in association with CPM but may occur in isolation as well. Extrapyramidal features and myoclonus of EPM are some of the symptoms that represent potentially treatable manifestations of the disease and should be differentiated from CPM.[83]

Signs and Symptoms

- Pseudobulbar palsy due to damage to corticobulbar tracts manifested as facial weakness, dysphagia, diplopia, and dysarthria.
- Spastic quadriparesis due to damage to corticospinal tracts: Spastic quadriparesis.
- This may eventually lead to "locked in syndrome", a condition characterized by complete paralysis of all voluntary muscles with preservation of vertical eye movement and blinking.

Treatment

There have been no trials or recommended guideline. At present, treatment is mainly supportive. Reports on small case series or single case reports of treatments including steroids, intravenous immunoglobulin, and thyrotrophin-releasing hormone have all shown good outcomes.

Alcohol withdrawal seizures (AWS) usually occur around 6-48 hours after major intake reduction. While they are often a single event, there is little knowledge on long-term evolution after AWS and risk factors for AWS relapse. Over 10% suffer from AWS relapses within the next 1 year after the first AWS. Risk factors for relapses generally are history of AWS, interictal epileptiform electroencephalogram (EEG) abnormalities, skull fractures, and presence of structural brain abnormalities in the initial neuroimaging.

SUBSTANCE ABUSE

There are five broad groups of recreational drugs mentioned in **Table 2**.

Emerging/new drugs: Production of new psychoactive substances (NPSs) such as synthetic cathinones (bath salts) and synthetic cannabinoids (spice). The three most common synthetic cathinones are mephedrone, methylone, and MDPV (3,4-methylenedioxypyrovalerone).

TABLE 2: Recreational drugs.

Drug class	Example
Stimulant	Cocaine/crack, amphetamine, 3,4-methylenedioxymethamphetamine ("Ecstasy"), ephedrine, phenylpropanolamine, and methylphenidate
Sedatives	Heroin and other opiates, barbiturates
Hallucinogens	Phencyclidine ("Angel dust"), cannabis, marijuana, and gamma hydroxybutyrate (GHB)
Organic solvents	Glue sniffers—toluene, hexane, and benzene
Athletic performance-enhancing drug	Anabolic steroids, growth hormone, erythropoietin, clenbuterol, cocaine, and amphetamine

Stroke

Cerebrovascular disorders, although less frequent, contribute to the morbidity and disability associated with illicit drug use. A few studies investigating the causes of stroke in the young adult found that drug abusers had an increased risk (6.5 times)[87] of both hemorrhagic and ischemic stroke.

In a cross-sectional study of hospital discharges, amphetamine increased the risk of hemorrhagic stroke, whereas cocaine increased the risk of both hemorrhagic stroke and ischemic stroke.[88]

Strokes can be caused by cocaine, amphetamines, heroin, morphine, cannabis, and the new synthetic cannabinoids, along with androgenic anabolic steroids.

Cocaine

Of all cocaine-associated strokes, 25-60% are ischemic.[89-91] The majority (50-80%) of infarcts involve the middle cerebral artery.[92] Patients with cocaine-related stroke tend to be young, in the fourth decade of life.[93]

The effects of cocaine in the central nervous system result from blocking of the reuptake of catecholamines such as dopamine, serotonin, norepinephrine, and epinephrine at nerve endings. These neuroanatomical actions result in a potentiation of sympathetic activity. Stroke can occur with both cocaine hydrochloride and alkaloid crack and following any method of administration.

Multiple overlapping mechanisms may be responsible for ischemic stroke related to cocaine. Acutely, cocaine can induce vasospasm, sudden onset of hypertension, and myocardial infarction[94] with cardiac arrhythmias. In the longer term, cocaine may induce cardiomyopathy,[95] endothelial dysfunction toward a prothrombotic condition and accelerated atherosclerosis,[96] increased platelet activation,[97] and vasculitis.[98]

Most ischemic strokes related to cocaine occur in the first few hours after cocaine consumption, but there may be a delay of up to several hours between cocaine intake and onset of stroke, delayed effects of vasoconstriction of cocaine metabolites and to an extended endothelial dysfunction.[96,99] Ischemic strokes related to cocaine have been found to have markedly elevated serum creatine kinase levels probably due to rhabdomyolysis associated with hyperthermia, adrenergic stimulation, or direct toxic action in muscular metabolism.[100]

In a recent retrospective and prospective study of ischemic stroke in the young, cocaine addicts had a higher rate of complications and mortality.[100]

Regarding treatment, thrombolysis seems to be safe in cocaine-associated stroke. A retrospective study found no complications in patients with cocaine-associated stroke treated with tissue plasminogen activator. Cocaine-positive and cocaine-negative treated patients had similar stroke severity and safety outcomes.[101]

Cocaine users have a higher frequency of intracranial hemorrhages (ICHs) than noncocaine users.[93] ICH is more common in those actively consuming cocaine, perhaps owing to acute spikes in blood pressure.

Cocaine use has been associated with several types of ICH, including intraparenchymal hemorrhage, intraventricular hemorrhage, and subarachnoid hemorrhage (SAH).[87] There are four proposed mechanisms by which cocaine can induce a hemorrhagic stroke **(Table 3)**:

1. A sudden increase in arterial pressure may enhance the rupture of a vessel, often in association with an underlying aneurysm or arteriovenous malformation,[93,102] which provides weak sites. Intra-aneurismal pressure can equal mean systemic arterial pressure[103] and become many times greater than that registered in the cerebral arteries. Up to 41% of patients presenting with a cocaine-associated cerebral hemorrhage were reported to have evidence of vascular abnormalities such as aneurysms or arteriovenous malformations. Arteriography should therefore be a part of the investigation of young patients who are suspected of being drug abusers.
2. Hemorrhagic transformation of ischemic infarcts related to multifocal vasoconstriction[104]
3. Vasculitis

TABLE 3: Mechanism of stroke with other drugs.

Drug	Stroke type	Mechanism
Opioids	Ischemic	• Cardioembolism—infective endocarditis, arrhythmias • Embolization of foreign substances • Global hypoperfusion and hypoxia—hypotension, bradycardia, and respiratory depression • Compression of carotid artery • Vasculitis
Pentazocine	Ischemic	Bacterial endocarditis
	Hemorrhagic	Embolization of foreign substances
LSD	Ischemic	Carotid vasoconstriction
Phencyclidine	Hemorrhagic	Sympathomimetic effect—acute hypertension
Anabolic steroid	Ischemic	• Enhanced atherogenesis • Prothrombotic effect, impaired endothelial function, and increased viscosity

4. Changes in cerebrovascular autoregulation. Cocaine causes vasodilatation and increases cerebral blood flow at blood pressures substantially higher than those resulting in vascular rupture in normotensive patients.[105]

Aneurysms have been reported to be significantly smaller and rupture at a younger age among cocaine users compared with nonusers.[106]

Simpson et al.[107] documented that patients who consumed cocaine intravenously and had an SAH had a poorer outcome than other patients with SAH. This was hypothesized to be due to an increased intensity and duration of vasospasm related to the use of cocaine.

Amphetamines and Related Agents

Hypertension, vasoconstriction,[108,109] and focal myocytes necrosis[110] are the major cardiovascular responses caused by binge administration of methamphetamine. Amphetamine use increases the risk of stroke by almost four times as compared to nonusers.[111] Most case series report a disproportionate rate of hemorrhagic stroke with amphetamine use, up to twice the risk with cocaine use.[84] Cerebral vasculitis is a commonly described histologic and radiological finding in abusers of methamphetamine with either hemorrhagic or ischemic stroke.[112] Pathologically, there is extensive medial necrosis of medium- and small-sized cerebral vessels with minimal inflammatory response.[113,114]

Some authors proposed the use of immunosuppressants in vasculitis associated with methamphetamine.[110]

Brain hemorrhages occur due to the combined effects of hypertension and vasculitis. Both subcortical and lobar hematomas have been described.[115] Patients with intracerebral hemorrhage related to the short-term use of amphetamine-like psychostimulants may present with fever and acute hypertension. Infarcts caused by ecstasy are frequently seen in the occipital cortex and globus pallidus.[104]

Cannabis

Altered cerebral autoregulation, hypotension, vasospasm, cerebral vasoconstriction syndrome, vasculitis, and cardioembolism (resulting from arrhythmia, namely atrial fibrillation or myocardial infarction are the possible mechanism of stroke in cannabis users.[116] In a prospective cohort of 48 consecutive young patients with ischemic stroke, 13 patients consumed cannabis. Ten of these patients showed a specific pattern of multifocal intracranial stenosis that seemed to be associated with cannabis use.[117] The main radiological characteristics of the angiopathy were involvement of multiple intracranial arteries and reversibility of vasoconstriction after cannabis withdrawal. In this study, ischemic strokes were more frequent in the vertebrobasilar territory.[117]

Reversible cerebral vasoconstriction syndrome (RCVS) is a rare neurological condition characterized by a thunderclap headache and angiographic evidence of reversible multifocal narrowing of cerebral vessels. A wide variety of illicit drugs being implicated in the development of RCVS.[118-120] However, aside from cannabis, other drugs such as cocaine, ecstasy, amphetamine, and methamphetamine showed distinct lack of evidence. Heroin and lysergic acid diethylamide (LSD) have not been found to be associated with any confirmed case of RCVS.[118-120]

Movement Disorder[121-123]

Table 4 summarizes briefly various movement disorders associated with substance abuse drugs.

TABLE 4: Movement disorders associated with drugs.

Drug	Movement disorder
MPTP	Parkinsonism—irreversible
MDMA	Tremor and serotonin syndrome
Cocaine	Tremor, tics, dystonia, and chorea
Amphetamines	Tremor and ataxia
Opioids	Myoclonus, hiccups, parkinsonism, and chorea

(MDMA: 3,4-methylenedioxymethamphetamine; MPTP: 1-methyl-4-phenyl-1,2,3,6-tetrahydropyridine)

Headache

Headaches are frequently reported by cocaine abuser. These headaches have migrainous character associated with acute use or drug withdrawal. Cocaine abusers have these headaches during acute phase possibly due to sympathomimetic action/vasoconstrictive action of cocaine whereas during withdrawal phase it is attributed to alteration of serotonergic system.[124]

Headaches may also be related to vasculitis or hypertensive encephalopathy or RCVS. Dissection of the carotid and vertebral arteries, ischemic stroke, or hemorrhagic stroke may also give rise to headaches.

Doxepin may be particularly helpful in those suffering from headaches due to cocaine withdrawal. Doxepin may hinder transient hypoactivity of norepinephrine and serotonin during the cessation of cocaine by preventing presynaptic reuptake of these neurotransmitters.[124]

Amlodipine has been found to decrease the rate of migraine in cocaine abusers possibly because they improved cerebrovascular tone. It has also been shown to reduce blood pressure and headache frequency in cocaine-dependent patients.[125]

Myelopathy/Acute Transverse Myelitis

Acute transverse myelopathy is an uncommon complication of heroin or cocaine intake. In this context, it usually has an abrupt onset, catastrophic presentation and poor outcome leading to severe long-term disability.[126]

According to one study,[127] drug abuse-related myelopathy was more frequent in men. The offending drugs were nitrous oxide (NO) in 43% of the cases, heroin in 29%, and heroin plus cocaine in 29% of the case. They usually had an acute-subacute presentation characterized by weakness, sphincter dysfunction, and numbness with sensory level and bladder and bowel involvement. MRI spine in all patients had hyperintense lesions on T2W images distributed in the posterior (43%), anterior (43%), and central (28%) cord. Posterior and central patterns were distinctive of NO and heroin overdose, respectively. Lesions were mostly longitudinally extensive with a predominant cervical localization. On cerebrospinal fluid (CSF) analysis, three patients had pleocytosis, elevated protein or both. The etiology was spinal cord strokes in four cases and vitamin B12 deficiency in three. Most of the patients were treated with IV methylprednisolone for the initial diagnosis of transverse myelitis without significant response.[127]

Myelopathy associated with heroin use mainly involves ventral pons and lateral and posterior column of cervical and upper thoracic cord specially. In most of the cases, myelopathy occurs on restarting the offending agent after a period of abstinence. The possibility of hypersensitivity mechanism has thus been suggested. Other suggested mechanisms include direct toxicity, embolism, and hypotension.[128-131] CSF findings are normal or show mild pleocytosis.[126,129,130]

Acutely, MRI can be normal[132] or show multilevel T2 hyperintensities with patchy gadolinium contrast enhancement and evidence of cord edema.[133] Histopathologically, the spinal cord demonstrates extensive necrosis of both gray and white matter with significant myelin loss as well as expansion of the spinal cord. Spinal cord blood vessels showed endothelial hyperplasia without evidence of arteritis.[126]

Treatment is largely supportive. Use of IV corticosteroids or plasma exchange may be tried but has not proven to be effective.[134] The prognosis for recovery is often poor, although some patients may recover completely.

Nitrous oxide is an anesthetic drug but it also has been used as a recreational drug. It is available in aerosol delivery systems for whipped cream. NO causes irreversible inactivation of vitamin B12 that can lead to an acute or subacute myelopathy identical to subacute combined degeneration of the spinal cord.[135]

Myelopathy, myeloneuropathy, peripheral neuropathy, and cognitive problems have been reported to occur with NO toxicity.[136,137] MRI may show changes identical to those that may be seen in patients with vitamin B12 deficiency: High T2 signal intensity in the posterior and lateral columns of the cervical and thoracic spinal cord.[138] Treatment is with high doses of cobalamin intramuscularly along with cessation of NO use. Improvement in clinical symptoms and MRI studies usually follow treatment.[135]

CONCLUDING REMARKS

Alcohol and substance abuse disorder can cause significant neurological complication with high morbidity and sometimes incomplete recovery or death. Abstinence from the same is primary prevention and prevents disease and its associated complications. Early diagnosis with high index of suspicion helps in early timely intervention and better outcome.

LEARNING POINTS

- Prevalence of alcohol-related central complications are frequently under diagnosed or delayed in diagnosis.
- In patients presenting with altered sensorium or acute dementia or seizures, injectable thiamine should be considered after ruling out hypoglycemia and other correctable factors with early brain imaging.
- In young patients presenting with stroke or stroke like illness, early imaging and history of substance abuse should be sought and sending urine for screening of the same helps in ruling one of the important etiology. Management of stroke in both group of patients remains the same.

REFERENCES

1. Alozai UU, Sharma S. Drug and Alcohol Use. In: StatPearls [Internet]. Treasure Island (FL): StatPearls Publishing; 2023.
2. Zhao J, Stockwell T, Naimi T, Churchill S, Clay J, Sherk A. Association between daily alcohol intake and risk of all-cause mortality: A systematic review and meta-analyses. JAMA Netw Open. 2023;6(3):e236185.
3. Paton A. Alcohol in the body. BMJ. 2005;330(7482):85-7.
4. Cederbaum AI. Alcohol metabolism. Clin Liver Dis. 2012;16(4):667-85.
5. Kerr WC, Stockwell T. Understanding standard drinks and drinking guidelines. Drug Alcohol Rev. 2012;31(2):200-5.
6. US Department of Agriculture and US Department of Health and Human Services. (2020). Dietary Guidelines for Americans, 2020-2025, 9th edition. [online] Available from https://www.dietaryguidelines.gov/sites/default/files/2020-12/Dietary_Guidelines_for_Americans_2020-2025.pdf [Last accessed June, 2024].
7. Millwood IY, Walters RG, Mei XW, Guo Y, Yang L, Bian Z, et al.; China Kadoorie Biobank Collaborative Group. Conventional and genetic evidence on alcohol and vascular disease aetiology: a prospective study of 500,000 men and women in China. Lancet. 2019;393(10183):1831-42.
8. Choi YJ, Myung SK, Lee JH. Light alcohol drinking and risk of cancer: A meta-analysis of cohort studies. Cancer Res Treat Off J Korean Cancer Assoc. 2018;50(2):474-87.
9. Hartz SM, Oehlert M, Horton AC, Grucza RA, Fisher SL, Culverhouse RC, et al. Daily drinking is associated with increased mortality. Alcohol Clin Exp Res. 2018;42(11):2246-55.
10. GBD 2016 Alcohol Collaborators. Alcohol use and burden for 195 countries and territories, 1990–2016: a systematic analysis for the Global Burden of Disease Study 2016. Lancet. 2018;392(10152):1015-35.
11. Dubowski K. (1977). Manual for analysis of ethanol in biological liquids. [online] Available from https://rosap.ntl.bts.gov/view/dot/1185/dot_1185_DS1.pdf [Last accessed June, 2024].
12. Harper C. Thiamine (vitamin B1) deficiency and associated brain damage is still common throughout the world and prevention is simple and safe! Eur J Neurol. 2006;13(10):1078-82.
13. Burns EM, Naseem H, Bottle A, Lazzarino AI, Aylin P, Darzi A, et al. Introduction of laparoscopic bariatric surgery in England: observational population cohort study. BMJ. 2010;341:c4296.
14. Todd KG, Hazell AS, Butterworth RF. Alcohol-thiamine interactions: an update on the pathogenesis of Wernicke encephalopathy. Addict Biol. 1999;4(3):261-72.
15. Thomson AD, Cook CC, Touquet R, Henry JA; Royal College of Physicians, London. The Royal College of Physicians report on alcohol: guidelines for managing Wernicke's encephalopathy in the accident and Emergency Department. Alcohol Alcohol. 2002;37(6):513-21.
16. Sechi G, Serra A. Wernicke's encephalopathy: new clinical settings and recent advances in diagnosis and management. Lancet Neurol. 2007;6(5):442-55.
17. Feinberg I, Fein G, Price LJ, Jernigan TL, Floyd TC. Methodological and conceptual issues in the study of brain-behavior relations in the elderly. In: Poon LW (Ed). Aging in the 1980s: Psychological Issues. US: American Psychological Association; 1980. pp. 71-7.
18. Butters N, Brandt J. In: Galanter M (Ed). Recent Developments in Alcoholism, volume 3. New York: Plenum Publishing; 1985. pp. 207-26.
19. Chandrakumar A, Bhardwaj A, Jong GW. Review of thiamine deficiency disorders: Wernicke encephalopathy and Korsakoff psychosis. J Basic Clin Physiol Pharmacol. 2018;30(2):153-62.
20. Jung YC, Chanraud S, Sullivan EV. Neuroimaging of Wernicke's encephalopathy and Korsakoff's syndrome. Neuropsychol Rev. 2012;22(2):170-80.
21. Manzo G, De Gennaro A, Cozzolino A, Serino A, Fenza G, Manto A. MR imaging findings in alcoholic and nonalcoholic acute Wernicke's encephalopathy: a review. Biomed Res Int. 2014;2014:503596.
22. Clark DD, Sokoloff L. Circulation and energy metabolism of the brain. In: Siegel GJ (Eds). Basic Neurochemistry: Molecular, Cellular and Medical Aspects, 6th edition. Philadelphia, PA: Lippincott; 1999.
23. Phypers B, Pierce JM. Lactate physiology in health and disease. CEACCP. 2006;6:128-32.
24. McCandless DW, Schenker S. Encephalopathy of thiamine deficiency: studies of intracerebral mechanisms. J Clin Invest. 1968;47:2268-80.
25. Cabezas R, Avila M, Gonzalez J, El-Bachá RS, Báez E, García-Segura LM, et al. Astrocytic modulation of blood brain barrier: perspectives on Parkinson's disease. Front Cell Neurosci. 2014;8:211.
26. Stokum JA, Kurland DB, Gerzanich V, Simard JM. Mechanisms of astrocyte-mediated cerebral edema. Neurochem Res. 2015;40(2):317-28.
27. Hazell AS, Pannunzio P, Rama Rao KV, Pow DV, Rambaldi A. Thiamine deficiency results in downregulation of the GLAST glutamate transporter in cultured astrocytes. Glia. 2003;43(2):175-84.
28. Arundine M, Tymianski M. Molecular mechanisms of calcium dependent neurodegeneration in excitotoxicity. Cell Calcium. 2003;34:325-s37.

29. Ota Y, Capizzano AA, Moritani T, Naganawa S, Kurokawa R, Srinivasan A. Comprehensive review of Wernicke encephalopathy: Pathophysiology, clinical symptoms and imaging findings. Jpn J Radiol. 2020;38(9):809-20.
30. Thomson AD, Cook CC, Guerrini I, Sheedy D, Harper C, Marshall EJ. Wernicke's encephalopathy: 'Plus ça change, plus c'est la même chose'. Alcohol Alcohol. 2008;43(2):180-6.
31. De Wardener HE, Lennox B. Cerebral beriberi (Wernicke's encephalopathy); review of 52 cases in a Singapore prisoner-of-war hospital. Lancet. 1947;1(6436):11-7.
32. Zahr NM, Kaufman KL, Harper CG. Clinical and pathological features of alcohol-related brain damage. Nat Rev Neurol. 2011;7(5):284-94.
33. Victor M, Adams R, Collins G (Eds). The Wernicke-Korsakoff syndrome and related neurologic disorders due to alcoholism and malnutrition. Philadelphia, Pa: FA Davis; 1989. pp. 142-5.
34. Harper CG, Giles M, Finlay-Jones R. Clinical signs in the Wernicke-Korsakoff complex: a retrospective analysis of 131 cases diagnosed at necropsy. J Neurol Neurosurg Psychiatry. 1986;49(4):341-5.
35. Galvin R, Bråthen G, Ivashynka A, Hillbom M, Tanasescu R, Leone MA; EFNS. EFNS guidelines for diagnosis, therapy and prevention of Wernicke encephalopathy. Eur J Neurol. 2010;17(12):1408-18.
36. Caine D, Halliday GM, Kril JJ, Harper CG. Operational criteria for the classification of chronic alcoholics: identification of Wernicke's encephalopathy. J Neurol Neurosurg Psychiatry. 1997;62(1):51-60.
37. Tallaksen CM, Bohmer T, Bell H, Karlsen J. Concomitant determination of thiamin and its phosphate esters in human blood and serum by high-performance liquid chromatography. J Chromatogr. 1991;564(1):127-36.
38. Lu J, Frank EL. Rapid HPLC measurement of thiamine and its phosphate esters in whole blood. Clin Chem. 2008;54(5):901-6.
39. Kono S, Miyajima H, Yoshida K, Togawa A, Shirakawa K, Suzuki H. Mutations in a thiamine-transporter gene and Wernicke's-like encephalopathy. N Engl J Med. 2009;360(17):1792-4.
40. Weidauer S, Nichtweiss M, Lanfermann H, Zanella FE. Wernicke encephalopathy: MR findings and clinical presentation. Eur Radiol. 2003;13(5):1001-9.
41. Murata T, Fujito T, Kimura H, Omori M, Itoh H, Wada Y. Serial MRI and (1)H-MRS of Wernicke's encephalopathy: report of a case with remarkable cerebellar lesions on MRI. Psychiatry Res. 2001;108(1):49-55.
42. Zuccoli G, Santa Cruz D, Bertolini M, Rovira A, Gallucci M, Carollo C, et al. MR imaging findings in 56 patients with Wernicke encephalopathy: nonalcoholics may differ from alcoholics. AJNR Am J Neuroradiol. 2009;30(1):171-6.
43. Kornreich L, Bron-Harlev E, Hoffmann C, Schwarz M, Konen O, Schoenfeld T, et al. Thiamine deficiency in infants: MR findings in the brain. AJNR Am J Neuroradiol. 2005;26(7):1668-744.
44. Thomson AD, Marshall EJ. The treatment of patients at risk of developing Wernicke's encephalopathy in the community. Alcohol Alcohol. 2006;41(2):159-67.
45. Rolland S, Truswell AS. Wernicke-Korsakoff syndrome in Sydney hospitals after 6 years of thiamin enrichment of bread. Public Health Nutr. 1998;1(2):117-22.
46. Victor M, Adams RD, Collins GH. The Wernicke-Korsakoff syndrome. A clinical and pathological study of 245 patients, 82 with post-mortem examinations. Contemp Neurol Ser. 1971;7:1-206.
47. Gerridzen IJ, Goossensen MA. Patients with Korsakoff syndrome in nursing homes: characteristics, comorbidity, and use of psychotropic drugs. Int Psychogeriatr. 2014;26(1):115-21.
48. Friese SA, Bitzer M, Freudenstein D, Voigt K, Küker W. Classification of acquired lesions of the corpus callosum with MRI. Neuroradiology. 2000;42(11):795-802.
49. Johkura K, Naito M, Naka T. Cortical involvement in Marchiafava-Bignami disease. AJNR Am J Neuroradiol. 2005;26(3):670-3.
50. Ellison D, Love S, Chimelli L, Harding BN, Lowe J, Vinters HV. Neuropathology: A reference text of CNS pathology, 2nd edition. Mosby: Philadelphia; 2004. pp. 489-90.
51. Lechevalier B, Andersson JC, Morin P. Hemispheric disconnection syndrome with a 'crossed avoiding' reaction in a case of Marchiafava–Bignami disease. J Neurol Neurosurg Psychiatry. 1977;40(5):483-97.
52. Arbelaez A, Pajon A, Castillo M. Acute Marchiafava-Bignami disease: MR findings in two patients. AJNR Am J Neuroradiol. 2003;24(10):1955-7.
53. Kakkar C, Prakashini K, Polnaya A. Acute Marchiafava-Bignami disease: clinical and serial MRI correlation. BMJ Case Rep. 2014;2014:502-4.
54. Marchiafava E, Bignami A. Sopra un alterazione del corpo calloso osservata in soggetti alcoolisti. Riv Patol Nerv. 1903;8:544-9.
55. Leong ASY. Marchiafava-Bignami disease in a non-alcoholic Indian male. Pathology. 1979;11(2):241-9.
56. Kosaka K, Aoki M, Kawasaki N, Adachi Y, Konuma I, Iizuka R. A non-alcoholic Japanese patient with Wernicke's encephalopathy and Marchiafava-Bignami disease. Clin Neuropathol. 1984;3(6):231-6.
57. Hillbom M, Pyhtinen J, Pylvänen V, Sotaniemi K. Pregnant, vomiting, and coma. Lancet. 1999;353(9164):1584.
58. Heinrich A, Runge U, Khaw AV. Clinicoradiologic subtypes of Marchiafava-Bignami disease. J Neurol. 2004;251(9):1050-9.
59. Hillbom M, Saloheimo P, Fujioka S, Wszolek ZK, Juvela S, Leone MA. Diagnosis and management of Marchiafava-Bignami disease: a review of CT/MRI confirmed cases. J Neurol Neurosurg Psychiatry. 2014;85(2):168-73.
60. Sehgal V, Kesav P, Modi M, Ahuja CK. Acute Marchiafava-Bignami disease presenting as reversible dementia in a chronic alcoholic. BMJ Case Rep. 2013;2013:bcr2012008286.
61. Singh S, Wagh V. Marchiafava Bignami disease: A rare neurological complication of long-term alcohol abuse. Cureus. 2022;14(10):e30863.
62. Canepa C, Arias L. Partial interhemispheric disconnection syndrome (P-IHDS) secondary to Marchiafava-Bignami disease type B (MBD-B). BMJ Case Rep. 2016;2016:bcr2016216823.
63. Staszewski J, Macek K, Stepień A. Odwracalna demielinizacja ciała modzelowatego w przebiegu choroby Marchiafavy-Bignamiego [Reversible demyelinisation of corpus callosum in the course of Marchiafava-Bignami disease]. Neurol Neurochir Pol. 2006;40(2):156-61.
64. Carrilho PE, Santos MB, Piasecki L, Jorge AC. Marchiafava-Bignami disease: a rare entity with a poor outcome. Rev Bras Ter Intensiva. 2013;25(1):68-72.
65. Kawarabuki K, Sakakibara T, Hirai M, Yoshioka Y, Yamamoto Y, Yamaki T. Marchiafava-Bignami disease: magnetic resonance imaging findings in corpus callosum and subcortical white matter. Eur J Radiol. 2003;48(2):175-7.
66. Tung CS, Wu SL, Tsou JC, Hsu SP, Kuo HC, Tsui HW. Marchiafava-Bignami disease with widespread lesions and complete recovery. AJNR Am J Neuroradiol. 2010;31(8):1506-7.

67. Bano S, Mehra S, Yadav SN, Chaudhary V. Marchiafava-Bignami disease: Role of neuroimaging in the diagnosis and management of acute disease. Neurol India. 2009;57(5):649-52.
68. Kumar KS, Challam R, J N, Singh WJ. Marchiafava-bignami disease: a case report. J Clin Diagn Res. 2014;8(8):RD01-2.
69. Yadala S, Luo JJ. Marchiafava-bignami disease in a nonalcoholic diabetic patient. Case Rep Neurol Med. 2013;2013:979383.
70. Garcia-Santibanez R. Marchiafava-Bignami disease presenting as acute dysarthria and ataxia. Alcohol Alcohol. 2015;50(2):256-7
71. Rosa A, Demiati M, Cartz L, Mizon JP. Marchiafava-Bignami disease, syndrome of interhemispheric disconnection, and right-handed agraphia in a left-hander. Arch Neurol. 1991;48(9):986-8.
72. Parmanand HT. Marchiafava-Bignami disease in chronic alcoholic patient. Radiol Case Rep. 2016;11(3):234-7.
73. Dong X, Bai C, Nao J. Clinical and radiological features of Marchiafava-Bignami disease. Medicine (Baltimore). 2018;97(5):e9626.
74. Bellido S, Navas I, Aranda MA, Ginestal R, Venegas B. Unusual MRI findings in a case of Marchiafava Bignami disease. Neurology. 2012;78(19):1537.
75. Gimeno MJ, Lasierra R, Pina JI. Marchiafava-Bignami disease. Four case reports. Rev Neurol. 2002;35(6):596-8.
76. Helenius J, Tatlisumak T, Soinne L, Valanne L, Kaste M. Marchiafava-Bignami disease: two cases with favourable outcome. Eur J Neurol. 2001;8(3):269-72.
77. Lee H, Roh S, Kim DJ. Alcohol-induced blackout. Int J Environ Res Public Health. 2009;6(11):2783-92.
78. Adams RD, Victor M, Mancall EL. Central pontine myelinolysis: a hitherto undescribed disease occurring in alcoholic and malnourished patients. AMA Arch Neurol Psychiatry. 1959;81(2):154-72.
79. Wright DG, Laureno RO, Victor MA. Pontine and extrapontine myelinolysis. Brain. 1979;102(2):361-85.
80. Lim L, Krystal A. Psychotic disorder in a patient with central and extrapontine myelinolysis. Psychiatry Clin Neurosci. 2007;61(3):320-2.
81. Kumar S, Fowler M, Gonzalez-Toledo E, Jaffe SL. Central pontine myelinolysis, an update. Neurol Res. 2006;28(3):360-6.
82. Laureno R, Karp BI. Myelinolysis after correction of hyponatremia. Ann Intern Med. 1997;126(1):57-62.
83. Martin RJ. Central pontine and extrapontine myelinolysis: the osmotic demyelination syndromes. J Neurol Neurosurg Psychiatry. 2004;75(Suppl 3):iii22-8.
84. Ashrafian H, Davey P. A review of the causes of central pontine myelinosis: yet another apoptotic illness? Eur J Neurol. 2001;8(2):103-9.
85. Mochizuki H, Masaki T, Miyakawa T, Nakane J, Yokoyama A, Nakamura Y, et al. Benign type of central pontine myelinolysis in alcoholism--clinical, neuroradiological and electrophysiological findings. J Neurol. 2003;250(9):1077-83.
86. Norenberg MD. A hypothesis of osmotic endothelial injury. A pathogenetic mechanism in central pontine myelinolysis. Arch Neurol. 1983;40(2):66-9.
87. Kaku DA, Lowenstein DH. Emergence of recreational drug abuse as a major risk factor for stroke in young adults. Ann Intern Med. 1990;113(11):821-7.
88. Westover AN, McBride S, Haley RW. Stroke in young adults who abuse amphetamines or cocaine: a population-based study of hospitalized patients. Arch Gen Psychiatry. 2007;64(4):495-502.
89. Daras M, Tuchman AJ, Koppel BS, Samkoff LM, Weitzner I, Marc J, et al. Neurovascular complications of cocaine. Acta Neurol Scand. 1994;90(2):124-9.
90. Brown E, Prager J, Lee HY, Ramsey RG. CNS complications of cocaine abuse. Prevalence, pathophysiology, and neuroradiology. AJR Am J Roentgenol. 1992;159(1):137-47.
91. Levine SR, Brust JC, Futrell N, Ho KL, Blake D, Millikan CH, et al. Cerebrovascular complications of the use of the "crack" form of alkaloidal cocaine. N Engl J Med. 1990;323(11):699-704.
92. Bartzokis G, Goldstein IB, Hance DB, Beckson M, Shapiro D, Lu PH, et al. The incidence of T2-weighted MR imaging signal abnormalities in the brain of cocaine-dependent patients is age-related and region-specific. AJNR Am J Neuroradiol. 1999;20(9):1628-35.
93. Klonoff DC, Andrews BT, Obana WG. Stroke associated with cocaine use. Arch Neurol. 1989;46(9):989-93.
94. Brust JC. Clinical, radiological, and pathological aspects of cerebrovascular disease associated with drug abuse. Stroke. 1993;24 (12 Suppl):I129-33.
95. Sauer CM. Recurrent embolic stroke and cocaine-related cardiomyopathy. Stroke. 1991;22(9):1203-5.
96. Sáez CG, Olivares P, Pallavicini J, Panes O, Moreno N, Massardo T, et al. Increased number of circulating endothelial cells and plasma markers of endothelial damage in chronic cocaine users. Thromb Res. 2011;128(4):e18-23.
97. Pereira J, Sáez CG, Pallavicini J, Panes O, Pereira-Flores K, Cabreras MJ, et al. Platelet activation in chronic cocaine users: effect of short term abstinence. Platelets. 2011;22(8):596-601.
98. Daras M, Tuchman AJ, Marks S. Central nervous system infarction related to cocaine abuse. Stroke. 1991;22(10):1320-5.
99. Havranek EP, Nademanee K, Grayburn PA, Eichhorn EJ. Endothelium-dependent vaso relaxation is impaired in cocaine arteriopathy. J Am Coll Cardiol. 1996;28(5):1168-74.
100. Carcelén-Gadea ME, Pons-Amate JM, Climent-Díaz B, García-Escrivá D, Guillén-Fort C. Implicación de la cocaína en la patología vascular cerebral [Involvement of cocaine in cerebral vascular pathology]. Rev Neurol. 2012;54(11):664-72.
101. Martin-Schild S, Albright KC, Misra V, Philip M, Barreto AD, Hallevi H, et al. Intravenous tissue plasminogen activator in patients with cocaine-associated acute ischemic stroke. Stroke. 2009;40(11):3635-7.
102. Oyesiku NM, Colohan AR, Barrow DL, Reisner A. Cocaine-induced aneurysmal rupture: an emergent factor in the natural history of intracranial aneurysms? Neurosurgery. 1993;32(4):518-25.
103. Ferguson GG. Direct measurement of mean and pulsatile blood pressure at operation in human intracranial saccular aneurysms. J Neurosurg. 1972;36(5):560-3.
104. Case records of the Massachusetts General Hospital. Weekly clinicopathological exercises. Case 27–1993. A 32-year-old man with the sudden onset of a right-sided headache and left hemiplegia and hemianesthesia. N Engl J Med. 1993;329(2):117-24.
105. Kibayashi K, Mastri AR, Hirsch CS. Cocaine induced intracerebral hemorrhage: analysis of predisposing factors and mechanisms causing hemorrhagic strokes. Hum Pathol. 1995;26(6):659-63.
106. Vannemreddy P, Caldito G, Willis B, Nanda A. Influence of cocaine on ruptured intracranial aneurysms: a case control study of poor prognostic indicators. J Neurosurg. 2008;108(3):470-6.
107. Simpson RK Jr, Fischer DK, Narayan RK, Cech DA, Robertson CS. Intravenous cocaine abuse and subarachnoid haemorrhage: Effect on outcome. Br J Neurosurg. 1990;4(1):27-30.
108. Salanova V, Taubner R. Intracerebral haemorrhage and vasculitis secondary to amphetamine use. Postgrad Med J. 1984;60(704):429-30.

109. Varner KJ, Ogden BA, Delcarpio J, Meleg-Smith S. Cardiovascular responses elicited by the "binge" administration of methamphetamine. J Pharmacol Exp Ther. 2002;301(1):152-9.
110. Petitti DB, Sidney S, Quesenberry C, Bernstein A. Stroke and cocaine or amphetamine use. Epidemiology. 1998;9(6):596-600.
111. McGee SM, McGee DN, McGee MB. Spontaneous intracerebral hemorrhage related to methamphetamine abuse: autopsy findings and clinical correlation. Am J Forensic Med Pathol. 2004;25(4):334-7.
112. Shibata S, Mori K, Sekine I, Suyama H. Subarachnoid and intracerebral hemorrhage associated with necrotizing angitis due to methamphetamine abuse. An autopsy case. Neurol Med Chir Tokyo. 1991;31(1):49-52.
113. Brust JCM. Vasculitis associated with substance abuse. Neurol Clin. 1997;15(4):945-57.
114. Ho EL, Josephson SA, Lee HS, Smith WS. Cerebrovascular complications of methamphetamine abuse. Neurocrit Care. 2009;10(3):295-305.
115. Thanvi BR, Treadwell SD. Cannabis and stroke: is there a link? Postgrad Med J. 2009;85(1000):80-3.
116. Renard D, Taieb G, Gras-Combe G, Labauge P. Cannabis-related myocardial infarction and cardioembolic stroke. J Stroke Cerebrovasc Dis. 2012;21(1):82-3.
117. Wolff V, Lauer V, Rouyer O, Sellal F, Meyer N, Raul JS, et al. Cannabis use, ischemic stroke, and multifocal intracranial vasoconstriction: a prospective study in 48 consecutive young patients. Stroke. 2011;42(6):1778-80.
118. Ducros A, Boukobza M, Porcher R, Sarov M, Valade D, Bousser MG. The clinical and radiological spectrum of reversible cerebral vasoconstriction syndrome: a prospective series of 67 patients. Brain. 2007;130(pt 12):3091-101.
119. Mirchandani N, Khan I, Wajnsztajn F. Recreational drug use and RCVS: should toxicity screens become standard in RCVS diagnostics? Neurology. 2015;84(14):2.284.
120. Short K, Emsley HCA. Illicit drugs and reversible cerebral vasoconstriction syndrome. Neurohospitalist. 2021;11(1):40-4.
121. Neiman J, Haapaniemi HM, Hillbom M. Neurological complications of drug abuse: pathophysiological mechanisms. Eur J Neurol. 2000;7(6):595-606.
122. Deik A, Saunders-Pullman R, Luciano MS. Substance of abuse and movement disorders: complex interactions and comorbidities. Curr Drug Abuse Rev. 2012;5(3):243-53.
123. Montoya-Filardi A, Mazón M. The addicted brain: imaging neurological complications of recreational drug abuse. Radiologia. 2017;59(1):17-30.
124. Dhuna A, Pascual-Leone A, Belgrade M. Cocaine-related vascular headaches. J Neurol Neurosurg Psychiatry. 1991;54(9):803-6.
125. Malcolm R, Liao J, Michel M, Cochran K, Pye W, Yeager D, et al. Amlodipine reduces blood pressure and headache frequency in cocaine-dependent outpatients. J Psychoactive Drugs. 2002;34(4):415-9.
126. Richter RW, Rosenberg RN. Transverse myelitis associated with heroin addiction. JAMA. 1968;206(6):1255-7.
127. Monsalve GP, Ocazionez F, Barreras P, Saidha S, Pardo-Villamizar C. Drug-abuse related myelopathies: A rising neurological problem (P2. 343). 2017;88 (16_supplement).
128. Malik MM, Woolsey RM. Acute myelopathy following intravenous heroin: a case report. J Am Paraplegia Soc. 1991;14(4):182-3.
129. Ell JJ, Uttley D, Silver JR. Acute myelopathy in association with heroin addiction. J Neurol Neurosurg Psychiatry. 1981;44(5):448-50.
130. McCreary M, Emerman C, Hanna J, Simon J. Acute myelopathy following intranasal insufflation of heroin: a case report. Neurology. 2000;55(2):316-7.
131. Kumar R, West DM, Jingree M, Laurence AS. Unusual consequences of heroin overdose: rhabdomyolysis, acute renal failure, paraplegia and hypercalcaemia. Br J Anaesth. 1999;83(3):496-8.
132. Riva N, Riva N, Morana P, Cerri F, Gerevini S, Amadio S, et al. Acute myelopathy selectively involving lumbar anterior horns following intranasal insufflation of ecstasy and heroin. BMJ Case Rep. 2009;2009:bcr08.2008.0669.
133. Sahni V, Garg D, Garg S, Agarwal SK, Singh NP. Unusual complications of heroin abuse: Transverse myelitis, rhabdomyolysis, compartment syndrome, and ARF. Clin Toxicol (Phila). 2008;46(2):153-5.
134. Goodman BP. Metabolic and toxic causes of myelopathy. Continuum (Minneap Minn). 2015;21(1):84-99.
135. Thompson AG, Leite MI, Lunn MP, Bennett DLH. Whippits, nitrous oxide and the dangers of legal highs. Pract Neurol. 2015;15(3):207-9.
136. Garakani A, Jaffe RJ, Savla D, Welch AK, Protin CA, Bryson EO, et al. Neurologic, psychiatric, and other medical manifestations of nitrous oxide abuse: A systematic review of the case literature. Am J Addict. 2016;25(5):358-69.
137. Li HT, Chu CC, Chang KH, et al. Clinical and electrodiagnostic characteristics of nitrous oxide-induced neuropathy in Taiwan. Clin Neurophysiol. 2016;127(10):3288-93.
138. Ramalho J, Nunes RH, da Rocha AJ, Castillo M. Toxic and metabolic myelopathies. Semin Ultrasound CT MR. 2016;37(5):448-65.

Visual Illusions and Hallucinations of Central Origin and their Differentials

Ambar Chakravarty

INTRODUCTION

Visual illusions and hallucinations of central origin are almost always binocular in distribution, usually involving the corresponding halves of the two visual fields. However, not too uncommonly, the entire visual fields of both eyes may be involved. The visual disturbance may be very short lasting or may be prolonged depending on the nature of the pathology causing the disturbance. A visual seizure would be an important differential for the former group of patients with very short-lasting visual illusions and hallucinations. In the first part of the chapter, we shall elaborate on binocular hemifield illusions and hallucinations and in the second part, illusions and hallucinations involving the entire fields of both eyes would be discussed.

DEFINITIONS

We should start by quoting the standard definitions of these two terms from standard psychiatric literature:

Hallucination: "*A sensory experience which occurs in the absence of corresponding external stimulation of the relevant sensory organ, has sufficient sense of reality resemble a veridical perception, over which the subject does not feel direct and voluntary control, and which occurs in the awake state.*"[1]

Illusion: These are false perceptions of a real external stimulus, e.g., a change in shape, size, color, or texture. In some cases, where the external stimulus is minimal, the differentiation nosologically from hallucination can be difficult, although illusions carry different etiological and diagnostic implications.

It would be of some interest to flash back on the definition of the much used term *delusion* in this context, though not directly related to the topic of this chapter. Delusions are abnormalities of thought rather than perception (although they may develop from the latter) and may be defined as "*fixed false beliefs, strongly held and immutable in the face of refuting evidence, that are not consonant with the person's education, social, and cultural background.*"[2] Its exact meaning and usage have evolved continuously, reflecting trends in psychology. Delusional themes commonly include guilt, worthlessness, ill health, persecution, reference, grandeur, love, jealousy, poverty, infestation, and religion. A range of beliefs are also recognized that lie somewhere between the delusional and nondelusional, these "overvalued ideas" are often best considered as sustained and unreasonable preoccupations, the unlikely validity of which the holder has little insight into.

VISUAL ILLUSIONS AND HALLUCINATIONS

Binocular Hemifield Illusions or Hallucinations

Binocular hemifield illusions or hallucinations have three possible causes: Migraine, occipito-parieto-temporal lesions, or vertebrobasilar transient ischemic attack (TIA).

Binocular illusions confined to a hemifield are usually caused by unilateral lesions of the occipito-parieto-temporal region. The lesions are tumors, infarcts, dysplasias, or inflammations. In most cases, they also cause a hemianopic visual field defect. Vertebrobasilar TIA must be considered as another cause. Finally, migraine may cause transient illusions of this sort (the "Alice in Wonderland syndrome"),[3,4] especially in children.

Illusions

Illusions caused by occipito-parieto-temporal lesions consist of alterations in shape, position, motion, and duration of a perceived object, often in combination. These striking illusions suggest a fresh, large, or expanding lesion or one that is causing seizures.

Altered Shape

Patients typically describe elongations of forms along one plane with overlapping of one object onto another ("cerebral metamorphopsia" or "illusory spread"[5]; "coneheads" may grow out of shoulders and gigantic fingers from elbows, rather like a Cubist image). Such illusions may be episodic or persistent, but they usually disappear spontaneously within days to weeks of onset. They often coexist with palinopsia (see further) or visual hallucinations (VHs).

Altered Position

Patients see the image of a previously viewed object as displaced into the opposite hemifield ("visual allesthesia").[6] For example, a figure standing to the right of fixation will, a moment later, appear to be standing to the left of fixation. When the inciting visual stimulus for allesthesia is still within view, patients report double vision ("cerebral diplopia") or multiple vision ("cerebral polyopia for stationary objects"). The allesthetic image is almost always displaced into a partial homonymous hemianopic field.

This altered visual experience may be an epileptic phenomenon. During the episode, patients often have either an altered sensorium, focal tonic-clonic movements, or a focal discharge on electroencephalogram (EEG). Antiepileptic medications may be effective.[6]

Preservation

Patients with this visual illusion report seeing a previously viewed scene, such as a household setting or a highway signpost, suddenly "played back" before their eyes. This is a form of visual preservation in time, or "palinopsia" (palinopsia, paliopia). The preservative illusion may occur immediately after the object has been viewed or hours later. The longer the interval, the more likely it is to be considered a hallucination rather than an illusion.

In some patients, the palinopsic experience appears to be part of a focal seizure.[7,8] Right posterior hemisphere lesions have outnumbered left hemisphere lesions. Whereas the episodes generally subside within weeks, they sometimes persist. In such cases, anticonvulsant therapy is worth a try.

Altered Motion

Patients who have occipital lesion may see objects that move smoothly across their path of vision like a sequence of snapshots or as trailed by a comet-like tail. Called "cerebral polyopia for moving objects,"[9] it differs from "cerebral polyopia for stationary objects," an illusion that results from visual allesthesia (see section Altered Position). A lesion in the same region may also give rise to the sensation of continuous or episodic motion of stationary viewed objects.[10]

Hallucinations

Like illusions, hemifield hallucinations are produced by migraine, vertebrobasilar TIA, or an occipito-parieto-temporal lobe lesion. Transient hemifield hallucinations are usually produced by migraine, and less commonly by vertebrobasilar TIA. On the other hand, persistent hemifield hallucinations always reflect an occipito-parieto-temporal lobe structural lesion.

Migraine

It is a prevalent episodic neurological condition characterized primarily by headache. In classic migraine (migraine with aura), the headache is preceded by a temporary neurological disturbance known as an "aura." The auras can manifest as positive or negative visual phenomena, paresthesias, aphasia, and hemiparesis, with visual disturbances being the most common among migraineurs.[11,12] Notably, migraine accounts for the majority of episodes involving binocular unformed VHs, not only in young individuals but also among the elderly.[13]

The most frequent type of aura experienced by migraineurs is unformed VHs, encompassing various visual patterns. One particular pattern, observed in approximately 30% of cases, is referred to as a "scintillating scotoma"—a twinkling zigzag shape resembling the outline of a medieval Roman fortress. This phenomenon is also known as a "fortification" or "teichopsia," derived from the Greek word "teichos," meaning city wall.[14] The scintillating scotoma is transient in nature and has been described as a "fortification spectrum" due to its spectral or ghostly appearance.[15] Approximately 25% of migraineurs with visual aura report the scotoma's gradual migration or expansion across one hemifield, at a speed of 3-5 mm/minute, similar to the cortical spreading depression associated with hallucinations caused by cortical hypoperfusion.[15]

The marching scintillating scotoma is rarely reported in vertebrobasilar TIAs[16] and is uncommon during posterior hemispheric surface electrode stimulation[17] or electrographically documented spontaneous seizures.[18,19] However, it has been documented in single case reports of individuals with occipito-parieto-temporal lesions, particularly arteriovenous malformations (AVMs).[20-23] Among 70 patients with occipital lobe AVMs, 21% experienced "migraine-like visual phenomena".[24] In two cases involving occipital AVMs, the migraine-like episodes ceased after surgical excision of the AVM.[20,21]

Thus, the marching scintillating scotoma is primarily considered a reaction pattern that occurs predominantly in the idiopathic disorder of migraine and rarely in cases of focal injury to the primary visual cortex.

While the marching scintillating scotoma is common in migraine, many patients with classic migraine also report other visual phenomena, such as stationary sparkling lights or pinwheels.[25,26] These scintillations are often not limited to one hemifield. In a significant proportion of migraineurs, particularly those above 50 years of age, the headache does not follow the visual hallucination, resulting in what is known as acephalgic or dissociated migraine.

Distinguishing migraine from vertebrobasilar TIA and occipito-parieto-temporal lesions can be aided by considering additional auras such as "marching paresthesia".[26] The marching paresthesia typically begins 5–30 minutes after the onset of the visual aura, followed by aphasia. In contrast, sensory auras in seizures have a much shorter latency period, and vertebrobasilar TIAs often present with multiple simultaneous neurological manifestations. Migraine rarely causes formed hallucinations, and when focal pathology is responsible, partial seizures originating from injured or deafferented parietal or temporal cortex may occur.

The visual aura experienced in migraine is subjective, and the individual's unique experiences are not directly accessible to others. However, sufferers can occasionally provide glimpses into their visual perceptions through graphic representations, allowing insights into the transiently dysfunctional brain.[27] Illustrations, particularly those capturing scotomas and fortification spectra experienced during migraine attacks, have played a vital role in understanding the mechanisms underlying visual aura.[27] These illustrations have revealed the uniform nature of many hallucinations, suggesting a consistent repertoire of processes generating the occipital cortex's hallucinations. The specific characteristics of the fortification spectrum, including the appearance of zigzag lines, shimmering effects, and the speed of peripheral spread, all rely on visual representation for elucidation. Such illustrations have contributed to understanding underlying pathophysiological mechanisms, including the involvement of spreading cortical depression.[27]

Illustrations have also shed light on rare and unusual VHs, which are not well understood in terms of their underlying processes. Migraine art exhibitions have showcased various perceptual visual disturbances, such as metamorphopsia, altered shapes or distorted contours of objects, out-of-body experiences, coronas around objects, Lilliputian hallucinations, illusory splitting, and macro- and microsomatognosia.[28,29] These illustrations have allowed the recording and characterization of these visual auras, providing valuable insights into differential diagnosis and nonmigrainous causes of VHs.

A multitude of illustrations has documented the wide array of VHs associated with various nonmigrainous disorders. These disorders can be classified into those affecting the visual pathways and those involving the brainstem/cholinergic system. The former group includes ocular diseases, occipital infarcts, epilepsy, and migraine, while the latter is associated with factors such as anticholinergic drugs, Parkinson disease (PD), narcolepsy, and peduncular lesions. Some disorders, such as dementia, psychoses, and delirium, may implicate both groups. Matching the syndrome to its etiology suggests that the hallucination palette observed in a patient reflects the location and extent of the susceptible cortex.[30] When VHs result from visual system disorders, self-illustration becomes an invaluable tool for identification and understanding.

For instance, in the context of occipital epilepsy in children, self-made illustrations have revealed distinct differences between epileptic hallucinations and those occurring in migraine. Epilepsy-related hallucinations tend to involve colors and circular or spherical shapes, whereas migraine-related hallucinations are typically jagged and often lack color.[31] The visual representation made during mescaline intoxication also highlights how illustrations can differentiate between hallucinations caused by different factors.[32] The unique contribution of self-made illustrations during an attack remains an underutilized scientific method that allows subjective experience to inform objective analysis.

In the Indian population, migraine with visual aura is relatively uncommon, occurring in only 2–3% of cases. Distinguishing it from epileptic visual aura, with or without headache, is often necessary. A commonly mentioned distinguishing feature is that migraine visual aura is usually monochromatic (black and white), while epileptic aura tends to be colored. This rule of thumb generally holds true in routine clinical practice.

Vertebrobasilar Transient Ischemic Attacks

Vertebrobasilar TIAs may cause transient negative or positive visual phenomena. The visual manifestations may be the only abnormality;[32] in one series, they were the first or only symptoms in 10% of cases.[33] The hallucinations take many forms; tadpoles, soapflakes, snowflakes, sparklers, pinwheels, or glowing light.[34] As in migraine, they may occupy the whole visual field or be restricted to a hemifield, depending upon whether the hypoperfusion affects one or both posterior cerebral arteries.[14,35]

Vertebrobasilar TIAs rarely produce the zigzag shape or the 20- to 30-minute march across the hemifield that is typical of migraine.[36] The visual disturbance usually lasts only seconds. If it lingers beyond a few hours, expect to find a persistent homonymous visual field defect and imaging evidence of occipital infarction.[37,38] After occipital infarction, the hallucinations usually regress within weeks, although some field loss usually persists.

Distinguishing vertebrobasilar TIA from migraine depends in part on the presence of features of brainstem ischemia, such as vertigo, disequilibrium, drop attack, diplopia, altered consciousness, nausea, extremity weakness, and numbness.[39] These symptoms, one or more of which are present in 90% of patients suffering a vertebrobasilar TIA,[40] are infrequent in migraine. There is, however, an adolescent form of migraine (basilar migraine and Bickerstaff migraine) that can also produce many of these symptoms.[41]

Occipito-parieto-temporal Lesion

Lesions in this posterior region of the cerebrum often give rise to episodic or persistent binocular VHs, sometimes as isolated manifestations. Three mechanisms have been proposed to explain these events: (1) Classic migraine auras triggered by the lesion, (2) partial seizures triggered by the lesion, and (3) release phenomena in visual association cortex disinhibited by lack of input from primary visual cortex.

Partial seizures with unformed VHs originate in primary visual cortex. Typically, the hallucination begins in one hemifield, but sometimes it spreads quickly over the entire field. Anatomic abnormalities are usually evident on brain imaging, the exception being benign childhood epilepsy with occipital paroxysms (CEOP), a self-limited condition that mostly affects preadolescent girls.[42,43]

Our knowledge of the visual experiences produced by partial seizures comes from patients' description during surface electrode stimulation[44-46] and during EEG recordings of spontaneous seizures.[37,38,47,48] The VHs consist of stationary lines, squares, stars, circles, disks, sparkling dots, and zigzags.[49] They last longer than those caused by vertebrobasilar TIA, and, in contrast to migraine, marching zigzags are rare. In a series of 20 patients with occipital seizures, no one described zigzags.[50]

Identifying partial seizures (or complex partial seizures) as cause of VHs depends on finding nystagmus, frequent blinking or eyelid fluttering, staring or other automatisms, tonic-clonic movements, or loss of consciousness. In one series of 25 patients with occipital lobe partial seizures,[51] eye deviation was present in 16 (64%) and repeated blinking in 14 (56%).

In the Indian context, partial seizures with visual aura (with or without generalization), especially in children and young adults, are often caused by cysticercal lesions in the occipital region. However, the visual aura is often binocular probably due to rapid spread of epileptic discharge to the other side. In children, presentation is often with only visual aura (generally colored) associated with a vascular type of headache, mimicking classical migraine. Response to antiepileptics is generally very satisfactory.

Visual hallucinations associated with occipito-parieto-temporal lesions are not always manifestations of focal seizures. Such lesions can block input to vision-related cortex and allow the emergence of endogenous visual activity as release phenomena. In one large series of patients with VHs following occipital infarctions, EEG failed to document any seizures. VHs developed only in those patients whose posterior hemispheric lesions spared much of visual association cortex and nearby white matter. The inference is that, for VHs to occur, association visual cortex must be intact and cut off from normal visual inputs by a lesion in the primary visual cortex region.[52]

Among patients who are not exposed to psychoactive agents and who have intact mentation and adequate vision, formed hallucinations (images of animate objects or scenes) always originate in parietal or temporal vision-related cortex. They may be manifestations of a partial seizure or release phenomena.[53]

Surface electrode stimulation of the cerebral cortex shows that partial seizures originating in temporal cortex often cause a dreamlike state.[54] The hallucinations evoke feelings of fear, pleasure, strangeness, or familiarity.[55,56] By comparison, partial seizures of parietal origin create formed hallucinations whose details are so vivid and realistic that patients temporarily believe that they are actually seeing them.[57,58]

Even though they are generated in a damaged hemisphere, formed hallucinations generally do not remain confined to the contralateral hemifield. In general, right posterior hemisphere lesions are more likely than left ones to produce formed hallucinations.[47]

Localizing Value of Epileptic Visual Aura: Recent Concepts

Visual auras of different kinds are well known in partial epilepsies. The possible significance of attributing those auras to the site of seizure onset, however, has not been extensively studied. The best known examples are visual phenomena such as elementary hallucinations or visual loss, which occur in occipital lobe epilepsy. This had been known since the time of Wilbur Penfield in 1950s. However, visual phenomena may also occur in temporal lobe seizures and erroneously lead to the assumption of an occipital origin. In addition to complex VHs, occipital like elementary visual experiences in temporal lobe seizures have also been described. A detailed study of areas of onset of different types of visual seizures has been reported by Bien et al.[48] from Bonn, Germany. The study was based on 20 operated cases where the morphological correlate of the epileptogenic zone could be demonstrated by intracranial ictal EEG recordings made pre- or perioperatively. Detailed structural changes were also made by magnetic resonance (MR) or computed tomography (CT) scanning in the preoperative period.

Elementary hallucinations, illusions, and visual loss were reported not only by all patients with occipital lobe epilepsy but also by patients with occipitotemporal and anteromedial temporal seizure onset. Complex hallucinations never occurred in occipital lobe seizures but were present in the latter two groups. Concentric changes in visual fields (tunnel vision) were also noted with seizure onset from the occipitotemporal and anteromedial temporal regions. Epileptologists and surgeons need to be appraised of the fact that though elementary VHs and visual loss, in general, are suggestive of seizure onset from the occipital lobe, they are by no means inconsistent with seizure onset from the occipitotemporal and anteromedial temporal regions. On the other hand, complex VHs and concentric changes in visual fields almost always are suggestive of seizure onset from the latter two regions.

Binocular Full-field Illusions or Hallucinations

Illusions or hallucinations involving both eyes and not confined to the hemifield may be initiated by the same focal processes identified earlier as causes of hemifield illusions or hallucinations. They can also result from nonlocalizing processes such as exposure to a psychoactive agent or an impaired mental or visual state. These nonlocalizing conditions should be ruled out first.

Exposure to Psychoactive Agent

When the patient has been exposed to a psychoactive agent, visual illusions and hallucinations must initially be considered pharmacologically induced. Virtually every psychoactive medication or drug has been associated with the production of visual illusions and hallucinations.[59-61] The medications most often implicated are those with anticholinergic, dopaminergic, or serotoninergic properties. Among hallucinogenic street drugs, mescal, psilocybin, lysergic acid, and amphetamines are most cited. Withdrawal from habitual use of some of these agents, as well as from alcohol, may cause prominent illusions and hallucinations, often of animals (zoopsia).[62] Although drug-induced or withdrawal-associated VHs may be accompanied by auditory hallucinations, psychotic thought disorder, or delirium, it is critical to recognize that the visual aberrations may be the most prominent, or the only, manifestation.

Abnormal Mental State or Impaired Vision Present

Inflammatory or Metabolic Encephalopathy

Visual illusions and hallucinations are frequent manifestations of delirium, an altered behavioral and autonomic state brought on by infection, fever, metabolic imbalance, or hypoxia.[63]

Dementia

Visual hallucinations are widely reported in the advancing stages of all dementing processes.[64] Usually formed, and often reminiscent of earlier life experiences, they may arise spontaneously and are exacerbated when the patient is left alone in a darkened room or treated with psychoactive medications (sundowning). Any type of dementia can produce VHs, but they are especially common in diffuse Lewy body disease.[65]

Psychosis

The VHs of psychosis are distinctive in being complex, delusional, and paranoid, and they are often integrated with auditory hallucinations.[66]

Sleep-like States

Visual hallucinations usually occur just before sleep (hypnagogic hallucinations) or upon awakening (hypnopompic hallucinations). They are also a prominent feature of narcolepsy.

Vivid animate hallucinations associated with a sleeplike state may arise from lesions of the midbrain (peduncular hallucinosis). Because sleep-wake cycle disturbances are always present, these hallucinations probably represent dream intrusions generated by a damaged reticular activating system.[67,68]

Trance-like States

Visual illusions and hallucinations are often reported during hypnosis, intense emotional stress, and religious rituals.[64] The fertile imaginations of children quite normally conjure up imaginary playmates they regard as real.[69]

Impaired Vision

When sight is poor, external visual stimuli can no longer shield the brain from its internal visual memories. Elderly patients who have 20/200 visual acuity or worse in the better eye often report seeing detailed floral or wallpaper patterns and unfamiliar faces (Charles Bonnet syndrome).[60,70] Although these figments are usually pleasant, they sometimes have a paranoid component that frightens the patients. This phenomenon is more likely to occur against a background of dementia, but it can also occur in persons in a normal cognitive state. Social isolation is a prominent feature. Low-dose haloperidol, 0.5–1.0 mg/day, or another antipsychotic medication often relieves the symptoms.

Abnormal Mental State or Impaired Vision not Present

When full-field binocular illusions or hallucinations cannot be attributed to the effects of a psychoactive agent, abnormal mental state or blindness, clues to precise localization come from the nature of the visual experience and the neuro-ophthalmologic findings.

Altered Color

Patients suffering digitalis toxicity may report a yellowish green tinge or frosting to their vision (xanthopsia), a manifestation of retinal photoreceptor damage.[71]

Achromatopsia, the inability to sort or match colors, may result from inferior occipital lobe lesions involving the lingual and fusiform gyri.[72] Patients also have superior altitudinal visual field defects to achromatic stimuli. Bilateral posterior cerebral infarctions are the most common cause.

Altered Spatial Relationships

Patients who have medullary ischemia from vertebrobasilar vascular insufficiency may see their environment as tilted or even upside down.[73] Infarction of the dorsolateral medulla (Wallenberg syndrome) may cause this illusion to persist for days to weeks. The diagnosis is based on eliciting other manifestations of brainstem damage.

Bilateral parieto-occipital lobe lesions may lead to great difficulty in judging the relative distances of objects in space and manifest as misreaching under visual guidance, bumping into furniture, or getting lost.[74] Although patients may complain that objects appear displaced, their problem is not that they are experiencing illusions but rather that they cannot function within space (topographic agnosia). Their deficit is believed to result from disconnection between visual cortex and parietal cortex, where multiple sensory inputs are integrated.[75]

Altered Motion

Illusions of motion may be caused by unilateral (or markedly asymmetric) optic neuropathy. When affected patients view a pendulum swinging in a place, they perceive its path as describing an ellipse (counterclockwise rotation if the right optic nerve is affected; clockwise rotation if the left optic nerve is affected). Called "Pulfrich stereo-illusions," this misperception is believed to result from unequal conduction rates in the two optic nerves.[76] Some patients who demonstrate the Pulfrich stereo-illusion also complain that they can no longer tell how fast the ball is moving or judge its distance from them. A ball thrown at them appears to curve as it approaches. Whether these complaints and the Pulfrich stereo-illusion are related is not known.

The most frequent illusions of motion do not arise from visual pathway lesions but from the oculomotor pathway. Oscillopsia is the name given to the illusion of movement of stationary objects. Oscillopsia is most clearly described by patients who have large-amplitude nystagmus. If the nystagmus is pendular (both phases are slow eye movements), patients perceive to-and-from movement. If the nystagmus is jerk (one phase is fast), they perceive the objects as moving only in the direction of the fast phase. Sometimes patients cannot clearly distinguish movement and report a "shimmery" sensation that may be misinterpreted as a scintillation.

Oscillopsia may also be described by patients who do not have nystagmus but instead have a defective vestibuloocular reflex (VOR).[74] When the VOR is functioning normally, head and body movements are synchronized perfectly with eye movements in the opposite direction, but when the VOR is defective, this synchrony is disturbed and the eyes cannot be held immobile in space during slight head or body movements. The result is that the patient sees stationary objects as blurred or "jiggling".[75] The offending lesion lies in the vestibular pathways, in either the end organs, nerves, or brainstem connections.

Patients who have chronic lesions adapt quite well to VOR defects. Oscillopsia occurs more frequently in acute processes such as aminoglycoside ototoxicity and brain stem infarct, demyelination, or tumor. A simple way to verify that the VOR is the cause of the symptom is to have the patient read a Snellen near card while moving the head rapidly from side to side. Under normal circumstance, the VOR compensation ensures continued clear vision; if the VOR is defective, acuity is degraded by at least two Snellen lines.

Oscillopsia is never a complaint of patients with congenital nystagmus, even when the ocular oscillations are very large. Those persons report blurred vision but are not aware of movement.

Visual Hallucinations in Psychotic States

Visual hallucinations are prevalent in psychotic states. While auditory hallucinations are considered cardinal symptoms of schizophrenia across cultures,[76-78] VHs are more frequent in schizophrenia than commonly believed. Affective disorders, including bipolar disorder, may also exhibit psychotic symptoms such as hallucinations and delusions. The presence of VHs in psychosis indicates a severe psychopathological profile and a less favorable prognosis. In bipolar disorder, individuals with hallucinations tend to have longer hospitalizations compared to those without hallucinations. Both younger patients with psychosis and older patients with neurodegenerative diseases experience poorer functioning and outcomes when VHs are present. Negative emotions, as indicated by studies linking stress and bereavement to VHs, play a role in their occurrence. For example, hallucinating about a deceased spouse is a common grief reaction among the elderly.

In schizophrenia, VHs often co-occur with hallucinations affecting other sensory modalities. Reports suggest that visual and auditory hallucinations co-occur in up to 84% of individuals with schizophrenia. Similar observations have been made in severe depression and mixed psychiatric diagnoses, although not necessarily simultaneously. Furthermore, when simultaneous auditory/VHs do occur, they are generally unrelated, suggesting potential differences in the underlying mechanisms of auditory and VHs in these disorders.

Interestingly, a different pattern is observed in organic neurological diseases. In PD, VHs are more predominant than auditory hallucinations. In ocular diseases, the absence of hallucinations in other sensory modalities is a diagnostic criterion. However, with ocular disease coexisting with dementia, auditory hallucinations and delusions may appear as the dementia progresses, as seen in PD or Alzheimer's disease. It is important to note that auditory hallucinations and VHs rarely occur simultaneously.

Overall, the relative proportion of auditory hallucinations to VHs differentiates the psychosis spectrum from organic neurological conditions. Fully formed VHs are more common than unformed visual experiences and distortions in psychotic conditions compared to conditions like migraine or epilepsy. Complex VHs often involve images of people, faces, animals, objects, or events occurring in front of the individual. In contrast to organic neurological conditions, frightening content (e.g., bugs, dogs, snakes, and distorted faces) is a common theme in VHs associated with distress. Visions of deceased individuals are rare, but visions of religious figures, such as God, angels, the devil, saints, and fairies, are common. VHs are perceived as real and "definitely present," with individuals often engaging in related activities, such as moving toward or hitting at the visions. Lack of control over the content and appearance is a prominent feature of VHs in psychosis. Individuals are often surprised by VHs and feel helpless in changing or stopping them. VHs may be attributed to external supernatural sources. Visioning images of influential religious figures are often interpreted as signs or threats to the patients' physical or psychological well-being, impacting their belief system and serving as evidence for delusional beliefs.

Thus, the rich phenomenology of VHs in psychosis indicates true hallucinatory experiences rather than mere misperceptions. Close examination of VH characteristics reveals significant similarities with auditory hallucinations in terms of perceptual quality, content, lack of control, beliefs, appraisals, and reactions. In comparison to organic neurological disorders, the form and character of VHs in psychosis resemble those seen in eye diseases and neurodegenerative disorders like Alzheimer's disease. However, several characteristics distinguish VHs in psychotic disorders, including frightening content, emotional reactions, appraisals of personal significance, a lack of illusions (common in neurodegenerative diseases), and common occurrence of simple VHs in ocular diseases.

CONCLUDING REMARKS

In conclusion, this chapter synthesizes current knowledge on VHs in the psychosis phenotype and contrasts it with literature from neurodegenerative disorders and eye diseases. The evidence challenges the traditional view that VHs are atypical or uncommon in psychosis. VHs are generally associated with a more severe psychopathological profile and less favorable outcomes in psychosis and neurodegenerative conditions. Co-occurrence of auditory hallucinations with VHs in psychosis suggests a shared etiological cause. VHs in psychosis exhibit remarkable complexity, negative content, and personal relevance. While cognitive mechanisms of VHs in psychosis have received limited investigation, existing studies indicate source-monitoring deficits, distortions in top-down mechanisms, and a lack of evidence for visual processing deficits found in organic literature. Brain imaging studies demonstrate visual cortex activation during hallucinations, along with structural and connectivity changes within broader brain networks in both psychosis and common neurological disorders such as migraine and epilepsy. The relationship between VHs in psychosis, eye disease, and neurodegeneration remains unclear. However, the similarities and differences described in this chapter suggest that comparative studies may have important clinical and theoretical implications.

LEARNING POINTS

To recognize VHs and differentiate them from other conditions, the following principles are important to consider:
- VHs must be experienced in full consciousness, excluding sleep-related VHs, fever-induced VHs, VHs associated with delirium, and VHs induced by hypnosis.

- VHs should not be elicited by an external stimulus, excluding visual distortions and illusions.
- VHs should have a sense of reality resembling veridical perception, including physical properties of real perceptions and a location in external space. Note that this does not imply that VHs must be perceived as real or lack insight.
- The individual should not feel direct and voluntary control over VHs, ruling out visual illusions.

REFERENCES

1. David AS. The cognitive neuropsychiatry of auditory verbal hallucinations: an overview. Cognit Neuropsychiatr. 2004;9: 107-23.
2. Sadock BJ, Sadock VA (Eds). Kaplan & Sadock's Comprehensive Textbook of Psychiatry, Volume 1, 7th edition. Lippincott Williams & Wilkins; 2000. p. 800.
3. Hupp SL, Kline LB, Corbett JJ. Visual disturbances of migraine. Surv Ophthalmol. 1989;33(4):221-36.
4. Todd J. The syndrome of Alice in Wonderland. Can Med Assoc J. 1955;73(9):701-4.
5. Critchley M. Types of visual perserveration: "Palinopsia" and "illusory visual spread." Brain. 1951;74(3):267-99.
6. Jacobs I. Visual allesthesia. Neurology. 1980;30(10):1059-63.
7. Cummings JL, Syndulko K, Goldberg Z, Treiman DM. Palinopsia reconsidered. Neurology. 1982;32(4):444-7.
8. Michel EM, Troost BT. Palinopsia: Cerebral localization with computed tomography. Neurology. 1980;30(8):887-9.
9. Bender MB. Polyopia and monocular diplopia of cerebral origin. Arch Neurol Psychiatry. 1945;54:323-38.
10. Bender MB. Oscillopsia. Arch Neurol. 1965;49:489-504.
11. Davidoff RA. Migraine: Manifestations, pathogenesis, and management, Philadelphia: FA Davis; 1995.
12. Alvarez WC. The migrainous scotoma as studied in 618 persons. Am J Ophthalmol. 1960;49:489-504.
13. Fisher CM. Late-life migraine accompaniments as a cause of unexplained transient ischemic attacks. Can J Neurol Sci. 1980;7(1):8-17.
14. Monteiro LR, Hoyt WF, Imes RK. Puerperal cerebral blindness. Arch Neurol. 1984;41(12):1300-1.
15. Plant GT. The fortification spectra of migraine. Br Med J. 1986;293(6562):1613-7.
16. Hoyt WF. Transient bilateral blurring of vision. Considerations of an episodic ischemic symptom of vertebro-basilar insufficiency. Arch Ophthalmol. 1963;70:746-51.
17. Penfield W, Jaspor H. Epilepsy and the Functional anatomy of the Human Brain. Boston: Little, Brown; 1954.
18. Ludwig BI, Ajmone C. Clinical ictal patterns in epileptic patients with occipital electroencephalographic foci. Neurology. 1975;25(5):463-71.
19. Panayiotopoulos CP. Elementary visual hallucinations in migraine and epilepsy. J Neurol Neurosurg Psychiatry. 1994; 57(11):1371-4.
20. Troost BT. Mark LE, Maroon JC. Resolution of classic migraine after removal of an occipital lobe AVM. Ann Neurol. 1979;5(2):199-201.
21. Riaz G, Hennessey JJ. Meningeal lesions mimicking migraine. Neuro-ophthalmology. 1991;11:41-8.
22. Kattah JC. Luessenhop AJ. Resolution of classic migraine after removal of an occipital lobe AVM. Ann Neurol. 1980;7(1):93.
23. Weiskrantz L, Warrington EK, Sanders MD, Marshall J. Visual capacity in the hemianopic field following a restricted occipital ablation. Brain. 1974;97(4):709-28.
24. Kupersmith MJ, Vargas ME, Yashar A, Madrid M, Nelson K, Seton A, et al. Occipital arteriovenous malformations: visual disturbances and presentation. Neurology. 1996;46(4):953-7.
25. Hachinski VC, Porchawka J, Steele JC. Visual symptoms in the migraine syndrome. Neurology. 1973;23(6):570-9.
26. Lippman C. Certain hallucinations peculiar to migraine. J Nerv Mental Dis. 1952;116(4):346-51.
27. Schott GD. Exploring the visual hallucinations of migraine aura: the tacit contribution of illustration. Brain. 2007;130(Pt 6): 1690-703.
28. Wilkinson M, Robinson D. Migraine art. Cephalalgia. 1985;5(3): 151-7.
29. Podoll K, Robinson D. Out-of-body experiences and related phenomena in migraine art. Cephalalgia. 1999;19(10):886-96.
30. Ffytche DH. Visual hallucination and illusion disorders: a clinical guide. Adv Clin Neurosci Rehab. 2004;4:16-8.
31. Panayiotopoulos CP. Elementary visual hallucinations, blindness, and headache in idiopathic occipital epilepsy: differentiation from migraine. J Neurol Neurosurg Psychiatry. 1999;66(4):536-40.
32. Williams D, Wilson TG. The diagnosis of the major and minor syndromes of basilar insufficiency. Brain. 1962;85:741-74.
33. Minor RH, Kearns TP, Millikan CH, Siekert RG, Sayre GP. Ocular manifestations of occlusive disease of the vertebro-basilar arterial system. Arch Ophthalmol. 1959;62(1):112-24.
34. Fisher CM. The posterior cerebral artery syndrome. Can J Neurol Sci. 1986;13(3):232-9.
35. Newman DS, Levine SR, Curtis VL, Welch KM. Migraine-like visual phenomena associated with cerebral venous thrombosis. Headache. 1989;29(2):82-5.
36. Bickerstaff ER. The basilar artery and the migraine-epilepsy syndrome. Proc R Soc Med. 1962;55(3):167-9.
37. Panayiotopoulos CP. Benign childhood epilepsy with occipital paroxysms: A 15-year prospective study. Ann Neurol. 1989;26(1):51-6.
38. Gastaut H. Zifkin BG. Benign epilepsy of childhood with occipital spike and wave complexes. In: Andermann F, Lugaresi E (Eds). Migraine and Epilepsy. An Overview. Boston: Butterworths; 1987.
39. Penfield W. Perot P. The brain's record of auditory and visual experience. Brain. 1963;86:595-696.
40. Dobelle WH, Mladejorsky MG, Garvin JP. Artificial vision for the blind: Electrical stimulation of visual cortex offers hope for functional prosthesis. Science. 1974;183(4123):440-4.
41. Brindley GS, Lewin WS. The sensations produced by electrical stimulation of the visual cortex. J Physiol. 1968;196(2):479-93.
42. Engel JL. Seizures and Epilepsy. Philadelphia: FA Davis; 1989.
43. Lance JW, Smee RI. Partial seizures with visual disturbance treated by radiotherapy of cavernous hemangioma. Ann Neurol. 1989;26(6):782-5.
44. Williamson PD, Thadani VM, Darcey TM, Spencer DD, Spencer SS, Mattson RH. Occipital lobe epilepsy: clinical characteristics, seizure spread patterns, and results of surgery. Ann Neurol. 1992;31(1):3-13.

45. Anderson SW, Rizzo M. Hallucinations following occipital lobe damage: The pathological activation of visual representations. J Clin Exp Neuropsychol. 1994;16(5):651-63.
46. Hacaen H. Albert ML. Human Neuropsychology. New York: John Wiley & Sons; 1978.
47. Teunisse RJ, Zitman FG, Kaes DC. Clinical evaluation of 14 patients with the Charles Bonnet syndrome (isolated visual hallucinations). Compr Psychiatry 1994;35(1):70-5.
48. Bien CG, Benninger FO, Urbach H, Schramm J, Kurthen M, Elger CE. Localizing value of epileptic visual auras. Brain. 2000;123 (Pt 2):244-53.
49. Russel WR, Whitty WM. Studies in traumatic epilepsy. 3. Visual fits. J Neurol Neurosurg Psychiatry. 1955;18(2):79-96.
50. Kolmel HW. Complex visual hallucinations in the hemianopic field. J Neurol Neurosurg Psychiatry. 1985;48(1):29-38.
51. Assad G, Shapiro B. Hallucinations: Theoretical and clinical overview. Am J Psychiatry 1986;143(9):1088-97.
52. Cummings JL. Clinical Neuropsychiatry. Orlando, Fla: Grune & Stratton; 1985.
53. Drugs that cause psychiatric symptoms. Med Lett Drugs Ther. 1989;31(808):113-8.
54. Critchley M. Neurological aspects of visual and auditory hallucinations. Br. Med J. 1939;2(4107):634-9.
55. Lerner AJ, Koss E, Patterson MB, Ownby RL, Hedera P, Friedland RP, et al. Concomitants of visual hallucinations in Alzheimer's disease. Neurology. 1994;44(3 Pt 1):523-7.
56. McShane R, Gedling K, Reading M, McDonald B, Esiri MM, Hope T. Prospective study of relations between cortical Lewy bodies, poor eyesight, and hallucinations in Alzheimer's disease. J Neurol Neurosurg Psychiatry. 1995;59(2):185-8.
57. Dunn DW, Weisberg LA, Nadell J. Peduncular hallucinations caused by brainstem compression. Neurology. 1983;33(10): 1360-1.
58. Mckee AC, Levine DN, Kowall NW, Richardson EP. Peduncular hallucinosis associated with isolated infarction of the substantia nigra pars reticulata. Ann Neurol. 1990;27(5):500-4.
59. Schultz G, Melzack R. Visual hallucinations and mental state. A study of 14 Charles Bonnet syndrome hallucinators. J Nerv Ment Dis. 1993;181(10):639-43.
60. Damos J, Skelton M, Jenner FA. The Charles Bonnet syndrome in perspective. Psychol Med. 1982;12(2):251-7.
61. Robertson DM, Hollenhorst RW, Callahan JA. Ocular manifestations of digitalis toxicity: Discussion and report of three cases of central scotomas. Arch Ophthalmol. 1966;76(5): 640-5.
62. Weleber RG, Shults WT. Digoxin retinal toxicity: clinical and electrophysiologic evaluation of a cone dysfunction syndrome. Arch Ophthalmol. 1981;99(9):1568-72.
63. Schneider T, Dahlheim P, Zrenner E. Experimental investigations of the ocular toxicity of cardiac glycosides in animals. Fortschr Ophthalmol. 1989;86:751-5.
64. Hornsten G. Wallenberg's syndrome. I. General symptomatology, with special reference to visual disturbances and imbalance. Acta Neurol Scand. 1974;50(4):434-46.
65. Piltz JR, Wertenbaker C, Lance SE, Slamovits T, Leeper HF. Digoxin toxicity. Recognizing the varied visual presentations. J Clin Neuroophthalmol. 1993;13(4):275-80.
66. Meadows JC. Disturbed perception of colors associated with localized cerebral lesions. Brain. 1974;97(4):615-32.
67. Pearlman AL, Birch J, Meadows JC. Cerebral color blindness: An acquired defect in hue discrimination. Ann Neurol. 1979;5(3): 253-61.
68. Steiner I, Shahin R, Melamed E. Acute "upside down" reversal of vision in transient vertebrobasilar ischemia. Neurology. 1987;37(10):1685-6.
69. Charles N, Froment C, Rode G, Vighetto A, Turjman F, Trillet M, et al. Vertigo and upside down vision due to an infarct in the territory of the medial branch of the posterior inferior cerebellar artery caused by dissection of a vertebral artery. J Neurol Neurosurg Psychiatry. 1992;55(3):188-9.
70. Holmes G. Disturbances of visual orientation. Br J Ophthalmol. 1918;2(9):449-68.
71. Damasio AR. Disorders of complex visual processing: Agnosias, achromatopsia, Balint's syndrome, and related difficulties of orientation and construction. In: Mesulam MM (Ed). Principles of Behavioral Neurology. Philadelphia: FA Davis; 1985. pp. 259-88.
72. Sokol S. The Pulfrich stereo-illusion as an index of optic nerve dysfunction. Surv Ophthalmol. 1976;20(6):432-4.
73. Heron G, Dutton GN. The Pulfrich phenomenon and its alleviation with a neutral density filter. Br J Ophthalmol. 1989;73(12):1004-8.
74. Brickner R. Oscillopsia: A new symptom commonly occurring in multiple sclerosis. Arch Neurol Psychiatry. 1936;36:586-9.
75. Leigh RJ. Management of oscillopsia. In: Barber HO, Sharpe JA (Eds). Vestibular Disorders. St Louis: Mosby-Year Book; 1988. pp. 201-11.
76. Waters F, Collerton D, Ffytche DH, Jardri R, Pins D, Dudley R, et al. Visual hallucinations in the psychosis spectrum and comparative information from neurodegenerative disorders and eye disease. Schizophr Bull. 2014;40(Suppl 4):S233-45.
77. Bernardin F, Schwan R, Lalanne L, Ligier F, Angioi-Duprez K, Schwitzer T, et al. The role of the retina in visual hallucinations: A review of the literature and implications for psychosis. Neuropsychologia. 2017;99:128-38.
78. Oorschot M, Lataster T, Thewissen V, Bentall R, Delespaul P, Myin-Germeys I. Temporal dynamics of visual and auditory hallucinations in psychosis. Schizophr Res. 2012;140(1-3):77-82.

A Note on Auditory Hallucinations

Ambar Chakravarty

INTRODUCTION

Auditory hallucinations (AHs), like visual hallucinations, can be defined as sounds experienced by an awake individual in the absence of any auditory stimulus from the external world. AHs are in essence auditory percepts—experienced during the waking state but not during dreams, during falling asleep, or soon after waking from sleep (hypnagogic hallucinations). They need to be distinguished from auditory imagery (i.e., sounds imagined or remembered) and auditory illusions. The last hearing of actual sounds, which are either misperceived or misinterpreted like misinterpreting a calling bell sound to be a clock alarm sound. AH needs differentiation from thought insertions and obsessive thoughts in psychiatric practice.

The classification of auditory hallucinations has yielded numerous types and subtypes. It is uncertain whether tinnitus should be classified as AH or not. Similar would be the case with echo of reading, polyacousis, certain forms of auditory synesthesia, and palinacousis. As in none of these there is true auditory stimulus, these can be grouped under the common rubric of AH.

PHENOMENOLOGY

Auditory hallucinations could be external meaning sounds originating from an extracorporeal (out of the body) or internal when perceived to be originating from an internal source like in the head or elsewhere in the body (abdomen, extremities) or nonlocalizable.[1] In the latter situations, the term extracampine hallucinations (i.e., hallucinations occurring outside the regular field of perception) is used. These are very rare but always associated with psychosis.[2] Other internal types of hallucinations may be associated with borderline personality disorders. In cases with unilateral internal or external hallucinations, exclusion of a structural brain pathology is essential. Ménière's disease, of course, in the initial stage may present with unilateral tinnitus but some degree of hearing loss may be detected on audiometry.

VERBAL AUDITORY HALLUCINATIONS

Auditory hallucinations may be verbal or nonverbal. Verbal AHs consist of hallucinated sounds, which feature a linguistic content. That content may vary from hearing one's name spoken out to complete sentences or even clusters of multiple voices, which may be intermittent.

At times verbal AHs may take the form of commands which may or may not be continually present;[3] at times the sounds of flowing water or a gas pipe leaking,[4] and even hallucinated sounds, which are either recognized as one's own thoughts or literally echo one's conscious thoughts;[5] echo of reading (a condition in which the reading of words or sentences is accompanied by a hallucinated echo of the same linguistic content);[6] and psychomotor verbal hallucinations in which verbal AHs may co-occur with subtle instances of motor activity within the larynx and/or vocal cords. Psychotic individuals mostly experience command or echo hallucinations.

NONVERBAL AUDITORY HALLUCINATIONS

Nonverbal AHs lack the linguistic content characteristic of verbal AHs, consisting instead of sounds ranging from ticking, clicking, or humming to the barking of dogs, the drone of airplane engines, or all-out classic symphonies. Nonverbal AHs are in some way close to tinnitus. The differentiation may be complex when a noise-type tinnitus or a tonal tinnitus gradually takes on a musical quality. This indeed then becomes a musical AH. The Exploding Head Syndrome experienced by some people while going off to sleep may be considered a rare form of nonverbal AH. Nonverbal hallucinations are thus not always indicative of any form of psychiatric disease.

Musical Hallucinations

Musical hallucinations consist of songs, tunes, melodies, harmonics, etc., which are perceived in the absence of any actual music.

After an initial phase of surprise and disbelief, most people come to accept soon that the music originates in their head and stop expressing their concern to others.

ETIOLOGY

Box 1 summarizes the well-recognized neurological and psychiatric causes of AH.

Auditory hallucinations, notably those of the verbal type, tend to be associated primarily with psychosis, the most common being schizophrenia. AHs may also be experienced in the context of unipolar depressive disorder, bipolar disorder, dementia, dissociative disorder, borderline personality disorder, and occasionally other psychiatric disorders.[7]

Occurrence in the Absence of Pathology

Auditory hallucinations may be experienced by 10–15% of all individuals in the general population, that is, in the absence of any demonstrable pathology. A group of phenomena experienced by an even larger number of individuals in the healthy population are hypnagogic and hypnopompic hallucinations, together known as hypnagogia. These may take the form of being in an elevator feelings, geometric visual hallucinations, and facial hallucinations, but they may also feature nonverbal and even verbal auditory phenomena, such as repetitions of recent conversations, hearing one's name called out, the sound of one's child talking or crying, reading aloud from a book, and indistinct talking. Occasionally, musical hallucinations have also been described. Hypnopompic hallucinations, on the other hand, which occur during the transitional phase from sleep to awake state, would seem to be less prevalent, and to consist mainly of dream images that stay on during the first few seconds or minutes of awake state. Because of their association with sleep, neither hypnagogic nor hypnopompic hallucinations tend to be considered as "true" hallucinations, and in the absence of any additional indicators of parasomnia their clinical relevance remains undetermined.

PATHOPHYSIOLOGY: EVIDENCE FOR A FUNCTIONAL AUDITORY NETWORK

Functional magnetic resonance imaging (MRI) and BOLD studies have established aberrant activation in the auditory network in the brain consisting of the Broca area, the insula, the frontal operculum, the precentral gyrus, the middle temporal gyrus, the superior temporal gyrus (i.e., Wernicke's area), the contralateral bilateral inferior parietal lobule, and the hippocampal and parahippocampal regions. The functional imaging signal reflects local increases in cerebral oxygen consumption, and the neurovascular-coupling hypothesis stipulates that such increases are indicative of changes in brain function.[8]

When those changes co-occur with reported verbal auditory hallucinations, they are taken as reliable indicators of hallucinatory activity. Some structural abnormalities have also been detected using advanced MRI techniques such as diffusion tensor imaging and magnetic tractography. Similarly functional aberrations in the brain network for musical appreciation and creation may be responsible for musical hallucinations. The structures involved include auditory areas, motor cortex, visual areas, basal ganglia, brainstem, pons, tegmentum, cerebellum, hippocampi, amygdala, and perhaps even the peripheral auditory system.

Contrary to the situation in verbal AHs, the most prevalent clinical condition associated with musical hallucinations is auditory deprivation or deafness. Thus the musical hallucinations of—notably the elderly—deaf are considered analogous to the visual hallucinations of the visually handicapped, also known as Charles Bonnet syndrome. In that sense, most (although certainly not all) instances of musical hallucination would seem to

---

BOX 1: Causes of auditory hallucinations.

- *Psychiatric*: Psychotic disorders, bipolar disorders, depressive disorder, dissociative disorder, borderline personality disorder
- *Neurologic*: Delirium, delirium tremens, dementia, Parkinson disease, brain tumors, paraneoplastic syndromes, limbic encephalitis, prion diseases, arteriovenous malformation (AVM), exploding head syndrome
- *Otologic*: Presbycusis, tinnitus, severe deafness disorders
- *Systemic disease*: Neurosyphilis, acquired immunodeficiency syndrome (AIDS), thyrotoxicosis, hyperhomocysteinemia, sarcoidosis, chromosomal diseases
- *Substance intoxication and/or withdrawal*: Alcohol, cannabis, cocaine, amphetamine, hallucinogens, antidepressants, anticholinergic, antibiotics
- *Physiologic*: Idiopathic, hypnagogic, bereavement, social isolation, intensive meditation, sleep deprivation, aging

fulfill the criteria of deafferentiation phenomena. Very rarely though, musical hallucinations may form a part of an epileptic aura. Also, very rarely, some specific musical note may trigger a seizure attack.

PHARMACOTHERAPY

The sheet anchor for the symptomatic treatment of AHs is antipsychotic medication, especially when the hallucinations at hand are experienced in the context of psychotic disorder, mood disorder, or delirium. The EUFEST (European First Episode Schizophrenia Trial) compared of the effects of five antipsychotic agents on the severity of hallucinations experienced by patients diagnosed with psychotic disorder.[9] As suggested by the EUFEST data, there are no significant differences in efficacy between haloperidol, olanzapine, ziprasidone, quetiapine, and amisulpride in their potential to reduce the frequency or severity of hallucinations. They all yield a significant reduction in symptom severity during the first month, with further reductions taking place during the first 12 months of treatment.

Nonpharmacologic treatment methods for AHs include psychotherapy, various protocols aimed at teaching patients to cope with their voices, self-help groups, electroconvulsive therapy (ECT), and lastly transcranial magnetic stimulation.

In sum, our current knowledge of AHs has transcended the rich phenomenology and taxonomy inherited from classic neuroscientific discourses to encompass the even richer harvest of neuroimaging findings obtained during the past two decades. This has made possible to gain an impression of a structural as well as a functional auditory network in the brain, and to relate various aspects of the AH experience to important nodes and hubs located in those networks.

REFERENCES

1. Copolov D, Trauer T, Mackinnon A. On the non-significance of internal versus external auditory hallucinations. Schizophr Res. 2004;69(1):1-6.
2. Sato Y, Berrios GE. Extracampine hallucinations. Lancet. 2003;361(9367):1479-80.
3. Erkwoh R, Willmes K, Eming-Erdmann A, Kunert HJ. Command hallucinations: who obeys and who resists when? Psychopathology. 2002;35(5):272-9.
4. Jaspers K. General Psychopathology, volume 1. Baltimore, MA: Johns Hopkins University Press; 1997.
5. Sommer IE, Selten JP, Diederen KM, Blom JD. Dissecting auditory verbal hallucinations into two components: audibility (Gedankenlautwerden) and alienation (thought insertion). Psychopathology. 2010;43(2):137-40.
6. Morel F. Echo de la lecture. Contribution àl'étudedes hallucinations auditives verbales. l'Encéphale. 1933;28:169-83.
7. Larøi F, Sommer IE, Blom JD, Fernyhough C, Ffytche DH, Hugdahl K, et al. The characteristic features of auditory verbal hallucinations in clinical and nonclinical groups: state-of-the-art overview and future directions. Schizophr Bull. 2012;38(4):724-33.
8. Villringer A. Understanding functional neuroimaging methods based on neurovascular coupling. Adv Exp Med Biol. 1997;413: 177-93.
9. Kahn RS, Fleischhacker WW, Boter H, Davidson M, Vergouwe Y, Keet IP, et al.; EUFEST study group. Effectiveness of antipsychotic drugs in first-episode schizophrenia and schizophreniform disorder: an open randomised clinical trial. Lancet. 2008;371 (9618):1085-97.

Index

Page numbers followed by *b* refer to box, *f* refer to figure, *fc* refer to flowchart, and *t* refer to table.

A

Abacavir 259
Abduction, weakness of 21
Abductor
　laryngeal dystonia 123
　sign 21
Abnormal mental state 390, 391
Acalculia 52
Accidents 12
Acetabular rotation 21
Acetaldehyde 371
　dehydrogenase activity 337
　plasma clearance 337
Acetaminophen 203
Acetylcholine 268, 356
Achromatopsia 391
Acid maltase deficiency 213, 214
Acquired immunodeficiency syndrome 31, 230, 258, 259, 293
Activated partial thromboplastin time 140
Addenbrooke's cognitive examination 46, 55, 65
Addison's disease 74, 230
Adenosine
　deaminase 38
　triphosphate 373
Adipose tissue storage homeostasis 269
Adjustment disorder 24, 44
Adrenal disorders 33
Adrenomyeloneuropathy 305
Aedes aegypti mosquito 261
Aerophobia 260, 261
Aggression 259
　poststroke 153
　presence of 133
　prevalence of 131
Agnosia 54, 262
　types of 54
Agoraphobia 325, 328
Agraphia 52, 287
Agrypnia excitata 269
Airway 140
Akathisia 161, 362, 365
　acute 164, 363, 366
　subacute 164

Akinesia 157
Akinetic mutism 26, 262, 357
Alcohol 35, 176, 336, 371
　abuse 303, 371
　　disorder 381
　amblyopia 337
　intoxication 336, 346
　neuropsychiatric aspects of 34
　use disorder 337, 371
　withdrawal 337, 346
　　syndrome 337
Alcoholism 177*t*
　central neurological manifestations of 371
Alexia 288
Alkalosis 333
Allergic reaction, higher risk of 103
Almotriptan 203
Alopecia 213
Alpha-amino-3-hydroxy-5-methyl-4-isoxazolepropionic acid
　encephalitis 247
　receptor 245
Alternating hand movements test 49
Alzheimer's disease 24, 46, 52, 129, 147, 150, 227, 230, 276, 287, 289, 298, 298*f*, 299, 359, 392
Amantadine 160, 343
Amino acids 321
Amitriptyline 206, 208, 344
Amlodipine 381
Amnesia
　anterograde 59
　drug-related 58, 62
　functional 61
　post-traumatic 58, 61
　psychogenic 58, 60, 61, 61*t*
　retrograde 59
　syndrome, acute 59
　temporal period of 58
　transient
　　epileptic 58, 61, 61*t*, 145
　　global 58, 59, 61, 61*t*, 145
Amnestic deficits 375
Amphetamines 342, 344, 379, 380
Amygdala 45, 223, 329, 331, 350, 353, 356
　dopaminergic 268
　stimulation of 350

Amyloid angiopathy 298*f*
Analgesics 344
Anarithmetria 52
Anemia 263
Aneurysms 380
Angelman syndrome 320, 320*f*
Angiography 307, 309
Angiotensin-converting enzyme 214
Angular gyrus syndrome 52, 53, 306
Anopheles mosquito 261, 263
Anorexia 30
Anosognosia 52
Anterior cerebral artery 26, 137-141
　infarcts 306
　territory 26
Anterograde memory 47
　deficits 60
Antiacetylcholine receptor
　antibodies 218
Anti-alpha-amino-3-hydroxy-5-methyl-4-isoxazolepropionic acid
　receptor 30
Antibiotics 344
Antibody 218, 248
　detection 249
　response 244
Anticholinergics 341
Antidepressants 113, 344, 362
Antiemetic 344
Antiepileptic drugs 111, 111*t*
　side effects of 110
Antigen 244
Antimuscle specific kinase 218
Antineutrophil cytoplasmic
　antibody 214
Anti-N-methyl-D-aspartate 234
　receptor encephalitis 29
Antinuclear antibody 214, 229
Antipsychotic 362
　medication 28, 367
Antiretroviral drugs 30, 259
Antiseizure medicine 27, 95, 104, 104*t*, 106
Antisocial personality disorder 127, 129
Antithrombotic therapy 150
Antituberculous therapy 31
Anton's syndrome 140

Anxiety 5, 44, 99, 110, 180, 230, 259, 272, 323
  disorder 17, 40, 113, 201, 237, 316
    generalized 17, 110, 201, 325
    poststroke 151
    profiles 316
Apathy 32, 180
Aphasia 249, 255, 262, 278
  global 51
  impaired comprehension 149
  progressive nonfluent 289
  transcortical 51
  transient global 27
  types of 66
Apperceptive visual agnosia 54
Apraxia 52, 158, 262
Arboviral infections 261
Argentine hemorrhagic fever 263
Arginine vasopressin 352
Aripiprazole 342
Arithmetic operations 51
Arousal 43
Arrhythmia, cardiac 35, 331
Arterial aneurysms, rupture of 136
Arterial carbon dioxide, partial pressure of 330
Arterial dissection 136
Arteriovenous fistula 307
Arteriovenous malformation 307
Arteritis, temporal 197
Artery-to-artery embolism 136
Artificial intelligence 281
Asperger's disorder 314
Aspirin 203
Astasia-abasia 23, 170
Asthma, bronchial 325
Astrocytoma, low-grade 105
Ataxia 74, 255, 263, 362, 367
  syndrome 305
Atherothrombosis 136
Athetosis 161, 262
Atonic seizures, drugs resistant 96
Atrophy 257f, 279f, 281
  bilateral
    frontal 277f
    parieto-occipital 280f
    temporal 299
  frontal 299
Attacks,
  antibody mediated 249
  number of 199
Attention deficit hyperactivity disorder 95, 113, 130, 189, 316
Auditory hallucinations 392, 395
  causes of 396b
Auditory illusions 112
Australian bat lyssavirus 260

Autism 102, 321
  spectrum disorder 95, 130, 321
    neurological aspects of 314
Autistic disorder 314
Autoantibodies 273
Autoimmune 211, 292
  diseases 249
  disorders 210
  encephalitis 29, 39, 243, 244, 244b, 244t, 248, 249, 249b, 251, 253, 273, 281, 304, 318
    management of 250
    misdiagnosis of 249
    neuropsychiatric aspects of 29, 243
    salient features of 244t
    syndromes 251
  neuropathies 216
  psychosis 247, 248, 248b, 251
  thyroiditis 34, 293
Automatic movement, loss of 157
Automatisms 101
  epileptic 133
Autonomic disorders 40, 336
Autonomic dysfunction 365
  early 158
Autonomic manifestations 100
Autonomic nervous
  dysfunction 212
  system 327
Autonomic phenomenon 71
Autoscopy 112
Axial fluid-attenuated inversion recovery 250f, 257f, 260f, 265f, 276f, 279f, 302f
  sequence 298f-300f
Axial functional neurological disorders 23
Azathioprine 250

B

Babinski's concept 14
Baclofen 237
Ballism 161
Barbiturates 111, 208
Basal cell skin cancer 217
Basal ganglia 1, 30, 156, 223, 265f, 309
  bilateral 302f
  encephalitis 245
  microbleeds 298
Behavior
  abnormalities 30, 318
  self-harm 95
  therapy 24, 204
Behavioral addictions 188
  development of 189, 189f
Behçet syndrome 39
Benzene 379

Benzodiazepine 94, 111, 152, 208, 338, 340, 367
  refractory delirium tremens, treatment of 338t
Beta-blocker 365
Bhasmas 35
Bilateral mesial temporal hyperintensities 250f
Binocular
  full-field illusions 390
  hemifield illusions 386
Biparietal syndrome 287
Bipolar disorder 129, 181, 230, 237, 277, 325
  prevalence of 237
Bizarre phenomena 23
Black box warning 367
Bladder 226
Bleeding 136
  etiology of 137f
Blepharospasm 123
Blood
  alcohol
    concentration 336
    levels 372t
  brain barrier 235
    dysfunction 373
  level 372
  pressure 136, 330
  sugar 140
  vessel, blockage of 136
Body
  acute opisthotonus of 12f
  dysmorphic disorder 17, 18
  morphology, maintenance of 269
Borderline personality disorder 129
Borrelia burgdorferi 257
  culture of 257
Botulinum toxin 365
  course of 206
  injection 204
Botulism 211
Bowel dysfunction 226
Brachial plexitis 261
Bradykinesia 156, 157
Brain 6, 43f, 137f, 270
  anatomy of 2f
  development 315
  disorder of 88
  function 13, 46, 314
  hemorrhage 136, 142
  imaging of 72, 263, 321, 353
  injury 131
    moderate-to-severe 357
  interstitium of 269
  iron accumulation 157, 163, 302
  lesions 373
  lobes of 43f

magnetic resonance imaging of 38*f*, 250*f*, 257*f*, 375*f*
monism, concept of 8
networks 125
neurotransmitter localization 124
parenchyma 136, 255
posterior circulation of 138
regions of 255
structure 3, 314, 330
time-of-flight magnetic resonance angiogram of 307*f*
tumors 143
Brain's functional architecture 125
Brainstem 45, 199
encephalitis 39
strokes 333
syndrome 245
tumors 333
Breath holding spell 72
Breathing 140
shortness of 323
Brivaracetam 95, 104
Broca's aphasia 50, 51
Broca's area 51
Bromocriptine 343, 346
Brown-Séquard syndrome 144
Brucella melitensis 256
Brucellosis 256
Brudzinski's sign 255
Brugada syndrome 74
Bulbar dysfunction 158, 263
Bulbar weakness 213
Bupropion 367
Buspirone 344

C

Caffeine 371
Calcitonin gene-related peptide 225
Caloric stimulation 150
Calves, pseudohypertrophy of 212*f*
Cancer 244
Cannabis 303, 371, 380
Capgras' syndrome 28
Capillary endothelial cells 373
Carbamazepine 94, 103, 104, 106, 111, 324, 357, 362, 367
failure 103
Carbohydrate 231
Carbon
dioxide, arterial partial pressure of 325
monoxide 157, 305
clioquinol 39
poisoning 305
Cardiac conduction blockade 363, 366
Cardioembolism 380
Cardiorespiratory diseases 230
Cardiovascular disease 287

Carnitine
deficiency 213, 214
palmitoyltransferase 214
Carotid
artery, compression of 380
massage 74*f*
sinus syncope 74
vasoconstriction 380
Cartesian principles 6
Catalepsy 39
Catatonia 259, 363, 368
malignant 345, 346
Catecholamines 356
Category fluency test 49
Caudate 156
nuclei, lesions of 374
Causalgia 123
Celiac disease 305
Cell
clusters produce, parallel system of 268
surface antibodies 294
Central nervous system 23, 29, 39, 39*f*, 210, 255, 258, 259, 265*f*, 291
infections, neuropsychiatric aspects of 30, 255
lymphomas, primary 306
nature of 304
symptoms of 336
toxoplasmosis 264
viral infections of 258
Central pain modulating system 207
Central pontine myelinolysis 238, 336, 378
Centre for epidemiological studies depression scale 151
Centrotemporal spikes 96
Cerebellar
artery
anterior inferior 139
posterior inferior 139
superior 139
ataxia 245, 336
atrophy 300, 301*f*
cortex 352
dysfunction 177, 373, 374
signs 158
syndrome 138, 139*f*
Cerebellum 309
Cerebral
amyloid angiopathy 136, 148
arteriovenous malformation 307*f*
artery
infarct, posterior 306
posterior 26
autosomal recessive arteriopathy 291
blood flow 125, 299, 327
normal 135

circulation 1
cortex 55
anterolateral 137
creatine deficiency syndrome 320
dural arteriovenous fistula 308*f*
functions, localization related 50
hemispheres, bilateral 264*f*, 265*f*
lymphoma, primary 333
palsy 102
salt wasting syndrome 31
venous sinus thrombosis 143
Cerebrolysin 150
Cerebrospinal fluid 29, 136, 160, 173, 235, 244, 248, 249, 255, 264, 269, 276, 293, 318, 356
abnormal 38
analysis 381
biomarkers 312
examinations 197
pleocytosis 245
Cerebrotendinous xanthomatosis 305
Cerebrovascular disease 40, 147, 275, 276
neuropsychiatric aspects of 26, 147
Cerebrovascular disorders
cognitive effects of 147
psychiatric effects of 150
Cerebrovascular events, increased risk of 368
Cerebrovascular insufficiency, chronic 290
Cervical cord 305*f*
demyelinating lesion 144
Charcot's pupils 12
Charcot-Marie-Tooth disease 211, 213, 216
Charlson comorbidity index 110
Chemotherapy 39
Chest pain 328
Chikungunya virus 261
Childhood disintegrative disorder 314
Chloroform 11
Chlorpromazine 342, 362
Choking, feeling of 328
Cholinergic neurotransmitter systems 268
Cholinesterase inhibitor 150, 218, 357
therapy, initiation of 150
Chorea 161, 162, 168, 262, 289
Chromosomal microarray analysis 321
Chromosome 216
Chronic fatigue syndrome 222, 229, 229*fc*, 230, 230*b*, 231
management of 231*t*
Chronic pain 222, 231, 232*b*
borderlands of 230, 231*f*
pathophysiology of 222, 227
prevalence of 227
Cincinnati prehospital stroke scale 137

Cingulate cortex 350
Cingulate gyrus 110, 223, 351, 353
   anterior 350, 356
Cingulum 353
Circulation 140
Citalopram 344
Classic amnesic syndrome 48
Classic ovarian sign 11
Clenbuterol 379
Clindamycin 265
Clinical ischemic stroke 150
Clobazam 94, 95, 104
Clomipramine 344
Clonazepam 365
Clorgiline 344
Clozapine 342, 368
Cocaine 34, 303, 339, 342, 344, 379
Cognitive behavioral therapy 8, 15, 24, 119, 121, 226, 229, 357
Cognitive deficits 297, 357
   anatomical basis of 43
Cognitive disorder 280, 358
Cognitive domains 148, 357
   multiple tests of 68
   specific strategic regions 149
Cognitive estimates test 49
Cognitive functions 43, 357
   localizations of 43t
Cognitive impairment 68, 159, 182, 319, 321, 341, 363, 367
   mild 42, 66, 275, 298
   symptoms of 147
Collapsin response mediator protein 248
Coma 255, 372
Communication difficulties 319, 321
Complete blood count 341
Complex executive functions 43
Complex partial seizure 129, 145, 329
   clinical symptomatology of 129
Complex regional pain syndrome 227
Complex visual symptoms 280
   myriad of 280
Comprehensive cognitive assessment 149
Computed tomography 137
   findings 297-300, 307-309
Concentration 259
Conduct disorder 129, 130
Conduction aphasia 51
   lesion localization of 51
Conduction speech disturbance 288
Confusion 255, 372
Confusional arousals 100
Consciousness 28
   horizon of 12
   level of 136
   loss of 70
   transient loss of 67

Continuous positive airway pressure 183
Conventional tests 68
Conversion 15
   disorder 9, 15, 19
   hysteria 326
   reaction 165
Convulsions 367
Convulsive movements 100
Cornu ammonis 59
Coronary angiography 206
Coronavirus disease-2019 362
   central nervous system manifestation of 39
   neurologic complications of 143
Corpus
   callosotomy 105
   callosum 303
Cortical
   functions 4
   ribbon sign 302f
   sensory loss 158
   spreading depression 144
   subcortical lesions 244
Corticobasal
   degeneration 28, 29, 280, 289, 300
   syndrome 157, 159, 292
Corticobulbar tracts 378
Corticomedullary junction 265f
Corticosteroids, high-dose 377
Corticotropin-releasing factor 328
Couch potato syndrome 214
Coxiella burnetii 257
Cranial autonomic symptoms 200, 225
Cranial nerve 235
   injuries 356
   nucleus 374
   palsies 255, 257, 258
Cranial neuropathy 40, 304
C-reactive protein 198, 229
Creatine kinase 214
Creatine phosphokinase 229
Creutzfeldt–Jakob disease 32, 157, 289, 292, 293, 302, 302f
   clinical features of 292f
   diagnosis of 293t
   familial 32
   sporadic 32
Critical care units 336
Cryptochrome 271
Cryptococcal meningitis 32, 263
Cryptococcus neoformans 263
Cushing syndrome 230
Cyclobenzaprine 344
Cyclothymic mood disorders 270
Cystic inflammatory diseases 39
Cysticercal arachnoiditis 263
Cytidinediphosphocholine 150
Cytomegalovirus 260

D

Dangerous cardiac arrhythmias 74
Dantrolene 237, 346
Dawson fingers appearance 305f
Daytime somnolence, excessive 271
De novo psychosis 112
Death 368
Debrancher deficiency 213
Declarative memory, types of 58
Deep brain stimulation 299
Deep cerebellar nuclei 352
Degenerative diseases 281
Dehydration 336
Dehydrogenase 371
Delirium 46, 58, 130, 257, 338, 340, 341t, 342t, 346, 363, 367
   evaluation of 341
   poststroke 152
   tremens 269, 338
      management 337
Delusion 392
Delusional disorder 17
Dementia 28, 32, 42, 64, 67, 113, 147, 148, 157, 159, 182, 247, 275, 276, 279, 281, 287, 281, 284, 289, 297, 299, 302, 305, 390, 392
   alcohol-induced 303
   complex 31
   diagnosis of 64, 275, 297, 312
   early prominent 158
   frontotemporal 28, 213, 234, 247, 287, 289, 292, 299f
   human immunodeficiency virus-associated 258, 259b
   Lewy body 299
   modifiable risk factors for 148
   neurodegenerative 287
   preclinical stage of 275
   presenile 287
   progressive 281
   pugilistica 306, 359
   rating scale 55
   semantic 54, 288, 289
   studio 68
   symptoms 280
   traumatic 359
   vascular 147, 148fc, 276, 287, 290, 306
   young-onset 287, 289fc, 290
Demyelination disorders 234, 239f, 240t
Denbufylline 150
Depersonalization 112, 272
Depression 18, 32, 44, 109-111, 113, 235, 281, 284
   etiological factors for 236
   mild-to-moderate 219
   severe 277
   symptoms of 99

Depressive disorder 201, 357
 diagnostic criteria of 179b
Derealization 112
Dermatomyositis 213, 214
Desmin myopathy 213
Developmental coordination
 disorder 316
Dexmedetomidine 337, 338
Dextromethorphan 344
Diabetes mellitus 230, 270
Dichotomy 6
Diclofenac 203
Diencephalic injury 7
Dietary deficiencies 374
Diffuse axonal injury 356
Diffuse brain
 atrophy 281
 injury 46
Diffusion-tensor imaging 7, 146, 281,
 298, 299
Diffusion-weighted imaging 59, 291
Digit span 46
Digital subtraction angiography 307
Dilated pupils 35
Dipeptidyl aminopeptidase-like
 protein 245
Dipeptidyl-peptidase-like protein 6 30
Diplopia 74, 362, 367, 378
Disability, chronic 218
Disconnection syndrome 51
Disease-modifying therapies 236
Disk herniation 211
Disruptive mood dysregulation
 disorder 129
Dissociative disorders 15, 77
Dissolution, concept of 4
Distal myopathies 213
Distinctive syndrome 35
Distracted straight leg raise
 discrepancy 21
Distress, emotional 223
Divalproate 192, 208
Divine intervention 19
Dizziness 362, 367
Dizzy spells 70
Doose syndrome 91
Dopa-decarboxylase activity 302
Dopamine 189, 245, 314, 342, 352
 precursors 343
 receptor blocking agents 157
 reuptake, altered 342
 transporter scan 288f
Dopaminergic
 agent 343
 agonists 357
Dorsal root ganglion 223, 227
Dorsolateral frontal lobes 48
Dorsolateral prefrontal cortex 356

Doxepin 381
Dravet syndrome 95, 104
Dressing apraxia 53
Droperidol 337, 342
Drowsiness, rhythmic midtemporal theta
 bursts of 77
Drugs 203, 365, 380, 381
 abuse 344
 class 379
 overuse
  clinical manifestations of 339t
  treatment of 339t
Duchenne muscular dystrophy 212f, 213
Duloxetine 344
Dural arteriovenous fistula 307
 Borden classification of 308
Dysarthria 32, 74, 158, 238, 249, 258,
 376, 378
Dyscontrol 288
Dysembryoplastic neuroepithelial
 tumor 105
Dysexecutive syndrome 7
Dyskinesia 289
 abdominal 161
 paroxysmal 161
Dysmorphophobic disorders 15
Dysphagia 158, 238, 378
 severe 158
Dyspnea 323
Dysrhythmic 71, 133
Dysthymia 24
Dystonia 12f, 123, 161, 162, 263, 362
 acute 164, 365
 functional 165
 psychogenic 123
Dystonic reactions 362
 acute 164, 363, 366

E

Ebola viruses 262
Eccentric nodule 265f
Ecstasy 303, 339
Edema
 cytotoxic 377
 neurogenic pulmonary 333
 perilesional 264f, 265f
 vasogenic 308f, 373
Efavirenz 259
Elbow flex-ex sign 22
Electrical failure 135
Electroencephalogram 15, 72, 76, 87,
 102f, 112, 117, 126, 131, 145, 244, 246f,
 248, 292, 317f, 320f, 321, 323, 338
 abnormalities 250
 role of 102
 typical 95f, 97f
Electroencephalography 60, 245

Electromyography 215
Electrophysiological tests 22, 123
Eletriptan 203, 344
Embolism 136
Emery–Dreifuss muscular dystrophy 213
Emotion 325
 anatomical basis of 45
Emotional disturbance 152
Emotional incontinence 290
Encephalitides
 infectious 293
 parainfectious 293
Encephalitis 243-245, 255, 257, 260, 261,
 333
 hemorrhagic 261
 immune-mediated 293
 lethargica 5
 progressive 263
 viral 30, 39
Encephalomyelitis
 acute disseminated 39, 238, 304
 progressive 245
Encephalomyopathy, mitochondrial 214,
 291
Encephalopathy 58, 111, 261, 263, 293,
 304
 acute alcoholic 336
 chronic
  hepatic 302, 303
  hypertensive 298
  traumatic 287, 306, 359
 epileptic 93-95, 105
 inflammatory 390
 metabolic 249, 293, 390
 mitochondrial 39
 steroid-responsive 34
Endocarditis, bacterial 380
Endocrine disorders 33, 230
Endocrine myopathies 213
Energy, feeling of 271
Entacapone 343
Entorhinal cortex 59
Enzyme-linked immunosorbent assay
 257, 264
Ependymitis 263
Epigastric aura 331
Epilepsy 44, 71, 80, 81, 87, 88, 88b, 91,
 98f, 100b, 104, 106, 109-111, 113, 118,
 131, 132, 315
 autosomal dominant 94
 benign
  focal 96, 103
  occipital 89, 96
  rolandic 89, 96, 96f
 childhood absence 89, 91, 96
 classification 88, 89, 89fc
 correct diagnosis of 88
 cryptogenic focal 92

defense 132
development of 110
diagnosis of 102
differential diagnosis of 99
drug-refractory 110
drug-resistant 105
dysthymic-like disorder of 99
epidemiology of 87
etiology of 88f, 102
false diagnosis of 106
familial 94
focal 103, 104
frontal lobe 89
gelastic 93
genetic generalized 91, 96, 97, 104
holistic management of 102
hysteron 11
idiopathic generalized 96
imitators 79
insular 332, 333
juvenile
  absence 91, 96
  myoclonic 89, 91, 96, 97f
left medial temporal 102f
long-term prognosis of 110
management, broad aspects of 87
mesial temporal lobe 92, 105
neocortical 92
neuropsychiatric aspects of 27, 109
new-onset 87f, 88f
nocturnal frontal lobe 76, 76t
pattern sensitive 100
photosensitive 100
refractory temporal lobe 331
symptomatic
  focal 92, 93, 97
  generalized 95
syndrome 87-89, 90t, 104t, 105b, 106
  simplistic classification of 89fc
temporal lobe 27, 89, 97, 99, 100, 109, 112
treatment of 103
type 89
Epileptic phenomenon 129, 331
Epileptic seizure 73, 75, 100b, 119, 329, 331
diagnosis of 70, 123
disorders, treatment of 113
psychiatric mimics of 127, 131
Epileptic visual aura, localizing value of 389
Epileptiform hysteria 11
Episodic cerebellar dysfunction, drug-induced 100
Episodic dyscontrol
organic correlates of 128
syndrome 127-129
  current nosological status of 129

Episodic memory 46, 58
  form of 48
  loss 86
Epstein-Barr virus 235, 260
Erb's palsy 211
Ergot alkaloids 150
Erythrocyte
  sedimentation rate 40, 198, 214, 229, 273
  transketolase activity assay 374
Erythropoietin 379
Escitalopram 344
Ethanol blood levels 371
Ethosuximide 94, 104, 111
Euglycemic 145
Euphoria 339, 372
Extraocular muscle weakness 213
Extrapyramidal dysfunction 177t
Extrapyramidal symptoms 362, 363, 363b
  incidence of 362
  types of 365, 365t
Eye
  closure 76
  fluttering 76
  opening 76, 101
  patching 150
  sign 75, 374
Eyelid myoclonia 91, 100

F

Facial
  dyskinesias 293
  pain, atypical 225
  weakness 378
Facioscapulohumeral dystrophy 212f, 213, 214
Factitious disorder 9
Fasciculus, median longitudinal 235
Fatal insomnia, familial 269
Fatigue 180, 228-230, 230t
  borderlands of 230, 231f
  central 229
  peripheral 229
  poststroke 152
  related disorders 232b
  syndrome, chronic 222, 229, 229fc, 230, 230b, 231
Fatty acid 231
Fearfulness 279
Feel guilty 128
Felbamate 111
Fentanyl 344
Fever 226, 293
  prodromal stage of 30
  triad of 258
Fibrinoid material, deposition of 136
Fibromuscular dysplasia 136

Fibromyalgia 223
  complex symptomatology of 228f
  diagnosis of 228f
  management of 228f
Filoviruses 262
Finger
  abduction sign 22
  agnosia 52
Fistula, complete obliteration of 308f
Flaccid monoplegia 144
Floppy infant 212f
Fluid-attenuated inversion recovery 38f, 39, 244, 264f, 290, 297, 301f
  sequence 301f, 307f, 309f, 375f
Fluorodeoxyglucose 299
  positron emission tomography scan 298f, 299f
Fluoxetine 18, 344
Fluphenazine 342
Fluvoxamine 344
Focal cortical dysplasia 92, 99, 105
Focal epilepsy 103, 104
  treatment of 103
Focal motor neuron disease 211
Focal neurological deficits 249
Forgetfulness 279
Fractional anisotropy 298
Fragile X-associated tremor syndrome 305
Free-floating affective feelings 6
Froment sign 157
Frontal assessment battery score 143
Frontal lobe
  inhibitory functions of 45
  syndrome 277
Frontotemporal dementia 28, 213, 234, 247, 287, 289, 292, 299f
  behavioral variant of 289
Frontotemporal lobar degeneration 275, 279, 298
  diseases 359
  late-stage 298
Frovatriptan 203, 344
Fukuyama congenital muscular dystrophy 213
Full-length survival motor neuron protein 216
Functional auditory network 396
Functional disorders 18, 22, 143
Functional facial movement disorder 22
Functional hyperkinetic movement disorders 165
Functional memory disorder 23
  diagnosis of 23
Functional movement disorders 165, 165b
Functional upper limb weakness, signs of 21

Fungal infections 31, 263
Fusiform gyrus 54

G

Gabapentin 111, 206
Gadolinium 235, 374
Gait 167
  antalgic 167
  apraxia 168
  cautious 167
  cerebellar ataxic 167
  disorder 23, 167
    early 158
    functional 23, 165
    higher level 168
    psychogenic 167
  dyskinetic 167
  human 168
  hypotonic 167
  monoplegic 21
  paretic 167
  parkinsonian 290
  sensory ataxia 167
  spastic 167
  syndromes 167t
  vestibular 167
Galanin 268
Galen's teachings 9
Gamma hydroxybutyrate 339
Gamma-amino-butyric acid 109, 268, 328, 373
  A receptor 247
    encephalitis 247
  acid receptor 245
  B receptor 245
    encephalitis 247
  decreased synthesis of 336
Ganglioglioma 105
Ganglion block 204
Gastroesophageal reflux 72
Gastrointestinal disorders 33
Gene
  replacement therapy 216
  transfer, categories of 215
Genetic 215
  disorders 157
  generalized epilepsy 91, 96, 97, 104
    general features of 97b
    treatment of 104
  influences 315
  predisposition 117
  testing 319, 321
GeneXpert test 39
Genome, coding portion of 215
Geriatric seizure mimics 84
Gerstmann's syndrome 52
Ginkgo biloba 150
Glasgow coma scale 377

Gliomatosis cerebri 39, 305
Gliosis 299f, 307f
Globus pallidus 156, 301f
Glossopharyngeal neuralgia 224
Glucose 273
  derived neurotransmitters, production of 373
Glutamate 110
  regulation 314
Glutamatergic neurotransmitter systems 268
Glutamic acid 373
  decarboxylase 245
    encephalitis 247
Glycemic control 142
Glycine receptor 245
Glycogenoses 214
Go-no-go test 49
Gower sign 217
Grandiosity 237
Granular osmiophilic material, accumulation of 290
Growth hormone 379
Guillain–Barré syndrome 143, 213, 260, 261
Gyri, thinning of 298
Gyriform 303

H

Hachinski ischemic score 148
Hallucinations 152, 259, 277, 323, 386, 387, 390
  auditory 392, 395
  elementary 390
  lilliputian 388
  musical 396
  nonverbal auditory 395
  verbal auditory 395
  visual 60, 279, 386, 389, 391
Hallucinogens 340, 371, 379
Haloperidol 337, 338, 342, 362
Hamartoma, hypothalamic 93, 100, 333
Hamilton depression rating scale 110, 151
Hashimoto encephalopathy 34, 39, 293
Head
  injury 44
    repetitive 359
  trauma 50, 129, 287
    deserve, high rates of 360
Head, side-to-side movements of 117
Headache 29, 30, 40, 195-197, 198t, 200, 201, 201t, 202, 202t, 207, 210, 224, 293, 381
  characteristics 196, 197
  chronic 224t
  cluster 196, 200, 224
  cold-stimulus 196

  disorders 195
    classification of 195
    epidemiology of 195
  management 202
  primary 196, 198, 199, 204
    cough 196
    exercise 196
  secondary 198, 200, 204, 225
  sinus 200
  tension-type 195, 196, 199, 199t, 203, 207, 224
  triggers 197
  types of 224
Headlong flight 326
Head-turning sign 44
Hearing
  impairment 341
  test 321
Heart
  failure 45
  insufficient pumping action of 74
  rate, accelerated 328
Heavy metal poisoning 216
Heidenhain variant 292
Hematoma, subdural 143
Hemianopia 53
Hemiconvulsion-hemiplegia-epilepsy syndrome 93, 105
Hemicrania
  continua 200, 224
  paroxysmal 196, 199, 200, 224
Hemifacial spasm 161
Hemimegalencephaly 105
Hemimotor disturbances 144
Hemineglect 53
Hemiparesis 74
Hemispatial glasses 150
Hemisphere functions 50
Hemispherectomy 105
Hemogram 273
Hemorrhage
  intracranial 136
  subarachnoid 136
  thalamic 333
Hemorrhagic infarcts 259
Hepatic encephalopathy 292
Hepatitis 256
Hepatosplenomegaly 213
Heroin 380
  vapor inhalation 305
Herpes encephalitis 304
Herpes simplex
  encephalitis 260f, 303
  virus 30, 244
Herpes virus infections 259
Heterogeneity 239
Heteromodal association cortices 52
Hexane 379
Hippocampal injury 47

Histamine 268
Hockey stick sign 33
Holocranial headaches 144
Hoover's sign 19-21
Hospital anxiety and depression scale 110
Hot
  cross bun sign 301f
  spots 192
Human herpes virus 260
Human immunodeficiency virus 30, 39, 197, 229, 230, 258, 259, 265f, 293
  encephalitis 304
    marker of 304
  infection 30, 258
Human leukocyte antigen 250
Human sexual function 350t
Human sexuality, exploring neurobiology of 348
Human T-lymphotropic virus 39
Human visual cortex 280
Hummingbird sign 300, 300f
Huntington disease 7, 157, 287, 289, 300, 301f
Hurt minds, balm of 272
Hydergine 150
Hydrocephalus 356
  normal pressure 157, 173, 309, 309f
  pressure 281
Hydrophobia 260, 261
Hydrotherapy 15
Hyperammonemia 292
Hyperekplexia 72, 161
Hyperexcitable 128
Hyperglycemia 141
Hyperintense irregular rim 297
Hyperintensity 257f, 375f
  periventricular 276f
Hyperkinesia 156, 336
Hyperkinetic movement disorders 156, 161, 161b, 163fc
  treatment of 163
Hyperparathyroidism 213
Hyperreflexia 32
Hypersensitive 316
Hypersexuality 184
Hypersomnia 32
Hypertension 270
  arterial 336
Hyperthermia 35
  malignant 214, 333
Hyperthyroidism 34
Hyperventilation 117, 325
  physiological effects of 326
  syndrome 323
    treatment of 327
Hypnagogia 269
Hypnotics 362, 371
Hypochondria 15

Hypochondriasis 10
Hypodensities, subcortical 308
Hypoglycemia 143
Hypointensity 291
Hypokalemia 327
Hypokinesia 156
Hypokinetic rigid gait 167
Hypometabolism
  mild bilateral frontal 273
  occipital 299
Hyponatremia 249, 293
Hypoperfusion, global 380
Hyposensitive 316
Hypotension
  orthostatic 74, 336
  postural 363, 366
Hypothalamic involvement 255
Hypothalamic-pituitary-adrenal 119, 231
  axis 109
Hypothalamopituitary dysfunction 255
Hypothalamus 45, 223, 350, 353
  role of 350
Hypothyroidism 34
  symptoms of 34
Hypovolemia 74
Hypoxia 380
Hypsarrhythmic pattern, modified 82f
Hysteria 9, 12f, 14, 15, 19, 20, 325
  complex of 13
  frequency of 10
  pathology of 10
  treatment of 10
Hysterical paroxysms 13

I

Ibuprofen 203
Ictal behavior 98
Ictal fear 330, 331, 333
Ictal panic 330, 331, 333
Ictal psychosis 27, 111
Ictal semiology, types of 333
Ideal body weight 338
Ideomotor apraxia 52
  progressive 289
Illicit drugs, classes of 34b
Illness, acute 341
Illusions 272, 386
Immature enzyme activity 337
Immobility 32, 341
Immunoglobulin-like cell adhesion molecule 245
Immunotherapy 251
Impaired sensory input 342
Impaired vision 390, 391
Implantable loop recorder 75
Impulsive control disorders 188
  neural basis of 188
Impulsive-compulsive spectrum 188

Inclusion body myositis 213
Infections 260, 303, 304
  bacterial 31, 255
  chronic 230
  opportunistic 30
  parasitic 31, 263
  viral 250, 258
Inferior medial temporal lobe 306
Inflammatory amyloid angiopathy 291
Inflammatory bowel disease 230
Inflammatory disorders 304
  chronic 230
Injury
  free radical-induced 356
  neurologic 341
  vascular 356
Insomnia 32, 111, 246, 269, 273
  classification of 269
  diagnosis of chronic 270
Inspiratory stridor 158
Insufficient circulatory volume 74
Insufficient vascular tone 74
Insula 15, 223, 350, 351
Insular epilepsy 332, 333
  diagnosis of 332
Intellectual disability 315
Intelligence quotient 148
Intensive care unit 28, 230, 245
Intensive coronary care unit 206
Interictal psychosis 27, 112
Intermittent explosive disorder 129
Internal carotid artery 138, 139, 141
  meningeal branch of 308f
Interpersonal therapy 120
Intra-arterial thrombectomy 141t
Intracranial atherosclerosis 136
Intracranial bleeding 135
  post-thrombolysis, development of 136
Intracranial pressure 136
Intranuclear ophthalmoplegia 235
Intravascular lymphomatosis 306
Intravenous thrombolysis, profile of 144
Irritable bowel syndrome 223, 228, 231
Ischemia, hippocampal 60
Ischemic stroke 137
  localization of 142
  types of 136
Isoenzymes 371
Isolated neck extensor myopathy 213
Ixodes tick 257

J

Janet's view 12
Japanese encephalitis 30
Jeavons syndrome 91
Jerking 71
Jitteriness 72

Joint pains 213
Joubert's syndrome 325, 333

K

Kayser-Fleischer ring 192
Kearne-Sayre syndrome 214
Kennedy disease 216
Ketamine 337
Ketones, urinary elimination of 337
Ketoprofen 203
Kidney disease, chronic 287
Kinesigenic dyskinesia 119
Klüver-Bucy syndrome 350
Knife blade atrophy 299f
Korsakoff's psychosis 337, 372
Korsakoff's syndrome 33, 46, 47
Krebs cycle 373
Kugelberg-Welander disease 216
Kyphoscoliosis 213

L

Lacosamide 94, 104, 106
Lactate 214
Lactic acidosis 214, 291
Lacunar infarcts 136
Lambert-Eaton myasthenic syndrome 211, 213, 215
Lamotrigine 94, 103, 104, 106, 111, 362
Landau-Kleffner syndrome 104, 316
Language 50, 259
  difficulties 319, 321
  disorder, acquired 278
  functions 65
  impairments 318
  regression 317
Large vessel
  disease 306
  occlusion 141
Lasmiditan 203
Lassa fever 263
Lateral ventricles, enlargement of 298
Learning process 48
Leber's optic atrophy 39
Left posterior temporal gyrus 27
Leg signs 21
Leigh's syndrome 39
Lennox-Gastaut syndrome 89, 93, 95, 95f, 104, 105
Leptin 368
Leptomeningeal disease 305
Leptomeninges, enhancement of 257f
Lesions, peripheral enhancement of 265f
Leucine-rich glioma inactivated protein 30, 245, 246, 249, 293
  encephalitis 246, 250f
Leukoaraiosis 290
Leukodystrophies 39, 281

Leukoencephalopathy 39, 148, 290
  fulminant acute 339
  multifocal 31
  reversible posterior 39
Levetiracetam 94, 95, 104, 106, 111
Levodopa 156, 158, 160, 280, 343
  higher dose of 273
Lewy body 28, 147, 157, 159, 275, 287, 299
  dementia 299
    diagnosis of 67
  variant 299
Libman-Sacks endocarditis 40
Ligand-based positron emission tomography scan 276, 281
Lightheadedness 212
Limb
  focal dystonia 123
  girdle muscular dystrophy 213, 214
  movements, asynchronous 101, 117
Limbic
  encephalitis 29, 244, 245
  loops 156
  system, components of 45f
Linezolid 344
Lipid disorders 214
Lipoic acid 337
Lipoprotein, low-density 142
Lithium 237, 344, 362, 368, 369
  toxicity, acute 363, 366
Locked-in syndrome 337
Logopenic aphasia, progressive 288, 289
Long QT syndrome 74
Lorazepam 346
Low backache 225t, 226
Lower limb functional weakness, positive signs of 20
Lower motor neuron disorders 139, 210
  signs of 210t
  symptoms of 210t
Luria's three-step test 49
Lyme's disease 39, 257
Lymphadenopathy 256
  regional 256
Lymphocytic choriomeningitis virus 262
Lysergic acid diethylamide 340, 344, 380

M

Machado-Joseph disease 157
Mad cow disease 32
Magnesium 336
Magnetic resonance
  angiography 7
  findings 297, 298-300, 307, 309
  imaging 87, 160, 173, 235, 236, 239f, 243, 244, 248, 249, 290, 293, 298, 320
    functional 7, 119

  spectroscopy 298, 320
    studies 374
Magnetoencephalography 332
Major depressive disorder 129, 235
Major neurocognitive disorder 64, 130, 297
Major psychiatric disorders 109
Major vascular cognitive impairment 148fc
Malaria 32
  cerebral 32, 263
Malignancy 230, 248, 249
Mammillary bodies 375f
Manganese 157
Mania 246, 357
  corticosteroid-induced 237
Manic behavior 7
Manic syndromes 50
Marburg viruses 262
Marchiafava-Bignami
  disease 303, 376
  syndrome 337
Marching paresthesia 388
Marijuana 35
Medial forebrain bundle 188
Medial globus pallidus 298
Medial temporal hyperintensities 249
Medical disorders 128, 230, 230t
Medication overuse
  complications of 207
  headache 200, 206, 207
    pathophysiology of 208f
    vicious cycle of 208f
Medicine, category of 365
Mefloquine 32
Melancholic dreams 10
Melanocortin 268
Memantine 150
Membrane failure 135
Memory 43, 46, 275
  anatomical basis of 45
  anterograde 47
    nonverbal 47
  autobiographical 47
  deficits 336
  difficulty 44
  episodic 46, 58
  impairment 337, 374, 375
  nondeclarative 58
  personal semantic 58
  problems 44
  public semantic 58
  retrograde 47
  semantic 46, 48, 58, 64
  types of 58
Meningeal irritation, signs of 255
Meningeal signs 293
Meninges, infections of 255

Meningitis 255, 261
  aseptic 40
  infective causes of 255
Meningoencephalitis 255, 257, 261
Mental
  defect 132
  disorder 3, 129
    functioning, specific components of 42
  functions 55
    health disorders 231f
      borderlands of 230
    retardation 102
    slowing 258
    status, altered 365
Meperidine 344
Mesenchymal-like cells pericytes 373
Mesial structures 110
Mesocorticolimbic reward system, neuroanatomy of 188
Mesolimbic dopaminergic system 349
Mesolimbic reward system 350
Metabolic disorders 143, 210, 292
Metabolic syndrome 270
Metabolism, inborn errors of 305
Metabotropic glutamate receptor 245
Metadoxine 337
Metamorphopsia 388
  cerebral 387
Metamorphosis 272
Metastatic disease 291
Methamphetamines 339
Methotrexate 39
Methylenedioxymethamphetamine 340, 344, 381
Metoclopramide 342, 344
Meyer's words 4
Microbiome 235
Microhemorrhages, multiple 277f
Midbrain 374
  atrophy 160, 300f
  gray matter of 5
  tegmentum of 300f
Middle cerebral artery 26, 137-141
  infarcts 137, 138f
Middle frontal gyrus 53
Migraine 100, 113, 143, 196, 198, 199, 199t, 202, 203t, 208, 387, 389
  acute 224
  chronic 224
  equivalents 72
  treatments 203t
Mind, concept of 8
Mindfulness-based therapy 204
Minimal brain dysfunction 128
Mini-mental state examination 46, 65
Minor neurocognitive disorder 42
Mitochondrial disease, features of 249
Mitochondrial disorders 39, 214
Miyoshi myopathy 214

Mobilization 342
Modern neuroimaging techniques 144
Monoamine oxidase
  B 160
  inhibitors 344
Monoclonal gammopathy 216
Monomelic amyotrophy 211
Mononeuropathy 40
  multiplex 216
Montreal cognitive assessment 55
Mood
  disorder 40, 50, 99, 178, 259
  fluctuation 181
  stabilizers 362
Morbid anxiety, somatic-psychic continuum of 326
Morphological magnetic resonance imaging 15, 125
Morvan's chorea 269
Morvan's syndrome 244
Motivational circuits 353
Motor
  apraxia 288
  axonal neuropathy, acute 216
  functions 290
  manifestations 333
  movements 98
  neuron disease 213
  neuronopathy 211
  preparation 15
  sequencing 49
Movement disorders 22, 40, 124, 156, 166, 176, 177, 255, 262, 380, 381, 381t
  drug-induced 164, 164b, 166
  functional cranial 165
  paroxysmal 119
  psychogenic 15, 123, 124
Moyamoya disease 136
Multicore disease 213
Multifocal disease 105
Multiple blooming foci 307
Multiple carboxylase deficiency, biotin-dependent 333
Multiple punctate foci 291
Multiple sclerosis 39, 227, 229, 230, 234, 235, 235fc, 304, 305f
Multiple system atrophy 157, 159, 280, 300
Multisystem atrophy 301f
Muscle 215
  anatomy of 2f
  aryl hydrocarbon receptor nuclear translocator-like protein 1 270
  rigidity 337, 365
  stiffness 35
  weakness, pattern of 213
Muscular dystrophy 211, 213, 219
  congenital 217, 219

Musculoskeletal
  function 167
  pain, chronic 223
Mutism 376
Myalgic encephalomyelitis 229, 230, 230b, 231
Myasthenia
  congenital 215
  gravis 40, 213, 215, 230
Myasthenic crisis 218
Myasthenic syndrome, congenital 218
Mycobacterium 38
Mycophenolate mofetil 250
Myelin oligodendrocyte glycoprotein-associated disease 238
Myelitis, acute transverse 381
Myelopathy 40, 257, 381
  acute transverse 381
Myeloradiculitis 260
Myocardial infarction, acute 340
Myoclonic encephalopathy, early 93
Myoclonic jerks 100
Myoclonus 123, 161, 162, 245
  benign 72
  epilepsy, progressive 94
  functional 165
  slow 262
Myofibrillar myopathy 213
Myoglobinuria 212
Myokymia 161
Myopathy 211, 213, 213t, 217, 227
  central core 213
  centronuclear 213
  congenital 213
  inflammatory 213, 218
  mitochondrial 213
  types of 213
Myorhythmia 161
Myositis 261
Myotonia 217
Myotonic dystrophy 212f, 213, 214
  congenital 217
  protein kinase 217
Myotonic myopathy 213

N

Naproxen 203, 206
Naratriptan 203, 344
Nasal zolmitriptan 206
Neck
  extensor weakness 213
  vibration 150
Negative sensory manifestations 211
Nemaline myopathy 213, 214
Neningovascular syphilis 257f
Neoplasia 211
Neoplasms, benign 105
Neoplastic disease 305

Nephritis 256
Nerve
　biopsy 215
　conduction
　　studies 215
　　velocity electromyography 229
Nervous system, anatomy of 2f
Nervousness 323
Neural connectivity 314
Neural romanticism 2
Neuroasthenia 228
Neuroaxonal leukodystrophy 305
Neurobehavioral syndromes 45
Neurobiology, functional 272
Neuroblastoma 319
Neuroborreliosis 304
Neurocognitive disorder
　human immunodeficiency virus-
　　associated 31, 258
　mild 258
Neurocognitive dysfunction 66, 67
Neurocognitive impairment 65
　asymptomatic 258
Neurocysticercosis 31, 263, 264, 264f
　diagnosis of 264b
Neurodegeneration 157, 302, 392
　types of 163
Neurodegenerative disorder 210, 213, 249, 359, 392
　causes of 289fc
　neuropsychiatric aspects of 28
Neurodevelopmental disorder 316
Neuroleptic 163
　malignant syndrome 39, 164, 214, 341, 342b, 343b, 362-364, 365b
　disorders 371
Neurological disorder 87, 227, 230, 315, 316
　functional 19, 22, 23, 249
Neurological syndrome 248
Neurology 124
Neuromodulation 204
Neuromuscular diseases 210
Neuromuscular disorders 215, 219, 227
　broad categories of 211t
　treatment of 215
Neuromuscular junction 210
　disease 213
　disorders 211
Neuromyelitis optica 39, 237
　spectrum disorders 237, 238
Neuron, axons of 352
Neuronal structures 249
Neuroparenchyma 307f
Neuropathic pain 223
　management of 227fc
Neuropathy 211, 223, 227
　chronic peripheral 216
　inherited 213

Neurophenomenology 7
Neuropsychiatric symptoms 26, 28
Neuropsychiatry 1, 7, 355
　evolution of 1
Neuropsychological assessment 64, 65f
Neuropsychological tests 67, 68, 357
Neuropsychometry 61
Neurosarcoid 305
Neurosarcoidosis 39, 292
Neurosis 127
Neurosyphilis 32, 256, 304
Neurotransmitter 189
　contributions 352
　excitotoxicity 356
　glutamate 216
　level 329
　systems 314
Neurotropic viruses 30
Next-generation sequencing 215
Nicergoline 150
Night terrors 76
Nimodipine 150
Nitrous oxide 381
N-methyl-D-aspartate receptor 245, 249, 293
　encephalitis 29, 244, 246f
Nonaggressive violent automatisms 132
Nonatherosclerotic abnormalities 136
Nonbenzodiazepine hypnotics 362
Noncontrast enhanced computed tomography scans 298, 300
Nonepileptic attack disorder 116
Non-Hodgkin lymphoma 217
Noninvasive neuromodulation 204
Noninvasive vagal nerve stimulation 204
Nonkinesigenic dyskinesia 119
Nonorganic psychogenic disorders 18
Nonpharmacologic therapy 150
Nonpharmacological management 204, 240
Non-rapid eye movement 267
　sleep 101
　　parasomnias 75, 100
Nonsteroidal anti-inflammatory drugs 202, 226
Norepinephrine 268
Nosology 19
Novel focal neurological syndrome 143
Nuclear
　imaging techniques 310
　medicine studies 297
Nucleus accumbens 353
　location of 188f
Nucleus paragigantocellularis 349
Numbness, feeling of 332
Nutraceuticals 204
Nutrition 342
Nutritional disorders 33

O

Obesity 235
Obligatory intracellular protozoan 32
Obsessive compulsive disorder 5, 17, 189, 248
Obstructive sleep apnea 142, 230, 269
Occipital infarction 389
Occipital nerve stimulation 204
Occipital paroxysm 389
Occipito-parieto-temporal lesion 387, 389
Ocular movement 71, 293
Oculomotor 156
　apraxia 287
　disorders 336
Oculopharyngeal muscular dystrophy 214
Oculopharyngodistal myopathy 213
Ohtahara syndrome 93
Olanzapine 237, 337, 342, 368
Oligodendroglioma 105
Oligonucleotide 216
Ondansetron 344
Ophthalmoparesis 213
Opioids 208, 340, 341, 371, 380
　antagonist therapy 190
Opisthotonus 117
　posturing 101
Oppositional defiant disorder 130
Optic
　aphasia 54
　ataxia 287
　atrophy 213, 262
　chiasm 376
Optokinetic stimulation 150
Orbitofrontal cortex 50, 350, 356
Orexin 268
Organ failure 356
Organic
　amnesic syndrome 61, 61t
　brain syndromes 127
　movement disorder 123
　solvent 379
　　inhalation 305
Orphan nuclear receptor 271
Orthostatic intolerance
　features of 330
　symptoms of 212
Oscillopsia 391
Osmotic demyelination syndrome 39
Osteoarthritis 222
Ovarian sign 11
Ovarian teratoma 244, 250
Overreaction 21
Oxcarbazepine 94, 104, 362, 367
Oxytocin 352

P

Pain 15, 223, 238
  central neuropathic 227t
  chronic 222, 231, 232b
    visceral 226
  classification of 223fc
  neuropathic 223
  orofacial 224t
  peripheral neuropathic 227t
  poststroke 227
  source of 225
  task force 223
  thoracic 226
Palatal myoclonus 22
Palinopsia 387
Palpitations 328
Panayiotopoulos syndrome 75
Panencephalitis, subacute sclerosing 293, 304
Panic
  attacks 119, 325, 328, 329
  disorder 17, 201, 323, 325, 328, 329
Pantothenate kinase-associated neurodegeneration 302, 302f
Papez circuit, components of 45f
Paracetamol 141, 231
Paradoxical vocal cord dysfunction 123
Paralysis 71
  functional 21
  general 32
Paramedian thalamus 306
Paraneoplastic 157, 211
  disorders 210
  encephalitis 58, 244, 244t, 247, 292
    features of 248t
  syndrome 39, 249
Paraphasia
  phonemic 27
  semantic 27
Parasomnia 72, 100, 101, 101t, 362
Parathyroid abnormalities 157
Parietotemporal cortex 306
Parkinson's disease 8, 28, 68, 157, 172, 178, 179b, 183, 188, 227, 230, 288f, 289, 299, 388
  dementia 275, 287
  diagnosis of 67
  neuropsychiatric manifestations of 178
  rating scale 157
Parkinsonian disorder 156, 157b, 166
Parkinsonian syndromes 156
  atypical 158
Parkinsonism 157, 160fc, 263, 279, 288, 362, 363, 365
  atypical 157, 158b
  drug-induced 164
  functional 22, 165

  postencephalitic 157
  secondary 159
Paroxetine 344
Pathological gambling 184, 188
Pavlovian 58
Pedunculopontine nucleus 156
Pelvic thrusting 101, 117
Pentazocine 380
Pentoxifylline 150
Perampanel 95, 104
Periodic acid-Schiff 255
Periodic paralysis 214
Periostitis 256
Peripheral nerves 210
  block 204
Peripheral nervous system 210, 211, 262, 353
  components of 210
Peripheral terminals, heightened responsiveness of 223
Pes cavus 213
Pharmacologic therapy 150, 231, 341, 343
Pharmacoresponsiveness 96
Pharmacotherapy 397
Phencyclidine 340, 379, 380
Phenelzine 344
Phenobarbital 338
Phenobarbitone 94, 95, 103, 104
  doses of 324
Phenomenology 395
Phenytoin 94, 104, 111, 324
Pheromones, assessment of 350
Phobia 201
Phonological disorders 150
Phosphoglycerate kinase deficiency 213
Physical disorders 127
Picture naming test 64
Pilomatricomas 217
Pisa syndrome 158
Pithiatism 14
Plaque reduction neutralization test 261
Plasma exchange 215
Plasmodium falciparum 263
Plexopathy 40, 211
Plexuses 210
Poliomyelitis 211, 216
Polycystic ovarian syndrome 270
Polymerase chain reaction 255
Polymyositis 213, 214, 230
Polyneuropathy 40
  acute peripheral 216
Polyopia, cerebral 387
Polyradiculoneuropathy
  acute inflammatory demyelinating 40
  chronic inflammatory demyelinating 213
Polyradiculopathy, chronic immune sensorimotor 215

Polysomnography 76, 267
Polytrauma 356
Polyunsaturated fatty acid 231
Polyuria 237
Pompe disease 213
Pons
  severe atrophy of 301f
  sparing of 160
Positron emission tomography 7, 125, 190, 298, 321, 332
Posterior cortical atrophy 140, 141, 280, 280f, 289
  syndrome 138
Posterior reversible encephalopathy syndrome 261, 308, 308f, 309, 340
  types of 308
Postictal confusion 101
Postmalaria syndrome 32
Postorgasmic prolactin secretion 352
Poststroke depressive disorders 150
Poststroke mania 152
  prevalence of 152
Poststroke personality disorders 152
Post-traumatic stress disorder 201, 228, 325, 356, 358
Postural orthostatic tachycardia syndrome 143, 330
Postural reflexes, loss of 157
Posture, disorder of 23
Pramipexole 160
Praxis 29
Pregabalin 111
Prehospital stroke scales, loss of 137
Presynaptic dopamine terminals 288f
Primary headaches 196, 198, 199, 204
  disorders 196
Primary psychiatric
  disease 249
  disorder 26
  illnesses 277
Prochlorperazine 342
Progressive aphasia, primary 278, 279, 292
Progressive multifocal leukoencephalopathy 31, 262, 293, 303f, 304
Promethazine 342
Propentofylline 150
Propofol 337
  infusion 338
Propranolol 365
Propriospinal myoclonus 22
Prosopagnosia 54, 288
Protective reflex 222
Protein, contactin-associated 245, 249
Prothrombin time 140
Protozoal infections 263
Proximal limb girdle weakness 213
Pseudobulbar palsy 378

Pseudodementia 67, 283
Pseudodepression 283, 285
Pseudomovement disorder 9
Pseudo-pseudodementia 285
Pseudopsychopathic personality disorder 50
Pseudoseizure 9
Pseudosyncope 100
Psychiatric comorbidity 75, 95, 97, 99, 110
   treatment of 113
Psychiatric diseases, diagnosis of 26
Psychiatric disorder 44, 109, 128, 201, 201t, 202t, 230, 235, 238
   management of 238
Psychiatric dysfunction 272
Psychiatric emergencies 336
Psychiatric medications
   encompass 362
   overview of 362
Psychiatric rating scales 240
Psychiatric symptoms 193, 238, 244
   high incidence of 8
Psychiatry 124
   disorders, diagnosis of 202
   medicines, neurological side effects of 362, 363b
Psychic traumas, source of 13
Psychodynamic therapy 24
Psychoeducation 120, 357
Psychogenic disorders 127
Psychogenic gait disorder 167
   features suggestive of 168
Psychogenic nonepileptic seizures 1, 15, 22, 70, 72, 76b, 87, 100, 116-118, 121, 123-125, 328
   classification of 117t
   clinical features of 116
   diagnosis of 116
   differential diagnosis of 119b
   management of 113, 119, 120t
   multifactorial model of 118f
   psychobiology of 117
   semiology, features of 117b
Psychomotor regression 95
Psychosis 5, 35, 40, 99, 111, 127, 151, 181, 237, 246, 259, 358, 390
   chronic interictal 27
   epileptic 112
   management of 237
   steroid-induced 237
   types of 111
Psychostimulants 34, 35
Psychotherapy 15
   interpersonal 121
Psychotic disorder 26, 129, 151, 201, 202, 325, 374
Psychotic illness, chronic 358

Psychotropic 367
   drug 369
   medicines 15, 113
Ptosis 213
Pulmonary embolism 325
Pulse wave amplitude 173
Pulvinar sign 33
Punctate calcifications 297
Putamen 156, 350
Putaminal rim sign 301f
Putaminal volume loss 300
Pyramidal signs 376
Pyridoxine, pyrrolidone carboxylate of 337
Pyrimethamine 265
Pyruvate
   dehydrogenase deficiency syndrome 325, 333
   levels 214

Q

Quadriparesis, spastic 378
Quadriplegia, acute 238
Quetiapine 342

R

Rabies 260, 261f
Radiation necrosis 305, 306
Radiculopathy 211, 257
Radiofrequency ablation 204
Raimiste's leg sign 21
Raised intracranial tension, syndrome of 263
Rankin score, modified 141
Raphe nuclei 110
Rapid eye movement 76, 101, 183, 279
Rasagiline 160, 344
Rasmussen encephalitis 105
Reflex
   primitive 376
   saccadic eye movement 279
   syncope 74
Reflexive aggression 7
Reflexogenic parasympathetic activity 348
Refractory errors 200
Relaxation therapies 204
Remote memory, loss of 48
Reproductive organs, role of 19
Reserpine 342
Respiratory alkalosis 333
Restless legs 161
Retinal abnormalities 291
Retinal auras 199
Retinal photoreceptor damage 391
Retrograde amnesia 59
   degree of 59

Rett's syndrome 325, 333
Reversible cerebral vasoconstriction syndrome 291, 380
Reye's syndrome 325, 333
Rey-Osterrieth complex figure test 54
Rheumatoid arthritis 229, 230
Rheumatologic disorders 33
Rhombencephalitis 261
Rickettsia 257
   prowazekii 257
   rickettsii 257
   typhi 257
Right hemispheric lesions, detection of 52
Rigidity 157, 376
Riluzole 216
Rim enhancement patterns 303
Risperidone 342
Ritonavir 344
Rituximab 250
Rizatriptan 203, 344
Rocky mountain spotted fever 257
Rodent borne viruses 262
Romano-Ward syndrome 331
Ropinirole 160

S

Safinamide 160
Salivation 96
Sandifer syndrome 72
Scapuloperoneal dystrophy 213
Scars, atrophic 105
Schizophrenia 27, 44, 109, 277, 358, 392
   negative symptoms of 99
Sclerosis 13
   amyotrophic lateral 211, 227, 289
   hippocampal 92, 99b, 102f
Secondary headaches 198, 200, 204, 225
   disorders 196
Sedatives 341, 362, 371, 379
   benzodiazepines 337
Seizures 35, 40, 81, 86, 88, 89, 96, 132, 194, 246, 262, 337, 356, 363, 367
   acute symptomatic 103
   alcohol withdrawal 378
   amnesic 60
   anoxic epileptic 75
   atonic 96
   classification 89f
   complex partial 129, 145, 329
   dacrystic 100
   diagnosis 73, 80, 81
   disorder 72, 89
   drug-resistant polymorphic 95
   epileptic 73, 75, 100b, 119, 329, 331
   extratemporal 98, 98t
   focal 71, 106, 145
   frequency 76, 120

frontal lobe 101, 110*t*
gelastic 100
generalized 106, 144
hypermotor 100, 332
manifestations 76
migrating partial 92
myoclonic astatic 91
new-onset 105*fc*
opercular-insular 332
partial 389
psychogenic 101, 116
    nonepileptic 1, 15, 22, 70, 72, 76*b*, 87, 100, 116-118, 121, 123-125, 328
pure sensory 100
self-induced 100
semiology 132
    typical 96
temporal 98, 98*t*
tonic-clonic 72, 88, 91, 94
true 101
type 88-90
visual 386
Selective serotonin reuptake inhibitor 18, 113, 229, 231, 325, 344, 357
    early 151
Selegiline 344
Semantic memory 46, 48, 58, 64
    loss 48
Sensations, abnormal spontaneous 223
Sensitization, central 223
Sensorineural hearing loss 263
Sensorium 60
Sensory
    abnormalities 321
    extinction 53
    hypersensitivity 314
    issues 318
    motor peripheral polyneuropathy 216
    neglect 52, 53
    neuropathy 207, 211
    phenomenon 71
    processing issues 316, 318
    symptoms 22
Sepsis 39
Septic emboli 291
Seronegative autoimmune encephalitis 248
Serotonin 268, 314, 356
    norepinephrine reuptake inhibitor 151, 192, 226, 228, 229, 329
    pathways 356
    syndrome 344, 244*t*, 346, 362, 363, 365, 366*b*
Sertraline 344
Serum creatine phosphokinase 39
Severe acute respiratory syndrome coronavirus 2 261
Sex atypical amygdala connections 350

Sexual abuse, childhood 118
Sexual drive 13, 349
Sexual dysfunction 363, 368
Sexual neurobiology 352
Sexual self-stimulation 352
Sexual theory 13
Short-lasting unilateral neuralgiform headache attack 199, 200, 225
Sickle cell disease 136
Simultagnosia 287
Single gene disorders 215
Single-photon emission computed tomography 7, 144, 377
Site-specific demyelinating disorders 39
Sjögren syndrome 230
Sleep 267
    abnormality, types of 362
    apnea 158
    architectural disarray 271
    behavior disorder 101, 279
    benign epileptiform transients of 77
    biology of 267
    deprivation 81, 269
        effect of 81
    disorder 81, 100, 183, 245
        management 184*b*
    disturbance 237, 272, 362, 363, 367
    effect of 80
    electroencephalogram, typical 96*f*
    enhancing activity 270
    functions of 268
    hygiene optimal 271
    like states 390
    medicine, essentials of 267
    myoclonus, neonatal 72
    neuroanatomy of 267
    neuroscience of 273
    parasomnias 76*t*
    physiology 272
    slow wave 367
    supports 269
    terror 100
    utility of 80
    walking 100
Small arteriovenous malformation 136
Small vessel
    disease 306
        setting of 148
    ischemic changes 298*f*
Smell, assessment of 350
Social
    anxiety disorder 201
    communication disorder 314, 318
    interaction 321
    jetlag 270
    misconduct 29
    networks 148
    phobia 201
    stigma 368

Sodium valproate 104, 324
Solitary tract, nucleus of 352
Somatic symptom disorder 15, 17
Somatization 119, 325
    disorder 15, 201, 202
Somatosensory
    auras 332
    cortices 223
    misperceptions 272
Somnambulism 76
Spasmodic torticollis 13
Spastic paresis 288
Spatial dyscalculia 52
Speech 199, 259, 320
    disorders 51*fc*
    disturbance 249
    retardation 82*f*
    spontaneous 288
Sphenopalatine 204
    ganglion stimulation 204
Spinal
    cord 309, 349
    deformity 212*f*
    hemiplegias 144
    injury centre 21
    muscular atrophy 211
        severe forms of 212
    nerve roots 210
Spinocerebellar ataxia 39, 289
Spondylosis 211
Sporadic hemiplegic migraine 143
Standard electrodiagnostic studies 218
Statin therapy 150
Status epilepticus 214
    nonconvulsive 28
Stereoelectroencephalography 331
Stereotypic movements 39
Stereotypic paroxysmal event 331
Steroids 215
    anabolic 379, 380
    sparing agents 215
Stiff person syndrome 245
Stiffness 214
Stigmata 12
Stimulants 357, 371
Straight leg raise 226
Stress, psychological 9
Stressors 119
    disorders 15
Striatum 353
Stroke 44, 113, 135, 141, 144, 151, 230, 261, 287, 379
    acute 139, 140*b*, 142, 340
        ischemic 142, 340
    chameleon 144, 145
    classification of 135*fc*
    episodes 39, 214, 291
    facilities are 145
    hemorrhagic 135, 148

illness 382
ischemic 137
large vessel 306
localization 137, 138f, 140f
management of 382
mechanism of 380t
medicine 135
mimic 141, 143-145
posterior circulation 58
secondary prevention of 141
thrombotic 137
type 380
Stupor 372
Sturge-Weber syndrome 98f, 105
Subcortical infarcts 39, 148
Substance abuse 184, 189, 378
central neurological manifestations of 371
disorder 381
drugs 380
Substance intoxication 130
Substance use 34
disorder 188, 189
neuropsychiatric aspects of 34
Substantia nigra 156, 299
Suicidal attempts 110
Suicidal ideation 259
risk of 111
Sulci, widening of 298
Sulfadiazine 265
Sumatriptan 203, 344
Superficial tenderness 21
Superior parietal lobule 53
Supplementary motor area 125
Supportive therapy 343
Suprachiasmatic nucleus 270
Supramarginal gyrus 53
Supranuclear palsy, progressive nonfluent 157, 158, 173, 272, 277, 289, 300, 300f
Surgery 90
Sweating 327, 328
Sylvian fissures 309f
Sylvian segment 138
Synaptic function 315
Syncope 72, 73, 75, 100, 119, 123, 363, 366
cardiogenic 74
classification of 74b
clinical features of 100b
Valsalva maneuver-induced 75
vasovagal 74, 330
Syphilis
primary 256
secondary 256
Syringobulbia 333
Systemic disorders 33
neuropsychiatric aspects of 33
Systemic lupus erythematosus 33, 40, 230
neuropsychiatric 33, 40

T

Tabula rasa 2
Tachycardia 327, 330
Tactile naming 54
Taenia solium 263
Tardive
akathisia 164, 363, 364
chorea 164
dyskinesia 164, 362, 363, 365
dystonia 164, 363-365
myoclonus 164
stereotypies 164
syndromes 164
tics 164
tremor 164
Tassinari syndrome 91
Temporal disorientation 272
Temporal lobe 29, 324
anterior 43f
Temporal neocortex 353
Temporomandibular
joint 225
pain disorder 225
Temporo-occipital cortex 306
Tension 323
Testicular malignancies 217
Tetrabenazine 342, 365
Tetrahydrocannabinol 340
Thalamic infarcts 26
Thalamic lesions, bilateral 306
Thalamus 26, 30, 33, 110, 223, 350, 353
Thiamine 373, 377
deficiency 373
direct measurement of 374
pyrophosphate 373
Thrombocytopenia 263
thrombotic 143
Thrombolysis, benefit of 144
Thrombus, propagation of 136
Thymine diphosphate participates 373
Thyroid
antibody profile 294
disorders 34, 230
peroxidase antibodies 249
Tiagabine 111
Tics 72, 161, 162
disorders 22
functional 165
Tinnitus 356
Tissue plasminogen activator 140, 140b
Tizanidine 237
Toes, phenomenon of 20
Tolcapone 343

Toluene 379
Tonic-clonic seizure, generalized 72, 88, 91, 94
Tonsillar biopsy tissue 33
Topiramate 94, 103, 104, 111, 206, 208
Torticollis, benign paroxysmal 72
Tourette's syndrome 316
Toxic 211
encephalopathies 293
leukoencephalopathy 305
myopathies 213
Toxins 157, 216
neuropsychiatric aspects of 34
Toxoplasma gondii 32, 264
Toxoplasmosis 32, 265f
Trail-making test 49
Tramadol 344
Transcortical motor aphasia 51
Transcortical sensory aphasia 51
Transcranial direct current stimulation 204
Transcutaneous electrical nerve stimulation 150, 228
Transient global amnesia 58, 59, 61, 61t, 145
diagnostic criteria for 59b
Transient global aphasia 27
causes of 27
Transient global memory loss 145
Transient ischemic attack 74, 137, 139, 145, 150, 287, 325
Transverse
myelitis 39
sinus hypoplasia 146
Trauma 15, 306
neonatal 211
Traumatic brain injury 7, 113, 287, 355
neuropsychiatry of 355
neuropsychological aspects of 355
Traumatic encephalopathy syndrome 359, 360
Trazodone 344
Tremor 22, 161, 327, 337, 362
drug-induced 363, 364
essential 161
functional 22, 165
psychogenic 123
Treponema pallidum 256
Tricarboxylic acid 373
Tricyclic antidepressant 226, 228, 231
Trigeminal autonomic cephalalgia 196, 199, 200, 203, 224
Trigeminal neuralgia 224
Triggers 119
sexual motivation 350
Trihexyphenidyl 365
Triptan 203, 344
Trisynaptic circuit 59

Trombone tongue 32
Tropheryma whipplei 255
   deoxyribonucleic acid 255
Tryptophan 344
Tuberculous meningitis 31
Tumor necrosis factor alpha 368
Tunnel vision 390
Twitching 71

U

Ulcers 213
Ullrich myopathy 218
Uncinate fasciculus 125
Upper limb
   functional weakness, positive signs
      of 21
   jerks 96
Upper motor neuron disorders 210, 235
   signs of 210*t*
   symptoms of 210*t*

V

Vagus nerve stimulation 204
Valbenazine 365
Valproate 94, 104, 106, 111, 357
Valproic acid 344, 362, 368
Valsalva maneuver 75
Vapors 10
Varicella zoster virus 259
Vascular cognitive impairment 147
   concept of 147
Vascular lesions 135
Vascular malformations 105
Vascular origin 135
Vascular parkinsonism 157, 172, 173
   diagnosis of 172
   differential diagnosis of 173*fc*
Vasculitis 136, 292, 380
Vasculopathy, cerebral 144
Vasoactive intestinal peptide acts 348
Vasospastic angina 206
Veins, early draining 307
Venlafaxine 344
Ventricular cysts 263
Ventromedial prefrontal cortex 349
Verbal aggression 129
Verbal fluency tests 48
Verbal memory 47

Vertebrobasilar transient ischemic
   attacks 388
Vertical supranuclear gaze palsy 158
Vertigo 74, 143, 362
   benign paroxysmal 72
   episodic 119
Vestibular syndrome, acute 144
Vestibulo-ocular reflex 391
Video electroencephalogram 76, 102
Vigabatrin 82*f*, 94, 104, 111
Violence 132
   stemming 7
Visceral auras 332
Visceromotor 332
Viscerosensory 332
Visual agnosias 54
Visual allesthesia 387
Visual auras 100
Visual distortions 272
Visual field 390
   defect 262
      persistent homonymous 389
Visual hemineglect 53*f*
Visual illusions 112, 386
Visual impairment 341
Visual loss 390
   functional 22
Visual memory 148
Visual phenomenon 144
Visual presentation 292
Visual variant 288
Visuospatial deficits 159
Visuospatial disturbance 287
Visuospatial skills 29, 259
Vitamin
   B
      complexes 377
      group, eight forms of 377
   B12 337
      deficiency 33, 39
   D 235
   deficiencies 216
Voltage-gated
   calcium channels 218
   potassium channel antibodies 246, 249

W

Waddell's signs 21
Wakefulness 267, 268

Wallenberg syndrome 138
Weakness 255
   episodic 214
   unilateral 144
Wechsler memory scale 47
Weight
   gain 368
   loss 226
Werdnig-Hoffmann syndrome 216
Wernicke's aphasia 27, 50, 51
   problem of 27
Wernicke's area 51
Wernicke's encephalopathy 39, 281, 292,
      293, 303, 337, 372, 373, 375*f*
Wernicke's reduction 4
Wernicke-Korsakoff syndrome 33, 372
West Nile virus 211, 216, 262
West syndrome 82*f*, 89, 93, 95, 104
Westphal variant 289
Whipple's disease 39, 255
White matter
   diseases, differential diagnosis of 39*b*
   hyperintensities 297
Whole exome sequencing 215, 321
Whole genome sequencing 215
Wicket waves 77
Willis circle 2*f*
Wilson's disease 157, 160, 162, 192, 281,
      302
   diagnosis of 192
Wisconsin card sorting test 49
Working memory 48
   deficit 48
   preservation of 145

X

Xanthine derivatives 150

Z

Zidovudine 259
Zika virus 261
Ziprasidone 342, 368
Zolgensma 215
Zolmitriptan 203, 206, 344
Zolpidem 367
Zonisamide 94, 103, 104, 111
Zoopsia 390
Zopiclone 367
Zoster virus infection 293

Other Best-selling Books

NEUROLOGY & INTERNAL MEDICINE: A CASE-BASED STUDY

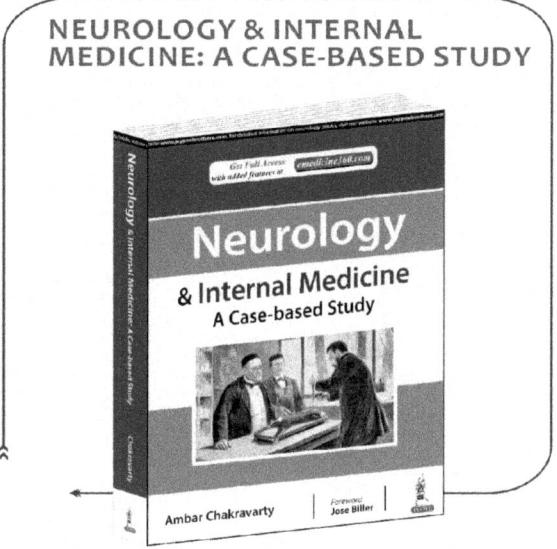

Ambar Chakravarty
Two Color | Hard Cover | 1/e, 2021
8.5" x 11" | 636 Pages | 9789354652066

MIMICS OF EPILEPTIC SEIZURES

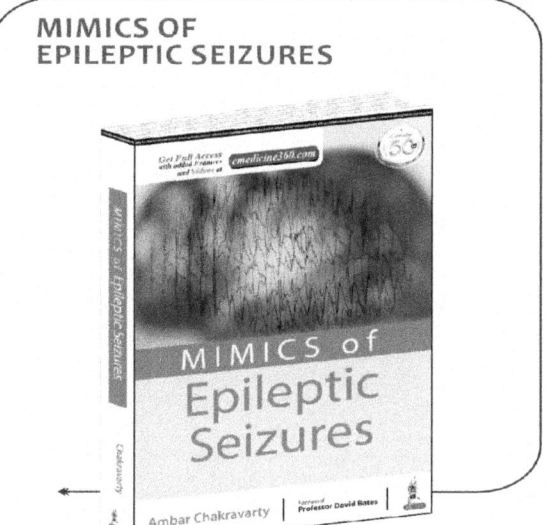

Ambar Chakravarty
Two Color | Soft Cover | 1/e, 2020
6.25" x 9.5" | 394 Pages | 9789390020966

CLINICAL NEURO-OPHTHALMOLOGY

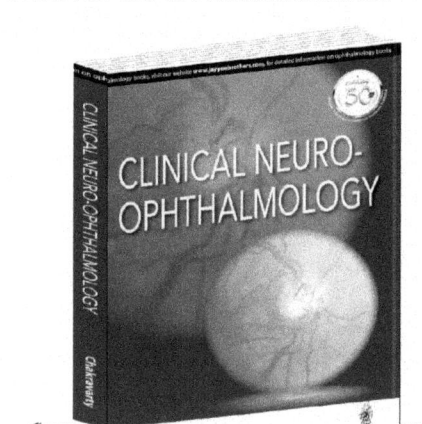

Ambar Chakravarty
Two Color | Hard Cover | 1/e, 2019
6.75" x 9.5" | 306 Pages | 9789352705573

JAYPEE
The Health Sciences Publisher

Please visit our website
www.jaypeebrothers.com or Scan the QR Code

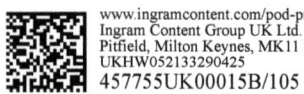